ADVANCES IN NEPHROLOGY

From the Necker Hospital

VOLUME 14

ADVANCES IN NEPHROLOGY

VOLUMES 1 through 5 (out of print)

VOLUME 6

VOLUME 7

VOLUME 8

VOLUME 9

VOLUME 13

ADVANCES IN NEPHROLOGY

From the Necker Hospital

FRENCH EDITORS

JEAN-FRANÇOIS BACH, M.D., D.Sc.
JEAN CROSNIER, M.D.
JEAN-LOUIS FUNCK-BRENTANO, M.D.
JEAN-PIERRE GRÜNFELD, M.D.

Department of Nephrology, Necker Hospital, Paris, France

AMERICAN EDITOR

MORTON H. MAXWELL, M.D.

*Clinical Professor of Medicine, University of California (Los Angeles)
Medical Center*

VOLUME 14 • 1985

YEAR BOOK MEDICAL PUBLISHERS, INC.
CHICAGO

Library of Congress Catalog Card Number: 73-154325

International Standard Serial Number: 0084-5957

International Standard Book Number: 0-8151-4137-8

Contributors

GINETTE ALBOUZE, M.D.
Department de Néphrologie, Hôpital Necker, Paris

P. ALLAIN, M.D.
Laboratory of Pharmacology, C.H.U. Angers, France

KONRAD ANDRASSY, M.D.
Department of Internal Medicine, University of Heidelberg, Heidelberg, West Germany

K. S. ANG, M.D.
Service of Medicine E - Nephrology, La Beauchée Hospital, Saint-Brieuc, France

R. A. ASHERSON, M.B., CH.B., F.C.P. (SA)
Department of Rheumatology, The Royal Postgraduate Medical School, Hammersmith Hospital, London, England

JEAN-FRANÇOIS BACH, M.D.
INSERM U-25, Department de Néphrologie, Hôpital Necker, Paris

JÜRGEN BOMMER, M.D.
Department of Internal Medicine, University of Heidelberg, Heidelberg, West Germany

EDWIGE BOURSZTYN, M.D.
Service de Chirurgie Digestive, Hôpital Paul Brousse, Villejuif

M. BROYER, M.D.
Service de Nephrologie Pediatrique et Clinique Urologique, Hôpital Necker, Enfants Málades, Paris

G. CAM, MD.
Service of Medicine E - Nephrology, La Beauchée Hospital, Saint-Brieuc, France

H. CAMPOS, M.D.
Department de Néphrologie (Unité de Transplantation Rénale) et INSERM U-25, Hôpital Necker, Paris, France

LUCIENNE CHATENOUD, M.D.
INSERM U-25, Department de Néphrologie, Hôpital Necker, Paris

N. CHKOFF, M.D.
Department de Néphrologie (Unité de Transplantation Rénale) et INSERM U-25, Hôpital Necker, Paris

J. F. CLOIX, M.D.
U7 and U90 INSERM Research Units, Department of Pharmacology, Hôpital Necker, Paris

M. CRABOS, M.D.
U7 and U90 INSERM Research Units, Department of Pharmacology, Hôpital Necker, Paris

J. CROSNIER, M.D.
Department de Néphrologie (Unité de Transplantation Rénale) et INSERM U-25, Hôpital Necker, Paris

ALAIN DANA, M.D.
Service de Radiologie des Maladies de l'appareil Urinaire, Hôpital Necker

H. DE THÉ, M.D.
U7 and U90 INSERM Research Units, Department of Pharmacology, Hôpital Necker, Paris

M. A. DEVYNCK, M.D.
U7 and U90 INSERM Research Units, Department of Pharmacology, Hôpital Necker, Paris

ALAIN DOUCET, M.D.
Laboratoire de Physiologie Cellulaire, College de France, Paris

DOMINIQUE DROZ, M.D.
Laboratoire Central d'Anatomie Pathologique, Hôpital Necker, Paris

MICHAEL J. DUNN, M.D.
Department of Medicine, Case Western Reserve University and Division of Nephrology, University Hospitals of Cleveland, Cleveland, Ohio

J. L. ELGHOZI, M.D.
U7 and U90 INSERM Research Units, Department of Pharmacology, Hôpital Necker, Paris

L. FAVRE, M.D.
Division of Endocrinology, Department of Médecine, University Cantonal Hospital, Geneva, Switzerland

DOMINIQUE FRANCO, M.D.
Service de Chirurgie Digestive, Hôpital Paul Brousse, Villejuif

F. BUFFET GACOIN, M.D.
Service de Néphrologie Pediatrique et Clinique Hôpital Necker Enfants Malades, Paris

A. GERBER, M.D.
Medizinische Poliklinik, University of Berne, Switzerland

G. GOLDSTEIN, M.D.
Ortho-Pharmaceutical Corporation, Raritan, New Jersey

HUGO GONZALEZ-DETTONI, M.D.
Unité de Recherches sur les Maladies Renales, INSERM U25 Hôpital Necker, Paris

HERMAN-JOSEF GROENE, M.D.
Department of Medicine, Case Western Reserve University and Division of Nephrology, University Hospitals of Cleveland, Cleveland, Ohio

JEAN-PIERRE GRÜNFELD, M.D.
Department de Néphrologic, Hôpital Necker, Paris

G. GUEST, M.D.
Service de Néphrologie Pediatrique et Clinique Hôpital Necker Enfants Malades, Paris

G. HAMON, M.D.
Centre de Recherches Roussel-Uclaf, Romainville, France

G. HENNING, M.D.
U7 and U90 INSERM Research Units, Department of Pharmacology, Hôpital Necker, Paris

G. R. V. HUGHES, M.D., F.R.C.P.
Department of Rheumatology, The Royal Postgraduate Medical School, Hammersmith Hospital, London, England

PAUL JUNGERS, M.D.
Department de Néphrologie, Hôpital Necker, Paris

L. A. KAMAL, M.D.
U7 and U90 INSERM Research Units, Department of Pharmacology, Hôpital Necker, Paris

JEROME P. KASSIRER, M.D.
Professor and Associate Chairman, Department of Medicine, Tufts University School of Medicine, Boston, Massachusetts

H. KREIS, M.D.
Departement de Néphrologie (Unité de Transplantation Rénale) et INSERM U-25, Hôpital Necker, Paris

CALVIN M. KUNIN, M.D.
Pomerene Professor of Medicine, Department of Medicine, Ohio State University College of Medicine, Columbus, Ohio

L. C. LACERDA-JACOMINI, M.D.
U7 and U90 INSERM Research Units, Department of Pharmacology, Hôpital Necker, Paris

M. LACOMBE, M.D.
Department de Néphrologie (Unité de Transplantation Rénale) et INSERM U-25, Hôpital Necker, Paris

K. LAEDERACH, M.D.
Medizinisch Poliklinik, University of Berne, Switzerland

BERNARD LAFFORGUE, M.D.
Centre de l'A.U.R.A., Rue des Peupliers, Paris

PAUL LANDAIS, M.D.
Department de Néphrologie, Hôpital Necker, Paris

F. LESTAGE, M.D.
Service de Néphrologie Pediatrique et Clinique Urologique Hôpital Necker Enfants Malades, Paris

MORTON H. MAXWELL, M.D.
UCLA School of Medicine, Los Angeles, California

Y. MAURAS, M.D.
Laboratory of Pharmacology, C.H.U. Angers, France

DAVID A. McCARRON, M.D.
Division of Nephrology and Hypertension, Oregon Health Sciences University, Portland, Oregon

P. MEYER, M.D.
U7 and U90 INSERM Research Units, Department of Pharmacology, Hôpital Necker, Paris

CYNTHIA D. MORRIS, PH. D.
Division of Nephrology and Hypertension, Oregon Health Sciences University, Portland, Oregon

A. M. MOURA, M.D.
Centre de Recherches Roussel-Uclaf, Romainville, Paris

ANNE MOYNOT, M.D.
Centre de l'A.U.R.A., Rue du Bessin, Paris

M. G. PERNOLLET, M.D.
U7 and U90 INSERM Research Units, Department of Pharmacology, Hôpital Necker, Paris

A. PRUNA, M.D.
Departement de Néphrologie (Unité de Transplantation Rénale) et INSERM U-25, Hôpital Necker, Paris

EBERHARD RITZ, M.D.
Department of Internal Medicine, University of Heidelberg, Heidelberg, West Germany

J. B. ROSENFELD, M.D.
U7 and U90 INSERM Research Units, Department of Pharmacology, Hôpital Necker, Paris

MICHAEL R. RUDNICK, M.D.
The Graduate Hospital, Philadelphia, Pennsylvania

FRANÇOISE RUSSO-MARIE, M.D.
INSERM U90, Hôpital Necker, Université Rene Descartes, Paris

P. SIMON, M.D.
Service of Medicine E - Nephrology, La Beaudhée Hospital, Saint-Brieuc, France

ALFRED D. STEINBERG, M.D.
Chief, Section on Cellular Immunology, ARB, NIADDK, National Institutes of Health; Medical Director, U.S. Public Health Service, Bethesda, Maryland

FRANÇOIS TRON, M.D.
Unité de Recherches sur les Malades Renales, INSERM U25, Hôpital Necker, Paris

M. B. VALLOTTON, M.D.
Division of Endocrinology, Department of Médecine, University Cantonal Hospital, Geneva, Switzerland

Ph VIGERAL, M D
Departement de Néphrologie (Unité de Transplantation Rénale) et INSERM U-25, Hôpital Necker, Paris

ABRAHAM U. WAKS, M.D.
   UCLA School of Medicine, Los Angeles, California

P. WEIDMANN, M.D.
   Medizinische Poliklinik, University of Berne, Switzerland

M. WORCEL, M.D.
   Centre de Recherches Roussel-Uclaf, Romainville, France

Table of Contents

Liver Changes and Complications in Adult Polycystic Kidney Disease

JEAN-PIERRE GRÜNFELD,* GINETTE ALBOUZE,*
PAUL JUNGERS,* PAUL LANDAIS,* ALAIN
DANA,† DOMINIQUE DROZ,‡ ANNE MOYNOT,§
BERNARD LAFFORGUE,‖ EDWIGE BOURSZTYN¶
AND DOMINIQUE FRANCO.¶

*Départment de Néphrologie, Hôpital Necker, Paris; †Service de Radiologie des
maladies de l'appareil urinaire, Hôpital Necker; ‡Laboratoire Central d'Anatomie
Pathologique, Hôpital Necker; §Centre de l'A.U.R.A., Rue du Bessin, Paris; ‖Centre de
l'A.U.R.A., Rue des Peupliers, Paris; ¶Service de Chirurgie Digestive,
Hôpital Paul Brousse, Villejuif.

IT IS GENERALLY CONSIDERED that liver complications are exceptional in adult polycystic kidney disease (PKD). Liver cysts are usually asymptomatic and do not alter the liver function or the natural history of the disease.[13, 20, 21] Isolated cases of liver complications have, however, been occasionally reported.[6, 14, 15]

We recently studied the prognosis of dialysis patients with PKD[24] and were struck by the not-exceptional occurrence of severe liver complications. We have therefore attempted to estimate the prevalence of liver cysts in PKD. Today the detection of liver cysts is made far easier by the use of noninvasive methods, such as radioisotope liver scanning or ultrasonography. We used the latter technique, which is the more reliable.

Our study showed that liver cysts develop more slowly than kidney cysts. The incidence of liver cysts (and of their compli-

1

0084-5957/84/0014-0001-0020-$04.00

cations) is maximal in dialysis patients. It may be expected that the progressive enlargement of liver cysts in these patients leads to an increased incidence of liver complications. This is not surprising: dialysis and/or renal transplantation afford prolonged survival in patients with end-stage renal failure; extrarenal abnormalities, which accompany some renal diseases, may develop and produce certain clinical manifestations which, before 1960, were thought to be asymptomatic or benign.

Prevalence of Liver Cysts in Adult PKD

PATIENTS AND METHODS

In a prospective study in 1982, we studied the prevalence of liver cysts in 132 hemodialysis patients with PKD. Intermittent hemodialysis had been initiated between 1965 and 1982 and then subsequently performed either at home or in dialysis centers. Ultrasonography was performed in 124 patients (i.e., 6% of the patients were unavailable for follow-up).

In addition we studied the prevalence of liver cysts in non-hemodialyzed patients with PKD. This retrospective study was based on 120 patients who underwent liver ultrasonography, either routinely, together with renal ultrasonography, or less often, because of liver enlargement. Thus the prevalence of liver cysts in PKD before end-stage renal failure may have been slightly overestimated.

Liver ultrasonography was performed in various centers, especially in patients living far from Paris. However most patients were living in Paris or in suburbs, and the majority of ultrasound examinations were performed by one of us (A.D.). A B-mode machine was used equipped with 16 gray-scale levels. The sonographic examination was performed with a 2.25- or 3.5-mHz transducer. The studies were done with a standard compound scanning unit, and pictures were obtained in sagittal and transverse planes. When necessary, views in additional planes were obtained in order to achieve complete visualization of the liver. More recently, real-time sonography was used, which enables better detection of smaller cysts. Liver cysts were characterized by anechoic sonolucent areas with well-defined boundaries and posterior enhancement.

RESULTS

Liver cysts were found in 85 of 124 patients on dialysis. Liver cyst prevalence was identical in both sexes (χ^2 NS), and the mean ages were similar in both sexes (Table 1).

In the 120 nondialysis patients (Table 2), with similar mean ages, the prevalence of liver cysts was significantly higher in females (75%) than in males (44%; $\chi^2 = 10.6$). The prevalence of liver cysts was higher in female than in male nondialyzed patients in all age groups (Fig 1).

We pooled the data obtained in 244 patients with PKD, irrespective of their level of renal function, and examined liver cyst incidence by age group. The prevalence of liver cysts increased with age. In females it reached a peak in the 30- to 39-year-old age group and remained stable thereafter. In males it culminated in the 40- to 49-year-old age group (Fig 2). However, few young patients were investigated, and any definitive statement on the progression of liver cysts with age according to sex should be considered as preliminary. Further investigation is required to clarify this issue.

TABLE 1.—PREVALENCE OF
LIVER CYSTS (LC) IN 124
HEMODIALYZED PATIENTS WITH
ADULT POLYCYSTIC KIDNEY
DISEASE

PATIENTS	AGE (YR)*	% LC	
Females ($n = 74$)	56.9 ± 9.3	75	NS
Males ($n = 50$)	54.9 ± 8.8	62	

*Means $\pm$ 1 SD.

TABLE 2.—PREVALENCE OF LIVER CYSTS
(LC) IN 120 NONHEMODIALYZED PATIENTS
WITH POLYCYSTIC KIDNEY DISEASE

PATIENTS	AGE (YR)*	LC +	% LC	
Females ($n = 68$)	45.3 ± 14.3	50	73	NS
Males ($n = 52$)	44.7 ± 15.0	23	44	

*Means $\pm$ 1 SD.

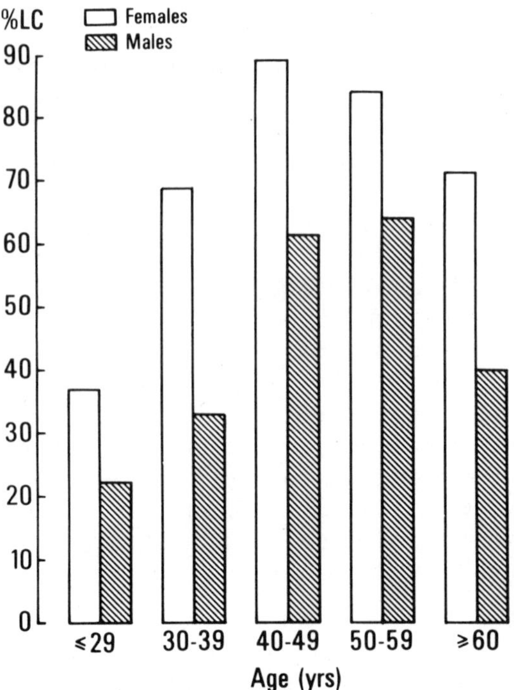

Fig 1.—Prevalence of liver cysts *(LC)* as detected by ultrasonography in 120 non-hemodialyzed PKD patients, according to age and sex.

COMMENT

The prevalence of liver cysts at autopsy in the general population is approximately 0.16%.[25] We have no evidence that it is higher in dialysis patients unaffected by PKD (unpublished data). To our knowledge, there have been no published accounts of the incidence of liver cysts as detected by ultrasonography in the general population. Holmes detected liver cysts in three of 115 subjects who had no renal cysts themselves but belonged to families with PKD.[23] It is to be expected that the prevalence of liver cysts would be higher in the latter group. Indeed, some families have been described in which certain members had PKD and others had solely polycystic liver,[12, 29] an observation anticipated by Dalgaard.[13]

In the published studies to date, the prevalence of liver cysts in PKD varies according to the series, the number of investi-

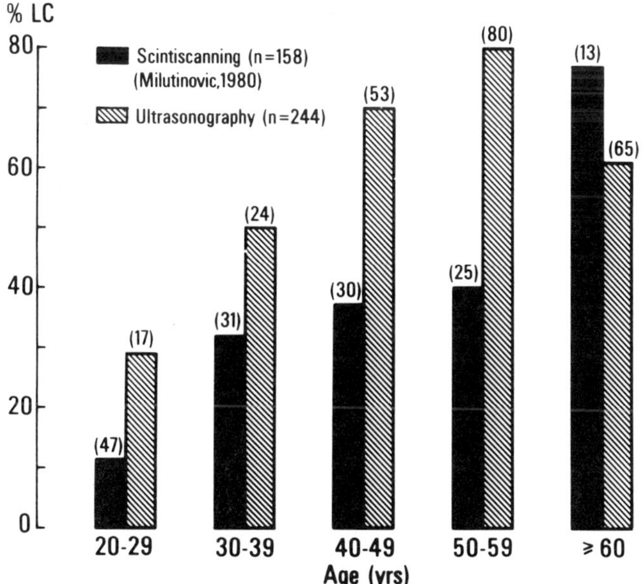

Fig 2.—Prevalence of liver cysts *(LC)* in PKD patients according to age and mode of detection: radioisotope liver scanning (from Milutinovic et al.[32]) or liver ultrasonography (present study).

gated patients, their ages (and thus, in part, the glomerular filtration rate), and the mode of detection used (autopsy, radioisotope scanning, or ultrasonography).

Of the studies based on autopsy data, that by Dalgaard is the most extensive. It includes 157 patients with "bilateral" PKD; liver cysts were found in 75 patients (a 48% prevalence). The prevalence differs with age: only 17% in the 18 patients aged 29–39 years; on average, 50% in the patients aged 40–69 years; and 75% in the 8 patients aged 70 years or older.[13] As in our study, the prevalence increased with age. It should be stressed that the study by Dalgaard was published in 1957, before the development of intermittent dialysis. It should therefore not be compared with data collected in patients with end-stage renal failure who have been on hemodialysis for 5–10 years or more. Most patients studied by Dalgaard died of renal failure or its consequences. The greatest number of deaths occurred in persons aged 40–59 years (106 of 157 cases), but some patients died in their sixth or seventh decades, demonstrating that in some patients PKD progresses only very slowly to renal failure. There is a strong inverse correlation between age and renal function, but this is not absolute. Other studies done before (cited by Dalgaard[13]) or after 1957[22] do not provide any more valuable additional information. The experience at the Clinique Néphrologique of Hôpital Necker was reported by Nézelof and Watchi in 1967. They do not stipulate the frequency of liver cysts in their series of 24 autopsy reports on PKD patients.[33] In a more recent autopsy study, we found liver cysts in 17 of 19 cases, a prevalence of approximately 90%. Such a prevalence might be explained by the longer survival of patients: in 17 of 19 cases, death occurred after 1 week to 10 years of hemodialysis (mean, 3.2 years).

Among the studies using radioisotope liver scanning, that by Milutinovic et al.[32] is the most valuable, dealing with 158 PKD patients (see Fig 2).[32] Liver scanning was performed with ^{99m}Tc-colloidal sulfur. The prevalence of liver cysts in the whole group was 29%. The following points should be noted. (1) Milutinovic et al.[32] included a larger proportion of younger patients than our own study; for example, their study included 47 patients aged 20–29 years, versus only 17 in our series. (2) The prevalence of liver cysts increased with age (see Fig 2) and with declining GFR: no liver cysts were found in patients less than 20 years of age, and 77% of the liver cysts were in patients aged 60 years or older.[32] (3) The prevalence of liver cysts was similar in both sexes. (4) In the younger patients, those aged 20–59 years, the prevalence of liver cysts was higher in our study, which used ultrasonography, than in the study by Milutinovic et al.[32] In contrast, the prevalence is identical (>60%) in patients aged 60 years or older. These discrepancies may be accounted for by two factors: (1) as was mentioned earlier, we have possibly overestimated the prevalence of liver cysts in our retrospective study in younger, nondialyzed patients. (2) The mode of liver cyst detection was different in the two studies. The lower limit of detection by liver scanning is 2.5 cm.[21] In contrast, it is presently 0.5 cm for sonography. Thus, liver scanning underestimates the prevalence of cysts in the younger patients, in whom the cysts are small, whereas both liver scanning and ultrasonography provide similar information in older patients, in whom the cysts are more voluminous.

Our study may be compared with that made by Holmes, who used sonography.[23] Holmes found liver cysts in 43.5% of the PKD patients, but his study was limited to patients with serum creatinine levels of 4 mg/dl or less.

In conclusion, the prevalence of liver cysts increases with age in PKD patients. It is more than 60% in the older patients, most of whom are dialyzed. Liver cysts develop more slowly than renal cysts and appear earlier in females than in males. This observation needs to be confirmed, however. In this regard, it may be recalled that polycystic liver, in the absence of renal involvement, predominates in females,[35] that congenital isolated liver cysts seem to be more frequent in females, and that estrogens may favor the development of certain histopathologic liver lesions. Thus, the hormonal status may modulate the rate of progression of liver cysts. This hypothesis requires further investigation.

Liver Histopathologic Changes in Adult PKD

Few studies have been devoted to the liver histopathologic changes found in large series of patients with adult PKD, although many publications have dealt with liver involvement in infantile PKD. Based on 19 autopsy reports, we attempted to analyze the liver lesions in adult PKD.

MATERIAL AND RESULTS

One of us (D.D.) analyzed the data collected from 19 autopsy reports (11 males and 8 females). Prior to death, all patients but two had been treated by hemodialysis; the diagnosis of adult PKD was confirmed at autopsy in all cases. Death was due to liver complications in five cases (two died of infections of liver cysts, two died of cholangiocarcinomas, and one died of cirrhosis).

Macroscopic examination showed that the liver weight was above 2 kg in 12 cases and above 3.5 kg in five; in the seven other cases, it ranged from 1.450 to 1.900 kg. Liver cysts were found in 17 cases, numerous and scattered diffusely in 14 and more localized and/or restricted to a single lobe in three cases. In two cases, the cysts contained pus, which was associated with intrahepatic abscesses in one case. Finally, a liver tumor was detected in two cases. In the first one, the tumor was localized to the upper part of the liver and was necrotic; in the second, it was solid, whitish, and massively invaded the liver parenchyma, only partially sparing the left lobe.

The results of the microscopic examination are summarized in Table 3. The changes were of various types.

LIVER CYSTS.—These are found either within or close to the portal tracts. The cavities are lined by cuboidal epithelium and are surrounded by a thin fibrous capsule. They do not communicate with the biliary tree. In only two cases were no cysts found on the sections examined. However, in one case there were dilated intrahepatic bile ducts in the large portal tracts. Liver cysts were usually associated with Von Meyenburg's complexes or with biliary fibroadenomatosis. Isolated liver cysts, in the absence of Von Meyenburg's complexes and fibroadenomatosis, were present in only two cases. In two other cases, suppurative cysts were found, accompanied in one case by acute angiocholitis involving the bile ducts of the portal tracts and the Von Meyenburg's complexes (Fig 3).

VON MEYENBURG'S COMPLEXES.—Von Meyenburg's complexes, or "biliary microhamartomas," are composed of a limited number of bile ducts lined by flattened epithelium and surrounded by fibrous tissue, and apparently unconnected to the portal tracts. These complexes were present in 11 cases and were numerous in five.

TABLE 3.—LIVER
HISTOPATHOLOGIC LESIONS IN
ADULT POLYCYSTIC KIDNEY
DISEASE*

LESION	NO.
Liver cysts	17
Von Meyenburg complexes	11
Biliary fibroadenomatosis	12
Other:	
Chronic hepatitis	7†
Cholangiocarcinoma	2
Infected liver cysts	2‡

*Data obtained from 19 autopsy studies.
†Of whom three were cirrhotic.
‡Of whom one showed angiocholitis.

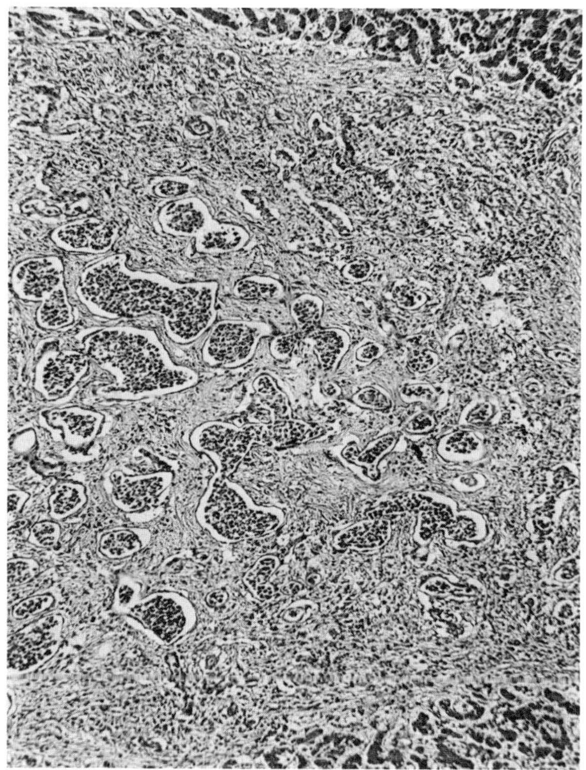

Fig 3.—Liver histopathology in adult-type polycystic kidney disease. Specimen shows acute angiocholitis involving the bile ducts in a Von Meyenburg complex (×450).

BILIARY FIBROADENOMATOSIS.—Biliary fibroadenomatosis is characterized by fibrosis of the portal tracts, which show an excessive number of more or less dilated bile ducts. No inflammatory cell infiltrate is found. In eight cases localized areas of fibroadenomatosis were seen (Fig 4). In four cases, the fibroadenomatosis was more diffuse, involving almost all the portal tracts examined. Von Meyenburg's complexes and fibroadenomatosis were observed concurrently in two cases.

LIVER CHANGES.—Various liver changes were also found. Severe lesions of chronic hepatitis were present in seven cases, with cirrhosis in three cases. Six of these seven patients had the hepatitis B surface antigen in their sera. No correlation was noted between the lesions of fibroadenomatosis and those

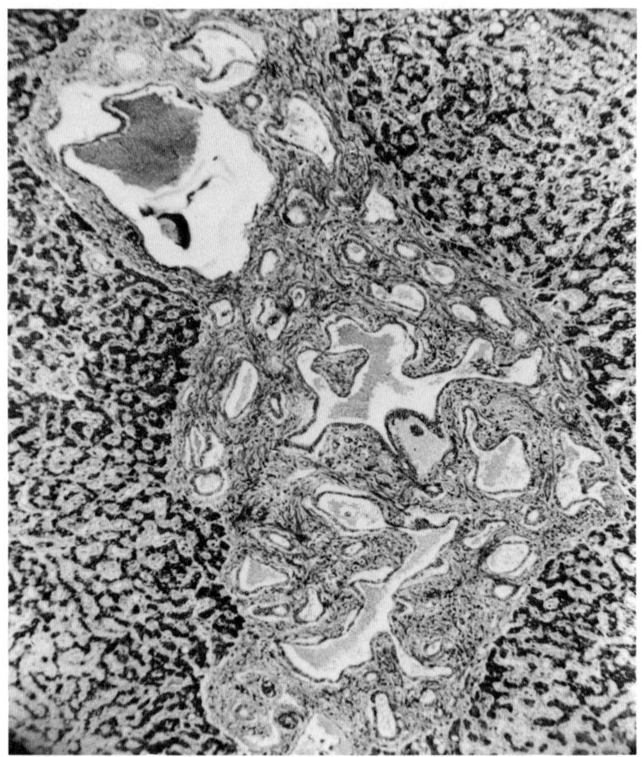

Fig 4.—Biliary fibroadenomatosis in adult-type polycystic kidney disease (Masson's trichrome stain, ×250).

of chronic hepatitis. Histopathologic study revealed the presence of cholangiocarcinoma in two cases; the tumor was well differentiated and mucosecreting in one case and poorly differentiated and necrotic in the other. In the former, for which multiple samples were available, we were able to show in situ carcinomatous transformation of the biliary epithelium in some Von Meyenburg's complexes (Fig 5). Such an aspect could not be found in the other 18 cases, either in the liver cysts or in the complexes.

COMMENT

Our results, based on the data collected from 19 autopsy reports, emphasize the high incidence of liver changes in adult

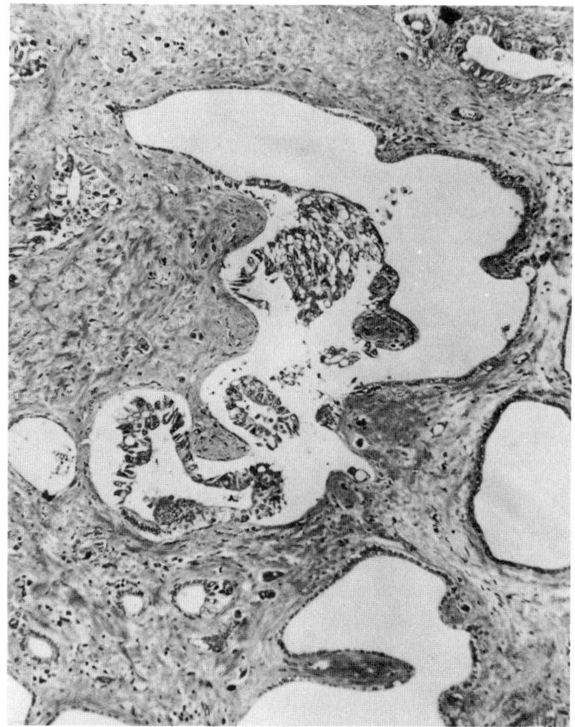

Fig 5.—Cholangiocarcinoma. Specimen shows in situ anaplastic transformation of biliary epithelium in Von Meyenburg complex (Masson's trichromic stain, ×650).

PKD.[33] Liver cysts, Von Meyenburg's complexes, and biliary fibroadenomatosis are the most characteristic lesions. They were not observed at autopsy in patients on hemodialysis who were unaffected by PKD.

The high incidence of liver cysts has already been mentioned. It is generally accepted that liver cysts are formed by the progressive segmentation and dilation of Von Meyenburg's complexes.[21] The complexes represent the remnants of intrahepatic bile ducts which were formed in excess and did not establish any connection with larger interlobular bile ducts, located in the portal tracts; normally, these complexes involute and disappear. Liver cysts do not generally communicate with the biliary tree, but their growth may cause them to rupture into adjacent bile ducts. This may then favor an infection of the cyst, as in one of our cases (see Fig 3). Liver cysts do not contain bile. The cyst fluid has been analyzed in a few studies in cases of polycystic liver or of solitary liver cysts, in the absence of kidney cystic involvement. It is stated that the constituents of the cyst fluid resemble the "bile salt-independent" fraction of human bile, and result from the secretory activity of the cyst epithelium.[35] It is not known whether or not this epithelium is sensitive to hormonal stimulation.

The lesions of biliary fibroadenomatosis and the Von Meyenburg's complexes have been observed in 60% of the cases investigated. It may be difficult to differentiate numerous Von Meyenburg's complexes from biliary fibroadenomatosis. Indeed, the apparent lack of continuity between complexes and portal tracts may be related simply to the site from which the histopathologic sections were taken.[18]

The liver histopathologic changes found in adult PKD are classically very different from those observed in congenital hepatic fibrosis, which is associated with infantile PKD.[1, 38] Congenital hepatic fibrosis consists of diffuse biliary fibroadenomatosis, so that the terms are considered synonymous by some authors.

In adult PKD the presence of liver cysts and Von Meyenburg's complexes is well recognized. On the other hand, the high incidence of biliary fibroadenomatosis lesions is surprising. Yet they are less diffuse and less important in adult PKD than in congenital hepatic fibrosis associated with infantile PKD. They are usually arranged as islets, but were diffuse in four cases. The clinical liver manifestations are different in infantile and adult PKD; the children predominantly develop portal hypertension with or without angiocholitis, and often early in the course of their disease; in adults, liver complications are less common and supervene later.[1, 38, 39] Until now, this difference has been explained by the contrasting liver histopathologic changes seen in the two forms of PKD. In fact, it should be questioned whether this difference could be related either to the distinct distribution of the biliary fibroadenomatosis lesions observed in these two conditions or to their associated lesions. The portal hypertension seen in congenital hepatic fibrosis may be caused by hypoplasia of the portal vein branches (or their compression by fibrous bands). Dilatation of the intrahepatic bile ducts (as in Caroli's disease) predisposes to episodes of angiocholitis.[17, 18, 39]

A few publications mention the coexistence of congenital hepatic fibrosis, without demonstrable portal hypertension, with adult PKD (case 17 reported by Clermont et al.,[10] cases 2 and 3 reported by Dupond et al.[15]). Such observations must be reinterpreted, taking into account the frequency of biliary fibroadenomatosis lesions seen in adult PKD.

There have been several recent animal studies on the induction of PKD, especially with the use of antioxidants.[19, 20] Intratubular obstruction has been proposed to explain the development and growth of the renal cysts. In such experimentally induced PKD in laboratory animals, the liver is never affected by cystic change, and therefore it is questionable whether one can extrapolate any reliable information from these studies with respect to human PKD, in which hepatic cysts or other lesions frequently appear in association with the renal cysts. A working hypothesis is needed to explain the development of both the hepatic and renal cysts. As noted by Grantham, the liver may be an important key to our understanding of the pathogenesis of renal disease.[20]

Liver Complications in Adult PKD

Quoting Fiessinger, Dalgaard stated the polycystic liver is "un foie énorme, silencieux et durable." This "dogma" remains true for most cases of hepatorenal polycystic disease preceding end-stage renal failure, but today needs to be revised to apply to those patients supported by dialysis.

STUDY POPULATION AND RESULTS

Between 1965 and 1982, we studied a group of 229 patients with polycystic kidney disease and end-stage renal failure. Most were on dialysis. The group included some patients also included in the studies discussed earlier in this chapter.

Of the 229 patients, 76 have died, 31 from cardiovascular complications (10 cerebrovascular accidents and 11 myocardial infarctions), 15 from complications related to polycystic disease (2 ruptured cerebral aneurysms, 5 renal cyst complications, and 8 hepatic-related deaths) and 30 from diverse causes (infection, cancer, aluminum encephalopathy, postoperative emboli, etc.). Thus, hepatic complications accounted for 10.5% of all causes of death in this group. Four deaths resulted from hepatic cyst infections; one patient had had coexisting portal hypertension thought to have been due to posthepatitic cirrhosis. One death was directly attributed to the voluminous polycystic liver which compressed adjacent viscera, rendering the patient grossly cachexic. One patient had HBsAg-positive chronic hepatitis with cirrhosis and died with hepatic encephalopathy. Finally, two patients died from cholangiocarcinoma, and at autopsy of one of these cases, it was shown that the carcinoma arose from hepatic cyst epithelium (see Fig 5; Table 4).

Apart from these fatal complications, we observed three cases of infection of hepatic cysts, which were adequately treated. A total of five female and six male patients suffered hepatic complications, whether or not fatal.

We are at present unable to give precise figures on the frequency of hepatic complications *prior* to end-stage renal failure. However, of almost 500 cases of PKD (including the 229 patients subsequently dialyzed) we found only three cases of hepatic cyst infection before end-stage renal failure, and all three were in women, aged 42, 48, and 61 years, respectively. It must be remembered that seven of the 229 dialyzed patients presented with liver cyst infection. However, the time span of observation was not the same in the two groups of patients. Indeed, patients seen prior to terminal uremia were observed for a longer period than those on dialysis. On the other hand,

TABLE 4.—LIVER COMPLICATIONS IN 229 PATIENTS WITH POLYCYSTIC KIDNEY DISEASE AND END-STAGE RENAL FAILURE*

COMPLICATION	DECEASED	SURVIVORS
Liver cyst infection	4†	3
Mechanical complications and cachexia related to liver cysts	1	
Liver encephalopathy	1‡	
Cholangiocarcinoma	2	

*Most were on dialysis.
†In one case, this was associated with portal hypertension probably related to posthepatitic cirrhosis.
‡Coexistence of posthepatitic cirrhosis and portal hypertension.

patients with the most complications, whether renal or extra-renal, tend to be referred preferentially to hospitals.

COMMENT

Complications of liver cysts, (for example, cyst rupture or torsion, intracystic hemorrhage, infection or compression) are considered to occur very rarely, whether the cysts are solitary or multiple or associated with PKD. However, this is not true of dialysis patients, in whom such complications represent almost 10% of the causes of death (7 of the 76 fatalities, excluding the single case in which posthepatitic cirrhosis probably played a significant role). Terminal renal failure may favor the development of certain complications, notably infections, but their frequency is probably proportional to increased survival of the patients due to dialysis, during which time liver cysts may appear and/or enlarge. While renal failure remains only moderate or is absent, these complications are hardly seen; only three women were affected, which indirectly supports the hypothesis stated earlier, that hepatic cysts develop earlier in women.

Liver cyst infection is the most alarming complication. In some cases, 1 or 2 L of pus have been evacuated from the cyst cavities.[34, 40] The infection may remain localized or may follow acute cholangitis or septicemia.[11] Fever (or septicemia) with hepatic cysts may falsely evoke various diagnoses: infected renal cysts, sigmoid diverticulitis, and all the other causes of fever in a patient on dialysis. Therefore, the possibility of hepatic cyst infection must be considered systematically in febrile patients with PKD and especially in those receiving hemodialysis. When cysts are infected, ultrasound examination may show a heterogeneous echo-dense area or a fluid level. Transcutaneous puncture, under ultrasound guidance whenever possible, relieves the associated pain, provides specimen material for microbiologic assessment, and yields informations on the diffusion of antibiotics into liver cysts.

Portal hypertension associated with hepatorenal polycystic disease has been discussed by several authors.[2, 4, 6–9, 14, 15] It appears that these patients do not constitute a single group. From the data available in the literature, the following statements can be made: (1) Portal hypertension may be due to liver cirrhosis following viral hepatitis.[25] (2) Portal hypertension may be caused by compression of the portal vein or its branches by the hepatic cysts. To support this explanation, the liver must show no evidence of fibrosis or cirrhosis on pathologic examination, and the portal pressure should normalize on drainage or ablation of the cysts. To our knowledge there are no reports of such findings in the literature.[2, 4, 16, 26] The case 1 dealing with a hemodialysis patient, reported by Del Guercio et al., causes most concern. The cause of death was gastrointestinal hemorrhage, and at autopsy hepatic cysts occupied 70% of the parenchyma, with no evidence of fibrosis.[14] (3) Certain publications have drawn attention to the unusual coexistence of PKD with biliary fibroadenomatosis, without firm proof of portal hypertension. These were the findings in case 7 reported by Clermont et al.[10] and cases 2 and 3 reported by Dupond et al.[15] In case 2 of Dupond et al. there were no hepatic cysts found at autopsy. Our histopathologic examination of liver autopsy specimens demonstrated that the lesions of biliary fibroadenomatosis were frequently observed in patients with PKD without any clinical liver manifestations.

A certain number of cases remain which are characterized by the association, in adults, of portal hypertension (often presenting with gastrointestinal bleeding), biliary fibroadenomatosis in the absence of large liver cysts, and renal cysts compatible with adult PKD. The cases described by Campbell et al. of three siblings aged 14–25 years are most frequently cited.[6] Such cases raise the question of how much overlap exists between the adult and infantile form of PKD, as illustrated by the following points: (1) Congenital hepatic fibrosis, with portal hypertension and gastrointestinal hemorrhage, was observed in a few adult patients with predominantly medullary renal cysts and collecting duct ectasia, findings which suggest the infantile or juvenile type of PKD than the adult type. The first case cited by Dupond et al. belongs to this group. In adult PKD it is rare for the renal failure to appear at 24 years and to reach an advanced stage by 32 years; furthermore, at autopsy the kidneys weighed only 170 gm and 240 gm.[15] (2) In other adult cases it was thought that the biliary fibroadenomatosis favored the development of episodes of acute cholangitis.[7, 30] (3) As stated by Alagille et al.[1] the distinction between juvenile and adult types of PKD is further complicated by reports of families in which some members had congenital hepatic fibrosis with infantile PKD, whereas others had apparently typical adult PKD (case 2 reported by Bradford et al.[5]). At the other end of the spectrum, adult PKD disease may present during childhood.[38]

The exact classification of these cases became increasingly difficult after Boichis et al.[3] and others described a possible association between hepatic fibrosis and medullary cystic disease of the kidney. Adults may be affected by this disease, which appears to show in this instance an autosomal dominant mode of inheritance. The cysts are well visualized on ultrasound and the kidneys are not enlarged.[28]

One particular case, not included in the present study, illustrates the difficulties in classification. A man had moderate impairment of renal function at age 36 years . Renal biopsy at age 40 showed chronic interstitial nephritis with medullary tubular ectasias. On intravenous urography the kidneys were small. The family history was negative. He died at age 49 of *E. coli* septicemia with jaundice, ascites, and cholestasis, but without any evidence of hepatocellular failure. Autopsy showed two atrophic kidneys weighing less than 100 gm and containing multiple cortical and medullary cysts surrounded by interstitial fibrosis. Pathologic examination of the liver showed widespread lesions of biliary fibroadenomatosis.

We have seen two cases of cholangiocarcinoma, one in a 54-year-old woman and one in a 57-year-old man after 1 and 9 years of hemodialysis, respectively.[27] In Europe, cholangiocarcinoma is considered extremely rare, being 8 times less common than hepatocellular carcinoma. Nine patients with liver cysts who subsequently developed cholangiocarcinoma have been described, of whom two had PKD. Moreover, the incidence of cholangiocarcinoma is greatly increased in two other closely related diseases, Caroli's disease and congenital hepatic fibrosis,[31] both of which show lesions of biliary fibroadenomatosis. It may be questioned whether the risk of cholangiocarcinoma is increased in dialysis patients with PKD. Further studies are needed to determine the true frequency of cholangiocarcinoma in PKD patients who are dialyzed for decades or who receive a renal transplant.[27]

Conclusion

In adult PKD, ultrasonography shows a high prevalence of liver cysts, reaching 60%–75% of those patients on dialysis. Liver cysts develop later than renal cysts and appear earlier in women than in men.

Histopathologic study based on 19 autopsy specimens confirmed the high frequency of liver cysts and showed various additional lesions: Von Meyenburg complexes (11 cases), lesions of biliary fibroadenomatosis, either diffuse or focal (12 cases), and cholangiocarcinoma (2 cases).

Complications of liver cysts were the cause of death in patients with PKD on dialysis, whereas such events were rare prior to end-stage renal failure. Liver cyst infection was seen in seven cases and was responsible for four deaths. Two patients died from cholangiocarcinoma, and in one, we were able to demonstrate in situ anaplastic transformation of the cyst epithelium in a Von Meyenburg complex.

It should be emphasized that the frequency of liver cyst complications is not negligible, and such complications may often be serious once patients are on dialysis. It may be questioned whether or not the incidence of these complications will increase in the future in proportion to the prolonged survival of these patients afforded by dialysis and/or renal transplantation.

Acknowledgments

We wish to express our gratitude to the physicians of dialysis units who cooperated in this study, and to Dr. Claude Degott for her advice. We also thank Mrs. Marie-Alice Monod for excellent secretarial help, Mrs. Lallemand for skillful technical assistance, Mrs. Lillié-Kadouche for photographs, and Miss Margaret Saunders for preparation of the manuscript.

REFERENCES

1. Alagille D., Odièvre M.: *Maladies du Foie et des Voies Biliaires chez l'Enfant.* Paris, Flammarion, 1978.
2. Bernard J.P., Béraud C., Loiseau P., et al.: Polykystose hépato-rénale de l'adulte: Documents splénoportographiques. *Arch. Mal. Appl. Dig.* 50:513–523, 1961.
3. Boichis H., Passwell J., David R., et al.: Congenital hepatic fibrosis and nephronophtisis. *Q. J. Med.* 42:221–233, 1973.

4. Boulard C., Suduca P., Gavalda J., et al.: Maladie polykystique hépato-rénale avec hypertension portale et dérivation spléno-cave spontanée. *Prev. Med.* 75:697–700, 1967.
5. Bradford W.D., Bradford J.W., Porter F.S., et al.: Cystic disease of liver and kidney with portal hypertension. *Clin. Pediatr.* 7:299–306, 1968.
6. Campbell G.S., Bick H.D., Paulsen E.P., et al.: Bleeding esophageal varices with polycystic liver. *N. Engl. J. Med.* 259:904–910, 1958.
7. Case records of the Massachusetts General Hospital: Case 18–1963. *N. Engl. J. Med.* 268:601–607, 1963.
8. Case records of the Massachusetts General Hospital: Case 16–1968. *N. Engl. J. Med.* 278:899–904, 1968.
9. Case records of the Massachusetts General Hospital: Case 11–1974. *N. Engl. J. Med.* 290:676–683, 1974.
10. Clermont R.J., Maillard J.N., Benhamou J.P., et al.: Fibrose hépatique congénitale. *Can. Med. Assoc. J.* 97:1272–1278, 1967.
11. Clinicopathological Conference: A case of polycystic disease of the liver and kidneys demonstrated at the Postgraduate Medical School of London. *Br. Med. J.* 4:1356–1358, 1965.
12. Comfort M.W., Gray H.K., Dahlin D.C., et al.: Polycystic disease of the liver: A study of 24 cases. *Gastroenterology* 20:60–78, 1952.
13. Dalgaard O.A.: Bilateral polycystic disease of the kidneys. *Acta Med. Scand.* 158(suppl. 328):1–255, 1957.
14. Del Guercio E., Greco J., Kim K.E., et al.: Esophageal varices in adult patients with polycystic kidney and liver disease. *N. Engl. J. Med.* 289:678–679, 1973.
15. Dupond J.L., Miguet J.P., Carbillet J.P., et al.: Polykystose rénale, principale expression de la fibrose hépatique congénitale. *Nouv. Presse Med.* 8:2885–2888, 1979.
16. Facci R.C., Milleo F.Q.: Tratamento cirurgico da policistose hepatica: Relato de un casa. *Nouv. Presse Med. Ediçao Brasileira* 1:423–424, 1982.
17. Fauvert R., Benhamou J.P., Meyer P.: Fibrose hépatique congénitale. *Rev. Fr. Et. Clin. Biol.* 9:375, 1964.
18. Fevery J., Tanghe W., Kerremans R., et al.: Congenital dilatation of the intrahepatic bile ducts associated with the development of amyloidosis. *Gut* 13:604–609, 1972.
19. Gardner K.D. Jr., Evan A.P.: Renal cystic disease induced by diphenylthiazole. *Kidney Int.* 24:43–52, 1983.
20. Grantham J.J.: Polycystic kidney disease: A predominance of giant nephrons. *Am. J. Physiol.* 244:F3–F10, 1983.
21. Hartnett M., Bennett W.: Extrarenal manifestations of cystic kidney disease, in Gardner K.D. Jr. (ed.): *Cystic Diseases of the Kidney.* New York, John Wiley & Sons, 1976, pp. 201–219.
22. Hatfield P.M., Pfister R.C.: Adult polycystic disease of the kidneys (Potter type 3). *JAMA* 222:1527–1531, 1972.
23. Holmes J.H.: Polycystic kidney disease, in Watanabe H., Holmes J.H., Holm H.H., et al. (eds.): *Diagnostic Ultrasound in Urology and Nephrology.* New York, Igaku-Shoin, 1981, pp. 39–48.
24. Jungers P., Albouze G., Aime F., et al.: Problèmes posés par l'hémodialyse périodique et la transplantation rénale chez les malades atteints de maladie polykystique rénale, in Küss R., Legrain M. (eds.): *Séminaires d'Uro-Néphrologie Pitié-Salpêtrière.* Paris, Masson, 1983, pp. 12–37.
25. Jungers P., Naret C., Zingraff J., et al.: Corrélations entre la persistance d'une antigénémie HB et la survenue d'une hépatite chronique chez les hémodialysés, Soulier J.P., Tacquet A., Jungers P., et al. (eds.): in *Hépatite à Virus B et Hémodialyse.* Paris, Flammarion, 1975, p. 45.

26. Katzen N.G.: Fatal hepatic polycystic disease. *Br. Med. J.* 2:839–840, 1964.
27. Landais P., Grünfeld J.P., Droz D., et al.: Cholangiocarcinoma in polycystic kidney and liver disease. *Arch. Intern. Med.,* to be published.
28. Landais P., Moreau J.F., Grünfeld J.P.: Case 48–1981: Ultrasound in the diagnosis of uremic disease in adults. *N. Engl. J. Med.* 306:995–996, 1982.
29. Longmire W.P. Jr., Mandiola S.A., Gordon H.E.: Congenital cystic disease of the liver and biliary system. *Ann. Surg.* 174:711–726, 1971.
30. Maillet P., Brette R., Bertrand J.L., et al.: Trois cas de polykystose hépato-rénale. *Lyon Med.* 230:439–442, 1973.
31. McCarthy L.J., Baggenstoss A.H., Logan G.B.: Congenital hepatic fibrosis. *Gastroenterology* 49:27–36, 1965.
32. Milutinovic J., Fialkow P.J., Rudd T.G., et al.: Liver cysts in patients with autosomal dominant polycystic kidney disease. *Am. J. Med.* 68:741–744, 1980.
33. Nézelof C., Watchi J.M.: Les maladies polykystiques hépatorénales. *Actualités Hépato-Gastro-Entérologiques de l'Hôtel-Dieu* 3:294–310, 1967.
34. Parneix M., Lotte P., Barandon E., et al.: La polykystose haépatique: À propos de 3 formes compliquées. *Chirurgie* 104:284–294, 1978.
35. Patterson M., Gonzalez-Vitale J.C., Fagan C.J.: Polycystic liver disease: A study of cyst fluid constituents. *Hepatology* 2:475–478, 1982.
36. Piering W.F., Hebert L.A., Lemann J. Jr.: Infantile polycystic kidney disease in the adult. *Arch. Intern. Med.* 137:1625–1626, 1977.
37. Proesmans W., Van Damme B., Macken J.: Nephronophtisis and tape to retinal degeneration associated with liver fibrosis. *Clin. Nephrol.* 3:160–164, 1975.
38. Royer P., Habib R., Mathieu H., et al.: Maladies kystiques des reins, in *Néphrologie Pédiatrique.* Paris, Flammarion, 1983, pp. 18–27.
39. Sherlock S.: Cysts and congenital biliary abnormalities, in Sherlock S. (ed.): *Diseases of the Liver and Biliary System.* Oxford, Alden Press, 1981, pp. 406–416.
40. Tenière P., Michot F., Testart J., et al.: La polykystose hépatique: Discussion thérapeutique à propos d'une observation. *J. Chir. (Paris)* 113:153–158, 1977.
41. Williams J.A., Price J.D.E.: Liver cysts in end stage uremia due to polycystic kidney disease. *Can. Med. Assoc. J.* 102:856–857, 1970.

Prenatal Diagnosis of Urinary Tract Malformations

M. BROYER, G. GUEST, F. LESTAGE, AND
F. BUFFET GACOIN

*Service de néphrologie pédiatrique et clinique urologique Hôpital Necker
Enfants Malades, Paris*

BIDIMENSIONAL ECHOGRAPHY introduced a new era of anatomical investigation, in nephrology as in numerous other areas. It was inevitable that fetal sonography would be used for the prenatal diagnosis of visceral malformations. Thus, in 1970 Garrett et al. reported the first prenatal diagnosis by ultrasound of renal polycystic disease.[25] Progress in ultrasound technology and the increased systematic use of ultrasound to follow the course of pregnancy today afford the possibility of prenatal diagnosis of kidney and urinary tract (UT) malformations. This possibility also raises a number of new questions concerning psychology and ethics, questions difficult to answer at the present time. In this chapter we report on a series of patients referred after birth to the Necker Enfants Malades Hôpital and in whom UT malformation had been made diagnosed in utero. This report will be followed by a discussion on this new chapter of medicine.

Material and Methods

Forty-four infants hospitalized at the Necker's Hospital between April 1978 and August 1983 were included in the study.

These patients were generally referred shortly after birth for further investigations and treatment, since the diagnosis of UT malformation had been made prenatally. Ultrasound examination during pregnancy usually was systematically performed in the obstetric department where the mothers were followed. The time of prenatal diagnosis was generally between weeks 30 and 35 of pregnancy, but some cases were screened earlier, between weeks 23 and 29.

The study included 32 male and 12 female infants, a sex ratio reflecting the increased incidence of UT malformations in males. The abnormalities detected were generally described as a dilation of the renal pelvis and/or as a liquid mass inside the kidney. The ureter was sometimes seen, allowing the diagnosis of megaureter. Unilaterality or bilaterality of the abnormalities was always mentioned and there were very few mistakes on this point, excepting some silent minor abnormalities. Finally, the bladder size was always noted, a dilation usually meaning a lower UT obstruction and/or a severe malformation.

UT Malformation According to Postnatal Diagnosis

The precise kind of UT malformation was determined after birth (Table 1). Malformations are described below.

MULTICYSTIC KIDNEYS.—This diagnosis was made in four patients after birth. In three, prenatal examination revealed a unilateral dilation of renal cavities, and in one, the diagnosis of prerenal liquid mass was suggested. The age at prenatal diagnosis was between 32 and 37 weeks' gestation. The postnatal

TABLE 1.—POSTNATAL DIAGNOSIS IN 44 INFANTS IN
WHOM SONOGRAPHIC EXAMINATION HAD DETECTED
URINARY TRACT ABNORMALITIES IN UTERO

DIAGNOSIS	NO.	UNILAT.	BILAT.
Multicystic kidney	4	4	0
Megaureter	9	7	2
Pelvoureteral junction stenosis	16	10	6
Urinary tract duplication	7	6	1
Massive reflux	3	0	3
Posterior urethral valves	1	. . .	. . .
Anterior urethral valves	1	. . .	. . .
Beckwith-Wiedemann syndrome	1	0	1
No abnormality	2	. . .	. . .

diagnosis was determined by histologic examination after nephrectomy.

MEGAURETERS.—This diagnosis was made in nine patients. In six, the lesion was unilateral, in two it was bilateral, and one patient had a megaureter on a single kidney. The in utero diagnosis of laterality was always correct, with the confirmation after birth of a normal kidney on the opposite side, except for the child with a megaureter on a single kidney. In this group of patients, the time of prenatal diagnosis was between weeks 27 and 37 of pregnancy (mean, week 33). The postnatal therapeutic approach varied according to the anatomical abnormalities. Nothing was done in children with a moderate dilation that spontaneously decreased. Five children underwent removal of the stenosed area of the ureter and replacement of the ureter in the bladder wall. Three of these five patients first underwent pyelostomy or a nephrostomy in the first month of life. Finally, one patient had severe bilateral dilation with impairment of renal function and died of renal failure and meningitis at age 4 months.

STENOSIS OF PELVIC URETERAL JUNCTION.—This abnormality was recognized after birth in 16 patients. Ten had a unilateral lesion, one a horseshoe kidney, and six cases were bilateral. Prenatal examination allowed a correct diagnosis of bilateral lesions in only two of these six patients; in fact, in three of the four misinterpreted cases the condition was asymmetric.

In the infant with a horseshoe kidney, the prenatal diagnosis hesitated between dilation of renal cavities and a colic abnormality. The time of prenatal diagnosis was for this group of patients between weeks 23 and 27 of pregnancy (mean, week 31). The therapeutic approach was again variable. Six of the ten with unilateral forms underwent surgical repair of the ureteral junction within the first 6 months, one child was nephrectomized, and nothing was done in three other patients. All these children with bilateral abnormalities were operated on (unilateral nephrectomy and/or surgical repair). Surgery was preceded in two cases by an early pyelostomy. Evolution was generally favorable in this group, and renal function improved in all the infants.

URINARY TRACT DUPLICATION.—Diagnosis of UT duplication was made in seven infants after birth, one of whom had bilateral lesions and three of whom had obstructive ureterocele.

Prenatal diagnosis had generally revealed a unilateral dilation of renal cavities, but in two cases the diagnosis was a paravertebral liquid mass whose renal origin was not obvious. This diagnosis was made between weeks 23 and 38 of pregnancy (mean, week 33). All these patients were operated on within the first 6 months: six underwent a partial nephrectomy and two a surgical repair of the ureterovesical junction. The course of all these patients continues favorable.

BILATERAL PASSIVE REFLUX WITH MEGACYSTIS.—Three cases of grade V reflux with megacystis without urethral obstruction were part of this series. The prenatal examination performed between weeks 30 and 35 of pregnancy revealed bilateral dilation of the renal cavities and megacystis. In two of these patients the bladder seemed to void satisfactorily. In one, it was decided to undertake premature delivery (see below). At birth renal function was impaired in these three patients and they underwent surgery, with good results. Presently their plasma creatinine level is between 60 and 90 μmoles/L.

POSTERIOR URETHRAL VALVES.—This diagnosis was made after birth in one patient. Bilateral dilation of renal cavities and megacystis had been found by echography at the 26th week of pregnancy. At this time a catheter was inserted in utero and subsequently the child was born after a premature delivery (see below). At birth posterior urethral valves with hypoplastic kidneys and renal insufficiency were found. Urine was diverted by a suprapubic permanent catheter and secondarily by means of a bilateral ureterostomy. Renal function remained poor in this child, who had a plasma creatinine value of 410 μmoles/L at 18 months.

ANTERIOR URETHRAL VALVES.—This diagnosis was made after birth in one child. Again, bilateral dilation of renal cavities was found in utero in week 36 of pregnancy, but the bladder looked normal. At birth renal functions were impaired but improved progressively after valve resection.

NEPHROMEGALY.—The diagnosis of Beckwith-Wiedemann syndrome was made in one infant after birth. Two enlarged kidneys had been found in utero in week 32 of pregnancy, and polycystic disease was thought likely. The correct diagnosis was made after birth on observance of facial abnormalities, macroglossy, and hypoglycemia.

FALSE ABNORMALITIES.—Two patients in our series were

found to be strictly normal after birth. Ultrasound examination had detected a bilateral dilation in one case and a unilateral dilation in the other in weeks 33 and 37 of pregnancy, respectively. In both cases the dilation was obvious but moderate.

Therapeutic Approaches After Prenatal Diagnosis

In Utero Maneuvers

The therapeutic approach remained generally a "wait and see" policy. In only two cases were in utero maneuvers attempted.

1. A right kidney dilation was detected in week 23 of pregnancy. The kidney was punctured in week 30 and 30 ml of liquid was withdrawn. After birth, the diagnosis of ureteral duplication with ureterocele and partial nephrectomy was made. In this case the puncture in utero was unjustified.

2. Bilateral dilation of the kidneys and ureters was found in week 26. A stent was inserted between the fetal bladder and the amniotic cavity. Flattening of the urinary tract persisted in week 29. By week 34 the stent was no longer in the right place and a premature delivery was elected. At birth the child had posterior urethral valves and renal insufficiency. The benefit to the child of in utero maneuver is far from obvious.

Premature Delivery

Premature delivery was undertaken in two other cases, as described below.

1. Dilation of the left kidney was noted in week 35. Unsuccessful attempt at premature delivery was made in week 38, followed by a cesarean section. The diagnosis of left pelvic ureteral stenosis was made after birth and the child operated on on day 10 of life. In this case the attempt at premature delivery was again unjustified and the cesarean section could have been avoided.

2. Bilateral dilation of renal cavities with megacystis was found in week 30, with a good voiding of the bladder after furosemide. Delivery was initiated in week 37. At birth the diagnosis of massive reflux and hypoplastic kidney was made and

a surgical operation was performed at 6 months. The benefit of premature delivery is again far from obvious.

In conclusion, none of the therapeutic manipulations undertaken in utero after prenatal diagnosis could be considered beneficial, and they may have been more dangerous than useful.

Discussion

KIDNEYS AND URINARY TRACT OF NORMAL FETUS

Nephrogenesis, which starts as early as week 4 of gestation, continues up to week 36. The metanephros from which the definitive kidney is formed appears in week 5. Nephronic differentiation occurs when the ureteral bud coming from the Wolffian duct meets the mesenchyme of the metanephros blastema, and any abnormality of this spatial meeting is thought to cause a defect in the normal development of nephrons.

Kidneys could be detected by sonography as small ovoid masses from the 15th week. Fetal kidney growth has been described according to gestational age. This growth is shown schematically in Figure 1, where the three dimensions of fetal kidney are represented from week 20 to week 41 of gestation,

Fig 1.—Evolution of the three dimensions of the fetal kidney according to gestational age.[37]

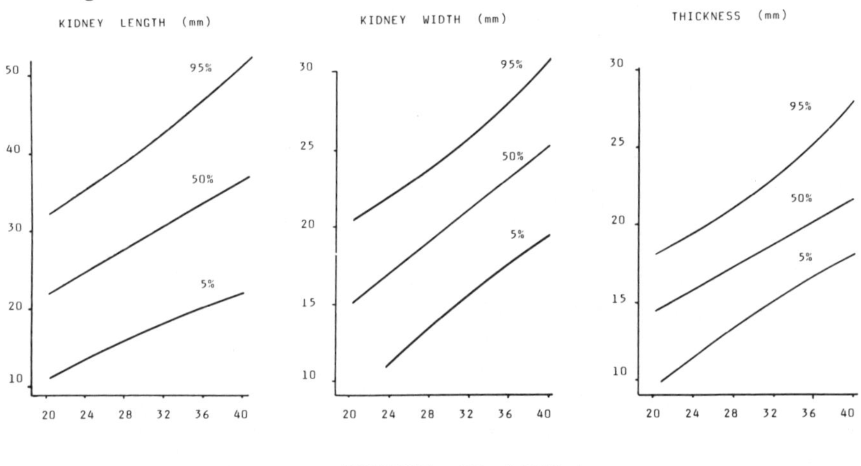

according to the study of Jeanty et al., based on fetal sonography.[37] Data from fetal autopsies are very similar.[30] The kidney size is a good marker of gestational age since it is not decreased by fetal hypotrophy. After week 20 sonography is able to show the details of kidney structure, including the strongly echogenic capsule, and can be used to measure the kidney size. At this time it is also possible to distinguish between the cortex and the medulla. The ureters are usually not seen, but sometimes their initial part can be detected. According to Gonzales,[29] the ureter diameter decreases in the last part of pregnancy, and some ureteral dilation in utero could be physiologic.

The bladder is detected by sonography from the 15th week. It is spherical and its volume varies with filling and voiding, which can be seen with real-time sonography. The maximal volume increases progressively with age from 10 ml in week 32 to 40 ml at birth. This volume can be calculated from the three diameters. Bladder filling and voiding are permanent and regular and occur at 110 ± 35 minute intervals (range, 55–155 minutes). This voiding is often incomplete, and it is not exceptional to find a residue in a normal fetus.

Urinary volume passed by the fetus can be calculated from the variation in bladder volume. This volume increases with gestational age from 0.6 ± 0.9 ml/hour in week 30 to 27 ± 2.3 ml/hour at birth.[63] It is decreased in hypotrophic fetuses and increased by 80%–150% after administration to the mother of 1 mg/kg of furosemide.[64] Although it is interesting to know the fetal urinary flow, it would be naive to estimate renal function based solely on this parameter, as was initially suggested. Finally, the urethra is usually not seen except in girls during voiding.

EFFECTS OF URINARY TRACT OBSTRUCTION ON THE DEVELOPMENT OF FETAL KIDNEY

The common association between obstructive uropathy and renal dysplasia led to the hypothesis of a causal relationship between in utero urinary tract obstruction and abnormal development of the kidney. Experimental studies on lambs have shown that ureter ligation before day 70 of fetal life leads to atrophic and hydronephrotic kidneys, with such classic features of dysplasia as primitive ducts, immature glomeruli, glomerular cysts, and mesenchyme excess. On the other hand, ligation after day 70 of gestation is followed by dilation of the pelvis and calices and by flattening of renal cortex, as can be seen in any postnatal obstruction.[5] Other studies on the lamb[56, 58] or on other species[7, 57] do not allow such clear-cut conclusions to be made, and the relationship between urinary obstruction and renal dysplasia remains speculative.

Whatever the mechanisms involved, it is clear that urinary tract malformation is currently associated with renal dysplasia. One common example is suggested by the abnormalities observed in the renal parenchyma in relation to ureteral and pelvic duplication with or without obstruction.[50] It could be hypothesized that these lesions appear early and are not reversible. That point constitutes a theoretical limitation to any in utero intervention, since the diagnosis is probably made too late. Irreversible renal lesion has been reported as early as week 14 of gestation in a case of urethral valves.[20]

RELATIONSHIP BETWEEN UT ABNORMALITIES AND AMNIOTIC FLUID VOLUME

Even if the mechanisms that control the volume of amniotic fluid are not fully understood,[60] it has been shown that a decrease in urinary secretion of the fetus is associated with oligoamnios.[12, 63] It is known that severe oligoamnios comes with bilateral renal agenesis. Oligoamnios can also be observed in severe UT obstruction with dysplasia. Oligoamnios leads to lung hypoplasia and respiratory distress at birth.

SONOGRAPHIC DIAGNOSIS OF FETAL UT ABNORMALITIES

Ten years has passed since the first in utero sonographic diagnosis of a renal disease by Garrett in 1970 and the routine use of this method in prenatal diagnosis. Of the 139 cases of in utero diagnosis of renal or urinary tract malformations reported in the literature, 123 have appeared since 1980. Sonographic examination is now systematically used in an increasing number of pregnant women and from week 22 may lead to the discovery of a urinary tract abnormality. This examination may also be performed intentionally in some situations, as in a pregnancy with oligoamnios or in a woman with a relevant family history (polycystic disease, renal agenesis, some dominant hereditary UT malformations,[15] and so forth). The risk of UT malformation is higher in a sibship in which one case has been already observed.[9]

The present series represents an incomplete list of the diagnoses that could be made by sonography, since it concerned essentially cases referred because of UT malformations. We will now try to give the complete list of kidney and UT abnormalities that could be detected in utero.

Bilateral Renal Agenesis

A number of cases have been reported.[19, 34, 38, 39, 41, 52] This diagnosis is possible after week 20 of pregnancy from the association of fetal hypotrophy, oligoamnios, absence of kidney, and absence of bladder. In some cases a small image of the bladder (less than 8 mm) is seen that does not increase after maternal furosemide administration. In fact, the diagnosis is established by administering a dose of 60 mg of furosemide, which normally increases fetal bladder size within 2 hours.

Polycystic Disease

Both forms of polycystic diseases could be detected in utero. In the infantile recessive type, the diagnosis is possible in weeks 20 to 22, but somctimes much later,[54] as the severity of the disease is variable, even in the same sibship. On sonographic examination the kidneys are grossly enlarged compared to the normal size at different fetal ages. The ratio of kidney diameter to abdomen diameter is also clearly increased, and in addition, kidney echogenicity is increased and the capsule is less easy to delimit.[22] The more severe forms are associated with oligoamnios. Several instances of prenatal diagnosis of recessive polycystic disease have been reported.[3, 25, 26, 32, 52] Some exceptional cases of dominant polycystic renal disease diagnosed in utero have also been reported.[15, 65] The feature could be similar to the infantile recessive type, but cysts could also be seen very early, although they were difficult to distinguish from obstructive uropathy. Trehalase assay in the amniotic fluid has been proposed for the in utero diagnosis of polycystic disease[46] but does not seem to have been confirmed as a valuable test. Finally, the key to prenatal diagnosis of dominant polycystic renal disease is provided by the family history and/or by kidney sonography of the parents. Some malformation syndromes could be associated with a severe polycystic renal disease—for instance, the Meckel syndrome with anencephaly and the Robert syndrome, including phocomely. These syndromes are easy to identify in utero with sonography.[39, 62]

Multicystic Kidney

This abnormality is one of those most frequently observed in utero.[3, 4, 23, 43, 45, 47, 49, 52] In typical cases the lesion is unilateral and appears as several round liquid images instead of the normal kidney. This feature is often difficult to differentiate from unilateral stenosis of the pelvoureteral junction, and the difficulty in interpretation sometimes persists after birth. The bladder and the contralateral kidney are normal, and sometimes hydramnios is noted. Bilateral forms may be seen which are in fact the equivalent of bilateral renal agenesis with absence of bladder and oligoamnios.

Urinary Tract Malformations

The images obtained with sonography in UT malformations depend on the site and the severity of the obstruction, but in general it is difficult to extrapolate a precise diagnosis from these sonographic images. Several types of abnormalities may be detected, as described below.

Ureteropelvic stenosis is associated with more or less marked dilation of pelvis and calices. It may be unilateral or bilateral. The dilated calices may mimic cysts. The ureter is not seen, and the bladder is normal. This diagnosis has been reported several times.[2, 8, 16, 40, 45, 47]

Ureteral duplicity with obstructive ureterocele is associated with unilateral or bilateral dilation of the renal pelvis, sometimes in the form of a laterovertebral liquid mass corresponding to the dilated supernumerous pelvis. Ureterocele may be elicited in some cases when the septum is seen in the bladder[1] but it is generally unrecognized and is detected after birth, as in the patients in the present series.

Megaureter is responsible for unilateral or bilateral dilation of the upper urinary tract. In fact it is difficult to ascertain a dilation of the ureter aside from the renal pelvis dilation, but it could be recognized in its retrovesical part. In this abnormality the bladder is normal, with normal voiding.

In urethral obstruction (posterior or anterior valves, etc.) the whole urinary tract is dilated and the bladder has poor voiding, as it appears at best after maternal furosemide administration. Some cases of in utero diagnosis have been reported,[11, 48, 55] but the polymorphism of this type of malformation must be emphasized.[27] It is a typical example of the malformation for which in utero relief of obstruction has been attempted.[6, 24, 35]

Certain syndromes, such as prune belly syndrome, are detectable in utero based on the association of megacystis, bilateral dilation of UT, and absence of testes in the scrotum in a male fetus.[14, 44, 53] Another syndrome with the association of megacystis and a microcolon with hypoperistaltism has also been reported in utero.[61]

The precise diagnosis of all UT malformations is usually made after birth, since in utero sonography does not allow one to describe exactly the anatomical lesions.

Tumors of the Fetal Kidney

It is theoretically possible to find a Wilms' tumor by means of sonography in utero, but to our knowledge no case had been yet reported. Other types of tumors, such as hamartoma and mesoblastic nephroma, have been found in utero.[10] These tumors result in an increase of the kidney size difficult to distinguish from that seen in infantile polycystic disease.

LIMITS OF IN UTERO SONOGRAPHY

In the present series there were only a few examples of conflicting data between the in utero and the postnatal examinations. We could note, for example, the absence of megacystis in the case with anterior urethral valves and the diagnosis of unilateral dilation in four infants with a bilateral pelvic ureteral junction stenosis, but in three of these four infants dilation was asymmetric with only the more dilated side seen in utero. More difficult to accept were the two cases of prenatal diagnosis of

UT dilation that were found to be normal after birth, but the dilation in utero was moderate. These vanishing dilations could be due to delayed maturation of muscular fibers of the ureters.[29] Conversely, some malformations discovered after birth could have escaped in utero diagnosis,[59] but again, these malformations were minor. Finally, if the accuracy of prenatal ultrasound is relatively poor, since a dilation could correspond to several types of malformation, on the whole we might question the viability of this method of investigation.

In Utero Intervention

The possibility of detecting obstructive UT malformation in utero led immediately to consideration of early therapy on the fetus itself. After the first attempt, reported in 1981, initial enthusiasm was followed by serious disillusionment. At the present time a small number of interventions have been performed on fetuses. Three types of approach have been used: percutaneous needle aspiration of the fetal UT, placement of a stent between the fetal bladder and the amniotic fluid, and fetal surgery.

Percutaneous Needle Aspiration

Several reports of this technique are available. In one case the percutaneous needle aspiration was performed in week 21 of pregnancy just after an obstructive uropathy was diagnosed.[24] Aspiration was followed by a clear decrease of the UT dilation, which remained stable up to week 37. A rapid increase in bladder volume at this time was treated by a second needle aspiration, and the decision was made to induce delivery. At birth prune belly syndrome with obstructive urethra was diagnosed. A urinary fistula was found on the abdomen related to the in utero needle aspiration. Renal function was normal. In this case it is possible that the needle aspiration and the subsequent fistula had protected renal function.

In another case the diagnosis of left major hydronephrosis was made in week 29. This UT dilation was said to be "threatening," and five needle aspirations were performed, removing 350–700 ml of fluid, representing half of the volume that had accumulated in the UT. At birth after the 36th week of gestation a left nephrectomy was performed and the child kept a right normal kidney.[42] One must wonder whether these aspirations were really necessary. Now they would be judged unnecessary in the case of unilateral abnormalities.

Insertion of a Stent Between the Fetal Bladder and the Amniotic Fluid

The first attempt to insert such a stent was made by a group in San Francisco.[28] It concerned a twin pregnancy for which sonography in the 17th week had revealed an ascitis in one of the fetuses. In week 23 dilation of the left UT was seen, and by week 30 the dilation was bilateral with megacystis. A first attempt to insert a stent failed, but a second one in week 32 succeeded, and the bladder was effectively drained. Spontaneous delivery took place 2 weeks later. The newborn had prune belly syndrome with ascitis. The stent was no longer effective, its distal tip having been covered over by the abdominal skin. Renal function remained satisfactory after ureterostomy. In this case it is difficult to say to what extent the stent insertion in utero was useful.

Another case reported at the same time by a group in New Haven[6] concerned a fetus with oligoamnios and a major dilation of the bladder and the UT. In week 24 a precurved stent was inserted under ultrasound guidance between the bladder and the amniotic fluid. This stent was immediately effective: UT dilation decreased and the amniotic fluid volume increased. But 3 weeks later the dilation returned and stabilized after needle aspiration of the bladder. Premature induction of labor in week 32 was followed by respiratory distress, and the newborn died at age 12 hours. At autopsy the stent was no longer permeable and was found in one of the ureters. The obstruction was related to urethral valves, and the kidneys were severely dysplastic with very few glomeruli. In this case the stent insertion was not useful. Two French groups also reported in 1982 an attempt at stent insertion. One case[21] concerned a predominantly unilateral hydronephrosis. A first catheter was inserted in the larger pelvis in week 30, but 3 weeks later the stent tip was covered over by fetal skin and the dilation developed again. Another attempt at stent insertion failed and early induction of labor was decided on in the 37th week. The newborn had a bilateral stenosis of the pelvoureteral junction and the more dilated side was rapidly operated on; the stent was found under the skin. No functional data were given in this case. The second case[17] also concerned a bilateral UT dilation for which a stent was inserted between the bladder and the amniotic fluid; unfortunately, no information was given on the time of this intervention or of the delivery 2 weeks later, and there is no reason to think that this stent insertion protected renal function, exactly as in the case we reported in the present series.

Fetal Surgery

The only in utero surgical intervention was reported in 1982 by the group in San Francisco,[35] who performed the first stent insertion. In that case severe oligoamnios was already known when bilateral UT dilation with megacystis was discovered in the 20th week. Surgical intervention was performed in the 21st week. After uterus section both ureters were derived to the abdomen fetal skin. Subsequently the UT dilation disappeared completely but the amniotic fluid volume did not increase. Spontaneous delivery occurred in the 35th week. The ureterostomy orifices were patent but passed little urine, and the newborn died at age 9 hours from respiratory distress. At autopsy the kidneys were hypoplastic and dysplastic. The authors concluded that despite a technically successful in utero intervention, the result had been totally nil because of early irreversible changes in the renal parenchyma.

Early Induction of Labor

There are several reports of early induction of labor with the aim of suppressing as soon as possible the UT obstruction. This decision was sometimes taken in a case of a rapidly increasing obstruction. It must always be preceded by checking the lecithine/sphingomyelin ratio in the amniotic fluid in order to assess pulmonary maturity, which could be accelerated with a corticosteroid.

Proposals for the Management of Fetal UT Abnormalities

Considering the poor or questionable results obtained after interventions on fetuses with UT abnormalities, the approach proposed by Harrison et al.[34] must be discussed, and other approaches proposed.

If a systematic sonographic examination leads to a diagnosis of UT malformation, it is necessary to perform this examination again after 1 or 2 weeks, using eventually a furosemide test. At this time several situations could be imagined. (1) The diagnosis of bilateral renal agenesis or bilateral severe renal dysplasia is made without any doubt. Interruption of the pregnancy could then be discussed. (2) The diagnosis of a unilateral UT abnormality with a normal contralateral kidney is made. In this case there is no indication for fetal intervention. (3) A bilateral obstructive uropathy is found. If severe oligoamnios is associated the situation is similar to bilateral renal agenesis and carries the risk of severe respiratory distress at birth. On the other hand, if the volume of amniotic fluid is within normal limits, the situation is less desperate but the severity of renal function impairment is difficult to assess and to follow. Therefore, it is not possible to codify the management of a fetus with such abnormalities.

Some workers believe that increasing bilateral UT dilation might be an indication to insert a stent between the fetal bladder and the amniotic fluid, but other groups are contesting the usefulness of such in utero intervention and instead suggest waiting until birth to release the obstruction. The question of whether to induce or not to induce premature labor could then be raised, taking into account the risks of such a decision on one hand and the hypothetical benefits of an earlier release of obstruction on the other hand. There is presently no basis for recommending one approach over the other. Progress in the assessment of fetal renal function and new observations are needed to go further. At present, most groups wait for spontaneous birth, and the most important question concerns postnatal management. There are no definitive rules, and the answer is different from one malformation to another one. Very generally it seems better to wait 4 or 5 days before performing the needed urologic investigations (sonography, IVP, or cystography). A major obstruction could then justify an external derivation through a transcutaneous stent. This derivation, when effective, is able to decrease the dilation and improve renal function. The surgical correction could be done in much better condition after some weeks or months of derivation as a preventive treatment of infections.

In conclusion, the in utero diagnosis of a UT abnormality allows early treatment of this abnormality after birth. It would be also relevant to discuss its negative features, and the psychic consequence of this diagnosis on the mother must be kept in mind. Because of the relative uncertainty of the diagnosis, it is better to remain very cautious.

REFERENCES

1. Athey P.A., Carpenter R.J., Hadlock F.P., et al.: Ultrasonic demonstration of ectopic ureterocele. *Pediatrics* 71:568–571, 1983.
2. Badlani G., Abrams H.J., Kunari S.: Diagnosis of fetal hydronephrosis in utero using ultrasound. *Urology* 16:315–316, 1980.
3. Bartley J.A., Golbus M.S., Filly R.A., et al.: Prenatal diagnosis of dysplastic kidney disease. *Clin. Genet.* 11:375–378, 1977.
4. Bateman B.C., Brenbridge A.N., Buschi A.: In utero diagnosis of multicystic kidney disease by sonography. *J. Reprod. Med.* 25:256–258, 1980.
5. Beck A.D.: The effects of intrauterine urinary obstruction upon the development of the fetal kidney. *J. Urol.* 105:784–789, 1971.
6. Berkowitz R.L., Grickman M.G., Walker Smith G.J., et al.: Fetal urinary tract obstruction: What is the role of surgical intervention in utero? *Am. J. Obstet. Gynecol.* 144:367–375, 1982.
7. Bernstein J.: Developmental abnormalities of the renal parenchyma, renal hypoplasia and dysplasia. *Pathol. Annu.* 3:213–247, 1968.
8. Blane C.E., Loff S.A., Bowerman R.A., et al.: Nonobstructive fetal hydronephrosis: Sonographic recognition and therapeutic implications. *Radiology* 147:95–98, 1983.
9. Bois E., Feingold J., Benmaiz H., et al.: Congenital urinary tract malformations: Epidemiology and genetic aspects. *Clin. Genet.* 8:37–47, 1975.
10. Bolande R.P.: Congenital mesoblastic nephroma of infancy, in Rosenberg H.S., Bolande R.P. (eds.): *Perspectives in Pediatric Pathology*. Chicago, Year Book Medical Publishers, 1973, vol. 1, pp. 227–250.
11. Busine A., Wesel S.: Diagnostic échographique anténatal des malformations foetales: À propos d'une cas d'agénésie uréthrale avec mégavessie. *Rev. Med. Brux.* 2:617–622, 1981.
12. Campbell S.: The antenatal detection of fetal abnormality by ultrasound B-scanning, in Murken J., Stengel-Rutkowski S., Schwinger E.: *Prenatal Diagnosis of Genetic Disorders*. Stuttgart, Enke, 1979, pp. 183–192.
13. Cass A., Smith S., Godec C., et al.: Prenatal diagnosis of fetal urinary tract abnormalities by ultrasound. *Urology* 18:197–202, 1981.
14. Christopher C.R., Spinelli A., Severt D.: Ultrasonic diagnosis of prune belly syndrome. *Obstet. Gynecol.* 59:391, 1982.
15. McCormack: Prenatal detection of the autosomal dominant type of congenital hydronephrosis by ultrasonography. *Prenat. Diagn.* 2:157–161, 1982.
16. Dantoine G., Leguern H., Boog G., et al.: Diagnostic prénatal par échotomographie d'une anomalie rénale complexe. *Ann. Radiol.* 23:585–588, 1980.
17. Dellenbach P., Msand I., Flori J., et al.: Uropathie malformative foetale: Traitement palliatif anténatal par drainage vésico-amniotique. *Nouv. Presse Med.* 11:1335, 1982.
18. Diament M.J., Fine R.N., Eurlich R., et al.: Fetal hydronephrosis: Problems in diagnosis and management. *J. Pediatr.* 103:435–440, 1983.
19. Dubbins P.A., Kurtz A.B., Warner R.J., et al.: Renal agenesis: Spectrum of in utero findings. *JCU* 9:189–193, 1981.
20. Duckett J.W., Harrisson M.R., de Lorimier A., et al.: Fetal intervention for obstructive uropathy. *Dialog. Pediatr. Urol.* 5:1–8, 1982.

21. Dumez Y., Vallancien G., Aubry M.C., et al.: La néphrostomie per cutanée in utero pour hydronéphrose foetale bilatérale. *Nouv. Presse Med.* 11:1787–1789, 1982.
22. Elkhazen N., Picard C., Schulman C.C.: Diagnostic prénatal de malformations urinaires chez le foetus par échographie. *Rev. Med. Brux.* 2:829–834, 1981.
23. Friedberg J.E., Milnick J.S., Davis D.A.: Antepartum ultrasonic detection of multicystic kidney. *Radiology* 131:198, 1979.
24. Gadziala N.A., Kawada C.Y., Doherty F.J., et al.: Intrauterine decompression of megalocystic during the 2d trimester of pregnancy. *Am. J. Obstet. Gynecol.* 144:355–356, 1982.
25. Garret W.J.: Prenatal diagnosis of fetal polycystic kidney by ultrasound. *Aust. NZ Obstet. Gynaecol.* 10:7, 1970.
26. Garret W.J., Kossoff G., Osborn R.A.: The diagnosis of fetal hydronephrosis, megaureter and urethral obstruction by ultrasonic echography. *Br. J. Obstet. Gynaecol.* 82:115–120, 1975.
27. Glazer G.M., Filly R.A., Callen P.W.: The varied sonographic appearance of the urinary tract in the fetus and newborn with urethral obstruction. *Radiology* 144:563–568, 1982.
28. Golbus M.S., Harrisson M.R., Filly R.A., et al.: In utero treatment of urinary tract obstruction. *Am. J. Obstet. Gynecol.* 142:383–388, 1982.
29. Gonzales J.: Le développement du haut appareil urinaire du foetus au cours du 3e trimestre de la grossesse. *Bul. Assoc. Anat.* 64:391–398, 1980.
30. Gonzales J., Gonzales M., Mary J.Y.: Size and weight study of human kidney growth velocity during the last three months of pregnancy. *Eur. Urol.* 6:37–44, 1980.
31. Gorf R.M., Callen P.W., Filly R.A., et al.: Prenatal percutaneous antegrade pyelography in posterior urethral valves: Sonographic guidance. *AJR* 139:994–996, 1972.
32. Habif D., Berdon W.E., Yeh M.N.: Infantile polycystic kidney diseases: In utero sonographic diagnosis. *Radiology* 142:475–477, 1982.
33. Hadlock F.P., Deter R.L., Carpenter R., et al.: Sonography of fetal urinary tract anomalies. *AJR* 137:261–267, 1981.
34. Harrison M.R., Filly R.A., Parer J.T., et al.: Management of fetus with a urinary tract malformation. *JAMA* 248:635–639, 1981.
35. Harrison M.A., Golbus M.S., Filly R.A., et al.: Fetal surgery for congenital hydronephrosis. *N. Engl. J. Med.* 306:591–593, 1982.
36. Harrison M.R., Ross N., Noall R., et al.: Correction of congenital hydronephrosis in utero: I. The model. Fetal urethral obstruction produces hydronephrosis and pulmonary hypoplasia in fetal lamb. *J. Pediatr. Surg.* 18:247–256, 1983.
37. Jeanty P., Dramaix-Wilmet M., Elkhazen N., et al.: Measurement of fetal kidney growth on ultrasound. *Radiology* 144:159–162, 1982.
38. Kaffe S., Godmilow L., Walker B.A., et al.: Prenatal diagnosis of bilateral renal agenesis. *Obstet. Gynecol.* 49:478–480, 1977.
39. Kaffe S., Rose J.S., Godmilow L., et al.: Prenatal diagnosis of renal anomalies. *Am. J. Med. Genet.* 1:241–251, 1977.
40. Kay R., Lee T., Tank E.: Ultrasonic diagnosis of fetal hydronephrosis in utero. *Urology* 13:286–288, 1979.
41. Keirse M., Meerman R.: Antenatal diagnosis of Potter syndrome. *Obstet. Gynecol.* 42(Suppl. 1):64–67, 1978.
42. Kirkinen P., Jouppila P., Tuonomen S., et al.: Repeated transabdominal renocentesis in a case of fetal hydronephrotic kidney. *Am. J. Obstet. Gynecol.* 142:1049–1052, 1982.
43. Legarth J., Verger H., Gronvall S.: Prenatal diagnosis of multicystic kidney by ultrasound. *Acta Obstet. Gynecol. Scand.* 60:523–524, 1981.
44. Loverro G., Putignano G., Loizzi P., et al.: Le syndrome de prune-belly, diagnostic prénatal. *J. Gynecol. Obstet. Biol. Reprod.* 10:695–697, 1981.

45. Mendoza S.A., Griswold W.R., Leopold G.R., et al.: Intrauterine diagnosis of renal anomalies by ultrasonography. *Am. J. Dis. Child.* 133:1042–1043,1979.
46. Morin P.R., Potier M., Dallaire L., et al.: Prenatal detection of the autosomal recessive type of polycystic kidney disease by trehalase assay in amniotic fluid. *Prenat. Diagn.* 1:75–79, 1981.
47. Moutard Codou M.L., Lejeune C.: Dépistage anténatal des anomalies de l'appareil urinaire par les ultrasons, in *Journée Parisienne de pédiatrie 1982* Paris, Flammarion Médecine Sciences, 1982, pp. 135–147.
48. Okulski T.A.: The prenatal diagnosis of lower urinary tract obstruction using B-scan ultrasound: A case report. *JCU* 5:268–270, 1977.
49. Older R.A., Hinman C.G., Crane L.M., et al.: In utero diagnosis of multicyctic kidney by gray scale ultrasonography. *AJR* 133:130–131, 1979.
50. Perrin E.V.: Renal dysplasia in anomalies of the urinary tract and chronic pyelonephritis. *Am. J. Pathol.* 43:18a, 1963.
51. Pope T.L., Alforo B.A., Buschi A.J., et al.: Nuclear scintigraphy and ultrasound in the diagnosis of congenital ureteropyelic junction obstruction. *J. Urol.* 124:917–918, 1980.
52. Schmidt W., Schoeder T.M., Buchinger G., et al.: Genetics, Pathoanatomy, and prenatal diagnosis of Potter syndrome and other urogenital tract diseases. *Clin. Genet.* 22:105–127, 1982.
53. Shih W.J., Greenbaum L.D., Baro C.: In utero sonogram in prune belly syndrome. *Urology* 20:102–105, 1982.
54. Simpson J.L., Sabbagha R.E., Eliap S., et al.: Failure to detect polycystic kidneys in utero by second trimester ultrasonography. *Hum. Genet.* 60:295, 1982.
55. Sweeny I., Kang B.H., Lin P., et al.: Posterior urethral obstruction caused by congenital posterior urethral valve. *NY State J. Med.* pp. 87–89, 1981.
56. Tanagho E.A.: Surgically induced partial urinary obstruction in the foetal lamb: I. Technique. II. Urethral obstruction. III. Ureteral obstruction. *Invest. Urol.* 10:19, 1972.
57. Thomasson B.H., Esterly J.H., Ravitch M.: Morphologic changes in the fetal rabbit kidney after intrauterine ureteral ligation. *Invest. Urol.* 8:261, 1970.
58. Vallancien G., Beurton D., Szemat M., et al.: Etude expérimentale comparée des conséquences rénales du reflux vésico-urétéral et de l'obstruction urétérale chez le foetus de brebis. *J. Urol. (Paris)* 88:27, 1982.
59. Van Regemorter N., Dudion J., Druart C., et al.: Major congenital malformations in 5448 newborns: Comments on genetic counseling and prenatal diagnosis. *Acta Paediatr. Belg.* 34:73–81, 1981.
60. Van Utterlo L.C., Wladimiroff J.W., Wallenburoh H.C.: Relationship between fetal urine production and amniotic fluid volume in normal pregnancy and pregnancy complicated by diabetes. *Br. J. Obstet. Gynaecol.* 84:205–209, 1977.
61. Vezina W.C., Morin F.R., Winsberg F.: Megacystic microcolon intestinal hypoperistalsis syndrome: Antenatal ultrasound appearance. *AJR* 133:749–750, 1979.
62. Wagner R.J., Kurtz A.B., Ross R.D., et al.: Ultrasonographic parameters in the prenatal diagnosis of Meckel syndrome. *Obstet. Gynecol.* 57:388–389, 1981.
63. Wladimiroff J.W., Campbell S.: Fetal urine production rates in normal and complicated pregnancy. *Lancet* 1:151–154, 1974.
64. Wladimiroff J.W.: Effect of furosemide on fetal urine production. *Br. J. Obstet. Gynaecol.* 82:221–224, 1975.
65. Zerres K., Weiss H., Bulla M., et al.: Prenatal diagnosis of an early manifestation of autosomal dominant adult type polycystic kidney disease. *Lancet* 2:988, 1982.

Use of Antimicrobial Agents in Treating Urinary Tract Infection

CALVIN M. KUNIN, M.D.

Pomerene Professor of Medicine, Department of Medicine, Ohio State University College of Medicine, Columbus, Ohio

TREATMENT of urinary tract infections can be one of the most gratifying experiences in clinical practice. Usually, the patient has a reasonably specific complaint, a definitive diagnosis can readily be made by microscopic examination of the urine and confirmed by culture, and a wide variety of effective antimicrobial agents are available for therapy. As with most infectious diseases, the efficacy of treatment or prophylaxis depend on (1) characteristics of the host, (2) the nature of the invading microorganism, (3) understanding the natural history of the disease, and (4) the efficacy of chemotherapy. The overall goal of management is to eradicate the invading organism from the entire system. Of almost equal importance is the necessity to anticipate, prevent, or treat recurrences. At times it is necessary to recognize failure and withhold antimicrobial therapy unless it is essential for treatment of sepsis.

General Considerations

The Host

Urinary tract infections are best categorized in relation to host factors. These are conveniently divided into simple or un-

0084-5957/84/0014-0039-0066-$04.00

complicated (medical) infections that occur in a patient with an otherwise normal tract and complicated (surgical) infections, in which the integrity of the voiding mechanism is impaired, or a foreign body is present. In addition, important considerations are age, sex, renal function, and such conditions as diabetes and polycystic disease, which predispose the kidneys to infection. Uncomplicated infections, most often encountered in females, are generally the most easy to treat, whereas those in which a foreign body such as a catheter or stone are present in the urinary tract are the most difficult. Because of the tendency of complicated infections to resist therapy or to recur soon after treatment, the microorganisms often become resistant to commonly-used antimicrobial agents. The ease of management of infections of the urinary tract according to type of patient, clinical characteristics, invading organism, and probability of tissue invasion is outlined in Table 1.

There has been considerable interest in the use of tests to localize the site of infection as a means of defining the need for more intensive or prolonged therapy. Theoretically, those infections that are associated with tissue invasion in some part of the urinary tract (a far more accurate description than "upper" versus "lower" tract infection) should be more difficult to manage and might be expected to indicate a greater potential for renal damage than those with "bladder bacteriuria."

This concept may be illusory. Various localizing procedures will show that as many as 50% of female patients with uncomplicated infections have evidence of upper tract infection. Yet, their ultimate prognosis remains excellent and urologic studies in similar populations rarely detect significant structural abnormalities. For these reasons, localization studies should be considered as research tools.

Instead of conducting these expensive tests and delaying decisions regarding therapy while awaiting results, I suggest that clinicians will be far better off simply to estimate the likelihood of tissue invasion from the clinical guides presented in Table 1.[1] The most that can be concluded at this time is that patients likely to have tissue invasion will respond poorly to single-dose therapy. This issue will be discussed in greater detail below.

TABLE 1.—GUIDELINES TO MANAGEMENT

GROUP	EASE OF MANAGEMENT SCALE	TYPE OF PATIENT	CLINICAL CHARACTERISTICS	ORGANISM	PROBABILITY OF TISSUE INVASION	THERAPY
I	Excellent	female, child or adult	Few previous episodes; reliable, with good follow-up available; less than 2 days between onset of symptoms and treatment	Usually *E. coli* sensitive to most agents	low	1 dose Amoxicillin, sulfonamide, TMP/SMZ, kanamycin
II	Good	female, child or adult	Few previous episodes, follow-up poor	Usually *E. coli* sensitive to most agents	high or low	3–10 days Prophylaxis for closely spaced recurrences
III	Fair	female, child or adult	Many previous episodes, history of early recurrence or diabetic, or postrenal transplant	Variable, tends to have more resistant bacteria, susceptibility tests essential	high	4–6 weeks Prophylaxis for closely spaced recurrences
IV	Fair	adult male	Recurrent infections, some underlying anatomic abnormality	Variable, susceptibility test needed	high often prostatic colonization	4–6 weeks Prophylaxis for closely spaced recurrences
V	Poor	male or female	Neurogenic bladder, large volume residual urine	Variable, susceptibility test needed	high	Intermittent catheterization (treatment for symptomatic infections only)
VI	Very Poor	male or female	Continuous drainage required	Variable, susceptibility test needed	very high	Indwelling catheter closed drainage (treatment for sepsis only)

The Microbe

Most urinary tract infections are due to the gram-negative enteric organisms found in the gut. Their common occurrence in urinary tract infections is used as one of the arguments to support the concept of the ascending route of infection. Anaerobic fecal flora, although present in 100 to 1000 times greater abundance in the stool than *E. coli,* rarely produce urinary tract infections. This is possibly because they do not grow well in urine. Anaerobes should not be discounted, however, because polymicrobial infections with these bacteria are now commonly encountered in patients with long-standing urolithiasis, renal and perirenal abscesses, and in patients with necrotizing genital lesions such as Fournier's disease.

The mechanism which anaerobic bacteria reach the kidney is not clear. They may move by means of the ascending route. Bollgren et al.[2] found that obligate anaerobic bacteria constituted 95% of the periurethral flora in young females. Most of these are gram-positive organisms. Girls prone to develop urinary tract infection often are colonized with gram-negative rods, primarily bacteroides. Although these organisms do not appear to produce infection, their presence may indicate specific ecologic changes in the periurethral zone in susceptible individuals. McDowall et al.[3] were able to isolate anaerobic bacteria in the urine of pregnant women with known or suspected renal disease by using suprapubic aspiration, when midstream cultures were not diagnostic. The most common organism isolated was Gardnerella vaginalis. Ureaplasma urealyticum was also frequently isolated. These studies emphasize that, although anaerobic bacteria do not commonly play a role in urinary tract infections, they are present in abundance in the urethra and can enter the bladder readily.

The most common organisms encountered in uncomplicated infections are *Enterobacteriaceae.* Of these, *E. coli* is the most frequent and accounts for roughly 80% of infections. The second most common organism in females with uncomplicated infection is *Staphylococcus saprophyticus,* accounting for 10%–15% of infections.[4-6] This has important implications for therapy, since most strains of *S. saprophyticus* are susceptible to penicillin G, ampicillin, trimethoprim/sulfamethoxazole, and cephalexin, but resistant to nitrofurantoin and nalidixic acid. Susceptibility to erythromycin varies.[7] Resistance to novobiocin is used as a marker of this group of organisms. In contrast, *E. coli* tend to be susceptible to many of the agents listed, depending largely on intensity of their use in a community. *E. coli* are not generally considered to be susceptible to erythromycin except under special circumstances in which the urine is alkalinized.

The finding of these two very different organisms—one a gram-negative rod encountered in the gut, the other a gram-positive coccus located on the skin surface—imply different mechanisms of infection. A reasonable explanation, based on current concepts of the pathogenesis of urinary tract infections in females is that certain strains of *E. coli*, staphylococci, and other bacteria are able to adhere well to the urothelial cells and therefore are more likely to invade the urinary tract.[8, 9]

Microorganisms more commonly encountered in complicated infections, are *Klebsiella, Proteus Enterobacter, Pseudomonas, Providencia, Serratia,* and *Morganella.* These organisms as well as *Acinetobacter* and *Candida,* are often recovered in patients subjected to instrumentation, particularly with indwelling catheters. Among the gram-positive bacteria, *Staphylococcus aureus* and groups B and D streptococci are particularly important. *S. aureus* infections tend to be much more invasive than those due to *S. saprophyticus.* Genitourinary infections with *S. aureus* may be either secondary to bacteremia from a nonurinary site producing metastatic abscesses in the kidney or they may arise primarily in the urinary tract following instrumentation.[10] The intensity and duration of therapy of infections due to *S. aureus* depends on whether one is dealing with uncomplicated urinary tract infection or a manifestation of a widespread systemic disease. These may be differentiated on the basis of the patient's history, clinical presentation, and associated clinical findings.

S. aureus should be considered to be resistant to penicillin G and ampicillin until proved otherwise. Infections caused by this organism are best treated with a penicillinase-resistant penicillin, such as methicillin or nafcillin, a first generation cephalosporin, such as cephalothin or cefazolin, or with vancomycin for seriously ill patients who are allergic to these drugs or when the bacteria are resistant to other agents.

Group B streptococci are a major cause of infections in the newborn. They also may produce bacteremic pyelonephritis, cellulitis, pneumonitis, and endometritis in adults. In one series,[11] seven of 24 patients with bacteremia due to this organism developed pyelonephritis and 45% of these patients were diabetic. These organisms are usually susceptible to penicillin G, ampicillin, cephalothin, erythromycin, and clindamycin, but resistant to aminoglycoside antibiotic.

Group D streptococci (including enterococci) tend to be found in individuals who are instrumented, particularly those with indwelling catheters. These organisms are a particular cause of concern because they may produce subacute bacterial endocarditis. Although of unproved value, prophylaxis for endocarditis must be considered in patients infected with these organisms who are to undergo urinary instrumentation. In animal models, penicillin plus an aminoglycoside antibiotic or vancomycin have been found to be the most effective agents for treatment or prophylaxis.

Occasionally, unusual or fastidious bacteria may produce urinary infections. These may at times be difficult to detect. For example, *H. influenza* does not grow well in the culture media commonly used to detect enteric bacteria and may go undetected unless suspected. This organism may be associated with bacteremia, prostatitis, and epididymo-orchitis in adults as well as children. Some of the strains are typical encapsulated group B, others may be *Hemophilus parainfluenza,* which are also associated with childhood respiratory disease; others may be less pathogenic untypable strains.[12–15] Other unusual organisms that have been reported to cause urinary tract infections include *Campylobacter, Legionella pneumophilia,*[16] *Corynebacterium, Salmonella,* and *Shigella.* Acid-fast organisms including *M. tuberculosis* and atypical *mycobacteria* also may invade the urinary tract, as well as such fungi as Blastomyces and Coccidiodomyces.

For these reasons, it is critical to perform gram and acid-fast stains of the urine sediment obtained from patients who exhibit pyuria when routine bacteriologic cultures are reported to be sterile. At times, suprapubic aspiration will be needed to confirm the presence of suspicious organisms, because the urinary outflow tract is heavily colonized with a variety of fastidious microorganisms. This subject will be considered in greater detail below when we discuss the urethral syndrome.

Birch et al.[17] used suprapubic aspiration in a study of patients with signs and symptoms suggestive of urinary tract infection, but with sterile routine cultures. They reported the frequent isolation of *Ureaplasma urealyticum,* particularly from individuals considered to have chronic atrophic pyelonephritis, recurrent urinary tract infections, and analgesic nephropathy. These findings may be difficult to interpret, but cannot be ignored.

Natural History

Our understanding of the natural history of urinary tract infections has undergone profound change in recent years.[18] Although urinary tract infections are common in the female, they rarely lead to renal damage sufficient to produce end-stage renal failure. The most important problem is management of morbidity, or the symptoms of infections. Most recurrent infections in females are due to reinfection with a new serotype of *E. coli* or a new bacterial species derived from the gut and transferred to the periurethral region, or local colonization with *S. saprophyticus.* The goal of therapy is therefore not only to eradicate infection, but also to anticipate and prevent reinfection. Most infections in males are acquired as a result of instrumentation, but they may appear without any discernible predisposing factor. Many recurrent infections in males are due to silent colonization of the prostate, usually with the same organism as in the previous infection, unless new organisms are introduced by instrumentation.

Renal disease in males and females is most often due to a long-standing combination of obstruction or foreign bodies and infection. As a generalization, to demonstrate the relative importance of risk factors, it is far more preferable to have a colonized, but well-functioning urinary tract than a sterile, obstructed system. The major exception is urinary tract infection in the diabetic. These individuals do not appear to acquire infections more often than others, but once acquired, infection tends to persist and may at times produce severe complications, such as renal papillary necrosis, xanthogranulomatous, emphysematous pyelonephritis, and perirenal abscesses.

Chemotherapeutic Agents

A wide variety of drugs are available treating urinary tract infections. These are listed in Table 2 according to whether they occur in nature (antibiotics) or are synthetic compounds,

TABLE 2.—ANTIMICROBIAL AGENTS COMMONLY USED IN THE TREATMENT OF URINARY TRACT INFECTIONS

ORAL THERAPY

Beta lactams
  Penicillin G
  Ampicillin
  Amoxicillin
  Carbenicillin
  Cephalexin
  Cephradine
  Cefaclor
	These agents are all active against the common coliform organisms found in urinary tract infections. Among these, ampicillin is about the least expensive. Amoxicillin has the advantage of less G.I. upset, and carbenicillin indanyl is useful for Pseudomonas. The oral cephalosporins are more expensive but no more effective.

Sulfonamides
Trimethoprim
TMP/SMZ
Nitrofurantoin
Nalidixic acid
Oxalinic acid
Cinoxacin
  hippurate
  mandelate
	These are synthetic compounds useful in treatment or prophylaxis of infection. Trimethoprim and nitrofurantoin are most useful in long-term prophylaxis. Sulfonamides are most useful in initial episodes of infection. The other agents are useful back-up drugs. The methenamine salts are used only for prophylaxis.

Tetracyclines
  Tetracycline
  Oxytetracycline
  Doxycycline
  Minocycline
	These are effective drugs, but may lead to overgrowth of Candida, and resistance may rapidly develop. They are useful in Chlamydia infections and prostatitis.

Chloramphenicol	This agent rarely needs to be used.
Other Agents	Staphylococcal infections are best treated with nafcillin, oxacillin, cloxacillin, or dicloxacillin. Anaerobic infections may be treated with clindamycin, metronidazole or chloramphenicol. Flucytosine may be used for Candida infections.

PARENTERAL THERAPY

Beta lactams
  Ampicillin
  First, second or third generation cephalosporins
	These agents are all equally effective if the organisms are susceptible. Second and third generation cephalosporins generally have a broader spectrum of activity against gram-negative bacteria, but have variable activity against Pseudomonas and are not effective against enterococci.

Carbenicillin
  Ticarcillin
  Mezlocillin
  Azlocillin
  Pipericillin
	These agents may be preferred over cephalosporins for treatment of urinary infection monas and enterococci. They may be of particular value in the patient with renal failure, to avoid aminoglycosides.

Aminoglycosides
  Streptomycin
  Gentamicin
  Tobramycin
  Amikacin
  Netilmicin
	Streptomycin is not commonly used because of the rapid development of resistance. Gentamicin and tobramycin are about equally effective; gentamicin is less expensive and probably no more nephrotoxic. Amikacin is preferred for multiresistant bacteria.

along with comments concerning their indications. I prefer not to use the term "urinary antiseptics," because it implies some special mode of action of the drugs. Rather, the most important predictors of efficacy are the concentration achieved in the urine and the microorganisms' susceptibility to the agent. The choice of drug depends on these factors as well as relative cost, ease of absorption from the gastrointestinal tract, rate of acquisition of resistance, and side effects.

One compound not mentioned in Table 2 is water. It can be shown that a brisk water diuresis accompanied by frequent emptying of the bladder can markedly lower bacterial concentrations in the urine and occasionally clear the tract of bacteria.[19] This probably accounts for the spontaneous clearing of bacteriuria in some females with uncomplicated infections. However, antimicrobial therapy is so much more powerful that for practical purposes the patient need not be instructed to drink large quantities of water when treated. Furthermore, there are anecdotal accounts of the value of a female voiding after intercourse, but this has not been subjected to clinical trial and is unnecessary when bed-time or postcoital antimicrobial prophylaxis is used.

An issue that has been repeatedly debated is the relative importance of urinary vs renal concentrations of drugs to treat infection. It is now clear that virtually all of the commonly-used drugs are concentrated to some extent in the tubules and renal interstitium. This depends on how well they are concentrated by the kidney and the extent of back diffusion that occurs. The latter is determined in part by the pKa of the drug and the pH of the urine. In general, the best guide to renal concentration is the concentration of the drug in the urine rather than in the blood.[20] The only exception to this generalization is with methenamine and its salts (hippurate or mandelate). Methenamine produces its antibacterial effect by breaking down in acid urine into formaldehyde and ammonia. This occurs primarily in the bladder. Therefore, these agents are reserved for prophylaxis and should not be used to attempt to eradicate infection, particularly if tissue invasion is suspected.

Alteration of the urine's pH may have a profound effect on the antimicrobial activity of a chemotherapeutic agent. For example, methenamine is much more active at acid pH. It is essential to adjust the pH of the urine to 6.0 or less by a high protein diet or by using acidifying agents, such as ascorbic acid or methionine. In contrast, streptomycin is much more active at alkaline pH. In general, drugs that are weak acids are more unionized and thereby more active at acid pH; the opposite is true of basic drugs. However, most of the currently available chemotherapeutic agents are so active against susceptible bacteria and achieve such high concentrations in the urine that pH adjustment is ordinarily not necessary. Furthermore, use of additional agents may inhibit patient compliance.

Another issue that has been considered to be of possible importance is the ability of a drug to diffuse into the periurethral mucosa and vaginal fluid. Stamey and coworkers[21] have proposed that urethral colonization with coliform bacteria is the major predisposing factor for recurrent infection in females. Although the issue has not been settled,[22] there appears to be some rationale for attempting to use agents that will concentrate in the vaginal and periurethral fluids and thereby eradicate potential invaders. It is clear, however, from several studies in which long-term prophylaxis has been used to prevent recurrent infections[23] that such agents as nitrofurantoin that do not alter the periurethral flora are just as effective as trimethoprim, which does. These results indicate that it makes little difference whether bacteria are killed before or after they enter the bladder urine.

Duration of Therapy

The duration of treatment needed to eradicate infection appears to be closely related to the likelihood that bacteria have invaded tissue. The less likely this possibility, the shorter the course of therapy. Thus, bladder bacteriuria can be readily eliminated by even a single dose of an effective agent, while long-standing pyelonephritis may require several weeks or longer.

Low-Dose Therapy

This approach is generally not recommended for therapy, but has proved useful in gaining an understanding of the mechanisms by which bacteria invade the urinary tract and to explain how antimicrobial agents might exert their effect. For example, very low doses of antimicrobial agents might be effective in treating urinary tract infections by inhibiting adhesion of the bacteria to the bladder mucosa.[24] Redjeb et al.[25] were able to eradicate bacteriuria temporarily, at least, in patients with only 10 mg per day of ampicillin, suggesting that even subinhibitory drug concentrations may be effective. In studies in experimental animals, globotetraose was shown to block attachment of *E. coli* to mouse bladder mucosal cells and to reduce recovery of bacteria in the kidney and bladder of treated animals.[9] It has also been shown that blockage of mannose receptor sites may prevent colonization of urethelial surfaces.[8]

It is important to recognize that the kinetics of growth of bacterial populations in bladder urine is a function of the number of organisms, the drug's concentration and mode of action, susceptibility to the agent, and the volume and frequency of voiding. This has been studied in detail by O'Grady.[19] These considerations are important, because dose schedules for treating urinary tract infections are often constructed from achievable levels of drug obtained in serum rather than urine.

Single-Dose Therapy

This approach has proved to be highly successful in selected populations. These are usually adult females who have uncomplicated infections due to *E. coli* who seek medical help shortly after becoming symptomatic.[26, 27] The rationale is based on the concept that many women will be colonized only with bacteria in their bladder urine and that an agent that inhibits growth combined with the natural washout effect of urination will cure the infection. Large doses of bactericidal agents are used to avoid regrowth of persisting organisms.

This concept is somewhat simplistic, since the presence of pus cells in most patients suggests that the bacteria have at least minimally invaded tissue. The high doses may be of value in eliminating this tissue phase. Single-dose treatment is much less effective in those who delay treatment or are believed to have more extensive tissue invasion. This may be assessed either on clinical grounds or by various localization tests, such as by determining the presence of antibody-coated bacteria in the urine, bladder washout tests, or high serum levels of C reactive protein.[28–30]

Single-dose therapy is not recommended in patients with highly recurrent infections, those whose follow-up might be poor, and patients with diabetes or structural abnormalities. Some studies suggest that it may be effective in pregnant women with urinary tract infection and older female children.[26] Nevertheless, careful follow-up is essential when single-dose therapy is used, particularly in pregnant women. There is evidence that pregnant women who do not respond to therapy are more likely to have premature infants. McCracken et al.[31] used a single dose of cefradoxil in children thought to have infection localized to the lower tract, as assessed by the C reactive protein test. Children receiving a single dose had more recurrences than those treated for 10 days. Until further studies are done that support the use of single doses in children, more prolonged courses of therapy are preferred.

Males should not be treated with single dose therapy because they may have prostatic involvement that will not respond. It should not be used for treatment of the urethral syndrome due to Chlamydia, and it has not been adequately tested for efficacy against infections due to *Staphylococcus saprophyticus*.

Proponents of single-dose therapy for treating patients with uncomplicated infection marshall the following arguments in its favor: (1) There are abundant clinical trials demonstrating that a single dose of an agent to which the organism is susceptible is equally as effective in eradicating infection as are standard treatments of 10–14 days. (2) Most recurrences in females are due to reinfection with a new organism, rather than to failure to eradicate the initial infection; more prolonged therapy does not prevent reinfection. (3) Single-dose therapy is less expensive. (4) It is less likely to be associated with adverse drug reactions and is less toxic to the fetus. (5) It is less apt to alter the bowel or vaginal flora and thereby less likely to select resistant strains. (6) It is much easier to achieve compliance. (7) It can be used, when combined with early follow-up cultures, to detect individuals who do not respond to treatment because of resistant organisms, tissue invasion, or because the infection is complicated.

For these reasons, the use of single-dose therapy is very attractive and is recommended for appropriate patients. It may be subject to abuse, however. Failure to respond may be misinterpreted as an indication for further urologic study.

Some of the issues that need to be considered are as follows: (1) Many physicians still diagnose and prescribe therapy for urinary tract infection over the telephone and provide no follow-up. (2) Many patients seen in emergency rooms or those not willing to return for follow-up studies would not qualify because they seek help only for their immediate problem. (3) The costs of management should include the costs of follow-up cultures for the compliant patient. In this regard, self-administered dip-slide cultures should be considered part of the therapeutic package. (4) Females with urinary tract infections are not a homogenous group. For example, in a cooperative study conducted by Rubin et al.,[32] about one third of the patients seen with acute uncomplicated infection had antibody-coated bacteria and would not be expected to respond well to a single dose. We still do not know whether women with recurrent infection will respond well to a single dose. (5) It is argued that failure to respond rapidly to single-dose therapy may define patients with tissue invasion and thereby identify a high risk, requiring further study. However, failure to respond must clearly be shown not to be due to resistant bacteria. This requires that in vitro susceptibility tests be done on positive follow-up cultures. This must be added to the cost of treatment. (6) It has not been clearly demonstrated that x-ray or urologic studies are productive in detecting correctable urologic abnormalities for those individuals in whom single-dose therapy fails when the organism is fully sensitive to the drug used. It is recognized that there is good agreement between "tissue invasion" and failure to respond to single-dose therapy as determined by bladder washout studies and the antibody-coated bacteria test.[30, 32]

However, it has not been shown, except in a small series,[33] that failure to respond to single-dose therapy provides an adequate basis for performing an intravenous pyelogram, voiding cystourethrograms, or cystoscopic studies. Two recent reports[34, 35] indicate that excretory urography and cystoscopy are not cost-effective in evaluating women with recurrent urinary tract infections. It is also important to emphasize that "tissue invasion" is not the same as complicated infection (as defined above) and does not necessarily carry the same risk of producing renal damage.

A wide variety of agents have been found effective when used for single-dose treatment. Ronald et al.[30] in 1976 originally used a single dose of 500 mg of kanamycin to demonstrate the efficacy of this approach. Since then, most studies have shown the following drugs to be highly effective: amoxicillin trihydrate, 3 grams; trimethoprim/sulfamethoxazole (320 mg of trimethoprim and 1,600 mg of sulfamethoxazole, or two double-strength tablets), trimethoprim alone (400 mg), sulfisoxazole or sulphafurazole (200 mg per kg body weight). The activity of cephalosporins has been erratic. Cephaloridine appears less effective than cefamandole when given by injection.[36, 37] Trials with the new so-called third generation cephalosporins and related compounds are underway, but it is too early to assess their efficacy. Cefaclor, given as a single oral dose of 2 g, cured seven of nine patients with negative antibody-coated bacteria tests.[38] The pediatric study using cefadroxil[31] was disappointing. To my knowledge, there are no evaluable studies of tetracyclines, nitrofurantoin, nalidixic acid, or cinoxacin as single-dose agents.

Intermediate Duration of Therapy

This is considered to be somewhere between three and 14 days of treatment. Most trials indicate that 10 days of therapy for uncomplicated infection are about as good as two weeks, and several studies indicate that three days are about as good as 10.[39, 40] Unfortunately, there are few comparative studies of single vs three and 10 days of treatment. There have also been trials using a single daily dose of trimethoprim given as 300 mg for seven days[41] as compared to more frequent doses, and of two courses of 3 g of amoxicillin given 12 hours apart compared to a seven-day course.[42] All of these studies have been reported as showing favorable responses.

Examination of this "mixed bag" of reports indicates that a variety of measures may be as effective as 10 days of treatment in uncomplicated infections in female patients. We might extrapolate, then, that three-day treatment may be more cost-effective for general populations in whom localization studies are not desired or needed. Even then, some patients will have relapses, but this can be detected by follow-up culture or recurrence of symptoms. Further comparative efficacy studies are needed in representative populations before therapy of three days, rather than 10 days, becomes standard management for uncomplicated urinary tract infections. My own bias is to use a conservative approach, recognizing the heterogeneity of the populations that investigators define for their studies. I prefer the 3–10 day method for most patients with uncomplicated infection, using follow-up cultures as a guide to relapse or the presence of resistant bacteria. It is important to realize, however, that many different approaches to dose and duration may be valid.

Long-term Therapy, With Special Reference to Infection in Men

Long-term treatment is defined as courses of 4–6 weeks or longer. It appears to be useful in individuals with marked tissue invasion, such as diabetics, patients with underlying structural abnormalities, and females who demonstrate early relapse after shorter courses,[43] and men with recurrent infection. Several studies have defined the potential for success and the limitations of treatment in men with longstanding infection. Gleckman et al.[44] conducted a controlled trial of two vs six weeks of treatment with trimethoprim/sulfamethoxazole in recurrent invasive urinary-tract infections in men. Most had infections complicated by diabetes and anatomic abnormalities, and many had suffered from bacteremia, epididymitis, and renal abscesses in the past. Gleckman's group confirmed previous studies that bacterial relapse rather than reinfection accounted for most recurrences. Using an endpoint of six weeks following treatment, they were able to demonstrate "cure" in six of 21 patients receiving two weeks of treatment as opposed to 13 of 21 treated for six weeks. It is possible that even longer therapy would have been more effective. Smith et al.[45] compared a 10-day course and a 12-week course of treatment with trimethoprim/sulfamethoxazole in men with urinary tract infections in whom the antibody-coated bacteria test was positive. At 12 weeks of follow-up the "cure" rate was nine of 15 for those treated for 12 weeks compared to only three of 15 treated for 10 days. The implications of prostatic colonization as a source of recurring infection in this population will be discussed below.

Long-term (prophylactic) therapy for chronic urinary tract infection in men was assessed in a large study by Freeman et al.[46] with follow-up to 10 years. They compared two years of continuous treatment with placebo vs sulfamethoxazole, nitrofurantoin, or methenamine mandelate. Continuous therapy with an effective drug delayed recurrence of bacteriuria and reduced clinical exacerbations of infection. Most infections relapsed when therapy was discontinued. Perhaps the most important observation was that males infected with *E. coli* who had minimal structural abnormalities had a good prognosis with short-term therapy alone. In the absence of severe urologic disease or concomitant noninfectious renal disease, no patients with persistent bacteriuria developed renal failure. This emphasizes the paramount importance of the presence of structural abnormalities rather than infection as the determinant of renal disease. The major value of long-term therapy in males was reduction in episodes of septic complications.

Prophylaxis

Prophylactic therapy is remarkably effective in female patients with frequent, closely spaced recurrent infection. Although it has been shown that the post-coital use of antimicrobial agents is effective in females with recurrent infections,[47] most trials use a regimen of small doses of an antimicrobial agent at bedtime. The preferred drugs are trimethoprim, alone or combined with sulfamethoxazole or nitrofurantoin, but other agents, such as methenamine salts or nalidixic acid and related drugs, may be used. It must be emphasized that regardless of the duration of prophylaxis (at least six months), recurrent infection, usually due to reinfection in females, will occur at about the same rate as that following a short course of treatment.[23, 48–50] Therefore, prophylaxis does not appear to affect host susceptibility. For this reason, prophylaxis must be considered only as a useful tactic for the patient with highly recurrent infection.

An alternate approach is to treat each infection as it occurs over time. In females, each course of therapy extracts about 20% of the population into long-term remission.[51] Multiple courses of treatment thereby reduce the population at risk of recurrence. Since each patient has an individual pattern of recurrence, the clinician should choose the most appropriate therapy for his patient. This, in practical terms, means that infections widely scattered in time may be treated intermittently, while closely spaced recurrences, particularly when symptomatic, respond better to continuous prophylaxis. In general it is recommended that prophylaxis be continued in females for about six months. If infection recurs, the patient can be managed either by intermittent treatment or a repeated course of prophylaxis.

Preoperative Prophylaxis

It is now clear that preoperative use of antimicrobial agents prior to urologic procedures will markedly reduce septic complications following surgery on the urinary tract. Treatment is most effective when used in those who have been shown to have bacteriuria and to be only of marginal benefit when the urine is sterile. An extensive critical review of the literature by Chodak and Plaut[52] found that most studies were flawed by being uncontrolled, not randomized, retrospective, or the drug was started postoperatively.

The need to provide adequate antimicrobial therapy prior to transurethral prostatectomy is well illustrated by the study of Cafferty et al.[53] Septicemia followed this procedure in only three of 206 operations (1.5%) in patients with initially sterile urine. In patients with infected urine preoperatively who did not receive appropriate antibiotics, septicemia developed in 11 of 169 (6.2%), whereas there was no septicemia following 180 operations in infected patients who received appropriate antibiotics 2–12 hours before operation. Clearly, this is a subject that requires considerable attention.

Treatment and Prophylaxis of Specific Conditions

ASYMPTOMATIC BACTERIURIA.—This is a laboratory finding, not a clinical entity. Patients in very different risk groups may not exhibit symptoms, yet have large numbers of bacteria in their urine. For example, young girls with asymptomatic bacteriuria are at very low risk of developing renal disease, while elderly individuals with the same findings but who have an indwelling catheter are at high risk of developing pyelonephritis and sepsis.

It is relatively easy to eradicate bacteriuria in young girls, yet virtually impossible in those with a catheter in place. For these reasons, asymptomatic bacteriuria should be considered as only an indicator of the presence of infection and as a guide to the efficacy of therapy.

The Urethral Syndrome

This is a clinical entity also known as the pyuria-dysuria syndrome. About half of the women complaining of dysuria seen in office practice will not be found to have significant bacteriuria by the usual criteria of 100,000 or more bacteria per ml of urine. About 75% of women with the urethral syndrome have pyuria. Stamm et al.[54] using suprapubic aspiration or urethral catheterization have presented evidence that these women are infected with either a coliform bacteria or *S. saprophyticus* present in low counts, or with *Chlamydia trachomatis*.

There has been considerable debate in the literature concerning the role of Lactobacilli, anaerobic streptococci and diphtheroids as a cause of the so-called urethral syndrome. Maskell et al.[55] favor an important role for these organisms. Brumfitt et al.,[56] however, have presented convincing evidence that most often these organisms are simply commensals representing the flora of the lower vagina and are not found on suprapubic aspiration. They were unable to confirm or deny the work of Stamm et al.[54]

The role of Chlamydia in this syndrome may be an important consideration for therapy, because these organisms are not sensitive to most of the drugs used to treat urinary tract infections. Instead, they require therapy with tetracyclines or trimethoprim/sulfamethoxazole. Since these agents are also effective against gonorrhea, another important cause of urethritis,[57] they may be of special value for treatment of the urethral syndrome. In a controlled trial, Stamm et al.[58] found that a 10-day course of doxycycline, given twice daily, was more effective than placebo in obtaining a clinical response and microbiologic cure of the urethral syndrome.

Urinary Tract Infections in Pregnancy

This subject has generated considerable controversy because of the potential role of such infections in producing low birthweight children. It is clear that bacteriuria of pregnancy is common; that it is usually asymptomatic in the early trimesters; and that it may become manifest during the last trimester. All studies have demonstrated that eradicating bacteriuria early in the course of pregnancy will prevent morbidity to the mother later on. Kass[59] and Elder et al.[60] have reported that bacteriuria in pregnancy is associated with prematurity and that it can be prevented by tetracycline therapy. However, it is possible that tetracycline may have prevented prematurity for reasons other than treatment of urinary tract infection. For example, Martin et al.[61] present evidence that treatment of Chlamydial infections may reduce prematurity. Many other trials of treatment of bacteriuria of pregnancy have not confirmed the initial reports. This is possibly because of sample size or because only those women who do not respond promptly to treatment are at high risk.

A large epidemiologic study (collaborative perinatal project) indicated that women who had symptomatic infections in pregnancy bore children more frequently with intellectual and motor defects.[62] Most people who have reviewed this subject tend to agree that if prematurity occurs in bacteriuric women, urinary tract infection can only account for a small proportion of the cases. Nevertheless, since bacteriuria is readily determined by simple culture methods and therapy is effective in preventing morbidity, it seems reasonable at the very least to detect and treat effectively bacteriuria of pregnancy.

Prostatic Infection

It is now believed that the prostate is often colonized in male patients with urinary tract infections and that bacteria released from this focus accounts for relapse in recurrent infections. For example, in the study by Smith et al.,[45] half the patients with recurrent infections had an identifiable prostatic infection. This subject was recently reviewed by Meares.[63] Despite elegant attempts to define how various antimicrobial agents enter the prostatic fluid and the attempt to use lipid soluble drugs (such as trimethoprim, minocycline, and rifampin) for this purpose, the response to therapy has been relatively poor.

For example, Meares found that only about one-third of men with chronic bacterial prostatitis were cured with trimethoprim/sulfamethoxazole. Trimethoprim does enter the prostate at therapeutic concentrations, so other factors must account for the failure. These failures may be due to the fact that—unlike the healthy dogs used in most studies in which the prostatic fluid is acidic—the fluid in infected men is characterized by an alkaline, solute-poor secretion. For this reason, I prefer to use long-term bedtime prophylaxis for periods up to a year or more when the patient does not respond to shorter and more intensive courses. The goal in these men is not necessarily to eradicate the prostatic focus, but to prevent recurrent infections and septic complications.

Prostatic colonization must be differentiated from acute bacterial prostatitis. Patients who are septic most likely have bacterial invasion into the tissue stroma. This is a very severe form of acute infection requiring aggressive management, usually with parenteral agents as in the treatment of generalized gram-negative sepsis. Penetration of drugs into the acutely-inflamed prostate does not appear to be a problem. These patients are generally treated with an aminoglycoside antibiotic for gram-negative bacteria plus additional agents that are effective against enterococci. Cephalosporin antibiotics and related "third generation" agents are not active against enterococci. Therefore, agents such as ampicillin, carbenicillin, ticarcillin, or the new acylamino penicillins are preferred.

ACUTE PYELONEPHRITIS.—This syndrome may be encountered in otherwise healthy young women as part of the natural history of uncomplicated infection, or it may be a serious complication in individuals with complicated infections. In either case, however, it seems reasonable, until bacteriologic information is available, to treat the patients with parenteral agents most likely to be effective against the invading organism. A useful guide to the choice of drug are the history of agents used in the past by the patient and antimicrobial susceptibility patterns in an individual institution.

For example, a young woman not previously treated with antibiotics may respond well to ampicillin or a first or second generation cephalosporin, while a patient who was treated on many occasions may require use of aminoglycosides, such as amikacin. I generally prefer to begin with an aminoglycoside antibiotic and ampicillin and then will change therapy depending on susceptibility tests. However, this is somewhat of a guessing game and a variety of agents and combinations would be likely also to be effective, depending on the frequency of susceptible strains.

Management of chronic pyelonephritis requires clear evidence that an active infection is present. There is no need to treat inactive, noninfected scarred kidneys. The presence of significant bacteriuria is an excellent guide to therapy. I prefer to monitor the urine for bacteria as an indicator of response or need for further treatment. The duration of therapy is then tailored to the patient (see Table 1).

Infection in the Presence of a Urinary Catheter

In most hospitals, a large proportion of patients with indwelling catheters will be found to be receiving antibiotics for other conditions. The rate of acquisition of infection is somewhat lower in these individuals.[64] However, it has repeatedly been shown that the favorable effect of antibiotics is limited to a few days and that the bacteria are soon replaced with resistant strains.[65] The addition of acidifying agents, such as ascorbic acid or methenamine salts, does not decrease the frequency of bacteriuria.[66] In recent reports, Warren et al.[67, 68] evaluated the common practice of using a short course of cephalexin in catheterized patients. They found that the frequency of fever was not reduced and that more cephalexin-resistant bacteria were isolated from treated patients. For these reasons, most investigators recommend that systemic antimicrobial therapy be limited to periods when the patient appears to be septic.

Bacteriuria in the Elderly

This condition should probably not be treated aggressively. It has been found in several surveys that 10% or more of women over 65 years of age will have asymptomatic bacteriuria, but maintain relatively normal renal function. Dontas et al.[69] reported that survival was decreased in elderly individu-

als found to have bacteriuria. However, it is difficult to assess
whether this finding was directly related, or an indicator of another factor. In any event, it is not clear that treatment will
delay mortality, nor that it will effectively prevent recurrence.
It seems reasonable, therefore, to reserve treatment in the elderly for symptomatic episodes.

Fungal Infections

Candida and Torulopsis infections of the urinary tract may
occur in patients on catheter drainage, in diabetics who are repeatedly treated with antibiotics, and in immunocompromised
patients with systemic candidiasis. This often presents a major
diagnostic problem in differentiating patients who only have
local infection from those with systemic disease.[70] Unfortunately, clinical criteria may not be helpful in distinguishing
reliably among these clinical entities. Various serologic and
gas chromatographic methods have been attempted, but there
is extensive overlap between patients who are colonized or infected. Blood cultures will also frequently be negative, even in
patients with *Candida endocarditis.* Occasionally, fungus balls
may obstruct the ureters. These patients may be managed with
oral flucytosine, with bladder irrigations with amphotericin B,
or with short courses of systemic amphotericin, in sequence, as
needed.[70–73]

Conditions in Which We Must Recognize Failure

Patients in whom there is a persistent foreign body, such as
a stone or catheter, will respond only transiently to chemotherapy. The objective in these patients is to remove the foreign
body whenever possible, or at least assure good urine flow.
Treatment should be reserved for episodes of sepsis. No one
really knows how long to treat such episodes, because the blood
stream frequently will clear spontaneously. In general, however, it seems best to treat the patients as though they had
acute pyelonephritis, as described above.

Future Therapy With New Antibiotics

In recent years, there has been a remarkable proliferation of
new semisynthetic beta lactam antibiotics. These can be

roughly divided into new broad spectrum penicillins (azlocillin, mezlocillin, and pipericillin); new beta lactamase stable cephalosporins (cefotaxime, cefmonoxime, cefoperazone, and moxalactam); a group of compounds in which a sulfur or oxygen atom is located outside of the dihydrothiazolidine ring (thienamycin); a group of simple compounds in which only the beta lactam ring is preserved (the monobactams); and beta lactamase inhibitors (clavulanic acid). Several recent trials have demonstrated that combinations of clavulanic acid with amoxacillin effectively treat urinary tract infections in which the organisms are resistant to amoxacillin by virtue of beta lactamase production.[74, 75] Two excellent review articles on the current status of these drugs in therapy have been published by Neu[76] and Eliopoulos et al.[77]

There are numerous reports in the literature of the efficacy of these drugs in the treatment of urinary tract infection, but they are difficult to evaluate because of the disparate nature of the populations treated and the difficulty in conducting comparative trials of so many agents. In general, the "gold standard" of therapy is the aminoglycoside antibiotics. Many of the trials attempt to demonstrate that a new beta lactam compound is equally effective, and less toxic than an aminoglycoside.[78] I am not aware of any study showing superiority except for organisms against which the aminoglycosides are not active. As with most forms of therapy for urinary tract infection, these new agents are effective in treating uncomplicated infections, are potentially useful in the initial treatment of gramnegative sepsis, but are disappointing in eradicating persistent tissue infection in the presence of foreign bodies or obstruction.

One potential disadvantage of the new beta lactamase-resistant drugs is their ability to induce the production of beta lactamases. This phenomenon is associated with the development of resistance during therapy.[79] Although the mechanism for resistance is still under investigation, one likely explanation is that relatively large amounts of induced enzyme may form complexes with the drugs in the periplasmic space of bacteria. Another problem with these agents is their high relative cost in relation to currently available effective agents.

In general, the new penicillins appear to offer more for the treatment of urinary tract infections than do the cephalosporins. The penicillins tend to be more uniformly active against Pseudomonas and many other gram-negative bacteria, and they are active against streptococci and many of the anaerobes. Nevertheless, they may not always be effective because they tend to be less active against high inocula. Another problem is that, despite their greater activity than many older drugs against gram-negative bacteria, they are used at higher doses than probably needed. This also adds to the cost of the agents. The characteristics of these agents are listed in Table 2.

My recommendation is that hospitals restrict the general use of these drugs, report information on susceptibility to physicians only when older agents are ineffective, and that only a single member of each group be available in the pharmacy when needed.

REFERENCES

1. Kunin C.M.: Duration of treatment of urinary tract infections. *Am. J. Med.* 71:849, 1981.
2. Bollgren I., Nord C.E., Pettersson L., et al.: Periurethral anaerobic microflora in girls highly susceptible to urinary tract infections. *J. Urol.* 125:715, 1981.
3. McDowall D.R.M., Buchanan J.D., Fairley K.F., et al.: Anaerobic and other fastidious microorganisms in asymptomatic bacteriuria in pregnant women. *J. Infect. Dis.* 144:114, 1981.
4. Jordan P.A., Iravani A., Richard G.A., et al.: Urinary tract infection caused by Staphylococcus saprophyticus. *J. Infect. Dis.* 141:510, 1980.
5. Marrie T.J., Kwan C., Noble M.A., et al.: Staphylococcus saprophyticus as a cause of urinary tract infections. *J. Clin. Microbiol.* 16:427, 1982.
6. Wallmark G., Arremark I., Telander B.: Staphylococcus saprophyticus: A frequent cause of acute urinary tract infection among female outpatients. *J. Infect. Dis.* 138:791, 1978.
7. Marrie T.J., Kwan D.: Antimicrobial susceptibility of Staphylococcus saprophyticus and urethral staphylococci. *Antimicrob. Agents Chemother.* 22:395, 1982.
8. Eisenstein B.I., Beachey E.H., Offek I.: Influence of sublethal concentrations of antibiotics on the expression of the mannose-specific ligand of Escherichia coli. *Infect. Immun.* 28:154, 1980.
9. Svanborg-Eden C., Fretere R., Hagberg L., et al.: Inhibition of experimental ascending urinary tract infection by epithelial cell-surface receptor analogue. *Nature* 298:560, 1982.
10. Demuth P.J., Gerding, D.N., Crossley K.: Staphylococcus auerus bacteriuria. *Arch. Intern. Med.* 139:78, 1979.
11. Bayer A.S., Chow A.W., Anthony B.F., et al.: Serious infections in adults due to group B streptococci. *Am. J. Med.* 61:498, 1976.
12. Albritton W.L., Hammond G.W., Ronald A.R.: Bacteremic haemophilus influenzae genitourinary tract infections in adults. *Arch. Intern. Med.* 138:1819, 1978.
13. Back E., Carlsson B., Hylander B.: Urinary tract infection from haemophilus parainfluenzae. *Nephron.* 29:117, 1981.
14. Goetz M.B., Craig W.A.: Haemophilus influenzae prostatitis. *J.A.M.A.* 247:3118, 1982.
15. Thomas D., Simpson K., Ostojic H., et al.: Bacteremic epididymo-orchitis due to hemophilus influenzae type B. *J. Urol.* 126:832, 1981.
16. Dorman S.A., Hardin N.J., Winn W.C. Jr.: Pyelonephritis associated with legionella pneumophila, Serogroup 4. *Ann. Intern. Med.* 93:835, 1980.

17. Birch D.F., Fairley K.F., Pavillard R.E.: Unconventional bacteria in urinary tract disease: Ureaplasma urealyticum. *Kidney Int.* 19:58, 1981.
18. Kunin C.M.: *Detection, Prevention, and Treatment of Urinary Tract Infection.* (Philadelphia: Third Edition, Lea and Febiger, 1979).
19. O'Grady F., Cattell W.R.: Kinetics of urinary tract infection: II. The Bladder. *Br. J. Urol.* 38:156, 1966.
20. Stamey T.A.: *Pathogenesis and Treatment of Urinary Tract Infections.* (Baltimore: The Williams & Wilkins Co., 1980.)
21. Stamey T.A., Sexton C.C.: The role of vaginal colonization with Enterobacteriaceae in recurrent urinary infections. *J. Urol.* 113:214, 1975.
22. Kunin C.M., Polyak F., Postel E.: Periurethral bacterial flora in women. Prolonged intermittent colonization with *E. coli. J.A.M.A.* 243:136, 1980.
23. Stamm W.E., Counts G.W., Wagner K.F., et al.: Antimicrobial prophylaxis of recurrent urinary tract infections. *Ann. Intern. Med.* 92:770, 1980.
24. Vosbeck K., Mett H., Huber U., et al.: Effects of low concentrations of antibiotics on Escherichia coli adhesion. *Antimic. Ag. Chemo.* 21:864, 1982.
25. Redjeb S.B., Slim A., Horchani A., et al.: Effects of 10 milligrams of ampicillin per day on urinary tract infections. *Antimicrob. Agents Chemother.* 22:1084, 1982.
26. Bailey R.R.: *Single dose therapy of urinary tract infection.* (Australia: ADIS Health Science Press, 1 Vol., p. 345, 1983.)
27. Souney P., Polk B.F.: Single-dose antimicrobial therapy for urinary tract infections in women. *Rev. Infect. Dis.* 4:29, 1982.
28. Fang L.S.T., Rubin N.E.T., Rubin R.H.: Efficacy of single-dose and conventional amoxicillin therapy in urinary-tract infection localized by the antibody-coated bacteria technic. *N. Engl. J. Med.* 298:413, 1978.
29. Mundt K.A., Polk B.F.: Identification of site of urinary-tract infections by antibody-coated bacteria assay. *Lancet* 2:1172, 1979.
30. Ronald A.R., Boutros P., Mourtada H.: Bacteriuria localization and response to single-dose therapy in women. *J.A.M.A.* 235:1854, 1976.
31. McCracken G.H. Jr., Ginsburg C.M., Namasonthi V., et al.: Evaluation of short-term antibiotic therapy in children with uncomplicated urinary tract infections. *Pediatrics.* 67:796, 1981.
32. Rubin R.H., Fang L.S.T., Jones S.T., et al.: Single-dose amoxicillin therapy for urinary tract infection. *J.A.M.A.* 244:561, 1980.
33. Bailey R.R., Abbott G.D.: Treatment of urinary-tract infection with a single dose of amoxycillin. *Nephron.* 18:316, 1977.
34. Engel G., Schaeffer A.J., Grayhack J.T., et al.: The role of excretory urography and cystoscopy in the evaluation and management of women with recurrent urinary tract infection. *J. Urol.* 123:190, 1980.
35. Fair W.R., McClennan B.L., Just R.G.: Are excretory urograms necessary in evaluating women with urinary tract infection? *J. Urol.* 121:313, 1979.
36. Brumfitt W., Faiers M.C., Franklin I.N.S.: The treatment of urinary infection by means of a single dose of cephaloridine. *Postgrad. Med. J.* 46(Suppl.):65, 1970.
37. Shaw P.G., Fairley K.F., Whitworth J.A.: Treatment of urinary tract infection with a single-dose intramuscular administration of cephamandole. *Med. J. Aust.* 1:489, 1980.
38. Greenberg R.N., Sanders C.V., Lewis A.C., et al.: Single-dose cefaclor therapy of urinary tract infection. *Am. J. Med.* 71:841, 1981.
39. Charlton C.A.C., Crowther A., Davies J.G., et al.: Three-day and ten-day chemotherapy for urinary tract infections in general practice. *Br. Med. J.* 1:124, 1976.
40. Fair W.R., Crane D.B., Peterson L.J., et al.: Three-day treatment of urinary tract infections. *J. Urol.* 123:717, 1980.
41. Iravani A., Richard G.A., Baer H.: Trimethoprim once daily *vs.* nitrofurantoin in treatment of acute urinary tract infections in young women, with special reference to periurethral, vaginal, and fecal flora. *Rev. Infect. Dis.* 4:378, 1982.

42. Brumfitt W., Hamilton-Miller J.M.T., Franklin I.N.S., et al.: Conventional and two-dose amoxycillin treatment of bacteriuria in pregnancy and recurrent bacteriuria: a comparative study. *J. Antimicrob. Chemother.* 10:239, 1982.
43. Turck M., Petersdorf R.G.: Optimal duration of treatment of chronic urinary tract infection. *Ann. Intern. Med.* 69:837, 1968.
44. Gleckman R., Crowley M., Natsios G.A.: Therapy of recurrent invasive urinary-tract infections of men. *N. Engl. J. Med.* 301:878, 1979.
45. Smith J.W., Jones S.R., Reed W.P., et al.: Recurrent urinary tract infections in men. *Ann. Inter. Med.* 91:544, 1979.
46. Freeman R.B., Richardson J.A., Thurm R.H., et al.: Long-term therapy for chronic bacteriuria in men. *Ann. Intern. Med.* 83:133, 1975.
47. Vosti K.L.: Recurrent urinary tract infections: Prevention by prophylactic antibiotics after sexual intercourse. *J.A.M.A.* 231:934, 1975.
48. Bailey R.R., Gower P.E., Roberts A.P., et al.: Prevention of urinary tract infection with low-dose nitrofurantoin. *Lancet* 2:1112, 1971.
49. Harding G.K.M., Ronald A.R., Nicolle L.E., et al.: Long-term antimicrobial prophylaxis for recurrent urinary tract infection in women. *Rev. Infect. Dis.* 4:428, 1982.
50. Stansfeld J.M.: Duration of treatment for urinary tract infections in children. *Br. Med. J.* 3:65, 1977.
51. Kunin C.M.: The natural history of recurrent bacteriuria in school girls. *N. Engl. J. Med.* 282:1443, 1970.
52. Chodak G.W., Plaut M.E.: Systemic antibiotics for prophylaxis in urologic surgery: a critical review. *J. Urol.* 121:695, 1979.
53. Cafferkey M.T., Falkiner F.R., Gillespie W.A., et al.: Antibiotics for the prevention of septicaemia in urology. *Br. Soc. Antimic. Chem.* 9:471, 1982.
54. Stamm W.E., Wagner K.F., Amsel R., et al.: Causes of the acute urethral syndrome in women. *N. Engl. J. Med.* 303:409, 1980.
55. Maskell R., Pead L., Allen J.: The puzzle of "urethral syndrome:" a possible answer. *Lancet* 1:1058, 1979.
56. Brumfitt W., Ludlam H., Hamilton-Miller J.M.T., et al.: Lactobacilli do not cause frequency and dysuria syndrome. *Lancet* 2:393, 1981.
57. Brunham R.C., Kuo C.C., Stevens C.E., et al.: Treatment of concomitant Neisseria gonorrhoeae and Chlamydia trachomatis infections in women: comparison of trimethoprim-sulfamethoxazole with ampicillin-probenecid. *Rev. Infect. Dis.* 4:491, 1982.
58. Stamm W.E., Running K., McKevitt M., et al.: Treatment of the acute urethral syndrome. *N. Engl. J. Med.* 304:956, 1981.
59. Kass E.H.: Bacteriuria and pyelonephritis of pregnancy. *Arch. Intern. Med.* 105:194, 1960.
60. Elder H.A., Santamarina B.A.G., Smith S., et al.: The natural history of asymptomatic bacteriuria during pregnancy: the effect of tetracycline on the clinical course and the outcome of pregnancy. *Am. J. Obstet. Gynecol.* 111:441, 1971.
61. Martin D.H., Koutsky L., Eschenbach D.A., et al.: Prematurity and perinatal mortality in pregnancies complicated by maternal Chlamydia trachomatis infections. *J.A.M.A.* 247:1585, 1982.
62. Sever J.L., Ellenbert J.H., Edmonds D.: Urinary tract infections during pregnancy: maternal and pediatric findings. Kass E.H., Brumfitt W. (eds.): *In infections of the Urinary Tract.* (Chicago: University of Chicago Press, pp. 19–21, 1978.)
63. Meares E.M. Jr.: Prostatitis: Review of pharmacokinetics and therapy. *Rev. Infect. Dis.* 4:475, 1982.
64. Garibaldi R.A., Burke J.P., Dickman M.L., et al.: Factors predisposing to bacteriuria during indwelling urethral catheterization. *N. Engl. J. Med.* 291:215, 1974.
65. Britt M.R., Garibaldi R.A., Miller W.A., et al.: Antimicrobic prophylaxis for catheter-associated bacteriuria. *Antimicrob. Agents Chemother.* 11:240, 1977.
66. Vainrub B., Musher D.M.: Lack of effect of methenamine in suppression of, or pro-

phylaxis against, chronic urinary infection. *Antimicrob. Agents Chemother.* 12:625, 1977.

67. Warren J.W., Anthony W.C., Hoopes J.M., et al.: Cephalexin for susceptible bacteriuria in afebrile, long-term catheterized patients. *J.A.M.A.* 248:454, 1982.
68. Warren J.W., Hoopes J.M., Muncie H.L., et al.: Ineffectiveness of cephalexin in treatment of cephalexin-resistant bacteriuria in patients with chronic indwelling urethral catheters. *J. Urol.* 129:71, 1983.
69. Dontas A.S., Charvati P.K., Papanayiotou P.C., et al.: Bacteriuria and survival in old age. *N. Engl. J. Med.* 304:939, 1981.
70. Fisher J.F., Chew W.H., Shadomy W., et al.: Urinary tract infections due to candida albicans. *Rev. Infect. Dis.* 1107, 1982.
71. Rohner T.J., Jr., Tuliszewski R.M.: Fungal cystitis: awareness, diagnosis and treatment. *J. Urol.* 124:142, 1980.
72. Wise G.J., Kozinn P.J., Goldberg P.: Flucytosine in the management of genitourinary candidiasis: five years of experience. *J. Urol.* 124:70, 1980.
73. Wise G.J., Kozinn P.J., Goldberg P.: Amphotericin B as a urologic irrigant in the management of noninvasive candiduria. *J. Urol.* 128:82, 1982.
74. Ball A.P., Davey P.G., Geddes A.M., et al.: Clavulanic acid and amoxycillin: A clinical, bacteriological, and pharmacological study. *Lancet* 1:620, 1980.
75. Martinelli R., Lopes A., Oliveira M., et al.: Amoxicillin-clavulanic acid in treatment of urinary tract infection due to gram-negative bacteria resistant to penicillin. *Antimicrob. Agents Chemother.* 20:800, 1981.
76. Neu H.C.: The new beta-lactamase-stable cephalosporins. *Ann. Intern. Med.* 97:408, 1982.
77. Eliopoulos G.M., Moellering R.C. Jr.: Azlocillin, mezlocillin and piperacillin: new broad-spectrum penicillins. *Ann. Intern. Med.* 97:755, 1982.
78. Abbruzzese J.L., Rocco L.E., Laskin O.L., et al.: Prospective randomized double-blind comparison of moxalactam and tobramycin in treatment of urinary tract infections. *Am. J. Med.* 74:694, 1983.
79. Sanders C.C.: Novel resistance selected by the new expanded-spectrum cephalosporins: a concern. *J. Infect. Dis.* 147:585, 1983.

Life-Threatening Acid-Base Disorders

JEROME P. KASSIRER, M.D.

Professor and Associate Chairman, Department of Medicine, Tufts University School of Medicine, Boston, Mass.

EXTREME DEVIATIONS in acid-base equilibrium are frequent accompaniments of many serious illnesses and in themselves can be a threat to survival. The threat derives not only directly from the severe acidity or alkalinity, but also from secondary effects on ventilation and electrolyte balance. The measures that can be taken to protect against extreme acid-base imbalance and those that reverse it are based on sound physiologic principles. To provide a framework for comprehending therapeutic issues, these principles are considered first.

The Henderson Equation

All acid-base derangements can be formulated in terms of the Henderson equation (Fig 1). This relation between Pa_{CO_2}, plasma bicarbonate concentration, and hydrogen ion concentration (i.e., pH) of the plasma asserts a simple truism about the acidity of body fluids at any given moment: the acidity of the plasma is a linear function of two variables, the Pa_{CO_2} and the plasma bicarbonate concentration. It also identifies, with simple precision, the four classes of acid-base disturbances as primary alterations (either increases or decreases) in these two variables. Thus, the two metabolic acid-base disturbances, metabolic acidosis and metabolic alkalosis, are defined as primary

0084-5957/84/0014-0067-0086-$04.00

$$[H^+] = 24 \ \frac{PaCO_2}{[HCO_3^-]}$$

Fig 1.—The Henderson equation. The acidity of body fluids (hydrogen ion concentration) at any given moment is a function of two variables, the partial pressure of carbon dioxide (Pa_{CO_2}) and the plasma bicarbonate concentration (HCO_3^-).

decreases and increases, respectively, of plasma bicarbonate concentration; the two respiratory acid-base disturbances, respiratory acidosis and respiratory alkalosis, are defined as increases and decreases, respectively, of Pa_{CO_2}.

The Henderson equation can be represented in algebraic form, as in Figure 1, or in graphic form, as in Figure 2. Values on the ordinate represent the numerator of the equation (Pa_{CO_2}), values on the abscissa represent the denominator (bicarbonate), and isobars radiating from the origin represent values for acidity (hydrogen ion concentration, or pH). The curves in Figure 2 will be explained in the course of the discussion.

Simple Acid-Base Disturbances

Primary alterations in plasma bicarbonate concentrations or Pa_{CO_2} set into effect a series of physiologic alterations that yield secondary, or adaptive, adjustments in the countervailing variable (Pa_{CO_2} is the countervailing variable of plasma bicarbonate; bicarbonate is the countervailing variable of Pa_{CO_2}). Thus, when the plasma bicarbonate level falls, acidification of the plasma leads to acidification of the spinal fluid in the region of the medullary respiratory center, which in turn results in hyperventilation and a consequent reduction in Pa_{CO_2}. The opposite sequence occurs in metabolic alkalosis. Primary increases in Pa_{CO_2} lead to increases in plasma bicarbonate levels either through mechanisms involving tissue buffers in the short term and or through mechanisms involving renal acid excretion over the long term. An opposite change in plasma bicarbonate concentration occurs in respiratory alkalosis. By convention, a simple acid-base disturbance consists of both the primary disturbance in either plasma bicarbonate or Pa_{CO_2} and the secondary adaptation (sometimes termed compensation).

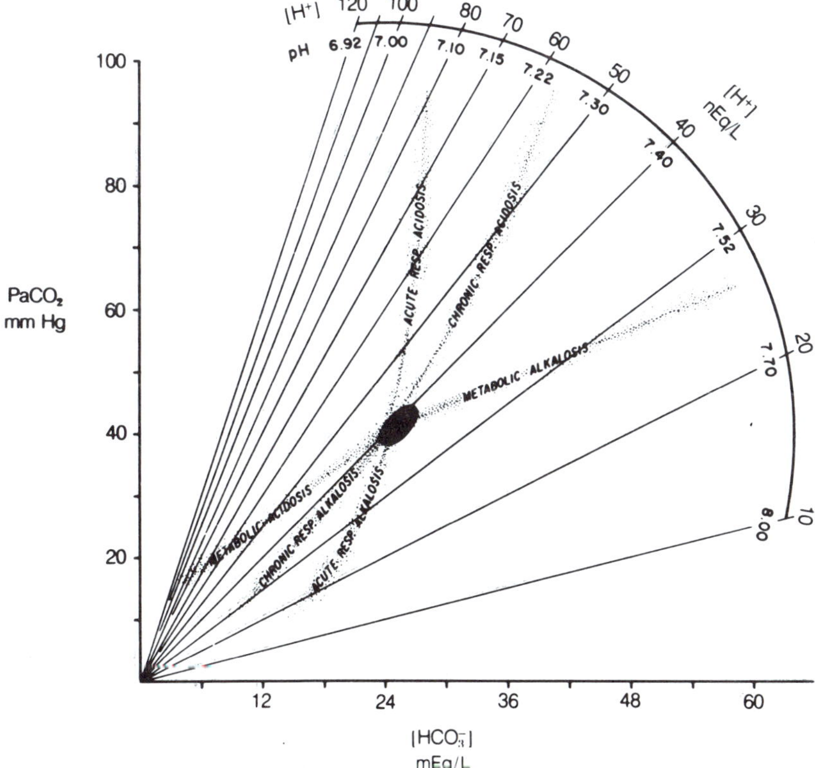

Fig 2.—Whole body titration curves in man. The coordinates of this Figure and its isobars are a graphic representation of the Henderson equation shown in Figure 1. The oval area in the center represents the limits of normal acid-base parameters. The labeled shaded areas represent the integrated responses to the primary acid-base derangements, metabolic acidosis, metabolic alkalosis, respiratory acidosis and respiratory alkalosis, and are the "whole body titration curves" for each of these disorders. The text contains an extensive explanation of these titration curves and a description of their use. (Modified from Cohen J.J., Kassirer J.P.: *Acid Base*. Boston, Little, Brown & Co., 1982. Reproduced by permission.)

Three Observations About the Adaptive Responses

The adaptations to primary acid-base disturbances are complex physiologic events, but several simple rules exist regarding their operation. First, the adaptive response always involves a change in the countervailing variable; a primary alteration in bicarbonate sets into motion an alteration in Pa_{CO_2}, and vice versa. Second, the secondary adaptive response is always in the same direction as the primary response: if the bicarbonate level falls, for example, the adaptation involves a reduction in Pa_{CO_2}; if Pa_{CO_2} rises, the adaptation involves an increase in bicarbonate. Third, the adaptive response is protective, that is, it prevents hydrogen ion concentration from reaching the height or nadir it would achieve if no adaptation had occurred. Nonetheless, the normal adaptive response is not sufficient, for any of the primary acid-base disturbances, to fully restore acidity to normal levels.

The extent of the adaptive response varies from one acid-base disturbance to another: even for a single primary disturbance, however, it depends on the duration of the disturbance. The extent of the adaptive response is a critical determinant of how one assesses and treats extreme acid-base derangements, and this issue is examined in detail in the next section.

The Concept of a Whole Body Titration Curve

To assess the extent of adaptation to acid-base disorders, studies have been directed at measuring the response to graded alterations in either the Pa_{CO_2} or the plasma bicarbonate level. In the same way that one might titrate a test tube containing a solution of alkali and buffers with an acid, studies of whole body titration are carried out by creating a graded acid-base challenge in the intact organism. This concept can be instantiated by reference to studies of the respiratory response to metabolic acidosis. To assess the extent of the respiratory response to metabolic acidosis, normal humans have been given ammonium chloride to lower plasma bicarbonate concentration. In a series of such studies, plasma bicarbonate has been lowered progressively in steps and allowed to attain a steady state at each new level. Once a steady state is achieved, the Pa_{CO_2} is measured as an index of the adaptive respiratory response. Such studies provide information about the adaptive response to metabolic acidosis across a wide range of plasma bicarbonate concentrations.

Extent of the Adaptive Responses: Whole Body Titration Curves in Man

The adaptive response to some of the primary acid-base disturbances (namely, acute respiratory acidosis, acute respiratory alkalosis, and metabolic acidosis) are rather well defined from experimental observations in man. The responses to the other disturbances are less well defined but can be inferred with reasonable certainty from observations in man and experiments in animals. The following sections describe the whole body titration curves for the four simple acid-base disturbances. Each section considers the physiology of the adaptive response, the implications of the response for the protection of normal acidity, and the limits of the response for each of the simple disturbances. Exploring these limits puts into focus the circumstances in which the simple disturbances can endanger a patient's health.

Metabolic Acidosis

Severe metabolic acidosis influences the peripheral circulation, the gastrointestinal tract, and electrolyte metabolism, but the most serious consequence of this disorder is its suppressive effect on cardiac contractility and its potentiation of ventricular arrhythmias. The mechanism of the adaptive respiratory response is well studied. A falling plasma bicarbonate level is reflected after several hours by a parallel, though not numerically comparable, fall in CSF bicarbonate level, which in turn acidifies the medullary respiratory center and leads to hyperventilation. The hyperventilation is the adaptive response that leads to the characteristic reduction in Pa_{CO_2} in metabolic acidosis. Several studies in man show that a progressive reduction in plasma bicarbonate is accompanied by a progressive reduction in Pa_{CO_2}, and that the relation between the fall in bicarbonate and the fall in Pa_{CO_2} is linear; for every 1 mEq/L fall in plasma bicarbonate, the Pa_{CO_2} falls approximately 1.2 mm Hg. This whole body titration curve for metabolic acidosis is illustrated in the lower left quadrant of Figure 2 ("metabolic acidosis"). Note that as the bicarbonate concentration falls progressively, even though the Pa_{CO_2} also declines concurrently, the acidity of body fluids increases progressively. In fact, even with the maximum normal respiratory adaptive response to a falling bicarbonate concentration, severe acidemia is an inescapable consequence of extreme reductions in bicarbonate concentrations (i.e., concentrations of 5 mEq/L or less).

The degree of normal respiratory adaptation to extreme reductions in bicarbonate has not been assessed, but if one assumes that the curve describing the adaptive response to metabolic acidosis at these low bicarbonate levels is the same as at higher levels (i.e., a fall in Pa_{CO_2} of 1.2 mm Hg accompanies every 1 mEq/L fall in bicarbonate), the disastrous consequences of bicarbonate reductions below 5 mEq/L become evident. As shown in Table 1, even with "appropriate" respiratory adaptation, acidity becomes extreme and life-threatening when bicarbonate concentrations reach these low levels. It is also apparent from Table 1 that, when plasma bicarbonate is severely reduced, a small further fall in bicarbonate yields remarkably large deviations in hydrogen ion concentration (and pH). When bicarbonate concentration is 4 mEq/L and falls only 1 mEq/L, for example, blood pH falls 0.1 unit, even with a normal respiratory adaptive response. The contrast between this situation and what is seen in severe metabolic alkalosis will become evident later.

It should be pointed out that the titration curve shown in Figure 2, describing the adaptive response to metabolic acidosis, does not describe the acute respiratory response to a falling bicarbonate level, only the relation several hours after a steady state of hypobicarbonatemia has been achieved. The significance of this observation will become evident later when correction of extreme acidosis is discussed.

METABOLIC ALKALOSIS

Extreme metabolic alkalosis is dangerous because it suppresses ventilation and usually is accompanied by severe potassium deficiency and volume contraction. The ventilatory adap-

TABLE 1.—EXTREME METABOLIC ACIDOSIS*

PLASMA BICARBONATE (mEq/L)	"APPROPRIATE" Pa_{CO_2} (mm Hg)	$[H^+]$ (nEq/L)	pH
5	17	82	7.09
4	16	96	7.02
3	15	120	6.92
2	14	168	6.77

*Assumes that the adaptive response to extreme reductions in bicarbonate is the same as that to lesser reductions, i.e., that Pa_{CO_2} falls 1.2 mm Hg for every 1 mEq/L fall in plasma bicarbonate.

tive response has been characterized only recently. Although it was thought for years that little or no respiratory adaptation occurred in response to an increase in plasma bicarbonate concentration, recent data, both in animals and in humans, provide convincing evidence that an adaptive increase in Pa_{CO_2} is an expected consequence of primary metabolic alkalosis. Evidence also indicates that the respiratory adaptive response is similar in mechanism, but opposite in direction, to that of metabolic acidosis. Unfortunately, few data are available on the response of normal individuals to graded increases in plasma bicarbonate. The best data suggest, however, that as in metabolic acidosis, the adaptive increase in Pa_{CO_2} in metabolic alkalosis is a linear function of the increase in plasma bicarbonate. Collected data from a variety of sources suggest that the respiratory response in metabolic alkalosis is not as vigorous as that in metabolic acidosis, yet it is sufficient to provide substantial protection against severe alkalemia when plasma bicarbonate increases remarkably. An increase in Pa_{CO_2} of 0.7 mm Hg for each increase in plasma bicarbonate of 1 mEq/L is a close approximation of the adaptive response, and this titration curve is shown in the upper right quadrant of Figure 2 ("metabolic alkalosis").

Several features of this titration curve are worth noting. Because of the relation between plasma bicarbonate and Pa_{CO_2}, extremely high plasma bicarbonate levels are not associated with extreme alkalemia as long as respiratory adaptation is appropriate. As shown in Table 2, blood pH does not exceed 7.7 even with bicarbonate levels as high as 70 mEq/L. The contrast with metabolic acidosis is striking; as noted above, small changes in bicarbonate at low plasma bicarbonate levels yield remarkably large changes in acidity, but large changes in bi-

TABLE 2.—EXTREME METABOLIC ALKALOSIS*

PLASMA BICARBONATE (mEq/L)	"APPROPRIATE" Pa_{CO_2} (mm Hg)	$[H^+]$ (nEq/L)	pH
36	48	32	7.50
48	57	29	7.54
60	65	26	7.59
72	74	25	7.61

*Assumes that Pa_{CO_2} increases 0.7 mm Hg for every 1 mEq/L increase in plasma bicarbonate.

carbonate at very high plasma bicarbonate levels provoke only small changes in alkalinity.

Although the respiratory adaptive response to metabolic alkalosis is remarkably protective, extreme alkalemia can be a serious threat to life; the circumstances in which this threat surfaces are several. First, the suppression of ventilation required to produce the adaptive response also produces hypoxemia, and with extreme elevations of plasma bicarbonate, Pa_{CO_2} values of 60–70 mm Hg are typically associated with Pa_{O_2} values of 40–50 mm Hg. This severe degree of hypoxia can be a danger to patients with lung and heart disease and is probably also a threat to the sick patient who has neither cardiac nor pulmonary disease. Another important consequence of extreme respiratory adaptation is potassium deficiency. Severe alkalosis is typically associated with severe potassium deficiency, and such deficits can impair renal, cardiac, and muscle function and produce important metabolic complications. Finally, the patient with appropriately adapted extreme metabolic alkalosis has excellent protection against severe alkalinity as long as the respiratory adaptive response remains appropriate; if for any reason the patient begins to ventilate more than is required for the appropriate adaptation (for example, because of anxiety, sepsis, or pulmonary embolism), severe alkalemia will ocurr. If a patient with a plasma bicarbonate level of 60 mEq/L, a Pa_{CO_2} of 65 mm Hg, and a blood pH of 7.59, for example, abruptly begins to hyperventilate and lowers his Pa_{CO_2} to 40 mm Hg, blood pH will immediately increase to approximately 7.80. Such an increase may lead to profound disturbances in CNS function, including seizures and coma.

RESPIRATORY ACIDOSIS

Severe hypercapnia in itself can produce serious CNS manifestations, including delirium, stupor, and coma. The adaptive responses to hypercapnia are conveniently separated into an acute and a chronic response on the basis of the mechanisms of these responses and the magnitude of their protective effects. The acute response involves only cell buffers; the kidney plays no role. This acute response yields only a modest increase in plasma bicarbonate concentration and thus provides little protection against the tendency of hypercapnia to acidify body fluids. The chronic response, on the other hand, includes both cell buffering and renal generation and preservation of high plasma bicarbonate levels. As a result of this greater increase in plasma bicarbonate in the long-term response, an individual will be less acidic for any specific level of Pa_{CO_2} (as compared to the response in acute hypercapnia). Because of the differences outlined here between acute and chronic hypercapnia, the acute adaptive response to hypercapnia and the chronic response will be discussed separately.

Acute Respiratory Acidosis

Studies of induced hypercapnia in humans show that plasma bicarbonate concentration increases several milliequivalents within minutes after the induction of hypercapnia. This increase occurs without an increase in renal acid excretion and is accounted for exclusively by extracellular buffering of the excess carbon dioxide. The graded response to increasing hypercapnia in humans has been characterized extensively. This response is represented in the upper right quadrant in Figure 2 (the titration curve labeled "acute respiratory acidosis"), and the algebraic relation between the increase in Pa_{CO_2} and the increase in hydrogen can be expressed as follows: for every 1 mm Hg increase in Pa_{CO_2}, plasma hydrogen ion concentration increases 0.75 nEq/L. As noted in Figure 2, the increase in plasma bicarbonate in acute hypercapnia is quite modest, even when hypercapnia is extreme; with acute increases in Pa_{CO_2} to levels of 90–100 mm Hg, the plasma bicarbonate level increases only 4 or 5 mEq/L. Although the increment in bicarbonate is indeed modest, it does provide some protection against severe acidity. For example, if Pa_{CO_2} suddenly increased to 100 mm Hg, blood pH would be 7.00 if there were no cell buffering and thus no increase in plasma bicarbonate. With a 4 mEq/L increase in bicarbonate level, however, pH falls to approximately 7.07.

Chronic Respiratory Acidosis

The chronic response to graded increases in Pa_{CO_2} in humans cannot be studied in the same fashion as the response to acute hypercapnia because humans cannot tolerate exposure to a high ambient Pa_{CO_2} for more than a few minutes. Studies in animals, however, demonstrate that the adaptive mechanisms that protect against severe acidity involve not only the tissue buffers (as in acute hypercapnia), but also adjustments in renal function. Aside from the modest increase in plasma bicarbonate level that derives from the tissue buffering of carbon dioxide, an increase in renal acid excretion and a concomitant increase in bicarbonate resorption add new bicarbonate to the plasma and thus contributes to the protection. Careful studies of graded degrees of chronic hypercapnia in animals show that the plasma bicarbonate level rises progressively with increasing levels of Pa_{CO_2}.

Although studies of chronic exposure to hypercapnia cannot be carried out in normal man, the response of humans to graded hypercapnia has been assessed by observations made in patients with chronic pulmonary disease who manifested sustained hypercapnia. When such patients are carefully selected so that they have no complicating acid-base disorders, they show virtually the same adaptive response to sustained hypercapnia as that seen in experimental animals. This titration curve is shown in the upper right quadrant in Figure 2 ("chronic respiratory acidosis"). The algebraic equivalent of this titration curve, that is, the relation between the increase in Pa_{CO_2} and the increase in hydrogen ion concentration, can be expressed as follows: for each 1 mm Hg increase in Pa_{CO_2}, the hydrogen ion concentration increases approximately 0.3 nEq/L.

It is useful to note the shape of both the acute and the chronic respiratory acidosis titration curves. For any given elevation of Pa_{CO_2}, a patient with chronic hypercapnia will have a higher plasma bicarbonate concentration, and thus a lower hydrogen ion concentration (higher pH), than the patient with acute hypercapnia. The difference in bicarbonate concentrations is accounted for exclusively by the renal response. The importance of this renal response in the management of chronic hypercapnia will become evident later. Note the shape of the chronic respiratory acidosis titration curve: despite an increasing renal contribution to body bicarbonate stores with higher levels of Pa_{CO_2}, acidity increases progressively with increasingly high values for Pa_{CO_2}; the curve veers progressively away from the isohydric line (pH 7.40). This curve is one of the lines of evidence referred to above that the normal adaptive response is not sufficient, for any of the primary acid-base disturbances, to fully restore acidity to normal levels.

RESPIRATORY ALKALOSIS

Severe respiratory alkalosis induces cerebral vasoconstriction and can impede higher cerebral function. The mechanism of the response of humans to hypocapnia is similar to that in hypercapnia, but the response is opposite in direction. It will be convenient, as was the case for hypercapnia, to consider the responses in terms of acute and chronic adaptive responses. As in hypercapnia, the acute response involves only buffering by tissues and the chronic response involves the additional contribution of the kidney in altering renal bicarbonate resorption. The acute response yields only a modest reduction in plasma bicarbonate concentration and thus provides little protection against the tendency of hypocapnia to alkalinize body fluids. The chronic response, on the other hand, includes both cell buffering and a suppression of renal bicarbonate resorption to preserve low plasma bicarbonate levels. As a result of this greater decrease in plasma bicarbonate levels, an individual with chronic hypocapnia will be less alkalotic at any specific level of Pa_{CO_2} (as compared to the response in acute hypocapnia). As with chronic respiratory acidosis, discussed previously, the early adaptive response to hypocapnia will be discussed separately from the late response.

Acute Respiratory Alkalosis

When acute hypocapnia is induced in humans, the plasma bicarbonate level falls within minutes. This reduction (as in acute hypercapnia) is unaccompanied by an alteration in renal acid excretion and is accounted for exclusively by tissue buffering. The graded response of humans to acute hypocapnia has been characterized extensively and the response is identified in Figure 2 in the lower left quadrant as the titration curve labeled "acute respiratory alkalosis." It is apparent that the titration curve for acute respiratory alkalosis is merely an extension of that for acute respiratory acidosis. Indeed, the algebraic description of the response to acute hypocapnia is quantitatively the same as that for the response to acute hypercapnia: in acute respiratory alkalosis, for each 1 mm Hg decrement in Pa_{CO_2}, the hydrogen ion concentration falls 0.75 nEq/L.

This fall in plasma bicarbonate does exert some protective influence on pH as Pa_{CO_2} falls acutely, but, as in acute hypercapnia, extreme reductions of Pa_{CO_2} acutely are associated with a severe degree of alkalemia. Acute reductions of Pa_{CO_2} to 15 mm Hg, for example, are accompanied by a fall in plasma bicarbonate to 17 mEq/L, yet blood hydrogen ion concentration still falls to approximately 21 nEq/L (pH, 7.68).

Chronic Respiratory Alkalosis

Few data are available from carefully controlled experiments on the adaptive response to chronic reductions in Pa_{CO_2}, and thus titration curves to chronic hypocapnia are drawn principally from observations made on humans living at high altitude. What is known about the response is that it bears striking similarities to the response to chronic hypercapnia, but in the opposite direction. Chronic reductions in Pa_{CO_2} induce the kidney to lower the rate of bicarbonate reclamation, and as a result, the plasma bicarbonate concentration remains low after a steady state has been achieved. Indeed, a progressive reduction in bicarbonate is the consequence of progressive chronic hypocapnia.

Of all the acid-base disorders, chronic respiratory alkalosis is perhaps the best "protected." In other words, as Pa_{CO_2} falls progressively, the plasma bicarbonate concentration falls sufficiently so that blood hydrogen ion concentration (pH) remains only slightly alkaline. The relation between Pa_{CO_2} and the plasma bicarbonate level in the chronic steady state of respiratory alkalosis is shown in the lower left quadrant of Figure 2 in the titration curve labeled "chronic respiratory alkalosis." The relation between the decrease in Pa_{CO_2} and the decrease in plasma bicarbonate concentration can be expressed as follows: for each 1 mm Hg decrease in Pa_{CO_2}, the plasma bicarbonate concentration decreases approximately 0.5 mEq/L. Note the difference in the chronic respiratory alkalosis titration curve and the one for chronic respiratory acidosis: in chronic respiratory acidosis, as described earlier, the curve veers farther and farther away from the isohydric line (normal pH) as the Pa_{CO_2}

rises. Although the same is true for chronic respiratory alkalosis, the deviation from the normal pH is quite modest even with severe chronic reductions in Pa_{CO_2}. This point is easily illustrated. Although an acute reduction in Pa_{CO_2} to 15 mm Hg, for example, is associated with a blood hydrogen ion concentration of approximately 21 nEq/L (pH nearly 7.70), in the setting of severe chronic hypocapnia and the same Pa_{CO_2} (15 mm Hg), the blood hydrogen ion concentration is typically not lower than 30 nEq/L (pH not higher than 7.52).

Combinations of Simple Disturbances

The coordinates in Figure 2 encompass virtually all possible combinations of Pa_{CO_2}, plasma bicarbonate level, and hydrogen ion concentration (pH) that can exist in humans, yet from a brief perusal of the six superimposed titration curves, it is apparent that only a minority of points on the coordinates lie on the titration curves and thus have acid-base parameters consistent with simple acid-base disturbances. By definition, points that lie off the curves represent combinations of the simple disturbances and are often referred to as mixed acid-base disorders. Because combinations of acid-base disturbances frequently can be even more hazardous than simple disorders, mixed disturbances will be considered here.

The Henderson equation (see Fig 1) provides the framework for understanding how mixed disturbances affect acid-base equilibrium. Because hydrogen ion concentration is a function of the two interacting variables, Pa_{CO_2} and plasma bicarbonate concentration, combinations of simple disturbances that change these two variables in *opposite* directions always conspire to move hydrogen ion concentration in the *same* direction and thus magnify the effect on acidity. For example, a concomitant increase in Pa_{CO_2} and fall in plasma bicarbonate level (mixed respiratory and metabolic acidosis) produces severe acidemia because both of the changes tend to increase hydrogen ion concentration; by the same token, a concomitant decrease in Pa_{CO_2} and increase in plasma bicarbonate level (mixed respiratory alkalosis and metabolic alkalosis) produces severe alkalemia because both of the changes tend to decrease hydrogen ion concentration.

It is also evident from the Henderson equation that combinations of simple disturbances that change Pa_{CO_2} and plasma bicarbonate in the *same* direction always conspire to move hydrogen ion concentration in the *opposite* direction and thus reduce the effect that either disturbance in itself has on acidity. Thus, a concomitant and independent increase in plasma bicarbonate in a patient with preexisting chronic respiratory acidosis (mixed respiratory acidosis and metabolic alkalosis) tends to yield hydrogen ion concentrations at normal or nearly normal levels because one disturbance (respiratory acidosis) increases acidity and the other (metabolic alkalosis) reduces it. By the same token, a concomitant reduction in Pa_{CO_2} in a patient with preexisting metabolic acidosis (mixed metabolic acidosis and respiratory alkalosis) also tends to yield normal or nearly normal hydrogen ion concentrations because of the offsetting influences of the two independent primary disturbances. It is apparent from this consideration of these mixed disturbances that the happenstance of a normal or nearly normal blood pH does not justify a complacent attitude toward a patient's acid-base status. Acidity alone is not the only criterion for judging the seriousness of an acid-base disturbance; this point is illustrated below for mixed chronic respiratory acidosis and metabolic alkalosis.

No attempt will be made to include all combinations of acid-base disorders; extensive analyses of these can be found elsewhere. In this section, however, many of the mixed acid-base disorders that endanger patient's lives are considered briefly. Complications of respiratory acidosis and metabolic acidosis are located in the upper left quadrant in Figure 2 in the area between the titration curve for acute respiratory acidosis and that for metabolic acidosis. This type of mixed acid-base disturbance is common in patients with cardiopulmonary emergencies, with acute hypercapnia from pulmonary failure and lactic acidosis from circulatory arrest. In such patients, even modest deviations from the normal Pa_{CO_2} and plasma bicarbonate level can produce severe acidemia. A patient with an increase in Pa_{CO_2} to only 50 mm Hg and a fall in plasma bicarbonate to only 18 mEq/L, for example, has a blood pH of 7.18. Obviously, more severe derangements of either Pa_{CO_2} or bicarbonate will have a profound effect on acidity.

Combinations of respiratory alkalosis and metabolic alkalosis are located in the lower right quadrant in Figure 2 in the area between the titration curve for acute respiratory alkalosis and that for metabolic alkalosis. This type of mixed acid-base disturbance is commonly found in patients with liver disease. Such patients frequently hyperventilate and thus have persistent hypocapnia, and often are given diuretics or lose acid gastric contents and develop superimposed metabolic alkalosis. In such patients as well, even modest deviations from the normal Pa_{CO_2} and plasma bicarbonate level can produce severe deviations in acid-base equilibrium. A patient with a persistent reduction in Pa_{CO_2} to only 30 mm Hg, whose plasma bicarbonate increases to only 30 mEq/L, for example, has a blood pH of 7.62. Once again, more severe derangements of either Pa_{CO_2} or plasma bicarbonate will produce extreme alkalemia.

Mixtures of metabolic acidosis and respiratory alkalosis, shown clustered around the isohydric line between the titration curves for metabolic acidosis and respiratory alkalosis in the lower left quadrant of Figure 2, are characteristic of salicylate intoxication and sepsis with shock. In such patients, reliance on only the blood pH as a screening test to assess the seriousness of the situation will be overly misleading, because in such patients the pH is normal or nearly normal despite grossly disordered acid-base status. Measurement of either Pa_{CO_2} or plasma bicarbonate quickly identifies the aberration and triggers appropriate management.

Combinations of respiratory acidosis and metabolic alkalosis, clustered in the upper right quadrant of Figure 2 around the isohydric line between the titration curves for metabolic alkalosis and respiratory acidosis, are frequently encountered in patients with chronic obstructive pulmonary disease given diuretics to treat edema. The superimposition of metabolic alkalosis on preexisting chronic hypercapnia may have profound effects. The normal adaptive response to metabolic alkalosis is a suppression of ventilation that raises Pa_{CO_2} and lowers Pa_{CO_2}; a similar suppression of ventilation in a patient who already has moderate to severe hypercapnia and hypoxia can be exceedingly dangerous. The optimal acid-base status for the patient with chronic hypercapnia is to be mildly to moderately acidemic; aggressive attempts should be made to eliminate superimposed metabolic alkalosis in patients with chronic hypercapnia whose blood pH is either neutral or akaline. Improvements in ventilation and oxygenation and reductions in Pa_{CO_2} frequently follow with such efforts.

Treatment and Its Pitfalls

The life-threatening acid-base disorders discussed here are amenable to corrective measures, and in most instances the physician can immediately eliminate the danger and then gradually correct the remaining offending disturbance. In the course of the corrective process, however, numerous complications may occur that, in themselves, can be threatening. These complications are predictable on the basis of the physiology of the acid-base disorder and the pharmacology of the agents used in therapy, making it possible to avoid a disastrous outcome of therapy.

Controversy exists concerning the need for alkali therapy in certain types of metabolic acidosis (particularly diabetic ketoacidosis), but few would argue with the need to avert the threat of extreme acidosis by administering small amounts of sodium bicarbonate. The example in Table 1 illustrates how little bicarbonate is required to lift the blood pH out of a dangerous range; assuming that the Pa_{CO_2} remains virtually unchanged during therapy, an increase in plasma bicarbonate concentration of only 3 mEq/L (from 2 to 5 mEq/L) raises blood pH from approximately 6.8 to approximately 7.1. Substantial note should be taken of the assumption that Pa_{CO_2} will remain low for several hours in the acidotic patient while the plasma bicarbonate level is increased by bicarbonate administration. This lag in restoration of Pa_{CO_2} is frequently observed during correction of metabolic acidosis and has been attributed to the delay in the alkalinization of CSF resulting from the sluggish movement of bicarbonate from blood into spinal fluid in the region of the medullary center that controls ventilation. This persistent reduction in Pa_{CO_2} during correction of metabolic acidosis accounts for the remarkable "alkaline overshoot" seen in some patients treated vigorously with exogenous bicarbonate. Only a small increase in plasma bicarbonate level is required to raise pH out of a dangerous range; a small additional increment raises pH to normal; and a further small increment produces profound alkalemia (in the example in Table 1, pH is 7.4

when plasma bicarbonate concentration is raised to approximately 10 mEq/L and 7.62 when bicarbonate concentration is 16 mEq/L). Obviously it is both unnecessary and undesirable to fully correct the pH, and even more undesirable to induce alkalosis during the correction process. Ordinarily only small amounts of bicarbonate need be given in the severely acidotic patient to eliminate the danger. Plasma bicarbonate concentration, pH, and Pa_{CO_2} should be monitored closely during the early part of the correction process; after the acute threat is alleviated, the plasma bicarbonate can be raised gradually to normal levels over several days by cautious bicarbonate administration.

Extreme metabolic alkalosis is most frequently the consequence of gastric fluid losses and is thus correctible by administration of a variety of chloride salts. Patients with extreme alkalosis typically are severely depleted of both sodium and potassium, and thus administration of both sodium and potassium chloride is a mandatory part of the correction process. When the plasma bicarbonate concentration is extremely elevated, however, these electrolyte replacements cannot be relied on to rapidly correct alkalosis because both depend on the capacity of the kidney to suppress renal acid excretion and to increase renal alkali excretion, processes that produce little change in plasma bicarbonate levels over a short period. For this reason, administration of a mineral acid or a mineral acid precursor frequently is required when the plasma bicarbonate level is above 50 mEq/L.

Each of the mineral acids available for intravenous infusion has its advantages and potential hazards. Ammonium chloride is available in a 2% solution that provides approximately 400 mEq/L of acid, and because it can provide a large quantity of acid in a small volume, it is highly effective in reducing plasma bicarbonate levels. Of course, its use is contraindicated in patients with liver disease, and even in patients with normal liver function, it must be given slowly (not faster than 500 ml/ hour) to avoid the CNS toxic effects induced by the ammonium ion. Arginine hydrochloride is another excellent acidifying agent. Because the 10% solution delivers approximately 0.5 mEq of acid per milliliter, it also is highly effective in treating severe elevations of bicarbonate concentration. Unfortunately, the cation arginine displaces potassium from cells and may lead to hyperkalemia during intravenous infusion even before alkalosis has been corrected. In addition, the tendency to produce hyperkalemia is exaggerated in the presence of renal insufficiency, and for this reason arginine is not recommended for use when renal function is impaired. Hydrochloric acid, 0.1N to 0.2N, is another highly effective acidifying agent that contains 100 or 200 mEq/L of acid, respectively. When given slowly by infusion into a large central vein it is safe. Commercial preparations are not available, so the solution must be prepared locally. Unless blood pH is dangerously high, none of these acidifying solutions should be given rapidly. A reasonable goal is to lower plasma bicarbonate levels by approximately 10 mEq/L over an 8–12-hour period. In contrast to the response to treatment in patients with extreme metabolic acidosis, rapid reductions of bicarbonate in patients with extreme metabolic alkalosis are not known to be hazardous.

The approach to extreme respiratory acidosis is dependent on the duration of hypercapnia. If hypercapnia has been present a few hours or less and if the acid-base parameters are consistent with acute respiratory acidosis (i.e., if the Pa_{CO_2}, plasma bicarbonate level, and blood pH are within the acute titration curve shown in Figure 2), then an abrupt enhancement of alveolar ventilation and consequent reduction of Pa_{CO_2} is the optimal strategy. Because the only increase in plasma bicarbonate in such patients results from buffering of carbon dioxide in the tissues, the abrupt reduction of Pa_{CO_2} will simply result in a reversal of this buffering process and in a restoration of normal acid-base parameters in a pattern that follows the acute respiratory acidosis titration curve from its extreme limits to the normal values. This rapid restoration of normal acid-base equilibrium in response to a rapid drop in Pa_{CO_2} does not occur in the patient with sustained hypercapnia and can produce dangerous posthypercapnic alkalosis. To understand the mechanism of this potentially life-threatening phenomenon it is necessary only to recall that the process of adaptation to chronic hypercapnia involves, in addition to the same tissue response as in acute hypercapnia, a substantial acceleration in renal bicarbonate resorption and a consequent sustained elevation of plasma bicarbonate to a level considerably greater than that which occurs in acute hypercapnia. When Pa_{CO_2} is abruptly lowered in a patient with sustained hypercapnia, the excess bicarbonate generated and maintained by the kidney is retained in the plasma; the kidney does not have the chance to excrete it and will not excrete it even over a period of days to weeks unless a chloride supplement is given to repair the chloride deficit incurred during the process of adaptation to the high Pa_{CO_2}. If Pa_{CO_2} is returned to normal and the plasma bicarbonate level remains markedly elevated, the chronic respiratory acidosis will be immediately converted into a moderate to severe metabolic alkalosis. If, instead, the Pa_{CO_2} happens to be lowered to below normal, the alkalosis will be even more severe. Posthypercapnic metabolic alkalosis can be prevented by reducing the Pa_{CO_2} slowly and at the same time providing a sufficient chloride source to repair any existing chloride deficit. If it does occur, severe alkalosis can be managed by the same technique described above.

The principles that apply to the correction of acute hypocapnia are the same as those considered earlier for acute hypercapnia. Because the acid-base changes during the adaptation to acute hypocapnia involve only tissue buffering, prompt restoration of a normal Pa_{CO_2} in a patient with acute respiratory alkalosis simply restores acid-base equilibrium to normal, with no adverse consequences. Although one might anticipate that some serious complications could occur during rapid restoration of a normal Pa_{CO_2} in the patient with chronic respiratory alkalosis, there is too little experience with this event to know whether it is a real or only theoretical problem. Nonetheless, when possible, it seems prudent to raise the Pa_{CO_2} gradually in any patient who has had a sustained reduction in Pa_{CO_2} for days or more.

Na-K-ATPase: General Considerations, Role and Regulation in the Kidney

ALAIN DOUCET, M.D.

Laboratoire de Physiologie Cellulaire College de France, Paris, France

Introduction

Since sodium-potassium adenosine triphosphatase (Na-K-ATPase) was discovered in crab nerve about 25 years ago, it has aroused the interest of large numbers of biochemists and physiologists. Found in all animal cells, in which it ensures the extrusion of sodium and the entrance of potassium at the expense of ATP hydrolysis, this enzyme plays a very special part in transporting epithelia. In this respect, the kidney is a particularly important organ because of its essential role in maintaining the hydromineral balance.

In view of the abundant literature dealing with Na-K-ATPase in general and its function in the kidney in particular, this review will only survey the major contributions that have helped to improve our understanding of the characteristics of this fundamental enzymatic system. Special attention has been devoted to the techniques permitting the study of the function and regulation of Na-K-ATPase.

Nature of the Sodium Pump

Our present conception of the sodium pump is mainly derived from the following two research strategies, which recently converged to provide a satisfactory definition of the pump and how it works: 1) Study of the physicochemical properties of an enzyme that hydrolyzes ATP and is found in cellular membranes, and 2) phenomenological analysis of sodium and potassium movements across cell membrane, chiefly erythrocyte membranes, or artificial membranes—for instance, liposomes.

ENZYMATIC OF THE SODIUM PUMP

Our knowledge of the molecular nature of the sodium pump goes back a quarter of a century to Skou's discovery[1] showing that the microsomal fraction of crab nerve contained an enzyme that hydrolyzes ATP and is specifically activated by the sodium concentration usually found inside the cells and the potassium concentration found outside them. Since this discovery, Na-K-ATPase has been studied in many laboratories and its properties are described below.

Purification of Na-K-ATPase

Kidney is the only mammalian tissue from which Na-K-ATPase has been purified in an active form.[2] It can also be purified from electric eel organs[3] and shark salt gland.[3, 4]

Na-K-ATPase is purified in its membrane-bound form from the plasma membranes of rabbit outer medulla. During the purification process, this enzyme's protein components remain in the lipid bilayer whereas the other proteins are selectively extracted with sodium dodecyl sulfate (SDS) in the presence of ATP.[5] The purified preparation consists of disk-shaped membrane fragments packed with Na-K-ATPase particles. Electron microscope observation after freeze-fracture indicates that Na-K-ATPase maintains its polarity throughout the purification process since the asymmetry of the particle distribution in the fractured surfaces is identical to that observed in native membranes.[6]

Selective protein extraction by SDS only provides pure Na-K-ATPase preparations with membranes of the outer medulla of mammalian kidney or of duck salt glands.[8] Such preparation from shark salt glands or electric eel organs are only 50%–60% pure,[4] but greater purification can be achieved by solubilization with non-ionic detergents and fractionation.[3]

Characteristics and Structure of Na-K-ATPase

The structural and functional properties of the Na-K-ATPase purified from kidney also apply to the Na-K-ATPase in tissues from which it cannot be purified, since even when derived from different sources, this enzyme displays similar properties.[9–12] Thus, immunological studies indicate that antibodies prepared against pure Na-K-ATPase cross-react with the Na-K-ATPase from other mammalian cells or tissues, e.g., human erythrocytes.[13, 14]

Purified renal Na-K-ATPase consists of two proteins in a molar ratio of 1:1. The α subunit, which is the largest, has a molecular weight of 104.000 d and constitutes nearly 70% of the total protein. The β subunit, a syaloglycoprotein, has a molecular weight of 40.000 d plus 17.000 d for its glucidic moiety.[15, 16]

The specific activity of pure Na-K-ATPase measured under optimal conditions of ionic strength, pH and temperature, is 32–37 μmoles of phosphate released per minute per mg of protein. Its maximal capacity for binding ouabain, ATP and vanadate, and for phosphorylation by ATP, is 3.5–3.7 nmoles per mg of protein, which corresponds to a minimal molecular weight of 270.000–280.000 d per binding site.[15, 17, 18] An Na-K-ATPase turnover rate of 10.000 min^{-1} or 170 s^{-1} may be computed from these data.

The presence of a single binding site per 270.000–280.000 d entity, the 1:1 molar ratio of the α and β subunits, and the molecular weight of 144.000 d of the $\alpha\beta$ complex suggest that functional purified Na-K-ATPase consists of an $\alpha_2\beta_2$ complex.[15, 17] The molecular weight of this complex is 314.000 d, including 280.000 d for the protein moiety and 34.000 d for the glucid one.

Enzymatic Properties of Na-K-ATPase

Although ATP is the preferential substrate for Na-K-ATPase, other nucleotides can be hydrolyzed at a slower rate (at 15%—0.5% of the rate obtained with ATP), in the following order of decreasing activity: CTP > ITP > GTP > UTP > TTP.[18a, 18b, 18c] In vitro, Na-K-ATPase has two apparent Km for the Mg-ATP complex : 0.48 mM and 1 μM. It is competitively inhibited by an excess of ATP (Ki = 4.8 mM) and non-competitively by an excess of Mg (Ki = 40 mM).[19] Its high affinity site for ATP is the enzyme phosphorylation site,[20] whereas the low affinity one probably serves as an allosteric activator of the phosphorylation and of the entire reaction.[21]

The Na-K-ATPase dependency on Mg^{2+} is not absolute and other divalent cations (Mn^{2+}, Co^{2+}) can replace Mg^{2+}, although less efficiently. Furthermore, Fe^{2+}, Ca^{2+}, Zn^{2+}, Cu^{2+}, Ba^{2+}, Sr^{2+}, and Be^{2+} all inhibit ATPase activity.[22]

Unlike the dependency on Mg^{2+}, the requirement of Na-K-ATPase for sodium and potassium is almost absolute and constitutes one of its fundamental properties.[1, 23] This enzyme is activated by intracellular sodium with a Km of 5–13 mM, depending on the systems.[23, 24] However, certain human erythrocytes can extrude lithium instead of sodium through the sodium pump,[25] although at a slower rate; renal tubules also transport lithium. The need for potassium (Km = 0.5–1.8 mM) is less imperative and it can be replaced by $T1^{+}$ (Km $\simeq$ 0.15 mM), Rb^{+}, Cs^{+} or NH_4^{+} (Km 0.7 - 6 mM). On the other hand, lithium is a poor agonist of the potassium site (Km $\simeq$ 11 mM).

Figure 1, redrawn from the work of Jorgensen[24] shows the influence of sodium and potassium on Na-K-ATPase activity at various ATP concentrations. The left portion of the curve characterizes the effect of intracellular sodium, and the right portion, of extracellular potassium. With a saturating ATP concentration of 3 mM, half-maximal activity is observed for a K:Na ratio of 1:149, and maximal activity is obtained with the usual concentrations of extracellular potassium and sodium, 5 mM and 145 mM, respectively. The left sigmoid portion of the curve indicates that half-maximal activity is obtained with an Na:K ratio of 37:113, which is close to the cytosolic concentration. The inset shows that this part of the curve shifts to the right when the ATP concentration is below 1 mM. However, at physiological ATP concentrations ($\simeq$ 2 mM), Na-K-ATPase activity is independent of ATP for a given Na:K ratio. Therefore, intracellular sodium constitutes the only physiological limiting factor.

Na-K-ATPase Inhibitors

This section will be confined to the two inhibitors mentioned in the following chapters, i.e., ouabain and vanadate. For infor-

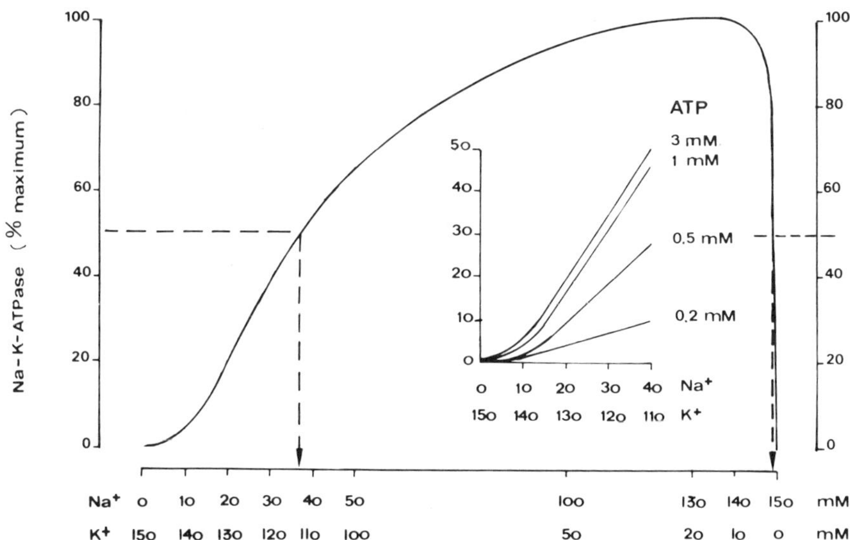

Fig 1.—Activity of purified renal Na-K-ATPase as a function of the Na$^+$, K$^+$ and ATP concentrations. ATP hydrolysis was measured at 37°C in a medium containing 3 mM MgCl$_2$ and 30 mM histidine, pH 7.5. The isotonicity of the medium was maintained by replacing NaCl with KCl. The principal curve was obtained in the presence of 3 mM ATP. (Reproduced from Jorgensen, P.L., et al. Antibodies to pig kidney Na-K-ATPase inhibit the NA-pump mechanism of the NA, K pump. Protein structure and conformations of the pure (Na$^+$ + K$^+$) ATPase. *Biochim. Biophys. Acta.* 694:27, 1982.)

mation regarding other Na-K-ATPase inhibitors (oligomycin, sulfhydryl reagents, butanedione, 7-chloro-4-dinitrobenzo-2-oxa-1, 3 diazole, ethacrynic acid, etc.) the reader is referred to the reviews by Schwartz et al.[26] and by Schuurmans-Stekhoven and Bonting.[27]

Digitalis glycosides form a group of natural substances that are specific Na-K-ATPase inhibitors. Therefore, they have been widely used in the study of this enzyme. Ouabain, or G-strophantin, is the most widely used of these substances because it is the most water-soluble. It has a molecular weight of 585 and consists of a glucid moiety, rhamnose, and a steroid moiety, ouabagenin. It is specific for Na-K-ATPase because it does not inhibit Ca-Mg-ATPase,[27a] K-H-ATPase[28] or anionic ATPase.[29]

Ouabain acts through the outer surface of the membrane[30] by inhibiting ATP binding[31] and Na-K-ATPase dephosphorylation.[32] Ouabain binding requires the presence of magnesium.[33] Na-K-ATPase phosphorylation by ATP or Pi markedly increases the ouabain association rate.[34] Lastly, ouabain binding is inhibited by internal sodium and potassium and by external potassium and is stimulated by external sodium through competition with external potassium.[35] It is now widely accepted that ouabain binds to phosphorylated Na-K-ATPase on or close to the external potassium binding site. Ouabain binding specificity probably depends on its steroid component and the stability of the ouabain-Na-K-ATPase complex on the glucid moiety.

The stability of this complex varies considerably among the different organs and species, owing to differences between dissociation rate constants.[36, 37] These constants range from 3×10^{-9} M for ox brain Na-K-ATPase to 1.5×10^{-7} M for that derived from guinea pig kidney.[38] Rat myocardium is the tissue whose Na-K-ATPase has the lowest affinity for ouabain, with a Kd of 1.2×10^{-5} M (1).

Vanadate, a vanadium oxide, is an essential trace element[39] that a few years ago was accidentally discovered to inhibit Na-K-ATPase. In 1975, Charney, Silva and Epstein reported that a renal Na-K-ATPase inhibitor was present in certain brands of commercial ATP extracted from horse muscle.[40] Later Josephson and Cantley,[41] Beauge and Glynn[42] and Hudgins and Bond[43] confirmed this observation and described a reciprocal action between potassium and the inhibitor concerned. Its chemical characterization as vanadate is due to Cantley et al.[44]

Although vanadate is a potent inhibitor, it is not specific for Na-K-ATPase.[45] Its action is modulated by various factors:

- Extracellular potassium at concentrations higher than 5 mM enhances inhibition by vanadate.[42, 46–49]

- This inhibition is also intensified by lowering the extracellular sodium concentration below physiological values.[42, 47]

- The presence of magnesium is required for vanadate inhibition to be effective.[46, 48, 50]

- The inhibitory action of vanadate is sensitive to the redox state of the system, i.e., vanadate reduction to vanadyl abolishes this action.

- Vanadate, unlike ouabain acts on the cytosolic side of the membrane[51] and must therefore enter the cell to be active.

Vanadate seems to inhibit Na-K-ATPase by binding to this enzyme's phosphorylation site[52] and blocking the protein in this configuration. Therefore, vanadate facilitates ouabain binding to Na-K-ATPase, thus potentiating its own effect and that of ouabain on intact cells.[53–55]

FUNCTIONING OF THE SODIUM PUMP

Various Stages in the Operation of the Pump

The interactions between Na-K-ATPase, its substrates, and the cations transported, as well as the intermediate reactions, have been characterized by studying sodium and potassium transport in erythrocytes, erythrocyte ghosts or artificial vesicles in which purified Na-K-ATPase was reconstituted. The model proposed by Karlish and coworkers[56, 57] incorporates most of the results so far obtained (Figure 2). The purified enzyme undergoes a series of reactions in which ATP binds to the high affinity site (E_1-ATP) and the Na-K-ATPase binds three intracellular sodium ions and is phosphorylated (E_1P-Na_3). A change in its conformation occurs at this stage ($E_1 \rightarrow E_2$), leading to a new configuration whose cationic sites display a low affinity for sodium and a high affinity for potassium. Therefore, sodium is released from the cell while two potassium ions bind the Na-K-ATPase (E_2P-K_2). After dephosphorylation, ATP binds to the low affinity site, inducing the reverse change of

Fig 2.—Model showing the interactions between cation movements, the phosphorylation of Na-K-ATPase, and the changes in its conformation when this enzyme functions normally (Na:K exchange). E_1 and E_2 represent two conformations of Na-K-ATPase. In the first, it has a high affinity for sodium and ATP, and in the second, for potassium.

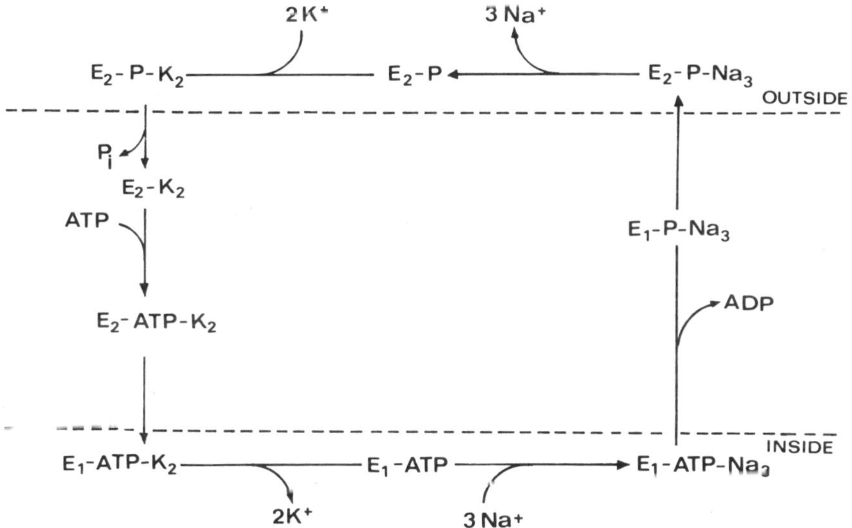

configuration as well as the release of potassium into the intra-cellular compartment.

This model, which resembles those of Post[58] and Albers,[59] does not provide any information regarding the molecular mechanisms of the cation translocation. Several important questions are still unanswered, despite the abundant literature they have generated.[10, 60–62] The two main outstanding problems are whether the pump operates as a channel or as a carrier and whether the $\alpha\beta$ complex is the functional unit or whether interactions between several $\alpha\beta$ entities are required for cation transport.

To account for the fact that, according to Karlish's model,[63] $\alpha_2\beta_2$ complexes bind a single molecule of ATP, ouabain or vanadate, it has been suggested that Na-K-ATPase operates as a dimer $(\alpha\beta)_2$, whose two $\alpha\beta$ moieties are out of phase,[64] thus preventing the simultaneous binding of a ligand to both of them.

Modes of Transport by the Erythrocyte Pump

Many investigations have attempted to define the properties of the sodium pump from erythrocytes.[26, 56, 60, 64, 65, 66] Depending on the experimental conditions, this pump is capable of transporting sodium and/or potassium in five different modes as follows (Fig 3):

- *Sodium-potassium exchange* is the normal operating mode of the pump. Under normal conditions, three intracellular sodium ions are exchanged for two extracellular potassium ions at the expense of the hydrolysis of one molecule of ATP. This transport is electrogenic.[67] When reconstituted in artificial vesicles, purified renal Na-K-ATPase also transports cations in the same ratio of 3 Na:2 K.[9, 67a] The Na:ATP ratios of 3.2:1 or 2.2:1 observed in these vesicles[9, 68] resemble those described for such transport in erythrocytes,[60] nerve cells,[69] or for transport by purified ATPase from electric eel organs or shark rectal gland.[70, 71] These results indicate that the stoichiometry Na:K:ATP is a fundamental property of Na-K-ATPase.

- *Sodium-sodium exchange* is observed when erythrocytes are incubated in a potassium-free medium. Intracellular sodium is exchanged against extracellular sodium in a 1:1 ratio, without ATP hydrolysis. The only requirement for Na:Na exchange is ADP. This abnormal operating mode of Na-K-ATPase does not

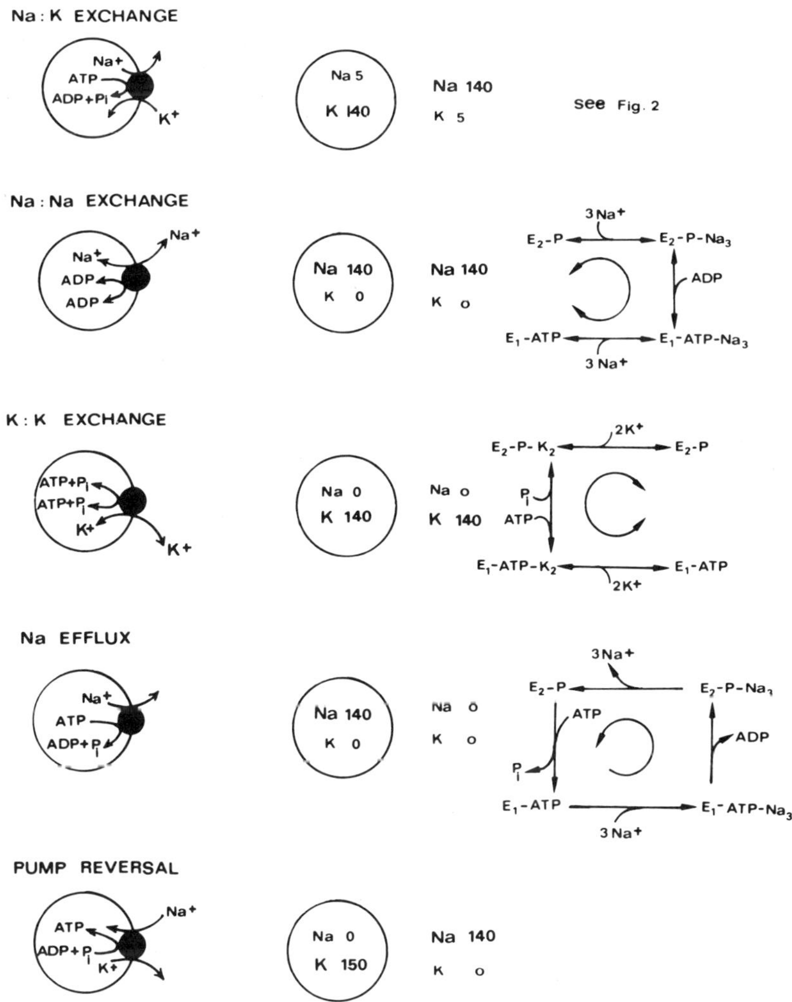

Fig 3.—Different modes of transport by the pump in erythrocytes. Left part of figure shows cation transfers and their dependence on nucleotides and phosphate. Central part indicates (in mM) the intra- and extracellular cation concentrations at which these modes of transport can be observed. Right part gives a schematic representation of the reactions involved.

lead to net cation transport across the cell membrane and consumes no metabolic energy. Such exchange proceeds by the reversible conversion of E_1ATP into E_2P through the pathways shown in the right part of Figure 2.

- *Potassium-potassium exchange* occurs when erythrocyte

ghosts are formed and incubated in a potassium-rich, sodium-free medium. This exchange operates in a $1:1$ ratio in the presence of ATP. It occurs by alternated conversion of E_2P into E_1ATP through the left portion of the cycle shown in Figure 2.

Na:Na and K:K exchanges are also observed with purified renal Na-K-ATPase in artificial vesicles.

- *A sodium efflux* is observed when erythrocyte ghosts are incubated in the absence of external sodium and potassium. Under such conditions, hydrolysis of one molecule of ATP leads to the extrusion of three sodium ions. This non-physiological functioning is inhibited by ouabain, indicating that Na-K-ATPase is involved in this efflux process. Transport occurs through the normal sodium efflux pathway (right side of Figure 2), the cycle being completed by a path proceeding from E_2P to E_1-ATP. This functioning has been observed with renal Na-K-ATPase in artificial vesicles.[68]

- *Reverse functioning* of the pump has been demonstrated by increasing the usual transmembrane concentration gradients and by choosing ADP and Pi concentrations permitting synthesis rather than hydrolysis of ATP. The steepness of the gradients required to make this synthesis possible depends on the energy of the γ-Pi binding of the ATP molecule. The observation that the pump is able to operate reversibly represents an important step forward in understanding the pump's functioning,[72, 73] and also demonstrates the reversibility of all the conversions in this cycle.

IDENTITY OF THE Na-K-ATPase AND THE SODIUM PUMP

Na-K-ATPase was originally suggested to play a part in cation transport on the basis of the similarities between the properties of this enzyme and the cation transport system. Both are located in the plasma membrane, preferentially use ATP as their source of energy, require the simultaneous presence of sodium and potassium on specific sides of the membrane, and are specifically inhibited by digitalis drugs. Furthermore, rearrangement of transmembrane cation gradients makes it possible to reverse the functioning of Na-K-ATPase and to synthetize ATP from ADP and Pi by a ouabain-sensitive process. Finally, sodium and potassium ions are transported in artificial vesicles into which Na-K-ATPase is incorporated.

Other observations suggest that Na-K-ATPase constitutes the molecular basis for active sodium transport. The sodium pump and this enzyme are similarly distributed in different tissues; moreover, in epithelia in which the pump is responsible for transcellular cation transport, Na-K-ATPase activity and the transport capacity develop in a parallel fashion during ontogenesis. Finally, certain antibodies prepared against purified renal Na-K-ATPase are able to inhibit Na-K-ATPase activity and sodium transport in a dose-dependent fashion.

This large body of evidence means that, with rare exceptions,[74] it is today generally accepted that Na-K-ATPase is responsible for active sodium and potassium transport, and that this enzyme is identical to the Na-K-pump. Finally, it should be stressed that the habitually-used term "sodium pump" is inadequate, since from the physiological view point potassium transport always accompanies that of sodium in this system.

Methods of Studying the Renal Sodium Pump

DETERMINATION OF THE Na-K-ATPase CONCENTRATION

The concentration of enzymatic sites can be evaluated by measuring the Na-K-ATPase activity, the rate of certain partial reactions or the binding capacity of certain ligands. The problems concerning substrate access to internal sites of action can be solved by the use of detergents under suitable conditions.

Measurement of Na-K-ATPase Activity

Any kinase-phosphatase reaction is an ATPase. Therefore, methods for measuring Na-K-ATPase activity are designed in such a way that potentially contaminating ATPases (Ca-Mg-ATPase, Mg-H-ATPase, etc.) can be distinguished from Na-K-ATPase. This can be done by subtracting the activity of non-specific Mg-ATPase from the ATPase activity measured after maximal stimulation of Na-K-ATPase. ATPase activity is determined as the amount of Pi released from ATP per unit of time under optimal conditions. Mg-ATPase activity is determined in a medium that is either devoid of sodium or potassium, or to which a maximal inhibitory concentration of ouabain (10^{-4} M) is added, usually with the simultaneous omission of potassium. The first type of control, which tests the cationic specificity of the pump, is especially used when the preparation is mildly sensitive to ouabain, as is the case for rat tissues.[36, 37] The second type, designed to test the molecular specificity of ATPase, avoids potential contamination of the preparation by an ouabain-insensitive Na-ATPase other than Na-K-ATPase, such as that found in many tissues.[23] Calcium is omitted from the mediums since it inhibits Na-K-ATPase.

Potassium-dependent Phosphatase Activity

Potassium-dependent phosphatase activity, an intrinsic activity of Na-K-ATPase (the latter is in fact an Na-kinase-K-phosphatase), is defined as the potassium-induced increase in magnesium-dependent phosphatase activity. Of the various organic phosphates serving as substrates for this reaction, para-nitrophenylphosphate (pNPP) is the most widely used. Hydrolysis of pNPP is studied by spectrophotometry at 420 nm, by the release of p-nitrophenyl.[37]

Ligand Binding Capacity

The density of the functional units with a molecular weight of 280.000 d ($\alpha_2\beta_2$) can be directly evaluated in binding studies, since each catalytic unit has a high affinity binding site for ATP, ouabain, and vanadate, as well as a phosphorylation site.[17, 18]

In vitro, Na-K-ATPase can be phosphorylated by ATP or Pi. Phosphorylation by ATP, the kinase component, is defined as the sodium-induced increase of the Mg-dependent phosphorylation. It is determined as the steady state amount of phosphoenzyme measured after phosphorylation by γ-32p ATP in the presence of sodium and magnesium.[75] The capacity of phosphorylation from Pi is defined as the Mg-dependent Pi incorporation into Na-K-ATPase,[76] and is stimulated by ouabain.

Localization of the digitalis binding site on the external surface of the membrane as well as the specificity and high affinity of such binding permit determination of the number of ^{3}H -ouabain binding sites on intact cells or tissues.[77, 78] Since ouabain binds the phosphorylated α subunit, ouabain binding is determined in the presence of Mg and Pi or of vanadate.[79] In addition to the saturable component constituting specific ouabain binding to Na-K-ATPase, there is usually a linear component that represents nonspecific ouabain binding and/or uptake.[77] Specific binding can be determined under equilibrium conditions, at various ouabain concentrations.[77, 78] Alternatively, this can be done by incubating the preparations with saturating concentrations of ouabain and measuring the bound radioactivity after a long period of cold rinsing,[78] since specific binding, unlike nonspecific binding, is not reversible in the cold. In addition to intact cells or tissues, the binding capacity of ouabain can also be determined on homogenates,[80] membrane fractions,[81] or purified Na-K-ATPase.[82]

ULTRASTRUCTURAL LOCALIZATION OF Na-K-ATPase IN RENAL CELLS

The ultrastructural location of renal Na-K-ATPase can be studied by the usual techniques of cell fractionation or by electron microscope observation. Such ultrastructural studies are based either on the cytochemistry of potassium-dependent phosphatase, or on immunoferritin labeling. These two techniques are the only ones possessing sufficient resolution. Nevertheless, they represent a compromise between the inevitable activation of Na-K-ATPase by fixatives and/or heavy metals on the one hand and the need to preserve the ultrastructure and fix the reaction products on the other.

Cytochemical Determination of Na-K-ATPase

The first cytochemical method for localizing Na-K-ATPase was developed by Ernst.[83, 84] This technique is derived from that of Wachstein and Meisel,[85] but differs from it in the use of formaldehyde as tissue fixative[86] and of strontium to fix the phosphate released by pNPP hydrolysis. This procedure prevents the Na-K-ATPase from being blocked by glutaraldehyde and inhibited by Pb^{2+}.[85] After the enzymatic reaction, the phosphate precipitate is stabilized by Pb^{2+} ions, which are then converted into lead sulfite. With this technique, the membranes are clearly visible in electron microscopy and the phosphate deposit can be precisely located. However, this method requires the labeling to be checked as potassium-dependent and ouabain-sensitive, in order to make sure that the material stained indeed corresponds to Na-K-ATPase. This is necessary because pNPP can be hydrolyzed non-specifically by many phosphatases; of these, alkaline phosphatase, is the most abundant in the kidney but its activity is selectively inhibited by cysteine.[83] Finally, the specificity of cytochemical Na-K-ATPase labeling is increased by dimethylsulfoxide, which stimulates the K-dependent phosphatase.[87] The phosphate released in the tissue can be quantified by X-ray microanalysis.

Immunoferritin Labeling of Na-K-ATPase

Antibodies against Na-K-ATPase or its α subunit can bind to their antigenic site without disrupting the cells when they are incubated into frozen sections of formaldehyde-fixed tissue.[88, 89] After washing, this initial binding is followed by the binding of ferritin-conjugated antirabbit-γ-globulin to the specific antibodies, and the formation of the resulting iron complex can be observed by electron microscopy. Immunoferritin binding occurs on the basolateral membrane of proximal and distal tubules. The use of anti-Na-K-ATPase antibody leads to slight staining of apical membranes. The high molecular weight of the Na-K-ATPase-Anti-Na-K-ATPase-Anti-Ig (around 800.000) makes the labeling difficult to quantify.

Cell Fractionation

The results obtained with various cell fractionation techniques suggest that Na-K-ATPase is exclusively located in the basolateral membrane in kidney cells. Thus, Kinne and colleagues[90] measured different enzymatic membrane markers in membrane fractions from rat renal cortex prepared by sucrose gradient centrifugation and electrophoresis. Their results indicate that the brush border, the lysosomes, and the endoplasmic reticulum were devoid of Na-K-ATPase activity. Schmidt and DuBach went further, and used a Na-K-ATPase micromethod to measure the enzyme's activity in cell fragments from proximal convoluted tubules, microdissected from freeze-dried sections of rat kidney.[91] Their results indicate that the pump is located on the basal side, because the brush border fragments were free of Na-K-ATPase activity.

This unilateral location of Na-K-ATPase in renal epithelial cells is responsible for the kidney's ability to reabsorb sodium and secrete potassium. Thus, the renal pump performs the double function of maintaining an Na/K ratio compatible with cell integrity and permitting active transepithelial transport that contributes to the homeostasis of the entire organism. Consequently, the specific activity of Na-K-ATPase is much higher in the kidney than in tissues that do not ensure any net ionic transport.

LOCALIZATION OF Na-K-ATPase ALONG THE NEPHRON

The precise contribution of Na-K-ATPase to cation transport under physiological or physiopathological conditions was not clear as long as the functioning and determination of the pump's activity were studied on the entire kidney, because whole kidney preparations contain a mixture of various nephron segments and non-tubular cells. In addition, reabsorption and secretion mechanisms along the nephron differ,[92] and the same nephron segment can have several functions.[93, 94]

Once it became possible to study the transport properties of structurally or functionally isolated nephron segments,[95, 96] a micromethod allowing Na-K-ATPase quantitation in homologous segments obviously had to be developed.

Techniques are now available permitting measurement of either Na-K-ATPase activity or of the number of enzymatic units in single nephron segments.

Determination of Na-K-ATPase Activity in Single
Nephron Segment

Schmidt and DuBach[97, 98] were the first to apply the methodology of Lowry and Passoneau[99] to developing a microassay of Na-K-ATPase activity at cellular level on freeze-dried sections of rat kidney. To determine this activity in samples with a dry weight of 5—25 ng, these authors used a recycling system designed to amplify the amount of Pi produced by the ATPase reaction. However, although this method has been fruitful over the past 15 years,[91, 100–102] it is extremely complex and has not been adopted by other laboratories. More recently, Schmidt and Horster, who fully grasped the problems inherent in the dissection of samples from freeze-dried sections, modified the original technique so that it became possible to dissect fresh tissue. After such dissection, samples are lyophilized and Na-K-ATPase activity is determined.[98, 103] This is the technique currently used in the United States for instance by Marver et al.[104]

Ten years after the original publication of Schmidt and Dubach's microassay,[97] we developed another micromethod[105] based on the technique of Burg et al.[96] for microdissection of tubule segments from collagenase-treated kidneys: Tubule segments (0.2–2.0 mm long) are isolated, and each one is individually submitted to a permeabilization procedure in order to facilitate the access of exogenous substrates to their internal catalytic sites. Enzyme activity is directly determined by measuring the ^{32}Pi released by hydrolysis of [γ-^{32}P] ATP. Results are expressed per unit of tubule length, thus allowing pump activity to be compared to the ionic fluxes measured in the isolated tubules.[106]

More recently, Garg and coworkers[107] developed another technique derived from that just described. Here again, the tubule segments are dissected and permeabilized but the enzyme assay is different, as it is based on a modified version of the method of Schoner et al.,[27] which combines ATP hydrolysis with NADH oxidation (the latter being studied by fluorometry).

Finally, Le Hir and colleagues[108] developed the most recent microtechnique. In it, radiochemical assay of ATPase was adapted to tubules dissected from freeze-dried sections.

The characteristic features of the different assays used at the present time are given in Table 1. Despite the subjective nature of any evaluation of the advantages and drawbacks of these assays, a few useful conclusions may be drawn. Although isolation of tubule fragments from kidney tissue sections certainly enables almost identical replicates to be obtained, the tiny size of the samples calls for an extremely sensitive assay. Amplification recycling systems give the necessary sensitivity, but are difficult to handle correctly. The technique developed by Le Hir and colleagues[108] appears to be a satisfactory compromise, since it permits direct determination of the Na-K-ATPase activity in these very small samples.

Nevertheless two problems are still outstanding. First, since results are expressed as a function of dry sample weight, difficult to determine on a quartz balance, direct comparison with ionic fluxes is difficult (although for certain nephron segments

TABLE 1.—CHARACTERISTICS OF THE VARIOUS MICROASSAYS FOR
Na-K-ATPase ON ISOLATED NEPHRON SEGMENTS

	SAMPLE PREPARATION		
	Dissection	Use of collagenase	NA-K-ATPASE ASSAY
Schmidt, DuBach[97]	on freeze-dried sections	−	recycling (Lowry & Passoneau)
Schmidt, Horster[103]	on fresh sections followed by freeze drying	−	id
Doucet et al.[105]	on fresh tissue	+	radiochemical (ATP-^{32}P)
Garg et al.[107]	on fresh tissue	+	direct (Schoner et al.)
Le Hir et al.[108]	on freeze-dried sections	−	radiochemical (ATP-^{32}P)

the relationship between dry weight and tubule length has been established). Second, the lyophilization step required to make the samples permeable affects the enzyme's activity considerably.[98] These reasons prompted us[105] and Garg et al.[107] to use fresh tissue and to express their Na-K-ATPase measurements in terms of tubule length. The large numbers of samples necessary for such determinations require collagenase treatment of the kidney tissue, but this treatment does not alter Na-K-ATPase activity.[105] Although fairly similar, those two methods give different results; the Na-K-ATPase activity measured by Garg et al.[107, 109] is 2—6 times higher than the level we observed.[110] This difference may be partly due to the fact that Garg et al. used NH_4^+ instead of K^+ ions to stimulate the pump.

Finally, it should be pointed out that whatever technique is used, Na-K-ATPase activity is measured under artificial optimal conditions. As we previously observed, internal sodium concentrations yielded to 50% stimulation of the maximal rate of enzyme activity; it is important to take this into consideration when comparing the Na-K-ATPase transport capacity to the sodium fluxes measured in homologous nephron segments.

Determination of Na-K-ATPase Units in Single Nephron Segments

To date, the only approach available to determine the number of catalytic units on well-defined nephron segments consists of measuring the specific binding of tritiated ouabain.

The first attempt to localize Na-K-ATPase by ouabain binding was made by Shaver and Stirling,[111] using autoradiography of rabbit kidney medulla slices previously incubated with ^{3}H-ouabain. Although this technique permitted localization of the pump in the cells of the thick ascending limb, rich in Na-K-ATPase, its lack of sensitivity has limited its scope for quantitative estimation.

We recently developed a microtechnique allowing the specific binding of tritiated ouabain to be measured on single nephron segments microdissected from collagenase-treated rabbit kidney. The use of vanadate to block the enzyme in the conformation in which it displayed a high affinity for ouabain enabled us to work with intact cells. Non-specific binding was reduced by post-incubating samples on ice after saturation of the specific sites. Under these conditions, we were able to determine in most nephron segments, the number of enzymatic sites $(\alpha_2\beta_2)$ (Table 2).

TABLE 2.—OUABAIN BINDING ALONG THE RABBIT NEPHRON

	fmol $.mm^{-1}$	10^6 SITES/ CELL	% TOTAL PROTEIN
PCT	11,0	25	1,4
PR	3,3	10	0,4
MAL	21,3	41	4,8
CAL	5,1	10	1,8
DCTb	31,5	50	5,5
DCTg	11,2	16*	2,5
CCT	6,8	8*	1,8
MCT	2,7	3*	0,6

PCT, proximal convoluted tubule; PR, pars recta; MAL, medullary portion of thick ascending limb of Henle's loop; CAL, cortical thick ascending limb; DCTb, bright portion of distal convoluted tubule; DCTg, granular portion of distal convoluted tubule; CCT, cortical collecting tubule; MCT, medullary collecting tubule. Number of sites per cell was calculated from the relationship between the number of cells and tubular length, according to Garg and colleagues (Mineralocorticoid effects on Na-K-ATPase in individual nephron segments. *Am. J. Physiol.* 240:F536, 1981). *, mean value for the different cell types constituting the nephron segment. Fraction of total protein constituted by Na-K-ATPase was calculated using the relationship between protein content and tubular length according to Vandewalle et al. (Distribution of hexokinase and phosphoenolpyruvate carboxykinase along the rabbit nephron. *Am. J. Physiol.* 240:F492, 1981).

The number of catalytic units along the nephron exhibited the same distribution pattern as Na-K-ATPase activity. This indicates that the enzyme turnover rate of ATP hydrolysis is identical in all nephron segments, and is close to 2.000 min^{-1} per ouabain binding site. It is worth noting that Na-K-ATPase rich cells, like the cells of the thick ascending limb of Henle's loop, contain over 40 million catalytic units, indicating that the pump is one of the main proteins in the basolateral membrane.

Determination of ouabain binding combined with the measurement of Na-K-ATPase activity should permit the characterization of the mechanisms regulating the pump, thereby indicating whether changes in this activity result from changes in the number or activity of the catalytic units. However, one of the major restrictions of this technique is that it cannot be applied to rats, owing to the low affinity of ATPase for ouabain in this species.[36, 37]

STUDY Na-K-ATPase SYNTHESIS

Study of the direct effect of hormones on Na-K-ATPase synthesis only became possible recently, thanks to the development of suitable analytical techniques. The recent elaboration of antibodies able to immunoprecipitate this enzyme's α and β subunits specifically[111, 112] now enables their relative biosynthesis rates to be determined. The post-transcriptional steps of β subunit glycosylation, first in the endoplasmic reticulum and then in the Golgi apparatus, can be studied by using treatment with tunicamycin and monensin, which respectively inhibit each of these steps.

This technique has been developed and used by Geering and colleagues[113] to study the effect of aldosterone on toad bladder Na-K-ATPase synthesis. After protein labeling by 30-minute ^{35}S-methionine pulses, the tissue extract is immunoprecipitated with either anti-α or anti-β γ-globulin prepared against purified toad kidney Na-K-ATPase.[112] This anti-α serum precipitates a single 96.000 d mol.wt. protein, which has been identified as the Na-K-ATPase α subunit[112, 114] and constitutes 0.3 to 0.8% of all the labeled proteins. The anti-β serum also precipitates a single 42.000 d m.w. protein, which is a non-glycosylated precursor of the β subunit.[114] After 18-hour labeling with ^{35}S-methionine the anti β serum immunoprecipitates the 60.000 d β subunit.

Antibodies against the subunits of renal mammalian Na-K-ATPase have also been prepared for determination of pump synthesis.[112]

Functions of Renal Na-K-ATPase

In contrast to the wealth of information available on the structure and the enzymatic and physiological properties of renal Na-K-ATPase, little was known until recently about the parameters governing its regulation. However two facts appear certain: 1) Na-K-ATPase is only responsible for part of renal sodium reabsorption, and 2) Na-K-ATPase is responsible for secondary active transport of solutes other than sodium. For a long time, the sodium pump's exact role in the various types of renal transport was studied in whole kidney. However, as already mentioned, such studies recently became possible in nephron segments, and attempts were made to define the respective roles of these segments in urine elaboration.

WHOLE KIDNEY STUDIES

The Na-K-ATPase-dependent Fraction of Sodium Reabsorption

Infusion of large doses of ouabain into dog renal artery inhibits 20–35% of total sodium reabsorption.[115–119] This effect reflects a fractional inhibition of the sodium pump. This is confirmed by the fact that such partial inhibition can be estimated after measurement of the animal's sodium excretion, since ouabain binding dissociates very slowly during the preparation of the homogenates or membrane fractions used to measure Na-K-ATPase activity[115, 116, 118–120] or ouabain binding.[120, 121] Na-K-ATPase measurements indicate that 10–30% of its activity is not inhibited by such large doses of ouabain. In vivo, doses of ouabain sufficient to inhibit Na-K-ATPase completely usually kill the animal, owing to the action of this drug on the myocardium. To circumvent this difficulty, the effect of higher doses of ouabain was tested on isolated perfused kidneys.[122] Under these conditions, complete inhibition of Na-K-ATPase inhibits sodium reabsorption by 45%. The ouabain-insensitive fraction of sodium reabsorption depends on the cell energy metabolism, since this reabsorption is completely abolished by cyanide or cooling.[123] These results indicate that at least half the sodium is reabsorbed by Na-K-ATPase-independent mechanisms.[123–126] Furthermore, when the reabsorbed sodium load shifts from the proximal to the distal tubule during saline loading or mannitol diuresis, the ouabain-induced natriuresis rises.[115, 127] Finally, urinary concentrating and diluting abilities are radically altered by ouabain.[116, 127] These findings suggest that the role of Na-K-ATPase in sodium reabsorption is quantitatively more important in the thick ascending limb and distal tubule than in the proximal tubule.

Vanadate has the same effects as ouabain, since its intravenous administration to rats induces dose-dependent diuresis and natriuresis.[128, 129] With a maximal dose of vanadate, 50% of the water and sodium-filtered loads are excreted into the urine.[129, 130] This effect of vanadate, observed in the absence of any change in the glomerular filtration rate, has been attributed to its inhibitory action on renal Na-K-ATPase. Clearance and micropuncture studies indicate that this action is both proximal and distal.[88, 128–133]

Reabsorption Capacity of Renal Na-K-ATPase

It is important to ascertain whether the Na-K-ATPase concentration in the kidney is sufficient to account for half this organ's reabsorption of sodium.

Measured in optimal conditions, the specific activity of Na-K-ATPase from rat kidney homogenates is 40–50 μmolPi/min/g of kidney.[134] Assuming that the stoichiometry is 3 Na^+/ATP and that the pump operates at 40% of its maximal rate, this activity corresponds to a reabsorption capacity of 48–60 μEq of Na/min/g. The glomerular filtration rate of the rat is 0.75 ml/min/g or 105 μEq of Na/min/g of which 98% or 100 μEq/min/g is reabsorbed. Under physiological conditions of functioning, Na-K-ATPase can insure 48–60% of the sodium reabsorption, which perfectly fits the data given above.

Na-K-ATPase Activity and ATP Synthesis

Another essential requirement for Na-K-ATPase activity is that the kidney must produce enough ATP to drive it. Renal oxygen consumption averages 3–6 μmoles O_2/min/g of kidney.[135, 136] Under aerobic conditions, this corresponds to a production of 18–36 μmoles ATP/min/g and a transport capacity of 46–108 μEq Na/min/g if all the ATP produced is used for active sodium transport. However, since only half the total ATP production is devoted to sodium transport,[118] renal oxidative metabolism seems sufficient to supply the energy required for Na-K-ATPase activity.

Na-K-ATPase and Renal Potassium Transport

The exact role of Na-K-ATPase is more difficult to understand in potassium reabsorption and secretion than in sodium transport, because Na-K-ATPase pumps potassium from the interstitial compartment to the tubular cells, which goes against reabsorption. This intracellular accumulation of potassium is not sufficient to explain potassium secretion, because potassium diffuses passively through the luminal or basolateral membrane, depending on the electrochemical gradients across these borders and on the relative permeability to potassium of these membranes. In the absence of a favorable gradient, potassium secretion through the apical border would be coupled to the entrance of sodium along its gradient, generated by Na-K-ATPase (i.e., sodium-potassium exchange would occur). [137] In any case, ouabain administration inhibits potassium secretion by the amphibian,[138] avian[139] and mammalian kidney,[140] and such inhibition of potassium reabsorption has been described in Amphiuma,[141] the bullfrog,[138] and the rat.[142, 143] Animals chronically loaded with potassium survive by increasing their renal potassium secretion.[33, 144–146] This renal adaptation to potassium secretion is also observed after the functional kidney mass is reduced by surgical ablation.[145–148] Silva and coworkers[33] were the first to suggest that Na-K-ATPase played a part in this adaptation after observing increased pump activity in kidney homogenates prepared from chronically potassium-loaded rats. Subsequent studies indicated that an increased potassium excretion capacity induced by chronic potassium loading or partial renal ablation, was accompanied by enhanced Na-K-ATPase specific activity in tissue homogenates obtained from kidney cortex, medulla or papilla,[140, 148, 149] and was almost completely inhibited by ouabain in isolated perfused rat kidneys.

These results underline the importance of Na-K-ATPase in renal potassium transport.

The Proximal Tubule

Initially, results for whole kidney indicated that only 30–50% of the sodium-filtered load is reabsorbed through Na-K-ATPase, but it was not possible at the time to characterize the pump's role in each segment of the nephron. Here again, the study of Na-K-ATPase activity and of the active transport capacity in single nephron segments has improved understanding of the pump's quantitative role. Through sodium transport, Na-K-ATPase is responsible for other important functions that have been studied in the proximal tubule, such as control of cell volume and various types of secondary active transport.

Na-K-ATPase and Proximal Sodium Reabsorption

The proximal tubule is morphologically heterogenous and has been divided into three consecutive segments (termed S_1, S_2, and S_3) in accordance with ultrastructural criteria.[150] This morphological segmentation corresponds to marked alterations in functional properties, such as glucose transport,[151] albumin uptake,[152] phosphate transport,[153] and possibly urea secretion.[154] The most striking of these changes is the gradual decrease in sodium reabsorption capacity along the proximal tubule,[155–158] which is accompanied by a decrease in the pump activity along this segment. Thus, Na-K-ATPase activity is 3–7 times greater in the proximal convoluted tubule (PCT) than in the pars recta (PR), the S_2 portion displaying an intermediate level of activity (Table 3). Similarly, the number of oubain binding sites in the rabbit was found to diminish from 11.0 fmol.mm^{-1} in the PCT to 3.3 fmol.min^{-1} in the PR (Table 2).

In addition to this axial heterogeneity, there are differences between the superficial and juxtamedullary nephrons. In the rabbit, the total length of the proximal tubule is similar in superficial and deep nephrons.[159] However, the respective lengths of the convoluted and straight tubules differ because juxtamedullary PCT are 25% longer and much wider than superficial PCT,[160] whereas superficial PR are much longer (4 mm) than juxtamedullary straight segments, which only measure 1 mm.[160] Functionally speaking, this heterogeneity is more

TABLE 3:—Na-K-ATPase Activity in Superficial
Proximal Tubule

		EARLY PCT (S_1)	LATE PCT (S_2)	PR (S_3)
Rabbit	Katz, Doucet, Morel[110]	2303	—	638
	Garg, Knepper, Burg[107]	6300	2400	1380
Rat	Ashton, Koepsell[100]	1207	—	184
	Katz, Doucet, Morel[110]	2450	—	505
	Garg, Mackie, Tisher[109]	14340	4080	1920
Mouse	Katz, Doucet, Morel[110]	1776	—	487

Activity is expressed in $pmol.mm^{-1}.h^{-1}$.

marked for the two types of nephrons. Thus, the glomerular fitration rate is 25% higher in juxtamedullary than in superficial nephrons,[159, 161, 162] as are the sodium and water reabsorption capacities per unit length, especially in the S_1 and S_2 segments.[163–166] These differences are reflected in the Na-K-ATPase activity, which is higher in deep PCT and PR (Table 4).

In microperfusion experiments in vivo, Fromter and coworkers[167] measured sodium reabsorption in rat proximal tubule, and found that 30% of proximal sodium reabsorption was active and directly dependent on Na-K-ATPase activity. From these findings, it is possible to calculate whether the Na-K-ATPase activity measured in isolated proximal tubules is sufficient to account for active sodium transport, estimated from the net sodium fluxes measured in tubules perfused in vivo in the rat and in vitro in the rabbit. At first sight, it might seem more logical to compare the Na-K-ATPase transport capacity to the unidirectional rather than the net sodium flux. However, measurement of the unidirectional flux using radioactive sodium results in overestimation of transport by the pump, since exchange diffusion fluxes are included in the evaluations made by this technique. Therefore, although measurement of the net sodium reabsorption flux may lead to underestimation of Na-K-ATPase function because of the existence of a passive backflux, this criteria seems more satisfactory. Comparison of sodium net flux and Na-K-ATPase activity is not reliable, either; these fluxes are measured under physiological conditions, whereas ATPase activity is determined under artificial condi-

TABLE 4:—Na-K-ATPase Activity in Superficial and Juxtamedullary Proximal Tubules

		EARLY PCT (S_1)		PR (S_3)	
		SUPERFICIAL	JUXTAMEDULLARY	SUPERFICIAL	JUXTAMEDULLARY
Rabbit	Schmidt, Horster[98]				
	-fresh tubules	3.3	6.3		
	-freeze-dried tubules	2.4	4.5		
Rat	Ashton, Koepsell[100]	1.7	2.4	0.4	0.7
	Schmidt, Horster[98]	1.8	3.8	0.3	0.8
Human	Schmidt, Horster[98]	2.1	4.1	0.2	0.3

Activity is expressed in $mol.kg^{-1}$ dry $wt.h^{-1}$

tions, including the absence of cation gradients, maximal rate, etc. Therefore, such estimations are necessarily approximate, and aim only at comparing orders of magnitude. The results in Table 5 indicate that when Na-K-ATPase activity is measured on fresh tissue,[107, 109, 110] it is sufficient to account for 30% of the net sodium reabsorption fluxes along the proximal tubule, even allowing for the fact that the pump operates physiologically at half its maximal rate. On the other hand, the values obtained with lyophylized segments [98, 100] are not sufficient to account for the active transport observed.

Na-K-ATPase and Control of Cell Volume

To maintain cell volume, the electro-osmotic gradient generated by the intracellular colloido-osmotic force ($\simeq$ 1–2 $mOsm.kg^{-1}$) has to be offset by ionic extrusion, which keeps the intracellular medium away from its electrochemical equilibrium. Therefore, it is of interest to find out whether the sodium pump is at least partly responsible for such cell volume control.

This controversial problem (see review by MacKnight and Leaf)[168] has been studied on several systems including the kidney, where attention has focused on the proximal tubule. One experimental approach consisted of examining the changes in the volume of cells exposed to a hypotonic medium and of characterizing the mechanisms causing these changes. In an early work, Dellasega and Grantham[169] described the response of isolated proximal tubules to a hypo-osmotic medium: The cells swelled rapidly during the first minute, but during the next 10 minutes their size diminished to a new steady state, close to their original volume. The swelling during the first phase occurred because water equilibrates through the membrane more quickly than solutes. The following volume regulation phase was apparently due to the extrusion of intracellular potassium, sodium, and chloride and to loss of water from the cell.[170]

Certain studies showed that the volume regulation phase persisted in the presence of ouabain concentrations, which completely inhibited Na-K-ATPase,[169, 170] suggesting that such regulation depended on an ouabain-insensitive sodium pump. The concept that a hypothetical ouabain-insensitive cation pump helps to control cell volume is supported by the results of Whit-

TABLE 5:—MAXIMAL TRANSPORT CAPACITY OF Na-K-ATPase AND SODIUM FLUX
IN THE PROXIMAL TUBULE

			PHYSIOLOGICAL MEASUREMENT	REFERENCE FLUX	SODIUM FLUX	Na-K-ATPase CAPACITY $(pEq.mm^{-1}.min^{-1})$	REFERENCES Na-K-ATPase
Lapin							
	S_1	superficial	IFR	[166]	104	56	[98]
			IFR	[343]	115	115	[110]
						315	[107]
		juxtamedullary	IFR	[166]	132	116	[98]
			IFR	[343]	158		
	S_2	superficial	IFR	[166]	134	120	[107]
			IFR	[163]	136		
	S_3	superficial	IFR	[344]	64	32	[110]
			IFR	[165]	66	69	[107]
Rat							
	S_1	superficial	AT	[345]	102	23	[98]
						60	[100]
			NF	[346]	505	122	[110]
						717	[109]

IFR, isoosmotic fluid reabsorption; AT, active sodium transplant; NF, net sodium flux.

tembury and colleagues,[126, 171, 172] who incubated kidney cortex slices in a chilled isotonic anaerobic medium and found that they lost potassium, accumulated sodium and chloride, and swelled. After rewarming under aerobic conditions, the slices extruded sodium chloride and regained their initial volume. This process was independent of the presence of ouabain, and was abolished by metabolic inhibitors such as 2,4-dinitrophenol. As mentioned above, these results were taken to indicate that cell volume is controlled by an energy-dependent, ouabain-insensitive cation pump,[126, 171, 172] and this interpretation has been extended to explain the volume regulation that occurs in response to a hypo-osmotic environment.[173–175]

More recently, Linshaw and coworkers[176] suggested that the volume control observed in the presence of ouabain, in response to an hypo-osmotic medium, might be due to the mechanical restraint exerted by the tubular basal membrane. This hypothesis is supported by Paillard et al.[177] and Linshaw and Grantham,[178] who showed that ouabain inhibits the volume regulation phase when renal tubules or cells are isolated after a collagenase treatment, which hydrolyzes the basal membrane. These results indicate that in a hypo-osmotic medium, proximal tubules are able to control their cellular volume in the absence of basal membrane, provided that Na-K-ATPase is functioning normally. In the absence of an operational pump, the basal membrane limits tubule cell swelling, although the latter process does not constitute true regulation. Lastly, it does not seem useful to incriminate a pump other than Na-K-ATPase to explain the volume regulation of proximal tubules described here.

Na-K-ATPase and Water Reabsorption

The results of in vitro microperfusion of rabbit proximal tubules indicate that Na-K-ATPase-dependent solute transport represents the driving force for water reabsorption, since the presence of ouabain[179] or absence of potassium[180, 181] in the peritubular bath reduces fluid reabsorption in both convoluted and straight segments of the proximal tubules. Residual fluid reabsorption after Na-K-ATPase inhibition varies from 10–40% in rabbit and hamster.[179, 182, 183]

Na-K-ATPase-dependent Solute Transport

Rabbit proximal convoluted tubules perfused in vitro are polarized with a negative lumen ($\simeq -3.8$ mV) when the perfusion medium contains sodium and glucose or aminoacids.[184] Since this potential difference is inhibited by the presence of ouabain[165, 184, 185] or absence of potassium in the bath,[181] it is dependent on Na-K-ATPase functioning. Similarly, proton secretion and bicarbonate reabsorption by the rabbit proximal tubule depend on the presence of luminal sodium and are inhibited by the addition of ouabain or the absence of potassium in the bath.[186] These results indicate that: 1) Sodium entrance through the luminal membrane depends on the presence of other solutes, such as glucose or aminoacids, and, 2) reabsorption of these solutes is due to Na-K-ATPase activity.

In the proximal tubule, transport of glucose[151] and aminoacids[187] across the luminal membrane is active, since they accumulate inside the cell. Such transport is also inhibited by ouabain, which suggests that it is secondary to Na-K-ATPase activity. The model proposed by Crane[188] for intestinal sugar transport can be applied to glucose and aminoacid transport in the proximal tubule. In this type of transport, Na-K-ATPase activity keeps the intracellular sodium far from its electrochemical equilibrium, and this cation, therefore, re-enters the cell along its downhill gradient through the apical or basolateral membrane. The energy dissipated during this diffusion can be used to transport other substances along their uphill electrochemical gradient, thanks to the coupling of uphill and downhill transport by specific membrane carriers. This secondary active transport may occur in the form of cotransport, i.e., in the same direction as sodium transport, as in the case of glucose, phosphate, and aminoacids, or as countertransport, i.e., in opposite directions, as for calcium and protons. This model requires the concomitant presence of both the entities to be transported.

The existence of sodium-dependent cotransport systems for glucose,[189, 190] aminoacids,[191] citrate and lactate,[192] and phosphate,[193] and of countertransport systems for protons[194] and calcium[195] has been demonstrated in vesicles from proximal tubule brush border. The sodium-glucose carrier has been solubilized and incorporated into liposomes[196] but none of these carriers has yet been purified.

Sodium-glucose and sodium-amino acid carriers are electrogenic, and negatively charged aminoacids are cotransported with several sodium ions.[197, 198] Phosphate might be similarly transported with two sodium ions.[193]

Proton secretion and bicarbonate reabsorption by the rat proximal tubule are active processes and are not abolished by ouabain,[183] suggesting that a luminal proton pump might account for proton secretion in this species.[194]

Figure 4 describes the various proximal transport systems, for which energy is supplied by Na-K-ATPase.

THE LOOP OF HENLE

The loop of Henle consists of two segments that have different diameters and functional properties.

Thin Limbs of the Loop of Henle

The thin loops of Henle can be divided into two types: short loops that have their hairpin bend in the outer medulla and are found in superficial nephrons, and long loops that form a bend at the tip of the papilla and are part of the juxtamedullary nephrons. The epithelia making up these two kinds of thin segment are very different, and have been classified into four groups.[195, 196] Garg and Tisher reported in a preliminary work[197] that the initial portion of the thin segment of the long loops (type II epithelium) was the only one to contain measurable Na-K-ATPase activity close to that of the pars recta. This portion is also the only one that displays the structural characteristic of a transporting epithelia, i.e., apical villosities, basolateral interdigitations and numerous mitochondria. These authors, therefore, suggested that this thin Na-K-ATPase-rich segment might be responsible for the potassium secretion described by Jamison et al. in the juxtamedullary descending limbs of Henle's loops.[198–200]

Except as regards type II epithelia, the low Na-K-ATPase activity measured in the thin segments of Henle's loop[100, 110, 197] is in agreement with in vitro microperfusion experiments that show the absence of active sodium transport in the thin

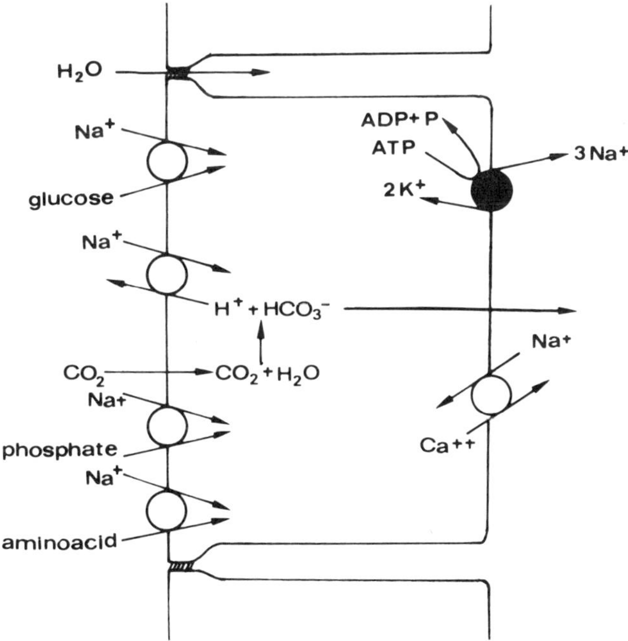

Fig 4.—Different modes of Na-K-ATPase-dependent transport in proximal tubule cells. Dissipation of the electrochemical sodium gradient generated by the pump is coupled with the reabsorption of glucose, phosphate, and aminoacids, and with the secretion of protons against their electrochemical gradient. Active calcium reabsorption by the basolateral membrane might also be coupled with the sodium gradient.

descending[201] and ascending[202–204] limbs of Henle's loop. Nevertheless, the low Na-K-ATPase activity measured in these segments might be sufficient to maintain a low intracellular Na/K ratio.

Thick Ascending Limbs of the Loop of Henle

There is no significant difference between the thick ascending segments in superficial and deep nephrons. On the other hand, there are gradual alterations in the cell ultrastructure along these segments, and it is now usual to separate them into medullary and cortical portions. The mechanism of the intense sodium reabsorption in both portions is probably similar, and only the factors regulating it differ.[205]

Active sodium chloride reabsorption by the thick ascending

limb of the loop of Henle is of capital importance to the control of urinary water excretion through the urea and NaCl gradients that sodium reabsorption generates, thanks to the specific permeability properties of the distal nephron segments. The physiological importance of these processes makes it important to understand the mechanism of active NaCl reabsorption in the thick ascending limb and the involvement of Na-K-ATPase in this absorption.

Until recently, it was generally admitted that Cl^- was actively transported along the thick ascending limb of the loop, since when segments of this limb were perfused in vitro at a high rate in the absence of a transepithelial gradient, their lumen was positive ($+ 7$ to $+ 9$ mV) in relation to the bathing solution.[205–216] This Cl^- transport was considered to be primarily active, on the basis of experiments showing that the substitution of choline for sodium did not alter the transepithelial potential difference.[208, 211, 213]

However, in a recent series of studies[209, 217–221] Greger re-examined the mechanism of Cl^- reabsorption in rabbit thick ascending limb, and demonstrated that:

1) - This reabsorption is sodium-dependent and has a half-stimulation constant of 3.4 mM.[217] According to Greger, previous contradictory results[208, 211, 213] were due to slight sodium contamination. His subsequent observation is suggestive of a secondary active Cl^- transport.

2) - Cl^- reabsorption depends on the presence of luminal potassium,[218] implying that it might occur through an Na^+-Cl^--K^+ luminal cotransport system.

3) - The luminal carrier is furosemide-sensitive, electroneutral and has a stoichiometry of $1Na^+ : 2Cl^- : 1K^+$.[221]

4) - Potassium is recycled through the luminal membrane by a barium-sensitive pathway.[219]

5) - Cl^- leaves the cell through the basolateral membrane in an electroneutral fashion with potassium and in a diffusional fashion.[220]

6) - The positive polarization of the tubular lumen is due to the specific conductance properties of luminal and basolateral membranes in relation to potassium and chloride respectively.[220]

7) - This transepithelial potential is the driving force for massive sodium reabsorption through the paracellular shunt pathway.

Greger's finding therefore indicates that it is sodium that is actively transported along the thick ascending limb, as could be presumed from the high Na-K-ATPase content of this segment[103, 107, 109, 110, 222] and by the inhibitory effect of ouabain on net NaCl reabsorption.[208, 213] Greger's model for secondary active Cl^- transport is depicted in Figure 5.

The sodium dependence of Cl^- reabsorption has been verified by Hebert and coworkers[205] on mouse medullary thick ascending limb. Eveloff and coworkers[223, 224] further showed that oxygen consumption by cells isolated from rabbit thick ascending limb[225] was dependent on the presence of both sodium and chloride and was inhibited by ouabain and furosemide. In addition, they demonstrated that ^{22}Na uptake by membrane vesicles pre-

Fig 5.—Model showing the mechanisms of active NaCl reabsorption in the thick ascending limb of Henle's loop in the rabbit. Filled circles indicate the Na-K-ATPase, which constitutes the primary active mechanism. Open circles represent the transport apical (Na^+, Cl^-, and K^+) and basolateral transport (K^+ and Cl^-) ion carriers. Other arrows indicate passive permeability. (Reproduced from Greger et al. Properties of the basolateral membrane of the cortical thick ascending limb of Henle's loop of rabbit kidney. A model for secondary active chloride transport. *Pflugers Arch.* 396:325, 1983.)

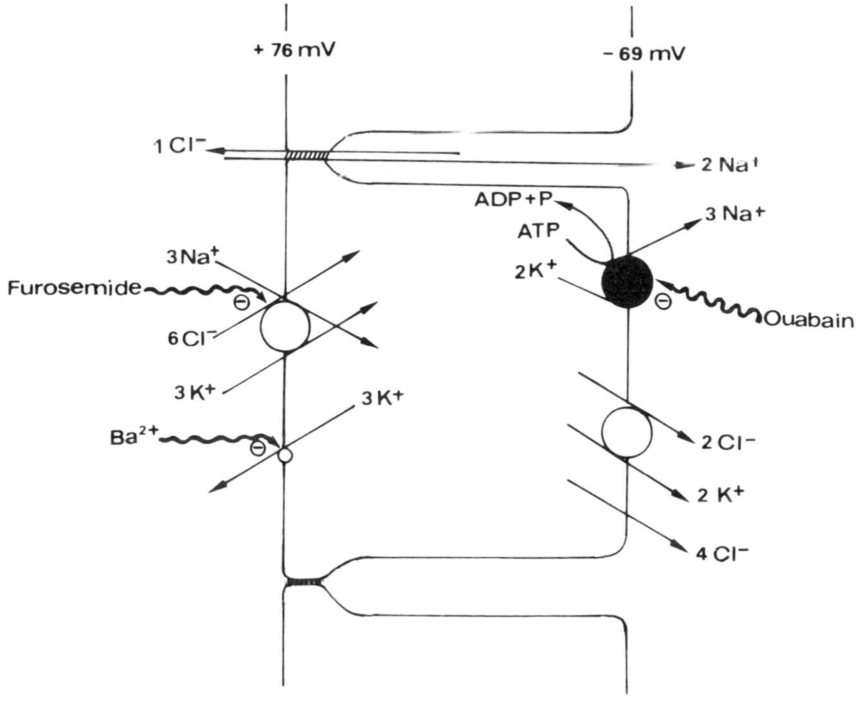

pared from these cells increased in the presence of a Cl^- gradient, diminished when nitrate was substituted for chloride, and was inhibited by furosemide in a dose-dependent fashion.[226] Finally, Koenig and Kinne[227] confirmed that sodium transport by membrane vesicles was potassium-dependent, implying the presence of Na^+-Cl^--K^+ cotransport system.

All of these results clearly indicate that Na-K-ATPase is the driving force for sodium chloride reabsorption by the thick ascending limb. Therefore, it is interesting to compare the sodium transport capacity of Na-K-ATPase measured on isolated segments of thick limb to the sodium flux determined by in vitro microperfusion. Greger's model (Fig 5)[220] indicates that three-fifths of the net sodium flux is directly driven by the pump, whereas the remaining two-fifths is reabsorbed through the shunt pathway. Assuming that Na-K-ATPase operates at half its maximal rate, the results in Table 6 indicate that the pump concentration found by various authors[98, 107, 109, 110] is sufficient to account for the pump-driven fraction of the sodium flux.

The Distal Convoluted Tubule and Collecting Duct

Unlike the homogeneous segments considered above, the distal convoluted tubule comprises several cell types with different functional properties. Works by Morel and colleagues,[93, 227–230] who determined the hormonal dependence of adenylate cyclase along the nephron, permitted a definition of the functional segmentation of the distal tubule, which accounts for the observations concerning its morphology and ultrastructure.[195, 231] These results prompted several studies that enabled the transport functions of each segment to be ascertained.[216, 232, 233] It is therefore necessary to recall briefly here the organization of the distal tubule before examining the role of Na-K-ATPase in each of its constituents.

Distal Tubule Segmentation

Physiologists usually define the distal convoluted tubule (DCT) as the nephron segment located between the macula densa and the first branching with another tubule. In the rabbit, the first part of this tubule, just beyond the macula densa,

TABLE 6:—MAXIMAL TRANSPORT CAPACITY OF Na-K-ATPase AND SODIUM FLUX IN THE THICK ASCENDING LIMB

		PHYSIOLOGICAL MEASUREMENT	REFERENCES FLUX	SODIUM FLUX	Na-K-ATPase CAPACITY ($pEq.mm^{-1}.min^{-1}$)	REFERENCES: Na-K-ATPase
Rabbit	MAL	NF	213	240	123 154 372	110 98 107
	CAL	NF NF	208 216	79 31	49 63 93	110 98 107
Rat	MAL	NF	215	66	90 227 417	98 110 109
Mouse	MAL	NF	210	94–134	185	110

MAL, medullary portion of the thick ascending limb; CAL, cortical portion of the thick ascending limb; NF, net reabsorption flux.

consists of thick ascending limb cells, the function of which has already been discussed. The next segment (DCTb) is 0.5 to 1 mm long and has a bright appearance under the microscope. This segment, considered the true distal convoluted tubule, consists of a single cell type, the DCT cells, which have tight junctions and are rich in mitochondria. After this segment comes a thicker one with a granular appearance (DCTg). In the midcortical and deep nephrons, several DCTg segments may combine to form a collecting duct with a uniform appearance that is called a granular cortical collecting tubule (CCTg). The DCTg and CCTg form the connecting tubule (CNT), which includes two cell types—connective and intercalated, or dark cells. Connective cells are fairly similar to DCT cells, except that they have fewer basolateral infoldings and mitochondria. In the intercalated cells, the basolateral surface area is not greatly increased by these infoldings, but the apical membrane is well developed and exhibits numerous microvilli. The collecting tubule following either the DCTg or the CNT also comprises two cell types: Intercalated cells similar to those found in the CNT, and principal or clear cells specific to this segment and similar to connective cells. The last two cell types are also found in modified form in the medullary collecting tubule. In the rat and mouse, the transition between DCTb and DCTg is less obvious, and cell types are more intricate.

Location of Na-K-ATPase

Na-K-ATPase activity was measured in the various segments of rabbit, rat and mouse distal convoluted tubule.[98, 102, 107, 109, 110] Although different techniques gave quite different values, all the results obtained indicate that the nephron segment with the highest Na-K-ATPase activity is the DCTb. Several studies show that this activity is higher in DCTb than in DCTg in rabbit[107, 110] and mouse (unpublished observations). In the latter segment, it is in turn higher than in the CCT and the MCT (Table 7). In rabbit nephrons, the number of ouabain binding sites in the segments extending from the DCTb to the MCT was found to decrease with the Na-K-ATPase activity (Table 2).[234]

Although Na-K-ATPase has not been quantified at cell level, a cytochemical study by Ernst[84] indicates that its activity is

TABLE 7:—Na-K-ATPase Activity in the Distal Nephron Segments

	DCTb	DCTg OR CNT	CCT	MCT	REFERENCES
Rabbit	—	—	1132	906	98
	3152*	1372*	822	514	110
	9120	7560	1380	1140	107
Rat	900	—	850	600	98, 102
	6679	—	769	750	110
	18900	—	4860	2460	109
Mouse	5897*	1529*	1071	265	110

Activity is expressed in $pmol.mm^{-1}.h^{-1}$. DCTb, bright portion of distal convoluted tubule; DCTg, granular portion of DCT; CNT, connecting tubule; CCT, cortical collecting tubule; MCT, medullary collecting tubule (outer stripe of the medulla). *, unpublished observations.

probably very low in intercalated cells. If true, this indication, which fits the ultrastructural data for intercalated cells, would explain the difference between the levels of Na-K-ATPase activity in the DCTb and DCTg.

This enzyme's activity in the distal convoluted tubule and collecting duct is modified by various factors like corticosteroids or sodium and potassium intake, which also alter the kidney's capacity for sodium reabsorption and potassium secretion. The results relating to these points are reviewed in the section on regulation of renal Na-K ATPase.

Role of Na-K-ATPase in Sodium and Potassium Transport

Micropuncture experiments on the rat indicate that Na-K-ATPase is responsible for sodium reabsorption by the distal convoluted tubule, since in this segment sodium is reabsorbed against a steep gradient concentration, and the tubular lumen is negatively polarized (−15 to −40 mV). Lastly, ouabain inhibits sodium reabsorption and the transepithelial potential difference in the distal convoluted tubule.[235-237] In the rabbit, sodium transport has been studied in the various distal segments by in vitro microperfusion. The lumen of the distal convoluted tubule and connecting tubule are negatively polarized at −30 mV[233, 238] and sodium reabsorption in these segments is active. In the cortical collecting tubule, the transepithelial potential difference depends on the mineralocorticoid status of the animals from which the tubule is dissected.[239] In the CCT, both the transepithelial potential difference and the sodium reabsorption are inhibited when ouabain is added to the perfusion bath.[240–242] In contrast, neither of these parameters in the outer medullary collecting tubule is sensitive to ouabain,[242] indicating that sodium reabsorption is diffusional in this segment. The last result correlates with the low Na-K-ATPase activity measured in the outer medullary collecting tubule.[98, 107, 109, 110]

In view of the true pumping rate of Na-K-ATPase determined under physiological conditions, the results in Table 8 indicate that Na-K-ATPase accounts for sodium transport in the distal convoluted tubule (DCTb), connecting tubule (DCTg), and cortical collecting duct. The values obtained by Garg et al.[107, 109] in the DCT and CNT greatly exceed the sodium fluxes measured in the rabbit or rat.

As already mentioned, potassium secretion depends on the intracellular activity of potassium ions and on the apical and basolateral membrane potentials. These parameters are in turn determined by the Na-K-ATPase activity and the relative membrane conductance to the major ions. During adaptation to augmented dietary potassium, the collecting tubule plays an important role in enhancing renal potassium secretion, and its Na-K-ATPase activity increases 2–3 fold.[243]

TABLE 8:—MAXIMAL TRANSPORT CAPACITY OF Na-K-ATPase AND SODIUM REABSORPTION IN THE DISTAL CONVOLUTED TUBULE AND COLLECTING TUBULE

		REFERENCES FLUX	SODIUM FLUX	Na-K-ATPase CAPACITY $(pEq.mm^{-1}.min^{-1})$	REFERENCES Na-K-ATPase
Rabbit	DCTb	216	82	158	110
		238	101	456	107
	CNT	216	62	69	110
		232	122	378	107
	CCT	239	34	41	110
		289	16	57	98
		281	52	69	107
Rat	DCT	236	99	334	110
		72	70	945	109
		235	114		

Regulation of Renal Na-K-ATPase

In order to maintain homeostasis, the kidney can adapt itself
to either acute or chronic environmental changes. Since Na-K-
ATPase activity makes a decisive contribution to the maintenance of renal transport functions and under normal conditions
is just sufficient to account for the capacity of the transports
involved, it seems desirable to identify the parameters controlling renal Na-K-ATPase activity.

Renal Na-K-ATPase activity is altered by numerous states,
such as adrenalectomy, mineralocorticoid or glucocorticoid administration, thyroidectomy, and the administration of thyroid
hormones, uninephrectomy, changes in the dietary intake of sodium or potassium, inducement of hypertension, or neonatal
development. To understand the functional relevance of these
observations, they must be correlated with the alterations in
cation transport occurring under such circumstances. Since Na-
K-ATPase activity in the different nephron segments varies,
these correlations have to be detected in the individual segments.

This activity can be regulated by changes in either synthesis
and/or degradation rates of the enzyme, or in the activation
constants of its various cofactors. As regards the adjustments
in the Na-K-ATPase concentrations in kidney tubules, a major
problem concerns the distinction between direct hormonal effects and effects secondary to changes in the intracellular sodium concentration. Certain potential factors of Na-K-ATPase
regulation have been studied from this point of view.

CONTROL OF THE Na-K-ATPase PUMPING RATE

Na-K-ATPase activity can be directly controlled by the availability of its substrates $-$Na$^+$, K$^+$, and ATP, and by certain
pharmacological substances, such as ouabain or vanadate. It is
important to consider whether these factors operate under normal or physiopathological conditions.

Control by Na-K-ATPase Substrates

Of the three Na-K-ATPase substrates just mentioned, only
the first can alter the functioning rate of the pump physiologi-

cally, since intracellular ATP concentrations are close to 2 mM, which is about the optimum required by this enzyme (See I-A-3). Similarly, the pump's affinity for extracellular potassium (0.5–1 mM) is such that when kalemia is normal (4–5 mM), the external potassium binding sites are almost saturated and the pump is totally activated from the external side. On the other hand, during severe hypokalemia, potassium might become rate-limiting when its concentration drops to below 2 mM.[244]

Intracellular sodium has a Km of 5–13 mM for purified Na-K-ATPase[23, 24] and of 15 mM for this pump in isolated tubules.[105] In these two preparations, maximal activity is reached for sodium concentrations of 120 mM and 70 mM, respectively. Although the intracellular sodium concentrations in kidney tubules are not precisely known, it is very likely that under normal conditions, sodium is rate-limiting. Therefore, changes in the intracellular sodium concentration occurring secondarily to alterations in membrane permeability (especially that of the apical membrane) may modify the functioning of the pump. This possibility might account for the instantaneous changes observed in active sodium transport, but no data are available to confirm such an explanation.

Vanadate

Agents able to modify the pump's affinity for sodium, potassium, or ATP are good candidates for fulfilling regulatory functions. Vanadate meets several criteria suggesting that it could be physiologically active.[245]

Vanadate, which is excreted in the urine, is accumulated by kidney cells prior to its elimination.[128, 246] When administered to rats, it induces marked diuresis and natriuresis in a dose-dependent fashion.[128, 130, 131, 131a,133] This effect, observed in the absence of changes in the glomerular filtration rate or blood pressure,[130, 131, 133] is attributed to the inhibition of renal Na-K-ATPase[44, 49] even though vanadate also inhibits several other enzymes.[247–249] Initial clearance[130, 131a] and micropuncture studies of the effects of vanadate[131] indicated reduced proximal reabsorption of sodium. More recently, Westenfelder and colleagues[133] have shown that vanadate also reduces sodium transport by the distal tubule.

In biological fluids, vanadium chiefly exists in two redox states: vanadate (HVO_4^{2-}) and vanadyl (VO^{2+}). Vanadate, the only form that inhibits Na-K-ATPase, is spontaneously formed by vanadyl oxidation. However, vanadyl can be stabilized in the presence of reducing agents like ascorbic acid or norepinephrine.[49] Furthermore, the existence of cellular vanadate reductase[250] suggests that vanadium is present as vanadate in extracellular fluids, and as vanadyl inside the cells,[49, 251] which seems to run counter to physiological inhibition by vanadate. However, the high vanadium concentration measured in the kidney implies that vanadate might be involved in the physiological control of water and electrolyte excretion. As stressed by Grantham,[245] it might act either by being constantly present in the cell and shifting from an active form (vanadate) to an inactive one (vanadyl), depending on the intracellular redox potential, or as a circulating hormone, with the kidney as its preferential target.

Ouabain

One of the most disturbing observations concerning Na-K-ATPase is the presence of specific binding sites for digitalis agents, a class of substance that is absent from the animal world. It is tempting to imagine that there are natural animal molecules possessing ouabain-like activity that might help to control pump activity and sodium excretion. In this connection, it has been suggested that "natriuretic hormone" (see IV-B-3) is one of these substances.[252–254] If such molecules really existed, the characterization of the factors rendering their action specific to the kidney would still constitute a major problem, because Na-K-ATPase is sensitive to ouabain in all mammalian tissues.

HORMONAL REGULATION

Mineralocorticoids are the most important of all the hormones affecting renal Na-K-ATPase activity, because the kidney is their main target and they control sodium and potassium excretion. A large number of studies aimed at defining the relationship between mineralocorticoids and Na-K-ATPase have been carried out on adrenalectomized animals, a condition

that raises doubts about the mineralo- or glucocorticoid origin
of the effects observed. This is why, in the present review, the
effects of these two types of corticoids will be considered together.

Adrenocorticosteroid

The study of aldosterone's action on toad bladder has provided important data that are applicable to the mammalian
kidney, and some of this information will be recalled here.

Numerous authors indicated that renal Na-K-ATPase activity decreases after adrenalectomy[101, 104, 255–266] and is at least
partially restored after the administration of mineralocorticoids and/or glucocorticoids.[102, 255, 259, 260–265, 267–271] This seems
to indicate Na-K-ATPase dependency on adrenocorticosteroids.
Owing to the great variety of experimental protocols used (normal or adrenalectomized animals, administration of mineralo-
or glucocorticoids, the different doses of hormones, periods of
treatment, types of kidney preparation and Na-K-ATPase assays, etc.), comparative analysis of these results is not feasible.
However, a study of the relevant literature gives rise to the
following questions:

—Are the respective actions of mineralo- and glucocorticoids
on Na-K-ATPase induced independently, by occupancy of the
specific receptors of these hormones, or do both types of steroid
act by occupying heterologous receptors that occur secondarily
to the high doses of hormone used?

—If each type of corticosteroid acts on Na-K-ATPase independently, are the effects identical (kinetics, mode of control,
localization along the nephron, etc.)?

—What are the corticosteroid target segments along the
nephron?

—Is the action of corticosteroids on Na-K-ATPase direct or
secondary to changes in the sodium load?

—Do corticosteroids act on the Na-K-ATPase synthesis rate,
its functioning rate, or both?

Our understanding of these problems greatly improved when
Schmidt and Dubach introduced the technique already mentioned allowing measurement of Na-K-ATPase activity in individual pieces of nephron segment.[97] Before this approach became available, it had been proposed that the stimulation of

Na-K-ATPase in target cells might be masked by the dilution of these cells with other cell types insensitive to aldosterone and outnumbering the target cells in the kidney.

Adrenalectomy reduces Na-K-ATPase activity in the proximal convoluted tubule (except in the rabbit[260]), in the thick ascending limb of Henle's loop, the distal convoluted tubule and the collecting duct[101, 102, 104, 258–260, 268] within several days.[258] However, the results of different experimental approaches indicated that only the collecting tubule is sensitive to mineralocorticoids. These approaches included localization of aldosterone receptors,[272, 273] measurement of changes in the transepithelial potential on in vitro microperfused tubules[233, 274, 275] and assay of the sensitivity to aldosterone of citrate synthetase (a target enzyme for mineralocorticoids) along the rabbit nephron.[276] The results of these investigations imply that the decline in Na-K-ATPase observed after adrenalectomy in segments other than the collecting tubule could be caused by glucocorticoid deprivation. In this connection, it is suggestive that specific glucocorticoid receptors are found all along the nephron.[277, 278] To evaluate the responsiveness of the various nephron segments to the two types of corticosteroids, hormonal dosage has had to be adjusted in such a way to avoid cross-reactions.

We attempted to distinguish between the effects of mineralo- and glucocorticosteroids by their location along the nephron, and by using specific antagonists.[260] In short, the results obtained on the adrenalectomized rabbit indicate that a single injection of 10 g/kg aldosterone restores Na-K-ATPase activity within three hours in the collecting tubule only. However, 100 μg/kg dexamethasone restores pump activity within the same period, in all nephron segments in which this activity is diminished by adrenalectomy (thick ascending limb, distal convoluted tubule and collecting tubule). Furthermore, previous administration of spironolactone (an antagonist of aldosterone receptors) blocks the effects of both the mineralocorticoid aldosterone and the glucocorticoid dexamethasone in the collecting tubule, but does not alter the response of other segments to glucocorticoids. These results suggest that the occupancy of glucocorticoid receptors controls Na-K-ATPase activity in the thick ascending limb and the distal convoluted tubule, whereas mineralocorticoid action is restricted to the collecting tubule.

Of these findings, the ones concerning the action of aldosterone on the collecting tubule are in agreement with previous observations by Horster et al.[268] and Petty et al.,[104] and those concerning the action of dexamethasone on the ascending limb are consistent with the results of Rayson and Edelman.[270]

What mechanisms underly Na-K-ATPase stimulation by both types of corticosteroids? Do they consist of activating pre-existent catalytic units, or of inducing the formation of new units?

In a recent study, Geering and colleagues[113] showed that aldosterone specifically stimulated synthesis of the α and β subunits of Na-K-ATPase from toad bladder. In their experiments, the synthesis rates of both subunits, measured by immunoprecipitation with polyclonal antibodies, were 2–3 fold higher in aldosterone-treated bladders than in the controls. The effect of aldosterone was blocked by spironolactone, but not by amiloride (which blocks the apical sodium entrance). These findings suggest that aldosterone has a direct effect on Na-K-ATPase expression at genome level. Recent observations made in our laboratory (unpublished results) indicate that administering aldosterone to the adrenalectomized rabbit raises the number of ouabain binding sites in the collecting tubule concomitantly with Na-K-ATPase activity. These results, showing that in mammalian kidney new Na-K-ATPase units appear as early as three hours after aldosterone administration, agree with the data for amphibians.[113] Using a different experimental approach, Nagel and Crabbe[279] reached the same conclusions after finding increased ionic conductance in the basolateral membrane of aldosterone-treated toad skins.

Glucocorticoids probably act through a different mechanism from that of mineralocorticoids. Thus, in the experiments already mentioned on adrenalectomized rabbits, we observed increased Na-K-ATPase activity in the thick ascending limb and distal convoluted tubule after administering dexamethasone, but we noted no change in the ouabain binding capacity. These results suggest that glucocorticoids might act through the activation of pre-existing catalytic units, either directly or via induced molecules. During long-term treatments with methylprednisolone, Hendler and colleagues[261] described parallel increases in Na-K-ATPase activity and ouabain binding in membrane fractions prepared from the cortex and medulla of adrenalectomized guinea-pigs. More recently, Sinha and colleagues[271] found that the Na-K-ATPase concentration rose after chronic or acute administration of dexamethasone to adrenalectomized rats. However, the latter authors also observed a change in the enzyme's affinity for ATP, suggesting that its rate of functioning might also be modified.

Another source of controversy is the question of whether corticosteroids induce Na-K-ATPase synthesis by acting directly on the genome, or whether this synthesis is induced secondarily to some effect of the hormones on the sodium load delivered to the nephron segment or on the intracellular sodium concentration.

Corticosteroids, especially glucocorticoids, are known to increase the glomerular filtration rate and therefore the filtered load of sodium. Consequently, it has been suggested that the action of these hormones on Na-K-ATPase is secondary to the increased sodium delivery.[263, 280] The following indications support this hypothesis: 1) - In the rat, renal Na-K-ATPase activity is not altered by the high circulating aldosterone levels induced by a dietary sodium depletion.[33, 255] 2) - Aldosterone-induced changes in the sodium and potassium concentrations in the plasma precede the corresponding changes in Na-K-ATPase activity.[263] 3) - The Na-K-ATPase stimulation induced by DOCA is abolished when animals are deprived of sodium,[255, 281] and conversely, saline loading stimulates pump activity in the cortex and medulla of adrenalectomized rats.[266] However, the arguments against this sodium-loading hypothesis are equally convincing: 1) - It has been clearly established that methyl-prednisolone,[282] dexamethasone,[265, 271] and aldosterone[259, 268] stimulate renal Na-K-ATPase activity in the absence of any change in the glomerular filtration rate. 2) - The localization of corticosteroid effects in specific nephron segments[259, 260] possessing hormone receptors is hard to reconcile with an extrarenal origin of the phenomenon, and 3) - Handler and colleagues reported that aldosterone-induced Na-K-ATPase activity in a cultured cell line derived from toad kidney.[283]

Another process through which sodium has been incriminated as a stimulant of Na-K-ATPase in response to corticosteroids is summarized by what is usually called the "permease theory."[284] According to this theory, interaction between aldosterone and the target cell genome induces the apical permease responsible for the entry of sodium into the cell, thus enhancing the intracellular activity of this cation. During the initial period, this would lead to activation by the substrate of the pre-existing catalytic units (see IV-A-1), and subsequently to the induction of new units, thus allowing the intracellular sodium to revert to its original steady state. This hypothesis is supported by observations showing that passage through the apical membrane of toad bladder cells is the limiting step in sodium reabsorption, as suggested by experiments with amphotericin B.[285] On the kidney, Petty and colleagues[104] showed that amiloride, which inhibits apical sodium entry into collecting tubule cells, abolishes the aldosterone-induced Na-K-ATPase stimulation, suggesting that sodium entry is required in order to induce pump activity.

On the other hand, Geering and colleagues[113] found that amiloride had no effect in the toad bladder on aldosterone-induced synthesis of pump subunits. In addition, it was shown that the sodium concentration did not change in toad bladder cells in response to aldosterone,[82, 286] suggesting that aldosterone induces the simultaneous formation of permease and Na-K-ATPase by pleiotropic action. Finally, we showed in a recent study that the kinetics of Na-K-ATPase induction in adrenalectomized rats resemble those of the inhibition of sodium excretion after aldosterone administration.[259] This similarity runs counter to the notion that the induction of Na-K-ATPase is secondary to increased apical sodium entry, and indicates that Na-K-ATPase induction may account for the increased sodium reabsorption.

The nature of the interactions between corticosteroids and Na-K-ATPase is a controversial subject, further complicated by the fact that these hormones have a trophic effect when administered chronically. This effect has been described in rabbits injected with 5 mg DOCA per day for several days. Wade et al.[287] first demonstrated an enlargement of the basolateral membrane in the principal cells of the collecting tubule of these animals, and their results were recently confirmed by Kaisling and Le Hir.[288] DOCA treatment also enhances the transepithelial potential difference and sodium and potassium transport measured in cortical collecting tubules perfused in vitro.[233, 274, 287, 289, 290] Recently, Garg and colleagues,[107] Le Hir et al.,[108] and ourselves[267] showed that Na-K-ATPase activity is stimulated in this nephron segment during chronic DOCA treatment. The kinetics of the DOCA-induced changes were similar for Na-K-ATPase activation, for the transepithelial potential difference, and for cation transport.[233, 289]

Studies by Kaissling, Le Hir, and DuBach[108, 288] clearly showed that during DOCA treatment, Na-K-ATPase activity in the collecting tubule increases with the surface area of the basolateral membrane. It is important to note that Na-K-ATPase is stimulated during this adaptation process in preference to other enzymes located in the same membrane, such as adenyl cyclase.[267] The mechanisms underlying these adaptive phenomena are not yet known.

2 - Thyroid Hormones

The renal Na-K-ATPase is reduced in hypothyroid animals and is stimulated by administering triiodothyronine (T_3),[291–293] indicating that thyroid status is related to the activity of the renal sodium pump. This stimulation is accompanied by changes in the glomerular filtration rate, the filtered load of sodium, and sodium reabsorption.[291, 293]

Like the steroids, T_3 acts at the DNA level by inducing or inhibiting specific genes that are subsequently expressed through the cell machinery.[294–296] The problem arises, therefore, of whether Na-K-ATPase is directly induced by T_3 or whether its activation is a result of the increase in the sodium-filtered load. This last hypothesis was proposed by Katz and Lindheimer[291] in the light of data indicating that Na-K-ATPase activity changes concomitantly with sodium reabsorption, and can be restored in thyroidectomized animals by increasing the filtered load of sodium. However, this hypothesis was convincingly refuted on a kinetic basis by Lo and colleagues.[293, 297] These authors showed that in thyroidectomized rats, Na-K-ATPase stimulation occurred as soon as 24 hours after T_3 was administered, whereas changes in the glomerular filtration rate were only observed 72 hours after.[293] They also showed that changes in transport functions were preceded by enhanced RNA synthesis.[297]

The stimulatory effect of T_3 results from the increase in the number of catalytic units, as indicated by the increments observed in the rate of subunit synthesis[298] and in the number of ouabain binding sites.[292]

It is widely accepted today that thyroid hormones stimulate

energy consumption in the kidney, as in many other organs, by acting directly on the pump, for thermogenic purposes.[299] In this respect, it is worth noting that thyroid hormones do not stimulate Na-K-ATPase synthesis in poikilothermic animals.[113]

No data are yet available concerning the exact areas in which T_3 is active along the nephron. All the authors agree that the cortex is one such region, but only some of them believe that this also applies to the medulla.[291, 292]

3 - Natriuretic Hormone

The existence of a "natriuretic hormone" or "third factor," was suggested more than 20 years ago by De Wardener and colleagues[300] on the basis of results showing that dogs acutely loaded with saline develop natriuresis despite reduced glomerular filtration and high levels of plasma aldosterone and antidiuretic hormone. It was recently proposed that natriuretic hormone might play a crucial role in the pathogenesis of essential hypertension, because it induces intracellular sodium enrichment.[301, 302] Despite the numerous attempts to purify it,[252, 303–307] the identity of this substance is still hypothetical, as its only known chemical characteristics are thermic stability and low molecular weight.

Detailed analysis of this problem is beyond the scope of the present review, and the discussion will be confined to evaluating the possible relationship between natriuretic hormone and the sodium pump, since several results strongly suggest that renal Na-K-ATPase might be a target for this hormone. Gonick and colleagues,[308] for instance, reported that renal Na-K-ATPase was inhibited by a circulating factor isolated from the plasma of volume-expanded rats. Their findings were confirmed by Gruber and colleagues,[254] who showed the presence of a plasmatic inhibitor of brain Na-K-ATPase in volume-expanded dogs, and by De Wardener et al.[253] and Cloix et al.[252] who reported that normal human plasma contained a substance inhibiting the renal pump of the guinea pig and dog. In this connection, it should be stressed that the properties of the fractions characterized by Gruber[254] and Cloix,[252] respectively, were to react with specific anti-digoxin antibodies, and to inhibit ouabain binding, thus implying that they contained a ouabain-like substance.

Chemical characterization of this third factor is necessary for correct interpretation of these observations, which are not unanimously accepted because some authors observe no inhibition of renal Na-K-ATPase during chronic or acute volume expansion.[255, 309]

4 - Other Hormones

The effects of several other hormones on renal electrolyte excretion have been attributed to the fact that these hormones help to regulate renal Na-K-ATPase activity.

Although quantitatively small, the effects of insulin on sodium and potassium excretion by the kidney are now well established. Using protocols that precluded the production by insulin of any extrarenal effects, Nizet et al.[310] and De Fronzo et al.[311] showed that physiological doses of this hormone stimulated sodium transport and inhibited potassium excretion. These effects were attributed to direct stimulation of this activity in the basolateral membranes of rabbit kidney by physiological doses of insulin.

Antidiuretic hormone is known for its effects on sodium reabsorption by the thick ascending limb of Henle's loop, and on the water permeability of the collecting tubule. On the basis of the fundamental part played by Na-K-ATPase in sodium transport along the thick ascending limb, Bayliss and colleagues recently proposed that the pump might be stimulated by vasopressin.[312] In their challenging work, these authors demonstrated that when whole kidney is exposed to vasopressin, Na-K-ATPase activity, measured by cytomicrodensitometry,[313] is specifically stimulated in the thick ascending limb. According to them, this activity rises when the dose of vasopressin varies from 2.10^{-15} to 2.10^{-12}M, and the maximal increase observed corresponds to an 80% enhancement of basal Na-K-ATPase activity. The molecular process underlying this vasopressin stimulation is not known.

C - PHYSIOPATHOLOGICAL ALTERATIONS IN Na-K-ATPase ACTIVITY

Alterations in renal Na-K-ATPase activity have been described under many different physiological or pathological conditions. Some are adaptive— for instance, those observed during renal compensatory hypertrophy or after adaptation to diets with modified cation or protein content. Other variations have been attributed to the genetic alterations in Na-K-AT-Pase expression that might accompany or cause certain types of pathology, such as hypertension or diabetes.

1 - Adaptation to Changes in Dietary Cation Intake

Adaptation to chronic alterations in dietary salt intake involves changes in the renal mechanisms of ionic transport. Thus, it has been shown that animals survived chronic potassium loading by increasing their urinary potassium excretion.[33, 144–146, 314] Micropuncture studies suggest that the terminal part of the nephron is responsible for adjusting cation excretion to altered cation intake.[315–318] However, these processes have only been precisely localized in isolated nephron segments. Furthermore, changes in sodium or potassium intake alter the level of plasma mineralocorticoids, which in turn can modify renal Na-K-ATPase activity. It is necessary, therefore, to dissociate the primary effects of cations from those of aldosterone.

The involvement of Na-K-ATPase in renal adaptation to altered potassium intake was suggested on the basis of experiments indicating that Na-K-ATPase activity in kidney homogenates was stimulated in chronically potassium-loaded animals[140, 148, 149] and that ouabain abolished the hypersecretion of potassium by these animals.[140] Studies on isolated nephron segments from potassium-loaded mice showed that Na-K-ATPase activity was stimulated in the collecting tubule only.[243] More recently, Garg and colleagues[109] showed that Na-K-ATPase activity in the rat collecting tubule specifically decreased during potassium depletion. These results contradict both those of Fine and colleagues,[319] who observed no alteration in Na-K-ATPase activity in the collecting tubule of potassium-loaded rabbits, and those of Linas and colleagues,[320] who observed stimulation of pump activity in the renal medulla of potassium-depleted rats.

Several arguments indicate that the changes in Na-K-ATPase during potassium adaptation occur independently of alterations in plasma aldosterone: First, the changes in the aldosterone level are moderate[243] compared to those observed, for example, after sodium depletion.[239] Second, as Silva et al. showed,[321] Na-K-ATPase activity can be stimulated in adrenalectomized potassium-loaded animals. And finally, administration of pharmacological doses of spironolactone does not affect the stimulation of Na-K-ATPase activity in the collecting tubule of potassium-adapted mice.[243]

Rodriguez and colleagues[149] have shown that stimulation of pump activity during this adaptation was due to an increase in the number of catalytic units. In addition, Evan et al.[322] reported a morphogenic effect on the principal cells of the collecting tubule, which displayed abnormal amplification of the basolateral membrane during potassium adaptation. The mechanisms governing these different alterations are not known.

In order to characterize the respective roles of aldosterone and of the sodium and potassium loads in the adaptive stimulation of renal Na-K-ATPase, Le Hir, Kaissling, and Du-Bach[108, 288] used an experimental protocol in which any changes in the plasma aldosterone of rabbits caused by a high K^+ and low Na^+ diet or the reverse were counterbalanced either by administering an antimineralocorticoid (e.g. potassium canrenoate) or by the injection of DOCA. These authors studied the resulting cell morphology (i.e., the amplification of the basolateral membrane) and the Na-K-ATPase activity in the distal segments of the rabbit nephron (DCT, CNT, and CCT). Their results suggest that, as already proposed, only the CCT is sensitive to mineralocorticoids, whereas all three segments respond to potassium loading. Their findings also indicate that the DCT responds more specifically to changes in sodium intake. Furthermore, there is perfect coordination between the factors that amplify the basolateral membrane and stimulate Na-K-ATPase activity, respectively.

2 - Renal Compensatory Hypertrophy

The effect of unilateral nephrectomy on the functioning of the remaining kidney and the resulting hypertrophy were described a long time ago.[323] Katz and Epstein[280] observed that after contralateral nephrectomy the glomerular filtration rate, sodium reabsorption, and Na-K-ATPase activity of a cortical microsomal fraction, expressed per g of tissue, increased gradually and concomitantly. In the rat, stimulation of Na-K-AT-Pase activity was also observed in microsomal fractions of medulla[324] and whole kidney homogenates[325] following unilateral nephrectomy, and in medullary homogenates after 75% reduction of the renal mass.[326]

Micropuncture studies[327] indicate that the sodium reabsorption capacity of proximal and distal tubules increases after unilateral nephrectomy. However, under these conditions, each structure behaves differently, because distal cells are less hypertrophied than proximal ones and take on proportionally higher additional work. Starting from this observation, Schmidt and Dubach[328] measured the Na-K-ATPase activity in proximal and distal convoluted tubules of heminephrectomized rats. Their results indicate that in the distal convoluted tubule, Na-K-ATPase activity is stimulated as early as the first day after surgery, whereas it takes about one week for a significant increase in this activity to appear in the proximal convoluted tubule. This finding suggests that adaptation to nephrectomy is controlled by separate mechanisms in the distal and proximal tubules. Here again, the nature of these mechanisms is not known.

In a recent study, Jacobsen et al.[329] showed that Na-K-ATPase stimulation after reduction of the renal mass was due to an increase in the number of catalytic units.

3 - Na-K-ATPase and Hypertension

Hypertensive subjects excrete sodium faster than normal subjects in response to infusion of hypertonic NaCl.[330] The same excessive natriuresis is observed in hypertensive rats.[331] Although the inhibition of renal Na-K-ATPase activity seems a logical explanation for this response, curiously, only a few studies in the literature have established any connection between hypertension and the renal pump (Table 9).

Malyusz et al.[332] were the first to report reduced Na-K-ATPase activity in the renal microsomal fractions of animals with Goldblatt's hypertension. Postnov and colleagues[333] confirmed this information for the medulla of the unclamped kidney, and also observed a decline in Na-K-ATPase activity in the outer medulla of spontaneously hypertensive adult rats. Young rats that were either prehypertensive or in an early stage of hyper-

TABLE 9:—Kidney Na-K-ATPase in Different Models of Hypertension in the Rat

MODEL	AGE	EXPERIMENTAL CONDITIONS		Na-K-ATPase	REFERENCE
Goldblatt's hypertension		Normal diet	Microsomes		Malyusz et al.[332]
Goldblatt's hypertension	8–11 weeks of treatment	''	Cortical and medullary microsomes	medulla	Postnov et al.[333]
Rats Kyoto vs. Wistar strain	6–8 weeks / 16–30 weeks	'' / '		No difference medulla	'' / ''
SHR vs. Wistar	?	''	Outermedullary homogenates		Dzurba et al.[334]
Normo and hypertensive Lyon	48 weeks	''	Outermedullary and Cortical homogenates	No difference	Biol et al.[335]
Okamoto vs. Wistar	16 weeks	''	Whole kidney Microsomes	No difference	Rodriguez-Sargent et al.[336]
	16 weeks	Na^+ depleted diet	''	No difference	
Normo and hypertensive Dahl	16 weeks	Normal diet	''		''
	16 weeks	Na^+ depleted diet	''		''
Normo and hypertensive Kyoto	10–12 weeks / 25 weeks	Normal diet / ''	Cortical and medullary homogenates	No difference cortex	Slegers, Forster[338]
Normo and hypertensive Sabra	10–12 weeks / 10–12 weeks	'' / Na^+ rich diet	Isolated tubules / ''	No difference / ''	Doucet et al.[337]

tension displayed no alteration in their renal Na-K-ATPase. Dzurba et al.[334] also observed reduced Na-K-ATPase activity in the renal medulla of spontaneously hypertensive rats, but did not state the age of these animals. On the other hand, Biol et al.[335] found no difference in the renal pump activity of spontaneously hypertensive rats of the "Lyon" strain compared to the activity in normal rats. This last result was confirmed by Rodriguez-Sargent et al.[336] in "Okamoto" hypertensive rats and by ourselves[337] in "Sabra" rats on normal or high sodium diets.

In a recent study, Slegers and Forster[338] showed that spontaneously hypertensive "Kyoto" rats already exhibited disturbed sodium excretion at the age of 10–12 weeks, at a time when they were hypertensive but their renal Na-K-ATPase had not changed. Only at 25 weeks did these authors observe reduced cortical Na-K-ATPase activity.

These results indicate that the development of essential hypertension is clearly dissociated from the decline in renal Na-K-ATPase since, in the first place, normal renal Na-K-ATPase was observed in spontaneously hypertensive rats of the Okamoto, Lyon, and Sabra strains, and secondly, in the strains displaying altered renal Na-K-ATPase (Dahl and Kyoto rats), the changes always came after the alteration in cation excretion and the development of hypertension. These results imply that hypertension is not due to a genetic alteration in Na-K-ATPase, nor by a dysfunction of the pump.

The data reported above were obtained by measuring Na-K-ATPase activity in vitro under optimal conditions. Consequently, they do not rule out the possibility that the "natriuretic hormone" might help to alter the functioning of the pump in vivo.

D - Development and Maturation of Renal Na-K-ATPase

1 - Pre- and Postnatal Development of Na-K-ATPase

Nature has provided an experimental model permitting the relationship between renal Na-K-ATPase and cation transport to be studied during kidney development. Since the development of kidney structure and function is centrifugal,[339] there is a certain degree of heterogeneity in that of individual nephrons.[340] Therefore, the study of renal growth brings to light the problems involved in locating and identifying the stage of evolution reached by the structures under study. The complexity of renal development processes probably explains the small number of studies dealing with this problem.

In an early work, Geloso and Basset[341] measured the Na-K-ATPase activity in rat kidney during fetal development. Their results indicated that pump activity, expressed per mg of proteins, remains low for the first 18 days of gestation, and that marked stimulation occurs between the 19th and the 20th days. In the newborn rat, Na-K-ATPase activity is about 40% of that measured in adult animals.

Postnatal phases of development were studied in the rat by Aperia et al.[342] and in the rabbit by Schmidt and Horster.[103] Aperia and colleagues[342] measured the Na-K-ATPase activity in the superficial cortex of 10-, 20-, and 40-day-old rats. Their tissue preparation comprised the most superficial 150 μm of the cortex and consisted of proximal convoluted tubules for 70%. Na-K-ATPase activity per mg of proteins was found to increase steadily for 10–40 days, when it became maximal. Maturation of the renal sodium pump exhibited the same time dependency as the development of the basolateral membrane and of the water reabsorption capacity of the proximal tubule.[343]

In the rabbit, Schmidt and Horster[103] measured the Na-K-ATPase activity in segments of proximal convoluted tubule, cortical, and medullary thick ascending limb, and collecting tubules, isolated from 2- to 5-day-old or adult rabbits. Their results indicate that Na-K-ATPase activity (expressed per kg of dry weight) displays the same distribution pattern along the nephrons of newborn and adult rabbits, and is 2–5 times higher in the latter. When these results are expressed per unit of length, the difference between the adult and newborn animals is greater. Since the substrate Km values are similar in both groups, the higher activity in adult animals is accounted for by a larger number of catalytic units. The results for the proximal tubule agree with the morphological and physiological data. Thus, the 2.6-fold expansion in the surface area of the basolateral membrane described for this segment in adults compared to neonates[344] is comparable to the 3.3-fold stimulation of Na-K-ATPase. Similarly, the NaCl reabsorption rate in proximal tubule is three times lower in neonate than adult rabbits.[345]

2 - Control of Development

Only the role of corticosteroids has been studied during the pre- and postnatal development of Na-K-ATPase.

In the rat fetus, Geloso and Basset[341] showed that suppression of adrenocorticoids by adrenalectomy of the mother and administration to the fetuses of metopirone (an antimineralocorticoid that penetrates the placental barrier) abolished the stimulation of Na-K-ATPase activity usually seen at 19 days *post coitum.* Administration of pharmacological doses of aldosterone to these 19-day-old fetuses restored pump activity. Although the gluco- or mineralocorticoid nature of the effect is not clear, these results indicate the important role of adrenocorticoids in the fetal development of renal Na-K-ATPase.

Aperia and colleagues[342] studied the actions of gluco- or mineralocorticoids on the cortical Na-K-ATPase activity of 10- to 40-day-old rats. Administration of either betamethasone or pharmacological doses of aldosterone markedly stimulated Na-K-ATPase activity in 10-, 20-, and 40-day-old animals. This stimulation was not blocked by the antimineralocorticoid canrenone, suggesting that betamethasone and aldosterone acted through the occupancy of glucocorticoid receptors. The results indicate that the Na-K-ATPase of immature proximal tubule cells is very sensitive to hormonal induction, and that this sensitivity persists at advanced stages of development.

Conclusion

The identical nature of Na-K-ATPase and the sodium-potassium pump is now generally accepted. However, despite thorough knowledge of the biochemical properties of this enzyme, the molecular processes underlying cation translocation remain unknown.

The role of Na-K-ATPase in kidney functions has been better understood since it became possible to measure this enzyme in morphologically and functionally defined individual nephron segments. Renal tubular Na-K-ATPase is not only responsible for large fractions of sodium reabsorption and potassium secretion, but it is also involved in other processes that help to ensure homeostasia, such as water reabsorption, control of cell volume, cell polarization, and secondary active transport.

It is now well established that tubular Na-K-ATPase activity can be acutely controlled by environmental parameters, such as sodium, glucocorticoids, mineralocorticoids, etc., thus allowing rapid changes in sodium transport. When environmental restrictions are maintained for long periods, the cell adapts itself by modifying the density of Na-K-ATPase units.

One of the major enigmas concerning Na-K-ATPase is the presence of specific binding sites for digitalis glycosides; these natural substances are not usually present in animal organisms.

REFERENCES

1. Skou J.C.: The influence of some cations on an adenosine triphosphatase from peripheral nerves. *Biochim. Biophys. Acta* 23:394, 1957.
2. Jorgensen P.L.: Isolation and characterization of the components of the sodium pump. *Q. Rev. Biophys.* 7:239, 1975.
3. Perrone J.R., Hackney J.F., Dixon J.F., et al.: Molecular properties of purified Na, K-ATPase and their subunits from the rectal gland of Squalus acanthias and the electric organ of Electrophorus electricus. *J. Biol. Chem.* 250:4178, 1975.
4. Esmann M., Skou J.C., Christiansen C.: Solubilization and molecular weight determination of the Na-K-ATPase from rectal glands of squalus acanthias. *Biochim. Biophys. Acta* 567:410, 1979.
5. Jorgensen P.L.: Isolation of Na,K-ATPase. *Methods Enzymol.* 32B:277, 1974.
6. DeGuchi N., Jorgensen D.L., Maunsbach A.B.: Ultrastructure of the sodium pump. Comparison of thin sectioning, negative staining, and freeze-fracture of purified, membrane bound (Na$^+$,K$^+$)-ATPase. *J. Cell Biol.* 75:619, 1977.
7. Jorgenson P.L.: Purification and characterization of Na,K-ATPase. III. Purification from the outer medulla of mammalian kidney after selective removal of membrane components by sodium dodecylsulfate. *Biochim. Biophys. Acta* 356:36, 1974.
8. Hopkins B.E., Wagner H., Smith J.W.: Na,K-ATPase of the nasal salt gland of the duck. *J. Biol. Chem.* 251:4365, 1976.
9. Goldin S.M.: Active transport of sodium and potassium ions by the sodium and potassium ion-activated adenosine triphosphatase from renal medulla. *J. Biol. Chem.* 252:5630, 1977.
10. Jorgensen P.L.: Mechanism of the Na$^+$,K$^+$ pump. Protein structure and conformations of the pure (Na$^+$+K$^+$)-ATPase. *Biochim. Biophys. Acta.* 694:27, 1982.
11. Peterson G.L., Hokin L.E.: Molecular weight and stoichiometry of the sodium and potassium-activated adenosine triphosphatase units. *J. Biol. Chem.* 256:3751, 1981.
12. Smith T.W., Wagner H., Jr.: Effects of (Na$^+$+K$^+$)-ATPase specific antibodies on enzymatic activity and monovalent cation transport. *J. Membr. Biol.* 25:341, 1975.
13. Jorgensen P.L., Hansen O., Glynn I.M., et al.: Antibodies to pig kidney Na,K-ATPase inhibit the Na-pump in human red cells provided they have access to the inner surface of the cell membrane. *Biochim. Biophys. Acta* 291:795, 1973.
14. McCans J.L., Lindenmayer G.E., Pitts B. Jr., et al.: Antigenic differences in (Na$^+$,K$^+$) ATPase preparations isolated from various organs and species. *J. Biol. Chem.* 250:7257, 1975.
15. Jorgensen P.L.: Purification and characterization of Na,K-ATPase. IV. Estima-

tion of the purity and of the molecular weight and polypeptide content per enzyme unit in preparation from the outer medulla of rabbit kidney. *Biochim. Biophys. Acta.* 356:53, 1974.

16. Kyte J.: Properties of the two polypeptides of Na,K-ATPase. *J. Biol. Chem.* 247:7642, 1972.

17. Jorgensen P.L.: Purification and characterization of Na,K-ATPase. VI. Differential tryptic modification of catalytic functions of the purified enzyme in presence of NaCl and KCl. *Biochim. Biophys. Acta.* 466:97, 1977.

18. Jorgensen P.L., Anner B.M.: Purification and characterization of Na,K-ATPase. VIII. Altered Na:K transport ratio in vesicles reconstituted with purified Na,K-ATPase that has been selectively modified with trypsin in presence of NaCl. *Biochim. Biophys. Acta* 555:485, 1979.

18a. Hegyvary C., Post R.L.: Binding of adenosine triphosphate to sodium and potassium ion-stimulated adenosine triphosphate. *J. Biol. Chem.* 246:5234, 1971.

18b. Matsui H., Schwartz A.: Purification and properties of a highly active ouabain sensitive Na^+, K^+-dependent adenosine triphosphatase from cardiac tissue. *Biochim. Biophys. Acta.* 128:380, 1966.

18c. Schoner W., Von Ilberg C., Kramer R., et al.: On the mechanism of Na^+ and K^+ stimulated hydrolysis of adenosine triphosphate. I. Purification and properties of a Na^+ and K^+-activated ATPase from ox brain. *Eur. J. Biochem.* 1:334, 1967.

19. Robinson J.D.: Nucleotide and divalent cation interactions with the $(Na^+ + K^+)$-dependent ATPase. *Biochim. Biophys. Acta* 341:232, 1974.

20. Robinson J.D.: Substrate sites of the $(Na^+ + K^+)$-dependent ATPase. *Biochim. Biophys. Acta* 429:1006, 1976.

21. Post R.L., Hegyvary C., Kume S.: Activation by adenosine triphosphate in the phosphorylation kinetics of sodium and potassium ion transport adenosine triphosphatase. *J. Biol. Chem.* 247:6530, 1972.

22. Dahl J.L., Hokin L.E.: The sodium-potassium adenosine triphosphatase. *Annu. Rev. Biochem.* 43:327, 1974.

23. Bonting S.L.: Sodium-potassium activated adenosine triphosphatase and cation transport. Bittar E.E. (ed.): In *Membranes and Ion Transport* (London: Wiley Interscience, vol. 1, pp. 257–363, 1970).

24. Jorgensen P.L.: Sodium and potassium ion pump in kidney tubules. *Physiol. Rev.* 60:864, 1980.

25. Dunham P.B., Senyk O.: Lithium efflux through the Na/K pump in human erythrocytes. *Proc. Natl. Acad. Sci. USA* 74:3099, 1977.

26. Schwartz A., Lindenmayer G.E., Allen J.C.: The sodium-potassium adenosine triphosphatase: pharmacological, physiological and biochemical aspects. *Pharmacol. Rev.* 27:1, 1975.

27. Schuurmans-Stekhoven F., Bonting S.L.: Transport adenosine triphosphatases: Properties and functions. *Physiol. Rev.* 61:1, 1981.

27a. Schatzmann H.J.: Active calcium transport and Ca^{2+}-activated ATPase in human red cells. *Curr. Top. Membr. Transp.* 6:125, 1975.

28. Ganser A.L., Forte J.G.: K^+-stimulated ATPase in purified microsomes of bullfrog oxynthic cells. *Biochim. Biophys. Acta.* 307:169, 1973.

29. Kasbekar D.H., Durbin R.P., Lindley D.: An adenosine triphosphatase from frog gastric mucosa. *Biochim. Biophys. Acta* 105:472, 1965.

30. Hoffman J.F.: The red cell membrane and the transport of sodium and potassium. *Am. J. Med.* 41:666, 1966.

31. Hansen O., Jensen J., Norby J.G.: Mutual exclusion of ATP, ADP and g-strophanthin binding to NaK-ATPase. *Nature* 234:122, 1971.

32. Sen A.K., Tobin T., Post R.L.: A cycle for ouabain inhibition of sodium- and potassium-dependent adenosine triphosphatase. *J. Biol. Chem.* 244:6596, 1969.

33. Skou J.C., Butler K.W., Hansen O.: The effect of magnesium, ATP, Pi, and so-

dium on the inhibition of the $(Na^+ + K^+)$-activated enzyme system by g-strophantin. *Biochim. Biophys. Acta* 241:443, 1971.

34. Van Winkle W.B., Allen J.C., Schwartz A.: The nature of the transport ATPase-digitalis complex. III. Rapid binding studies and effects of ligands on the formation and stability of magnesium phosphate-induced glycoside-enzyme complex. *Arch. Biochem. Biophys.* 151:85, 1972.

35. Hansen O., Skou J.C.: A study on the influence of the concentration of Mg^{2+}, Pi, K^+, Na^+, and Tris on $(Mg^{2+} + Pi)$-supported g-strophanthin binding to $(Na^+ + K^+)$-activated ATPase from ox brain. *Biochim. Biophys. Acta* 311:51, 1973.

36. Tobin T., Brody T.M.: Rates of dissociation of enzyme-ouabain complexes and $K_{0.5}$ values in $(Na^+ + K^+)$adenosine triphosphatase from different species. *Biochem. Pharmacol.* 21:1553, 1972.

37. Tobin T., Henderson R., Sen A.K.: Species and tissue differences in the rate of dissociation of ouabain from $(Na^+ + K^+)$-ATPase. *Biochim. Biophys. Acta* 274:551, 1972.

38. Erdmann E., Schoner W.: Ouabain-receptor interactions in $(Na^+ + K^+)$-ATPase preparations from different tissues and species. Determination of kinetic constants and dissociation constants. *Biochim. Biophys. Acta.* 307:386, 1973.

39. Schwartz K., Milne D.B.: Growth effects of vanadium in the rat. *Science* 174:426, 1971.

40. Charney A.N., Silva P., Epstein F.H.: An in vitro inhibition of Na-K-ATPase present in adenosine triphosphate preparation. *J. Appl. Physiol.* 39:156, 1975.

41. Josephson L., Cantley L.C.: Isolation of a potent (Na-K)ATPase inhibitor from striated muscle. *Biochemistry* 16:4572, 1977.

42. Beauge L., Glynn I.M.: A modified of $(Na^+ + K^+)$ ATPase in commercial ATP. *Nature* 268:355, 1977.

43. Hudgins P.M., Bond G.H.: $(Mg^{2+} + K^+)$-dependent inhibition of Na,K-ATPase due to a contaminant in equine muscle ATP. *Biochem. Biophys. Res. Commun.* 77:1024, 1977.

44. Cantley L.C., Josephson L., Warner R., et al.: Vanadate is a potent $(Na^+ + K^+)$ATPase inhibitor found in ATP derived from muscle. *J. Biol. Chem.* 252:7421, 1977.

45. Nechay B.R., Saunders J.P.: Inhibition by vanadium of sodium and potassium dependent adenosine triphosphatase derived from animal and human tissues. *J. Environ. Pathol. Toxicol.* 2:247, 1978.

46. Beauge L.A., Cavieres J.D., Glynn I.M., et al.: The effects of vanadate on the fluxes of sodium and potassium ions through the sodium pump. *J. Physiol.* 301:7, 1980.

47. Beauge L., Glynn I.M.: Commercial ATP containing traces of vanadate alters the response of $(Na^+ + K^+)$ATPase to external potassium. *Nature* 272:551, 1978.

48. Bond G.H., Hudgins P.M.: Kinetics of inhibition of Na-K-ATPase by Mg^{2+}, K^+, and vanadate. *Biochemistry* 18:325, 1979.

49. Grantham J.J., Glynn I.M.: Renal Na-K-ATPase: Determinants of inhibition by vanadium. *Am. J. Physiol.* 236:F530, 1979.

50. Karlish S.J.D., Beauge L.A., Glynn I.M.: Vanadate inhibits $(Na^+ + K^+)$ATPase by blocking a conformation change of the unphosphorylated pump. *Nature* 282:333, 1979.

51. Cantley L.C., Jr., Resh M.D., Guidotti G.: Vanadate inhibits the red cell $(Na^+ + K^+)$ATPase from the cytoplasmic side. *Nature* 272:552, 1978.

52. Cantley L.C., Jr., Cantley L.G., Josephson L.: A characterization of vanadate interactions with the $(Na^+ + K^+)$ATPase. *J. Biol. Chem.* 253:7361, 1968.

53. Hansen O.: Facilitation of ouabain binding to $(Na^+ + K^+)$ATPase by vanadate at in vitro concentrations. *Biochim. Biophys. Acta.* 568:265, 1979.

54. Myers T.D., Boerth R.C., Post R.L.: Effects of vanadate on ouabain binding and inhibition of (Na$^+$ + K$^+$)ATPase. *Biochim. Biophys. Acta.* 558:99, 1979.

55. Wallick E.T., Lane L.K., Schwartz A.: Regulation by vanadate of ouabain binding to (Na$^+$+K$^+$)ATPase. *J. Biol. Chem.* 254:8107, 1979.

56. Caveries J.D.: The sodium pump in human red cells. Ellory J.E., Lew V.L. (eds.): In *Membrane Transport in Red Cells* (New York: Academic Press, p. 1, 1977).

57. Karlish S.J.D., Yates D.W., Glynn I.M.: Elementary steps of the (Na$^+$+K$^+$)ATPase mechanism, studied with formycin nucleotides. *Biochim. Biophys. Acta.* 525:230, 1978.

58. Post R.L., Kume S., Tobin T., et al.: Flexibility of an active center in sodium-plus- potassium adenosine triphosphatase. *J. Gen. Physiol.* 54:306s, 1969.

59. Albers R.W.: Biochemical aspects of active transport. *Annu. Rev. Biochem.* 36:727, 1967.

60. Glynn I.M., Karlish S.J.D.: The sodium pump. *Annu. Rev. Physiol.* 37:13, 1975.

61. Kyte J.: Molecular considerations relevant to the mechanism of active transport. *Nature* 292:201, 1981.

62. Levitt D.G.: The mechanism of the sodium pump. *Biochim. Biophys. Acta* 604:321, 1980.

63. Karlish S.J.D., Yates D.W., Glynn I.M.: Conformational transitions between Na$^+$-bound and K$^+$-bound forms of (Na$^+$+K$^+$)ATPase, studied with formycin nucleotides. *Biochim. Biophys. Acta.* 525:252, 1978.

64. Robinson J.D., Flashner M.S.: (Na$^+$+K$^+$)-activated ATPase enzymatic and transport properties. *Biochim. Biophys. Acta.* 549:145, 1979.

65. Albers R.W.: The sodium plus potassium transport ATPase in the enzymes of biological membranes. *Enzymes Biol. Membr.* 3:283, 1976.

66. Dunham P.B., Hoffman J.F.: Na and K transport in red blood cells. Andreoli T.E., Hoffman J.F., Fanestil D.D. (eds.): In *Physiology of Membrane Disorders* (New York: Publishing Corps., pp. 255–272, 1978).

67. Hoffman J.F., Kaplan J.H., Callahan T.J.: The Na:K pump in red cells is electrogenic. *Fed. Proc.* 38:2440, 1979.

67a. Anner B.M., Lane L.K., Schwartz A., et al.: A reconstituted Na, K-pump in liposomes containing purified Na-K-ATPase from kidney medulla. *Biochim. Biophys. Acta.* 467:340, 1977.

68. Anner B.M.: Reconstitution of the Na-K-transport system in artificial membranes. *Acta Physiol. Scand.* (Suppl.) 1980.

69. De Weer P.: Aspects of the recovery processes in nerve. Hunt C.C. (ed.): In *MTP Int. Rev. Sci., Physiol. Ser.: Neurophysiology* (Baltimore: University Park Press, vol. 3, pp. 231–278, 1975).

70. Hilden S., Hokin L.E.: Active potassium transport coupled to active sodium transport in vesicles reconstituted from purified Na,K-ATPase from rectal gland of Squalus acanthias. *J. Biol. Chem.* 250:6296, 1975.

71. Hokin L.E., Dixon I.F.: Parameters of reconstituted Na$^+$ and K$^+$ transport in liposomes in which purified Na,K-ATPase is incorporated by "freeze-thaw-sonication". Skou I.C., Norby J.G. (eds.): In *Sodium, Potassium-ATPase: Structure and Kinetics* (New York: Academic Press, pp. 47–67, 1979).

72. Garrahan P.J., Glynn I.M.: Driving the sodium pump backwards to form adenosine triphosphate. *Nature* 211:1414, 1966.

73. Garrahan P.J., Glynn I.M.: The incorporation of inorganic phosphate into adenosine triphosphate by reversal of the sodium pump. *J. Physiol.* 192:237, 1967.

74. Ling G.N., Neguendank W.: Do isolated membranes and purified vesicles pump sodium? A critical review and reinterpretation. *Perspect. Biol. Med.* 23:215, 1980.

75. Post R.L., Sen A.K.: ^{32}P-labelling of a (Na$^+$+K$^+$)-ATPase intermediate. *Methods Enzymol.* 10:773, 1967.

76. Schuurmans-Stekhoven F.M.A.H., Van Heeswijk M.P.E., De Pont J.J.H.H.M., et

al.: Studies on $(Na^+ + K^+)$-activated ATPase. XXXVIII. A 100,000 molecular weight protein as the low energy phosphorylated intermediate of the enzyme. *Biochim. Biophys. Acta* 422:210, 1976.

77. Baker P.F., Willis J.S.: Binding of the cardiac glycoside ouabain to intact cells. *J. Physiol. (Lond.)* 224:441, 1972.

78. Clausen T., Hansen O.: Ouabain binding and Na-K-transport in rat muscle cells and adipocyte. *Biochim. Biophys. Acta.* 345:387, 1974.

79. Hansen O., Jensen J., Norby J.G., et al.: A new proposal regarding the subunit composition of Na,K-ATPase. *Nature* 280:410, 1979.

80. Hossler F.E., Sarras M.P., Barrnett R.J.: Ouabain binding during plasma membrane biogenesis in duck salt gland. *J. Cell Sci.* 31:179, 1978.

81. Zubler-Faivre L., Dunant Y.: Na,K-ATPase of electric organ: Interaction with ouabain in situ, in a membrane fraction and in solubilized form. *Mol. Pharmacol.* 12:1007, 1976.

82. Hansen O.: The relationship between g-strophanthin-binding capacity and ATPase activity in plasma membrane fragments from ox brain. *Biochim. Biophys. Acta.* 233:122, 1971.

83. Ernst S.A.: Transport adenosine triphosphatase cytochemistry. *J. Histochem. Cytochem.* 20:23, 1972.

84. Ernst S.A.: Transport ATPase cytochemistry: Ultrastructural localization of K-dependent and K-independent phosphatase activities in rat kidney cortex. *J. Cell Biol.* 66:586, 1975.

85. Wachstein M., Meisel E.: Histochemistry of hepatic phosphatase at a physiologic pH. *Am. J. Clin. Pathol.* 27:13, 1957.

86. Maunsbach A.B.: The influence of different fixatives and fixation methods on the ultrastructure of rat kidney proximal tubule cells. I. Comparison of different perfusion fixation methods and of glutaraldehyde, formaldehyde and osmium tetroxide fixation. *J. Ultrastruct. Res.* 15:242, 1966.

87. Guth L., Albers R.W.: Histochemical demonstration of Na-K-ATPase. *J. Histochem. Cytochem.* 22:320, 1974.

88. Kyte J.: Immunoferritin determination of the distribution of Na,K-ATPase over the plasma membrane of renal convoluted tubules. I. Distal segment. *J. Cell Biol.* 68:287, 1976.

89. Kyte J.: Immunoferritin determination of the distribution of Na,K-ATPase over the plasma membranes of renal convoluted tubules. II. Proximal segment. *J. Cell Biol.* 68:304, 1976.

90. Kinne R., Schmitz I.E., Kinne-Saffran E.: The localization of the Na,K-ATPase in the cells of rat kidney cortex: A study on isolated plasma membranes. *Pflügers Arch.* 329:191, 1971.

91. Schmidt U., Dubach U.C.: Na K stimulated adenosine triphosphatase: Intracellular localization within the proximal tubule of the rat nephron. *Pflügers Arch.* 330:265, 1971.

92. Jacobson H.R.: Functional segmentation of the mammalian nephron. *Am. J. Physiol.* 241:F203, 1981.

93. Morel F., Chabardes S., Imbert M.: Functional segmentation of the rabbit distal tubule by microdetermination of hormone-dependent adenylate cyclase activity. *Kidney Int.* 9:264, 1976.

94. Woodhall P.B., Tisher C.C.: Response of the distal tubule and cortical collecting duct to vasopressin in the rat. *J. Clin. Invest.* 52:3095, 1973.

95. Burg M.B.: Renal handling of sodium chloride. Brenner B.M., Rector F.C. (eds.): In *The Kidney* (Philadelphia: W.B. Saunders Co., vol. 1, pp. 272–298, 1976).

96. Burg M., Grantham J., Abramov M., et al.: Preparation and study of fragments of single rabbit nephrons. *Am. J. Physiol.* 210:1293, 1966.

97. Schmidt U., DuBach U.C.: Activity of (Na^+K^+)-stimulated adenosine triphosphatase in rat nephron. *Pflügers Arch.* 306:219, 1969.

98. Schmidt U., Horster M.: Sodium-potassium-activated adenosine triphosphatase: Methodology for quantification in microdissected renal tubule segments from freeze-dried and fresh tissue. Martinez-Maldonado M. (ed.): In *Methods in Pharmacology* (New-York: Publishing Corp., vol. 4B, pp. 259–296, 1978).

99. Lowry O.H., Passoneau J.V.: A flexible system of enzyme analysis. New York : Academic Press, 1972.

100. Ashton K., Koepsell H.: Measurement of Na-K-ATPase activity in segments of proximal tubules from superficial and juxtamedullary rat nephrons during antidiuresis. *Pflügers Arch.* 363:251, 1976.

101. Schmidt U., DuBach U.C.: Sensitivity of Na K adenosine triphosphatase activity in various structures of the rat nephron: Studies with adrenalectomy. *Eur. J. Clin. Invest.* 1:307, 1971.

102. Schmidt U., Schmid J., Schmid H., et al.: Sodium-and-potassium activated ATPase: A possible target of aldosterone. *J. Clin. Invest.* 55:655, 1975.

103. Schmidt U., Horster M.: Na-K-activated ATPase : Activity maturation in rabbit nephron segments dissected in vitro. *Am. J. Physiol.* 233:F55, 1977.

104. Petty K.J., Kokko J.P., Marver D.: Secondary effect of aldosterone on Na-K-ATPase activity in the rabbit cortical collecting tubule. *J. Clin. Invest.* 68:1514, 1981.

105. Doucet A., Katz A.I., Morel F.: Determination of Na-K-ATPase activity in single segments of the mammalian nephron. *Am. J. Physiol.* 237:F105, 1979.

106. Doucet A., Chabardes D., Imbert-Teboul M., et al.: Enzyme activity measurement in single nephron segments as an approach to physiological problems. Procedure of the 8th Int. Congr. Nephrol., Athens, 1981, pp. 958–964.

107. Garg L.C., Knepper M.A., Burg M.B.: Mineralocorticoid effects on Na-K-ATPase in individual nephron segments. *Am. J. Physiol.* 240:F536, 1981.

108. Le Hir M., Kaissling B., DuBach U.C.: Analysis of distal segment in the rabbit kidney tubule after adaptation to altered Na- and K-intake. II. Changes in Na-K-ATPase activity. *Cell Tissue Res.* 224:493, 1982.

109. Garg L.C., Mackie S., Tisher C.C.: Effect of low-potassium diet on Na-K-ATPase in rat nephron segments. *Pflügers Arch.* 394:113, 1982.

110. Katz A.I., Doucet A., Morel F.: Na-K-ATPase activity along the rabbit, rat, and mouse nephron. *Am. J. Physiol.* 237:F114, 1979.

111. Shaver J.L.F., Stirling C.: Ouabain binding to renal tubules of the rabbit. *J. Cell. Biol.* 76:278, 1978.

112. McDonough A.A., Hiatt A., Edelman I.S.: Characteristics of antibodies to guinea pig $(Na^+ + K^+)$-adenosine triphosphatase and their use in cell-free synthesis studies. *J. Membr. Biol.* 69:13, 1982.

112a. Girardet M., Geering K., Frantes J.M., et al.: Immunochemical evidence for a transmembrane orientation of both the (Na^+, K^+)-ATPase subunits. *Biochemistry* 20:6684, 1981.

113. Geering K., Girardet M., Bron C., et al.: Hormonal regulation of (Na^+, K^+)-ATPase biosynthesis in the toad bladder. Effect of aldosterone and 3,5,3′-triiodo-L-thyronine. *J. Biol. Chem.* 257:10338, 1982.

114. Geering K., Rossier B.C.: Purification and characterization of $(Na^+ + K^+)$ATPase from toad kidney. *Biochim. Biophys. Acta.* 556:157, 1979.

115. Nechay B.R.: Relationship between inhibition of renal Na, K-ATPase and natriuresis. *Ann. NY Acad. Sci.* 242:501, 1974.

116. Nelson J.A., Nechay B.R.: Effects of cardiac glycosides on renal adenosine triphosphatase activity and Na^+ reabsorption in dogs. *J. Pharmacol. Exp. Ther.* 175:727, 1980.

117. Robinson J.W.L., Mirkovitch V., Sepulveda F.V.: A comparison of the effects of ouabain and ethacrynic acid on the dog kidney in vivo and in vitro. *Pflügers Arch.* 371:9, 1977.

118. Sejersted O., Mathisen O., Kiil F.: Oxygen requirement of renal Na,K-ATPase dependent sodium reabsorption. *Am. J. Physiol.* 232:F152, 1977.
119. Vandewalle A., Wirthensohn G., Heidrich H.-G., et al.: Distribution of hexokinase and phosphoenolpyruvate carboxykinase along the rabbit nephron. *Am. J. Physiol.* 240:F492, 1981.
120. Saita H., Nishida H., Monma Y., et al.: Intrarenal distribution and ATPase inhibiting activity of ouabain in dogs. *Jpn. J. Pharmacol.* 26:171, 1976.
121. Torelli G., Milla E., Faelli A., et al.: Energy requirement for sodium reabsorption in the in vivo rabbit kidney. *Am. J. Physiol.* 211:576, 1966.
122. Epstein F.H., Silva P.: Role of sodium, potassium-ATPase in renal function. *Ann. NY Acad. Sci.* 242:519, 1974.
123. Besarab A., Silva P., Epstein F.H.: Multiple pumps for sodium reabsorption by the perfused kidney. *Kidney Int.* 10:147, 1976.
124. Kleinzeller A., Knotkova A.: The effect of ouabain on the electrolyte and water transport in kidney cortex and liver slices. *J. Physiol.* 175:172, 1964.
125. Ross B., Leaf A., Silva P., et al.: Na-K-ATPase in sodium transport by the perfused rat kidney. *Am. J. Physiol.* 226:624, 1974.
126. Whittembury G., Proverbio F.: Two modes of Na extrusion in cells from guinea pig kidney cortex slices. *Pflügers Arch.* 316:1, 1970.
127. Torretti J., Hendler E., Weinstein E., et al.: Functional significance of the Na-K-ATPase in the kidney: Effects of ouabain inhibition. *Am. J. Physiol.* 222:1398, 1972.
128. Balfour W.E., Grantham J.J., Glynn I.M.: Vanadate stimulated natriuresis in the rat. *Nature* 275:768, 1978.
129. Day H.A., Grantham J.J.: Effect of vanadate on renal tubular sodium and water reabsorption in conscious rats. *Clin. Res.* 27:413A, 1979.
130. Day H., Middendorf D., Lukert B., et al.: The renal response to intravenous vanadate in rats. *J. Lab. Clin. Med.* 96:382, 1980.
131. Higashi Y., Bello Rouss E · Effects of sodium orthovanadate on whole kidney and single nephron function. *Kidney Int.* 18:302, 1980.
132. Kumar A., Corder C.N.: Diuretic and vasoconstrictor effects of sodium orthovanadate on the isolated perfused rat kidney. *J. Pharmacol. Exp. Ther.* 213:85, 1980.
133. Westenfelder C., Hamburger R.K., Garcia M.E.: Effect of vanadate on renal tubular function in rats. *Am. J. Physiol.* 240:F522, 1981.
134. Jorgensen P.L.: Regulation of the $(Na^+ + K^+)$-activated ATP hydrolyzing enzyme system in rat kidney. II. The effect of aldosterone on the activity in kidneys of adrenalectomized rats. *Biochim. Biophys. Acta.* 192:326, 1969.
135. Cohen J.J., Kamm D.E.: Renal metabolism: Relation to renal function. Brenner B.M., Rector F.C. (eds.): In *The Kidney* (Philadelphia: W.B. Saunders Co., vol.1, pp.126–214, 1976).
136. Thurau K.: Renal Na-reabsorption and O_2 uptake in dogs during hypoxia and hydrochlorothiazide infusion. *Proc. Soc. Exp. Biol. Med.* 106:714, 1961.
137. Sachs G.: Ion pumps in the renal tubule. *Am. J. Physiol.* 233:F359, 1977.
138. Wilkinson H.L., Deeds D.G., Sullivan L.P., et al.: Effect of ouabain on potassium transport in the perfused bullfrog kidney. *Am. J. Physiol.* 236:F175, 1979.
139. Orloff J., Burg M.: Effect of strophantidin on electrolyte excretion in the chicken. *Am. J. Physiol.* 199:49, 1960.
140. Silva P., Ross B.D., Charney A.N., et al.: Potassium transport by the isolated perfused kidney. *J. Clin. Invest* 56:862, 1975.
141. Wiederholt W., Sullivan W.J., Giebisch G.: Potassium and sodium transport across single distal tubules of Amphiuma. *J. Gen. Physiol.* 57:495, 1971.
142. Duarte C.G., Chomoty F., Giebisch G.: Effect of amiloride, ouabain, and furosemide on distal tubular function in the rat. *Am. J. Physiol.* 221:632, 1971.

143. Strieder N., Khuri R., Wiederholt M., et al.: Studies on the renal action of ouabain in the rat. Effects in the non-diuretic state. *Pflügers Arch.* 349:91, 1974.
144. Berliner R.W., Kennedy T.J., Jr., Hilton J.G.: Renal mechanisms for excretion of potassium. *Am. J. Physiol.* 162:348, 1950.
145. Finkelstein F.O., Hayslett J.P.: Role of medullary structures in the functional adaptation of renal insufficiency. *Kidney Int.* 6:419, 1974.
146. Schon D.A., Silva P., Hayslett J.P.: Mechanism of potassium excretion in renal insufficiency. *Am. J. Physiol.* 227:1323, 1974.
147. Bank N., Aynedjian H.S.: A micropuncture study of potassium excretion by the remnant kidney. *J. Clin. Invest.* 52:1480, 1973.
148. Finkelstein F.O., Hayslett J.P.: Role of medullary Na-K-ATPase in renal potassium adaptation. *Am. J. Physiol.* 229:524, 1975.
149. Rodriguez H.J., Hogan W.C., Hellman R.N., et al.: Mechanism of activation of renal Na^+-K^+-ATPase in the rat: Effects of potassium loading. *Am. J. Physiol.* 238:F315, 1980.
150. Zimmerman K.W.: Zur Morphologie der Epithelzellen der Säugetierniere. *Arch. Mikroskop. Anat.* 78:199, 1911.
151. Tune B., Burg M.: Glucose transport by proximal renal tubules. *Am. J. Physiol.* 221:580, 1971.
152. Bourdeau J.E., Carone F.A.: Protein handling by the renal tubule. *Nephron* 13:22, 1974.
153. Greger R., Lang F., Marchand G., et al.: Site of renal phosphate reabsorption: Micropuncture and microinfusion study. *Pflügers Arch.* 369:111, 1977.
154. Kawamura S., Kokko J.P.: Urea secretion by the straight segment of the proximal tubule. *J. Clin. Invest.* 58:604, 1976.
155. Burg M.B., Orloff J.: Control of fluid absorption in the renal proximal tubule. *J. Clin. Invest.* 47:2016, 1968.
156. Fromter E., Gessner K.: Free flow potential profile along rat kidney proximal tubule. *Pflügers Arch.* 351:69, 1974.
157. Fromter E., Gessner K.: Active transport potentials. Membrane diffusion potentials and streaming potentials across rat kidney proximal tubule. *Pflügers Arch.* 351:85, 1974.
158. Schafer J.A., Patlak C.S., Andeoli T.E.: Fluid absorption and active and passive ion flows in the rabbit superficial pars recta. *Am. J. Physiol.* 233:F154, 1977.
159. Bankir L., de Rouffignac C.: Anatomical and functional heterogeneity of nephrons in the rabbit: Microdissection studies and SNGFR measurements. *Pflügers Arch.* 366:89, 1976.
160. Woodhall P.B., Tisher C.C., Simonton C.A., et al.: Relationship between para-aminohippurate secretion and cellular morphology in rabbit proximal tubules. *J. Clin. Invest.* 61:1320, 1978.
161. Bonvalet J.P., Bencsath P., de Rouffignac C.: Glomerular filtration rate of superficial and deep nephrons during aortic constriction. *J. Physiol.* 222:599, 1972.
162. Horster M., Thurau K.: Micropuncture studies on the filtration rate of single superficial and juxtamedullary glomeruli in the rat kidney. *Arch. Ges. Physiol.* 301:161, 1968.
163. Jacobson H.R.: Characteristics of volume reabsorption in rabbit superficial and juxtamedullary proximal convoluted tubules. *J. Clin. Invest.* 63:410, 1979.
164. Jacobson H.R., Kokko J.P.: Intrinsic differences in various segments of the proximal convoluted tubule. *J. Clin. Invest.* 57:818, 1976.
165. Kawamura S., Imai M., Seldin D.W., et al.: Characteristics of salt and water transport in superficial and juxtamedullary straight segments of proximal tubules. *J. Clin. Invest.* 55:1269, 1975.
166. Mc Keown W.J., Brazy P.C., Dennis V.W.: Intrarenal heterogeneity for fluid phosphate, and glucose absorption in the rabbit. *Am. J. Physiol.* 237:F312, 1979.

167. Fromter E., Rumrich G., Ullrich K.J.: Phenomenologic description of Na^+, and Cl^- and HCO_3^- absorption from proximal tubules of the rat kidney. *Pflügers Arch.* 343:189, 1973.
168. MacKnight A.D.C., Leaf A.: Regulation of cellular volume. *Physiol. Rev.* 57:510, 1977.
169. Dellasega M., Grantham J.J.: Regulation of renal tubule cell volume in hypotonic media. *Am. J. Physiol.* 224:1288, 1973.
170. Grantham J.J., Lowe C.M., Dellasega M., et al.: Effect of hypotonic medium on K and Na content of proximal renal tubules. *Am. J. Physiol.* 232:F42, 1977.
170a. Hughes P.M., MacKnight A.D.C.: The regulation of cellular volume in renal cortical slices incubated in hyposmotic medium. *J. Physiol.* 257:137, 1976.
171. Whittembury G.: Sodium extrusion and potassium uptake in guinea pig kidney cortex slices. *J. Gen. Physiol.* 48:699, 1965.
172. Whittembury G.: Sodium and water transport in kidney proximal tubular cells. *J. Gen. Physiol.* 51:303S, 1968.
173. Kleinzeller A.: Cellular transport of water in metabolic pathways. Hokin L.E. (ed.): In *Metabolic Transport* (New York: Academic Press, vol. 6, pp. 91–131, 1972).
174. MacKnight A.D.C.: Water and electrolyte contents of rat renal cortical slices incubated in potassium-free media and media containing ouabain. *Biochim. Biophys. Acta.* 150:263, 1968.
175. Whittembury G., Grantham J.J.: Cellular aspects of renal sodium transport and cell volume regulation. *Kidney Int.* 9:103, 1976.
176. Linshaw M.A., Stapleton F.B., Cuppage F.E., et al.: Effect of basement membrane and colloid osmotic pressure on renal tubule cell volume. *Am. J. Physiol.* 233:F325, 1977.
177. Paillard M., Leviel F., Gardin J.P.: Regulation of cell volume in separated renal tubules incubated in hypotonic medium. *Am. J. Physiol.* 236:F226, 1979.
178. Linshaw M.A., Grantham J.J.: Effect of collagenase and ouabain on renal cell volume in hypotonic media. *Am. J. Physiol.* 238:F491, 1980.
179. Burg M.B., Orloff J.: Effect of strophanthidin on electrolyte content and PAH accumulation of rabbit kidney slices. *Am. J. Physiol.* 202:565, 1972.
180. Burg M.B., Green N.: Role of monovalent ions in the reabsorption of fluid by isolated perfused proximal renal tubules of the rabbit. *Kidney Int.* 10:221, 1976.
181. Cardinal J., Duchesneau D.: Effect of potassium on proximal tubular function. *Am. J. Physiol.* 234:F381, 1978.
182. Imai M., Kokko J.P.: Transtubular osmotic pressure gradients and net fluid transport in isolated proximal tubules. *Kidney Int.* 6:138, 1974.
183. Ullrich K.J., Rumrich G., et al.: Coupling between proximal tubular transport processes. Studies with ouabain, SITS and HCO_3^--free solutions. *Pflügers Arch.* 368:245, 1977.
184. Kokko J.P.: Proximal tubule potential difference: Dependence on glucose, HCO^-_3, and aminoacids. *J. Clin. Invest.* 52:1362, 1973.
185. Lutz M.D., Cardinal J., Burg M.B.: Electrical resistance of renal proximal tubule perfused in vitro. *Am. J. Physiol.* 225:729, 1973.
186. Burg M.B., Green N.: Bicarbonate transport of isolated perfused rabbit proximal convoluted tubules. *Am. J. Physiol.* 233:F307, 1977.
187. Barfuss D.W., Schafer J.A.: Active amino acid absorption by proximal straight tubules. *Am. J. Physiol.* 236:F149, 1979.
188. Crane R.K.: Hypothesis for mechanism of intestinal active transport of sugars. *Fed. Proc.* 21:891, 1962.
189. Aronson P.S., Sacktor B.: Transport of D-glucose by brush border membranes isolated from renal cortex. *Biochim. Biophys. Acta.* 356:231, 1974.
190. Kinne R., Murer H., Kinne-Saffran E., et al.: Sugar transport by renal plasma

membrane vesicles: Characterization of the systems in the brush border microvilli and basal-lateral membrane. *J. Membr. Biol.* 21:375, 1975.

191. Evers J., Murer H., Kinne R.: Phenylalanine uptake in isolated renal brush border vesicle. *Biochim. Biophys. Acta.* 426:598, 1976.

192. Kinne R., Schwartz J.L.: Isolated membrane vesicles in the evaluation of the nature, localization, and regulation of renal transport processes. *Kidney Int.* 14:547, 1978.

193. Hoffman N., Thees M., Kinne R.: Phosphate transport by isolated renal brush border vesicles. *Pflügers Arch.* 362:147, 1976.

194. Murer H., Hopfer U., Kinne R.: Sodium/proton antiport in brush border membrane vesicles isolated from rat small intestine and kidney. *Biochem. J.* 154:597, 1976.

194a. Ullrich K.J., Fromter E., Gmaj P., et al.: What are the driving forces for proximal tubular H^+ and Ca^{++} transport? The electrochemical gradient for Na^+ and/or ATP. *Curr. Probl. Clin. Biochem.* 8:170, 1978.

195. Gmaj P., Murer H., Kinne R.: Calcium ion transport across plasma membranes isolated from rat kidney cortex. *Biochem. J.* 178:549, 1979.

195a. Kriz W.: Structural organization of the renal medulla: Comparative and functional aspects. *Am. J. Physiol.* 241:R3, 1981.

196. Fairclogh P., Malhthi P., Preiser H., et al.: Reconstitution into liposomes of glucose active transport from the rabbit renal proximal tubule. *Biochim. Biophys. Acta.* 553:295, 1979.

196a. Schwartz M.M., Venkatachalam M.A.: Structural differences in thin limbs of Henle: Physiological implications. *Kidney Int.* 6:193, 1974.

197. Garg L.C., Tisher C.C.: Na-K-ATPase activity in thin limbs of rat nephron. *Am. Soc. Nephrol.* (Abstract) Chicago, 1982, p. 162A.

197a. Kinne R., Haase W., Gmaj P., et al.: ATP hydrolysis as driving force for transport processes in isolated renal plasma membrane vesicles. *Curr. Probl. Clin. Biochem.* 8:178, 1978.

198. Battilana C.A., Dobyan D.C., Lacy F.B., et al.: Effect of chronic potassium loading on potassium secretion by the pars recta or descending limb of the juxtamedullary nephron in the rat. *J. Clin. Invest.* 62:1093, 1978.

198a. Sacktor B.: Transport in membrane vesicles isolated from the mammalian kidney and intestine. *Curr. Top. Bioenerg.* 6:39, 1977.

199. Dobyan D.C., Lacy F.B., Jamison R.L.: Suppression of potassium-recycling in the renal medulla by short-term potassium deprivation. *Kidney Int.* 16:704, 1979.

200. Jamison R.L., Lacy F.B., Pennell J.P., et al.: [illegible] secretion by the descending limb or pars recta of the juxtamedullary nephron. [illegible] 1976.

201. Kokko J.P.: Sodium chloride and water transport in the descending [limb of] Henle. *J. Clin. Invest.* 49:1838, 1970.

202. Imai M.: Function of the thin ascending limb of Henle of rats and hamsters perfused in vitro. *Am. J. Physiol.* 232:F201, 1977.

203. Imai M., Kokko J.P.: Sodium chloride, urea, and water transport in the thin ascending limb of Henle. Generation of osmotic gradients by passive diffusion of solutes. *J. Clin. Invest.* 53:393, 1974.

204. Imai M., Kokko J.P.: Mechanism of sodium and chloride transport in the thin ascending limb of Henle. *J. Clin. Invest.* 58:1054, 1976.

205. Hebert S.C., Culpepper R.M., Andreoli T.E.: NaCl transport in mouse medullary thick ascending limb. I. Functional nephron heterogeneity and ADH-stimulated NaCl transport. *Am. J. Physiol.* 241:F412, 1981.

206. Bourdeau J.E., Burg M.B.: Voltage dependence of calcium transport in the thick ascending limb of the Henle's loop. *Am. J. Physiol.* 236:F357, 1979.

207. Bourdeau J.E., Burg M.B.: Effect of PTH on calcium transport across the cortical thick ascending limb of Henle's loop. *Am. J. Physiol.* 239:F121, 1980.

208. Burg M., Green N.: Function of the thick ascending limb of Henle's loop. *Am. J. Physiol.* 224:659, 1973.
209. Greger R.: Cation selectivity of the isolated perfused cortical thick ascending limb of Henle's loop of rabbit kidney. *Pflügers Arch.* 390:30, 1981.
210. Hall D.A., Varney D.M.: Effect of vasopressin on electrical potential difference and chloride transport in mouse medullary thick ascendling limb of Henle's loop. *J. Clin. Invest.* 66:792, 1980.
211. Imai M.: Effect of bumetanide and furosemide on the thick ascending limb of Henle's loop of rabbits and rats perfused in vitro. *Eur. J. Pharmacol.* 41:409, 1977.
212. Imai M.: Calcium transport across the rabbit thick ascending limb of Henle's loop perfused in vitro. *Pflügers Arch.* 374:255, 1978.
213. Rocha A.S., Kokko J.P.: Sodium chloride and water transport in the medullary thick ascending limb of Henle: Evidence for active chloride transport. *J. Clin. Invest.* 52:612, 1973.
214. Rocha A.S., Magaldi J.B., Kokko J.: Calcium and phosphate transport in isolated segments on rabbit Henle's loop. *J. Clin. Invest.* 59:975, 1977.
215. Sasaki S., Imai M.: Effects of vasopressin on water and NaCl transport across the in vitro perfused medullary thick ascending limb of Henle's loop of mouse, rat and rabbit kidneys. *Pflügers Arch.* 383:215, 1980.
216. Shareghi G.R, Stoner L.C.: Calcium transport across segments of the rabbit distal nephron in vitro. *Am. J. Physiol.* 235:F367, 1978.
217. Greger R.: Chloride reabsorption in the rabbit cortical thick ascending limb of the loop of Henle. A sodium dependent process. *Pflügers Arch.* 390:38, 1981.
218. Greger R., Schlatter E.: Presence of luminal K^+, a prerequisite for active NaCl transport in the cortical thick ascending limb of Henle's loop of rabbit kidney. *Pflügers Arch.* 392:92, 1981.
219. Greger R., Schlatter E.: Properties of the lumen membrane of the cortical thick ascending limb of Henle's loop of rabbit kidney. *Pflügers Arch.* 396:315, 1983.
220. Greger R., Schlatter E.: Properties of the basolateral membrane of the cortical thick ascending limb of Henle's loop of rabbit kidney. A model for secondary active chloride transport. *Pflügers Arch.* 396:325, 1983.
221. Greger R., Schlatter E., Lang F.: Evidence for electroneutral sodium chloride cotransport in the cortical thick ascending limb of Henle's loop of rabbit kidney. *Pflügers Arch.* 396:308, 1983.
222. Schmidt U., Dubach U.C.: Activity of (Na^+K^+)-stimulated adenosine-triphosphatase in rat nephron. *Pflügers Arch.* 306:219, 1969.
223. Eveloff J., Bayerdorffer E., Haase W., et al.: Biochemical and physiological studies on cells isolated from the medullary thick ascending limb of Henle's loop. *Int. J. Biochem.* 12:55, 1980.
224. Eveloff J., Bayerdorffer E., Silva P., et al.: Sodium-chloride transport in the thick ascending limb of Henle's loop: Oxygen consumption studies in isolated cells. *Pflügers Arch.* 389:263, 1981.
225. Eveloff J., Haase W., Kinne R.: Separation of renal medullary cells: Isolation of cells from the thick ascending limb of Henle's loop. *J. Cell. Biol.* 87:672, 1980.
226. Eveloff J., Kinne R.: Sodium-chloride transport in the medullary thick ascending limb of Henle's loop: Evidence for a sodium-chloride cotransport system in plasma membrane vesicles. *J. Membr. Biol.* 72:173, 1983.
227. Koenig B., Kinne R.: The role of potassium in chloride transport of the thick ascending limb of Henle's loop. *Pflügers Arch.* 394:R23, 1982.
228. Bailly C., Imbert-Teboul M., Chabardes D., et al.: The distal nephron of rat kidney: A target site for glucagon. *Proc. Natl. Acad. Sci. USA* 77:3422, 1980.
229. Chabardes D., Gagnan-Brunette M., Imbert-Teboul M., et al.: Adenylate cyclase responsiveness to hormones in various portions of the human nephron. *J. Clin. Invest.* 65:439, 1980.

230. Chabardes D., Imbert-Teboul M., Montegut M. et al.: Catecholamine sensitive adenylate cyclase activity in different segments of the rabbit nephron. *Pflugers Arch.* 361:9, 1975.
231. Kaissling B., Kriz W.: Structural analysis of the rabbit kidney. *Adv. Anat. Embryol. Cell Biol.* 56:1, 1979.
232. Almeida A.J., Burg M.B.: Sodium transport in the rabbit connecting tubule. *Am. J. Physiol.* 243:F330, 1982.
233. Imai M.: The connecting tubule: A functional subdivision of the rabbit distal nephron segment. *Kidney Int.* 15:346, 1979.
234. El Mernissi G., Doucet A.: Quantitation of ^{3}H-ouabain binding and turnover of Na-K-ATPase along the rabbit nephron. *Am. J. Physiol.* (submitted for publication).
235. Costanzo L.S., Windhager E.E.: Calcium and sodium transport by the distal convoluted tubule of the rat. *Am. J. Physiol.* 235:F492, 1978.
236. Gertz K.H.: Transtubuläre Natriumchloridflüsse und Permeabilität für Nichtelektrolyte im proximalen und distalen konvolut der Ratteniere. *Pflügers Arch.* 276:336, 1963.
237. Hierholzer K., Wiederholt M., Stolte M.: Hemmung der Natrium resorption im proximalen und distalen Konvolut adrenalectomierter Ratten. *Pflügers Arch.* 291:43, 1966.
238. Lombard W.E., Kokko J.P., Jacobson H.R.: Ion transport in superficial distal convoluted tubule perfused in vitro. *Proceedings of the 8th Int. Congr. Nephrol.* Athens, 1981, p. 35.
239. Schwartz G.J., Burg M.B.: Mineralocorticoid effects on cation transport by cortical collecting tubules in vitro. *Am. J. Physiol.* 235:F576, 1978.
240. Burg M.B., Isaacson L., Grantham J., et al.: Electrical properties of isolated perfused rabbit renal tubules. *Am. J. Physiol.* 215:788, 1968.
241. Grantham J.J., Burg M.B., Orloff J.: The nature of transtubular Na and K transport in isolated rabbit renal collecting tubules. *J. Clin. Invest.* 49:1815, 1970.
242. Stokes J.B.: Na and K transport across the cortical and outer medullary collecting tubule of the rabbit: Evidence for diffusion across the outer medullary portion. *Am. J. Physiol.* 242:F514, 1982.
243. Doucet A., Katz A.I.: Renal potassium adaptation: Na-K-ATPase activity along the nephron after chronic potassium loading. *Am. J. Physiol.* 238:F380, 1980.
244. Sejersted O.M.: In vivo regulation of the Na-K-ATPase activity. Skou J.C., Norby J.G. (eds.): In Proceedings, 2nd International Conference on the Properties and Functions of Na,K-ATPase (New York: Academic Press, pp. 525–535, 1979).
245. Grantham J.J.: The renal sodium pump and vanadate. *Am. J. Physiol.* 239:F97, 1980.
246. Hopkins L.L., Tilton B.E.: Metabolism of trace amounts of vanadium 48 in rat organs and liver subcellular particles. *Am. J. Physiol.* 211:169, 1966.
247. Bowman B.J., Slayman C.W.: The effects of vanadate on the plasma membrane ATPase of Neurospora crassa. *J. Biol. Chem.* 254:2928, 1979.
248. O'Neal S.G., Rhoads D.B., Racker E.: Vanadate inhibition of sarcoplasmic reticulum Ca^{2+}-ATPase and other ATPases. *Biochem. Biophys. Res. Commun.* 89:845, 1979.
249. Simons T.J.B.: Vanadate—a new tool for biologists. *Nature* 281:337, 1979.
250. Erdman E., Krawietz W., Phillip G., et al.: Purified cardiac cell membranes with high $(Na^+ + K^+)$ATPase activity contain significant NADH-vanadate reductase activity. *Nature* 282:335, 1979.
251. Cantley L.C., Aisen P.: The fate of cytoplasmic vanadium. *J. Biol. Chem.* 254:1781, 1979.
252. Cloix J.-F., Miller E.D., Pernollet M.-G., et al.: Purification d'un inhibiteur en-

dogène de la sodium-potassium ATPase. *C. R. Seances Acad. Sc. Paris (D)* 296:III 213, 1983.

253. De Wardener H.E., McGregor G.A., Clarkson E.M., et al.: Effect of sodium intake on ability of human plasma to inhibit renal Na$^+$-K$^+$-adenosine triphosphatase in vitro. *Lancet* 1:411, 1981.

254. Gruber K.A., Whitaker J.M., Buckalen V.M., Jr.: Endogenous digitalis-like substance in plasma of volume expanded dogs. *Nature* 287:743, 1980.

255. Charney A.N., Silva P., Besarab A., et al.: Separate effects of aldosterone, DOCA, and methylprednisolone on renal Na-K-ATPase. *Am. J. Physiol.* 227:345, 1974.

256. Chignell C.F., Roddy P.M., Titus E.O.: Effect of adrenal steroids on a Na$^+$K$^+$-dependent adenosine triphosphatase. *Life Sci.* 4:559, 1965.

257. Chignell C.F., Titus E.: Effect of adrenal steroids on a Na$^+$- and K$^+$- requiring adenosine triphosphatase from rat kidney. *J. Biol. Chem.* 241:5083, 1966.

258. Doucet A., Katz A.I.: Short-term effect of aldosterone on Na-K-ATPase in single nephron segments. *Am. J. Physiol.* 241:F273, 1981.

259. El Mernissi G., Doucet A.: Short-term effect of aldosterone on renal sodium transport and tubular Na-K-ATPase in the rat. *Pflügers Arch.* 399:139, 1983.

260. El Mernissi G., Doucet A.: Short-term effects of aldosterone and dexamethasone on Na-K-ATPase along the rabbit nephron. *Pflügers Arch.* 399:147.

261. Hendler E.D., Torretti J., Kupor L., et al.: Effects of adrenalectomy and hormone replacement on Na-K-ATPase in renal tissue. *Am. J. Physiol.* 222:754, 1972.

262. Jorgensen P.L.: Regulation of the (Na$^+$ + K$^+$)-activated ATP hydrolyzing enzyme system in rat kidney. I. The effect of adrenalectomy and the supply of sodium on the enzyme system. *Biochim. Biophys. Acta* 151:212, 1968.

263. Jorgensen P.L.: The role of aldosterone in the regulation of (Na$^+$ + K$^+$)-ATPase in rat kidney. *J. Steroid Biochem.* 3:181, 1972.

264. Landon E.J., Jazab N., Forte L.: Aldosterone and sodium- potassium-dependent ATPase activity of rat kidney membranes. *Am. J. Physiol.* 211:1050, 1966.

265. Rodriguez H.J., Sinha S.K., Starling J., et al.: Regulation of renal Na$^+$-K$^+$-ATPase in the rat by adrenal steroids. *Am. J. Physiol.* 241:F186, 1981.

266. Westenfelder C., Arevalo G.J., Baranowski R.L., et al.: Relationship between mineralocorticoids and renal Na$^+$-K$^+$-ATPase: Sodium reabsorption. *Am. J. Physiol.* 233:F593, 1977.

267. El Mernissi G., Chabardes D., Doucet A., et al.: Changes in tubular basolateral membrane markers after chronic DOCA treatment. *Am. J. Physiol.* 245:100, 1983.

268. Horster M., Schmid H., Schmidt U.: Aldosterone in vitro restores nephron Na-K-ATPase of distal segments from adrenalectomized rabbits. *Pflügers Arch.* 384:203, 1980.

269. Knox W.H., Sen A.K.: Mechanism of action of aldosterone with particular reference to (Na$^+$K$^+$)-ATPase. *Ann. NY Acad. Sci.* 242:471, 1974.

270. Rayson B.M., Edelman I.S.: Glucocorticoid stimulation of Na-K-ATPase in superfused distal segments of kidney tubules in vitro. *Am. J. Physiol.* 243:F463, 1982.

271. Sinha S.K., Rodriguez H.J., Hogan W.C., et al.: Mechanisms of activation of renal (Na$^+$ + K$^+$)-ATPase in the rat. Effects of acute and chronic administration of dexamethasone. *Biochim. Biophys. Acta* 641:20, 1981.

272. Doucet A., Katz A.I.: Mineralocorticoid receptors along the nephron: (^{3}H)aldosterone binding in rabbit tubules. *Am. J. Physiol.* 241:F605, 1981.

273. Vandewalle A., Farman N., Bencsath P., et al.: Aldosterone binding along the rabbit nephron: An autoradiographic study on isolated tubules. *Am. J. Physiol.* 240:F172, 1981.

274. Gross J.B., Imai M., Kokko J.P.: A functional comparison of the cortical collecting tubule and the distal convoluted tubule. *J. Clin. Invest.* 55:1284, 1975.

275. Gross J.B., Kokko J.P.: Effect of aldosterone and potassium- sparing diuretics on electrical potential differences across the distal nephron. *J. Clin. Invest.* 59:82, 1977.
276. Marver D., Schwartz M.J.: Identification of mineralocorticoid target sites in the isolated rabbit cortical nephron. *Proc. Natl. Acad. Sci. USA,* 77:3672, 1980.
277. Farman N., Vandewalle A., Bonvalet J.P.: Aldosterone binding in isolated tubules. II. An autoradiographic study of concentration dependency in the rabbit nephron. *Am. J. Physiol.* 242:F69, 1982.
278. Lee S.-M.K., Chekal M.A., Katz A.I.: Corticosterone binding sites along the rat nephron. *Am. J. Physiol.* 244:F504, 1983.
279. Nagel W., Crabbe J.: Mechanisms of action of aldosterone on active Na^+ transport across toad skin. *Pflügers Arch.* 385:181, 1980.
280. Katz A.I., Epstein F.H.: The role of sodium-potassium-activated adenosine triphosphatase in the reabsorption of sodium by the kidney. *J. Clin. Invest.* 46:1999, 1967.
281. Stoner L.C., Burg M.B., Orloff J.: Ion transport in cortical collecting tubule; effect of amiloride. *Am. J. Physiol.* 227:453, 1974.
282. Fisher K.A., Welt L.G., Hayslett J.P.: Dissociation of Na-K-ATPase specific activity and net reabsorption of sodium. *Am. J. Physiol.* 228:1745, 1975.
283. Handler J.S., Preston A.S., Perkins F.M., et al.: The effect of adrenal steroid hormones on epithelia formed in culture by A6 cells. *Ann. N.Y. Acad. Sci.* 372:442, 1981.
284. Sharp G.W., Leaf A.: Mechanism of action of aldosterone. *Physiol. Rev.* 46:593, 1966.
285. Lichtenstein N.S., Leaf A.: Effect of amphotericin B on the permeability of the toad bladder. *J. Clin. Invest.* 44:1328, 1965.
286. Lipton P., Edelman I.S.: Effects of aldosterone and ADH on electrolytes of toad bladder epithelial cells. *Am. J. Physiol.* 221:733, 1971.
287. Wade J.B., O'Neil R.G., Pryor J.L., et al.: Modulation of cell membrane area in renal collecting tubules by corticosteroid hormones. *J. Cell. Biol.,* 81:439, 1979.
288. Kaissling B., Le Hir M.: Analysis of distal segments in the rabbit kidney tubules after adaptation to altered Na- and K- intake. I. Structural changes. *Cell Tissue Res.* 224:469, 1982.
289. O'Neil R.G., Helman S.I.: Transport characteristics of renal collecting tubules: Influences of DOCA and diet. *Am. J. Physiol.* 233:F544, 1977.
290. Stokes J.B., Ingram M.J., Williams A.D., et al.: Heterogeneity of the rabbit collecting tubule: Localization of mineralocorticoid hormone action to the cortical portion. *Kidney Int.* 20:340, 1981.
291. Katz A.I., Lindheimer M.D.: Renal sodium- and potassium- activated adenosine triphosphatase and sodium reabsorption in the hypothyroid rat. *J. Clin. Invest.* 52:796, 1973.
292. Lo C.-S., August T.R., Liberman U.A., et al.: Dependence of renal $(Na^+ + K^+)$-adenosine triphosphatase activity on thyroid status. *J. Biol. Chem.* 251:7826, 1976.
293. Lo C.-S., Lo T.N.: Time course of renal response to triiodothyronine in the rat. *Am. J. Physiol.* 236:F9, 1979.
294. Oppenheimer J.H., Koerner D., Schwartz H.L., et al.: Specific nuclear triiodothyronine binding sites in rat liver and kidney. *J. Clin. Endocrinol. Metab.* 35:330, 1972.
295. Oppenheimer J.H., Schwartz H.L., Surks M.I., et al.: Nuclear receptors and the initiation of thyroid action. *Recent Prog. Horm. Res.* 32:539, 1976.
296. Somjen O., Ismail-Beigi F., Edelman I.S.: Nuclear binding of T_3 and effects on QO_2, Na-K-ATPase, and -GPDH in liver and kidney. *Am. J. Physiol.* 240:E146, 1981.

297. Lo C.-S., Gerendasy D., Lo T.N.: Effect of triiodothyronine on renal growth and renal sodium reabsorption in hypothyroid rats. *Pflügers Arch.* 390:186, 1981.

298. Lo C.-S., Edelman I.: Effect of triiodothyronine on the synthesis and degradation of renal cortical ($Na^+ + K^+$)-adenosine triphosphatase. *J. Biol. Chem.* 251:7834, 1976.

299. Smith T.J., Edelman I.S.: The role of sodium transport in thyroid thermogenesis. *Fed. Proc.* 38:2150, 1979.

300. De Wardener H.E., Mills I.H., Clapham W.F., et al.: Studies on the efferent mechanism of the sodium diuresis which follows the administration of intravenous saline in the dog. *Clin. Sci. (London)* 21:249, 1961.

301. De Wardener H.E., MacGregor G.A.: Dahl's hypothesis that a saluretic substance may be responsible for a sustained rise in arterial pressure : Its possible role in essential hypertension. *Kidney Int.* 18:1, 1980.

302. Marx J.L.: Natriuretic hormone linked to hypertension. *Science* 212:1255, 1981.

303. Bourgoignie J.J., Klahr S., Bricker N.S.: Inhibition of transepithelial sodium transport in the frog skin by a low molecular weight fraction of uremic serum. *J. Clin. Invest.* 50:303, 1971.

304. Brown P.R., Koutsaimanis K.G., De Wardener H.E.: Effect of urinary extracts from salt-loaded man on urinary excretion by the rat. *Kidney Int.* 2:1, 1972.

305. Favre H., Hwang K.H., Schmidt R.W., et al.: An inhibitor of sodium transport in the urine of dogs with normal renal function. *J. Clin. Invest.* 56:1302, 1975.

306. Kramer H.J., Backer A., Krück F.: Antinatriferic activity in human plasma following acute and chronic salt-loading. *Kidney Int.* 12:214, 1977.

307. Sealey J.E., Kirshman J.D., Laragh J.H.: Natriuretic activity in plasma and urine of salt loaded man and sheep. *J. Clin. Invest.* 48:2210, 1969.

308. Gonick H.C., Kramer H.J., Paul W., et al.: Circulating inhibitor of sodium-potassium-activated adenosine triphosphatase after expansion of extracellular fluid volume in rats. *Clin. Sci. Mol. Med.* 53:329, 1977.

309. Katz A.I., Gonant H.K · Effect of extracellular expansion on renal cortical and medullary Na-K-ATPase. *Pflügers Arch.* 330:136, 1971.

310. Nizet A., Lefebvre P., Crabbe J.: Control by insulin of sodium potassium and water excretion by the isolated dog kidney. *Pflügers Arch.* 323:11, 1971.

311. De Fronzo R.A., Cooke C.R., Andres R., et al.: The effect of insulin on renal handling of sodium, potassium, calcium, and phosphate in man. *J. Clin. Invest.* 55:845, 1975.

312. Baylis P.H., Pitchfork J., Chayen J., et al.: A cytochemical bioassay for arginine vasopressin: Preliminary studies. *J. Immunoassay* 1:399, 1980.

313. Chayen J., Frost G.T.B., Dodds R.A., et al.: The use of a hidden metal-capture reagent for the measurement of Na^+-K^+-ATPase activity: A new concept in cytochemistry. *Histochemistry.* 71:533, 1981.

314. Wright F.S., Strieder N., Fowler N., et al.: Potassium secretion by distal tubules after potassium adaptation. *Am. J. Physiol.* 221:437, 1971.

315. Giebisch G., Stanton B.: Potassium transport in the nephron. *Annu. Rev. Physiol.* 41:241, 1979.

316. Hierholzer K., Wiederholt M.: Some aspects of distal tubular solute and water transport. *Kidney Int.* 9:198, 1976.

317. Wright F.S.: Sites and mechanisms of potassium transport along the renal tubule. *Kidney Int.* 11:415, 1977.

318. Wright F.S., Giebisch G.: Renal potassium transport: contribution of individual nephron segments and populations. *Am. J. Physiol.* 235:F515, 1978.

319. Fine L.G., Yanagawa N., Schultze R.G., et al.: Functional profile of the isolated uremic nephron: Potassium adaptation in the rabbit cortical collecting tubule. *J. Clin. Invest.* 64:1033, 1979.

320. Linas S.L., Peterson L.N., Anderson R.J., et al.: Mechanism of renal potassium conservation in the rat. *Kidney Int.* 15:601, 1979.

321. Silva P., Hayslett J.P., Epstein F.H.: The role of Na-K-activated adenosine triphosphatase in potassium adaptation: Stimulation of enzymatic activity by potassium loading. *J. Clin. Invest.* 52:2665, 1973.

322. Evan A., Huser J., Bengele H.H., et al.: The effect of alterations in dietary potassium on collecting system morphology in the rat. *Lab. Invest.* 42:668, 1980.

323. Addis T., Myers B.A., Oliver J.: The regulation of renal activity. IX. The effect of unilateral nephrectomy on the function and structure of the remaining kidney. *Arch. Intern. Med.* 34:243, 1924.

324. Wald H., Guy R., Gutman Y., et al.: Sodium, ammonium and unilateral nephrectomy: Differential effect on microsomal ATPase of kidney cortex and medulla. *Int. J. Biochem.* 8:33, 1977.

325. Jorgensen P.L.: Dissociation between compensatory renal growth and induction of $(Na^+ + K^+)$-ATPase in rat kidney after uninephrectomy. *Experientia* 27:527, 1971.

326. Silva P., Torretti J., Hayslett J.P., et al.: Relation between Na-K-ATPase activity and respiratory rate in the rat kidney. *Am. J. Physiol.* 230:1432, 1976.

327. Hayslett J.P., Kashgarian M., Epstein F.H.: Functional correlates of compensatory renal hypertrophy. *J. Clin. Invest.* 47:774, 1968.

328. Schmidt U., Dubach U.C.: Induction of Na-K-ATPase in the proximal and distal convolution of the rat nephron after uninephrectomy. *Pflügers Arch.* 346:39, 1974.

329. Jacobson M.P., Rodriguez H.J., Hogan W.C., et al.: Mechanism of activation of renal Na^+-K^+-ATPase in the rat: Effects of reduction of renal mass. *Am. J. Physiol.* 239:F281, 1980.

330. Lowenstein J., Beranbaum E.R., Chasis H., et al.: Intrarenal pressure and exaggerated natriuresis in essential hypertension. *Clin. Sci.* 38:359, 1970.

331. Stumpe K.O., Lowitz H.D., Ochwadt B.: Fluid reabsorption in Henle's loop and urinary excretion of sodium and water in normal rats and rats with chronic hypertension. *J. Clin. Invest.* 49:1210, 1970.

332. Malyusz M., Mehnert I., Radel R.: Interdependence of Na-excretion, plasma electrolytes, plasma volume and renal Na-K-ATPase activity in hypertensive rats. Bern : Huber, 1976.

333. Postnov Y., Reznikova M., Boriskina G.: Na-K-adenosine triphosphatase in the kidney of rats with renal hypertension and spontaneously hypertensive rats. *Pflügers Arch.* 362:95, 1976.

334. Dzurba A., Michajlovskij N., Ponec J., et al.: The effect of saline loading on Na^+-K^+ ATPase activity in the kidney of spontaneously hypertensive rats. *Physiol. Bohemoslov.* 27:241, 1978.

335. Biol M.C., Vincent M., Sassard J.: Ouabain-sensitive ATPase activities in the kidney and liver of spontaneously hypertensive rat. *Arch. Int. Physiol. Biochim.* 87:291, 1979.

336. Rodriguez-Sargent C., Cangiano J.L., Opava-Stitzer S., et al.: Renal Na^+-K^+-ATPase in Okamoto and Dahl hypertensive rats. *Hypertension* 3:II86, 1981.

337. Doucet A., Mekler J., El Mernissi G., et al.: Na-K-ATPase in single nephron segments of hypertension-prone rats. *J. Hypertension* 1:53, 1983.

338. Slegers J.F.G., Forster F.T.G.: Natriuresis and renal Na-K-ATPase activity in kidney of normotensive and spontaneously hypertensive rats. *Mineral Electrolyte Metab.* 8:21, 1981.

339. Potter E.L.: Normal and Abnormal Development of the Kidney. Chicago: Year Book Medical Publishers, 1972.

340. Horster M.: Principles of nephron differentiation. *Am. J. Physiol.* 235:F387, 1978.

341. Geloso J.-P., Basset J.-C.: Role of adrenal glands in development of foetal rat kidney Na-K-ATPase. *Pflügers Arch.* 348:105, 1974.

342. Aperia A., Larsson L., Zetterstrom R.: Hormonal induction of Na-K-ATPase in developing proximal tubular cells. *Am. J. Physiol.* 241:F356, 1981.

343. Aperia A., Larsson L.: Correlation between fluid reabsorption and proximal tubule ultrastructure during development of the rat kidney. *Acta Physiol. Scand.* 105:11, 1979.

343. Jacobson H.R.: Effects of CO_2 and acetazolamide on bicarbonate and fluid transport in rabbit proximal tubules. *Am. J. Physiol.* 240:F54, 1981.

344. Larson L., Horster M.: Ultrastructure and net fluid transport in isolated perfused developing proximal tubules. *J. Ultrastruct. Res.* 54:276, 1976.

344a. Schafer J.A., Troutman S.L., Andreoli T.E.: Volume absorption transepithelial potential differences, and ionic permeability properties in mammalian superficial proximal straight tubules. *J. Gen. Physiol.* 64:582, 1974.

345. Fromter E.: Electrophysiology and isotonic fluid absorption of proximal tubules of mammalian kidney. Thurau K. (ed.): In *Kidney and Urinary Tract Physiology* (London: Butterworths, pp.1–38, 1974).

345a. Horster M., Larsson L.: Mechanisms of fluid absorption during proximal tubule development. *Kidney Int.* 10:348, 1976.

346. Morel F., Murayama Y.: Simultaneous measurement of unidirectional and net sodium fluxes in microperfused rat proximal tubules. *Pflügers Arch.* 320:1, 1970.

Chemical, Experimental, and Clinical Studies on Endogenous Ouabain-Like Substance in Hypertension

J.F. CLOIX, M.D., M. CRABOS, M.D.,
M.A. DEVYNCK, M.A., M.D., J.L. ELGHOZI, M.D.,
G. HENNING, M.D., L.A. KAMAL, M.D.,
L.C. LACERDA-JACOMINI, M.D., P. MEYER, M.D.,
M.G. PERNOLLET, M.D., J.B. ROSENFELD, M.D.,
AND H. DE THÉ, M.D.

*U7 and U90 INSERM Research Units, Dept. of Pharmacology, Hôpital Necker,
161 rue de Sèvres, 75015 Paris, France*

A heat-stable, low molecular weight, anionic substance(s) capable of inhibiting ^{3}H-ouabain binding and Na^+-K^+-ATPase activity could be extracted from human urine and plasma. The level of the inhibitor was elevated in 40%–50% of essential hypertensives, compared to controls, and also in some of the offspring of hypertensive parents. Higher levels of the inhibitor were measured in patients treated with β-blocking agents than in those treated with diuretics.

The inhibitor extracted from plasma also appeared capable of (1) inhibiting the uptake of serotonin in human platelets, an Na^+-dependent mechanism, and (2) inducing an increase in blood pressure when injected intracerebroventricularly. From these various data, we propose that the increase in the endogenous inhibitor may play a role in essential hypertension and may modulate, at least partially, some of the various cell functions that depend on a transmembrane Na^+ gradient, including cellular excitability.

INCREASED renal excretion of Na^+ during extracellular volume expansion has been attributed in part to inhibition of the Na^+-

K^+ pump by an endogenous circulating inhibitor.[1-3] This inhibitor might, in addition to the renal effect, increase the intracellular concentration of Na^+ in excitable cells possessing a Ca^{2+}-Na^+ exchange, the resulting increase in intracellular Ca^{2+} triggering various events observed in essential hypertension.[4,5] It might also potentiate adrenergic stimuli through reuptake inhibition.[5] Several authors have proposed that the endogenous Na^+ pump inhibitor has a pathogenic role in this disease.[5,6]

In Na^+-dependent hypertension in animal studies, a circulating Na^+ pump inhibitor appears to be responsible for a reduction of ouabain-sensitive rubidium fluxes in blood vessels.[7] In plasma of essential hypertensives, an increase of an Na^+ transport inhibitor was detected with the use of a cytochemical method.[8] This finding was reinforced by studies on leukocytes Na^+ effluxes, which were found decreased in hypertensives.[9] A similar reduction in Na^+ effluxes was observed in leukocytes of normotensive subjects when incubated in sera from hypertensives.[10] The concentration of the Na^+ pump inhibitor appears higher in patients with low renin levels.[11]

Recent studies indicated that this inhibitor of Na^+ transport has the features of a digitalis-like compound. It was shown to inhibit the specific binding of ^{3}H-ouabain to the Na^+ pump digitalis sites[12] and the Na^+-K^+-ATPase activity, which is the enzymatic expression of the Na^+ pump; this inhibition appeared more pronounced in severe hypertension.[13]

Since ^{3}H-ouabain binding studies do not indicate the functional properties of the competitor, which may have agonist or antagonist characteristics, and since several compounds may inhibit Na^+-K^+-ATPase activity without having digitalis-like properties, a clear-cut conclusion necessitates the simultaneous use of several methods.

We used various technical procedures to answer the following questions: (1) Is it possible to confirm in human plasma and urine the presence of an endogenous compound with digitalis-like properties and an inhibitory effect on the Na^+ pump? (2) Is there any difference between normotensive controls and hypertensives? (3) What are the arguments giving the inhibitor a physiologic role? (4) What are the properties of the inhibitor suggesting its involvement in the pathogenesis of essential hypertension?

Several independent studies from our laboratory have already brought some answers to these questions.[12, 14–18] We shall try here to give an overall view of the basic and applied data obtained so far.

Methods

Chemistry of the Endogenous Na^+ Pump Inhibitor

It was previously reported that the endogenous Na^+-K^+-ATPase inhibitor was heat stable. Therefore, human plasma was boiled for 15 minutes. The supernatant was treated by filtration on AcA 54 ultrogel, followed by anion-exchange chromatography on DEAE-cellulose. Details of the procedures are given elsewhere.[15] The various fractions of gel filtration and ion exchange chromatography were examined for their ability to inhibit ^{3}H-ouabain binding and for Na^+-K^+-ATPase activity.[15]

The Na^+ pump endogenous inhibitor was also purified from plasma and urine using an affinity chromatography procedure. Semipurified dog kidney Na^+-K^+-ATPase was cross-linked with ovalbumin; this immobilized enzyme was used in batch affinity chromatography and 1M ammonium acetate was used as the washing off solution. The procedure is fully described elsewhere.[18] The experiments were performed in plasma and in urine from normal subjects and from subjects receiving an acute Na^+ load (346 mmoles) in 1 day.

Investigation of Human Hypertension

Analytic Procedures

Heat-stable plasma extracts from controls and patients were tested for their inhibitory effect on ^{3}H-ouabain binding to erythrocytes and on Na^+-K^+-ATPase activity.

Binding of ^{3}H-ouabain (17–37 Ci/mmole) to normal erythrocytes was performed at equilibrium, as described elsewhere.[12] Number of pump units and affinity were calculated from Scatchard plots. The inhibition by plasma extracts was expressed as the decrease in apparent affinity given as a percentage of the erythrocyte affinity in the absence of plasma.

164   J. F. CLOIX ET AL.

The Na^+-K^+-ATPase activity (EC 3.6.1.3., prepared from dog kidney) was determined by hydrolysis of $\gamma^{32}P$-ATP. To 80 μl of a medium containing 100mM NaCl, 2.5mM EGTA, 4mM $MGCl_2$, 2mM ATP sodium, 16 nCi ^{32}P-ATP, and 80mM tris-HCl buffered to 7.4 were added 10 μl of plasma extracts, corresponding to 190 μl of boiled plasma supernate or ionic plasma-like solution, and 10 μl of enzyme suspension (3 $\times$ 10^{-3} unit). After 30 minutes of incubation at 37° C, the reaction was stopped by placing the tubes at 0° C and adding 100 μl of 23% $HC10_4$. Liberated phosphates, separated from ATP adsorbed on acid-washed charcoal, were then counted.

Patients and Controls

One hundred subjects on a free Na^+ diet were studied. Their blood pressure was recorded with a mercury manometer in the sitting position. They were divided into six groups, as follows:

Group 1 consisted of 21 normotensive healthy volunteers with no known family history of hypertension (13 men and 8 women, aged 23–53 years; mean age, 32.1 $\pm$ 2.0 years); their mean blood pressure was 90.8 $\pm$ 1.9 mm Hg.

Group 2 consisted of 21 normotensive healthy volunteers who had at least one parent with high blood pressure (13 men and 8 women, aged 23–50 years; mean age, 34.4 $\pm$ 1.7); their mean blood pressure averaged 95.5 $\pm$ 2.0 mm Hg.

Group 3 consisted of 27 hypertensive patients untreated for at least 2 weeks (18 men and 9 women, aged 22–71 years; mean age, 46.1 $\pm$ 2.9). Essential hypertension was diagnosed after careful clinical investigation. Their mean blood pressure was 121.0 $\pm$ 2.1 mm Hg. In all patients, plasma Na^+ and K^+ were in the normal range.

Groups 4 and 5 consisted of 21 hypertensive patients who had been under antihypertensive therapy for at least 2 weeks. Seven (2 men and 5 women, aged 40–84 years) were on thiazide diuretics (group 4); their mean blood pressure was 120.0 $\pm$ 4.8 mm Hg. Fourteen (11 men and 3 women, aged 23–66 years; mean, 42.6 $\pm$ 3.6) were on β-blocking agents (group 5); their mean blood pressure was 115.1 $\pm$ 3.8 mm Hg. None of the patients had a significant change in plasma potassium.

Group 6 consisted of 10 patients with renal insufficiency and a serum creatinine level above 170 μmoles/L (mean, 434 $\pm$ 96

μmoles/L). No patient was dialyzed or had received a transplant. None was hypertensive. Their daily diet contained 6–10 gm of NaCl.

Platelet Serotonin Uptake

Twenty milliliters of venous blood withdrawn from normotensive subjects without a family history of hypertension were centrifuged at 300 g for 10 minutes. Aliquots of platelet-rich plasma containing $1–2 \times 10^8$ platelets were incubated with various concentrations of inhibitor-enriched fractions for 45 minutes at 37° C. Uptake was initiated by addition of ^{3}H-5-hydroxytryptamine (10.8 mCi/mmole), 4.4×10^{-7}M (final concentration), and continued for 30 seconds. Platelets were then filtered, washed with a buffer containing 150 mM NaCl, 1mM EDTA, and 10mM tris, pH 6.5, and counted.

Animal Experiments: Intracerebroventricular Injections of Plasma Fractions and Blood Pressure Recording

Male Wistar rats weighing 230–330 gm were anesthetized with urethane (1.25 gm/kg, i_2p_2) and the right iliac artery was cannulated to measure blood pressure and heart rate. Animals were placed in a stereotaxic frame and a stainless steel guide was inserted with its mandrel into the anterior part of the cerebral third ventricle. Plasma enriched fractions or vehicle, in 10-μl amounts, was infused over 10-minute periods and its effects compared with those of ouabain.

Results

Biochemical Analysis of Plasma and Urine Extracts

The gel filtration of supernatant of boiled plasma produced one peak capable of inhibiting the Na^+-K^+-ATPase activity. This peak, appearing just after the salt peak, was slightly adsorbed onto the gel.

This plasma extract was resolved by anion exchange chromatography in four peaks inhibiting Na^+-K^+-ATPase activity. The first one, not retained by the Cellex D resin, corresponded to plasma cations and particularly to calcium. The three peaks retained on the Cellex D were eluted with 150mM, 250mM, and 500mM ammonium acetate, respectively. When expressed as inhibitory potency per optical density (at 254 nm) units, their mean factor of enrichment as compared to crude plasma was estimated to reach 200.

These three fractions (named 1, 2, and 3) also inhibited ^{3}H-ouabain binding in an apparently competitive manner (Table 1). As indicated below, the three fractions were also capable of inhibiting active ^{3}H-serotonin uptake by human platelets.

Affinity chromatography experiments allowed detection in both plasma and urine of an endogenous substance capable of inhibiting the Na^+-K^+-ATPase activity. This substance was washed off from Na^+-K^+-ATPase crosslinked with ovalbumin by 1M ammonium acetate and was shown not to be a plasma cation or phosphate ion. Moreover, the degree of inhibition of urine extracts appeared to increase after Na^+ administration.

CLINICAL INVESTIGATION: ESSENTIAL HYPERTENSION; INHIBITION OF ^{3}H-OUABAIN BINDING AND Na^+-K^+-ATPase ACTIVITY

Plasma extracts from nearly half of the essential hypertensive patients and of the normotensive offspring of hypertensive parents exerted a marked inhibitory effect on the two biochemical parameters used as tests of interaction with Na^+-K^+ pumps. The mean inhibition in these two groups was significantly higher than that measured in the normotensive control group (Fig 1). A significant correlation ($r = 0.74$; $n = 44$) was obtained between the inhibition of ouabain binding to erythro-

TABLE 1.—OUABAIN-LIKE ACTIVITIES OF PLASMA FRACTIONS

INHIBITOR-ENRICHED FRACTIONS	INHIBITION OF Na^+-K^+-ATPase ACTIVITY* $(10^{-9}M)$	INHIBITION OF OUABAIN BINDING* $(10^{-9}M)$	INHIBITION OF PLATELET SEROTONIN UPTAKE* $(10^{-9}M)$
1	3.6 ± 1.5	8.0 ± 2.8	1.4 ± 0.4
2	2.4 ± 0.3	5.3 ± 1.9	6.5 ± 1.9
3	2.7 ± 1.7	6.4 ± 1.2	4.2 ± 1.7

*Expressed as ouabain-like concentration in whole plasma, based on an average of 3–10 independent determinations.

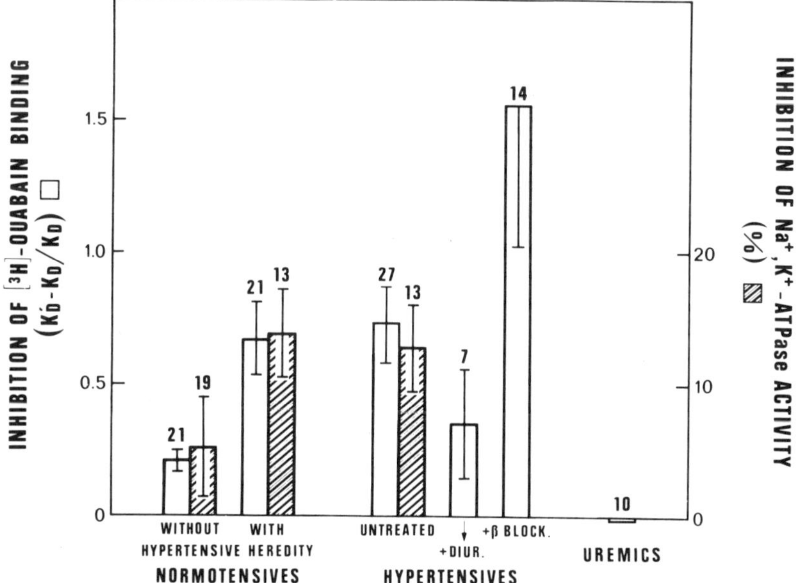

Fig 1.—In vitro inhibition by plasma extracts of ouabain binding and Na^+-K^+-ATPase activity. Inhibition of ouabain binding *(white bars)* is given as the decrease in the apparent affinity induced by plasma extracts $(K'_D$-$K_D)$ expressed as a percentage of its value in the absence of plasma (K_D). Inhibition of Na^+-K^+-ATPase activity *(shaded bars)* is given as a percentage of the ouabain-sensitive activity. Values are in means ± SEM. The number of subjects or patients is indicated.

cytes and that of ATP hydrolysis obtained in individual plasma extracts.

Figure 1 also shows that plasma from patients on thiazide therapy did not significantly inhibit ³H-ouabain binding, whereas plasma from patients receiving β-blockers exerted a marked inhibition.

Plasma extracts from patients with chronic renal failure did not decrease the affinity of the binding sites for ouabain but induced a small decrease in the number of binding sites, averaging 9.1% ± 1.9%.

INHIBITION OF PLATELET SEROTONIN UPTAKE

The uptake of serotonin in blood platelets is a sodium-dependent process that is inhibited by ouabain.[19] It has been recently reported to be modified in hypertensive subjects.[20] The effects of increasing concentrations of inhibitor-enriched fractions on ^{3}H-serotonin uptake by platelets of normotensive controls were studied. A dose-dependent inhibition was observed for the three fractions as for ouabain. Their concentration could thus be evaluated by the concentration of ouabain, giving a similar inhibition when expressed in ouabain-like units. Fraction 1, 2, and 3 activities in whole plasma were calculated to be in the 10^{-9}M range (see Table 1). This does not take into account the possible losses during isolation.

EFFECT ON BLOOD PRESSURE OF INTRACEREBROVENTRICULAR INJECTIONS OF PLASMA FRACTIONS

Na^+-K^+-ATPase inhibitors have been described in brain,[21] and intracerebroventricular administration of ouabain induces a sympathetic overactivity, with blood pressure and heart rate increases.[22] The effects on blood pressure and heart rate of intracerebroventricular injections of the three inhibitor-enriched fractions were therefore investigated. The most evident response was a slight but significant increase in blood pressure after fraction 2 injection. An amount equivalent to that extracted from 0.5 ml of whole plasma induced a 12 mm Hg ($n = 2$) increase, and that equivalent to 1.3 ml plasma resulted in a 16 ± 2 mm Hg increase in blood pressure ($n = 4$) within 9 ± 2 minutes after the beginning of injection.

Comment

Our investigation confirmed the existence of an endogenous compound possessing digitalis-like activities in human plasma and urine. In addition, we found that the Na^+ pump inhibitor levels are increased in essential hypertension (in approximately 50% of patients). Plasma extracts were capable of inhibiting serotonin uptake in platelets, a cellular process depending on Na^+ gradient, and of increasing blood pressure after central infusion, as ouabain does.

The endogenous inhibitor chemical characteristics reported in the present study are heat stability, anionic properties, and low molecular weight ($<$ 1,500 daltons); they are similar to those previously reported in other studies.[23–28] It is not clear whether the three inhibitory fractions isolated on anion exchange chromatography represent three independent inhibitions or three forms of a single inhibitor.

Plasma of only half of essential hypertensive patients were found to contain elevated levels of the inhibitor, a proportion smaller than that previously reported.[13] In addition, contrary to previous reports,[11, 13] no correlation was found between the inhibitor and blood pressure or plasma renin activity. It is possible that these discrepancies are related to differences in sex, severity of the disease, or ethnical characteristics. The absence of correlation between plasma renin activity and pump inhibition may be related to the fact that stimulation of renin release through Na^+ restriction might have been necessary to demonstrate a correlation, as previously shown.[11]

Increased inhibition values were also observed in 40% of the normotensives with a family history of hypertension, which confirms the presence of a sodium transport inhibitor in such subjects. Other changes of Na^+ cellular metabolism similar to those found in the hypertensives have also been reported in these subjects. These changes include an increase in intracellular Na^+,[29] an increase in net Na^+ efflux from erythrocytes,[30, 31] a reduction of Na^+-K^+ cotransport,[32] a reduction of leukocyte sodium effluxes in the absence[33] or presence of plasma,[34] and alteration of acute renal sodium excretion.[35–36]

The elevated inhibitory values found in the normotensives with a family heredity confirm the lack of relation between pump inhibition and blood pressure and show that the presence of the inhibitor is not secondary to established hypertension. It also suggests that this inhibitor does not per se induce an immediate rise in blood pressure.

In the treated patients, it was previously shown that diuretic therapy could correct some abnormal cellular finding such as intracellular Na^+ or sodium effluxes.[37–38] Our results extend these observations to sodium pump inhibitors. Thiazides could induce a reduction of the extracellular volume and suppress factor secretion as was suggested previously.[6] High levels of inhibitors were found in patients on β-blocking agents. Such patients tend to have a low renin concentration, a condition that has been associated with a high inhibition value.[11]

The reduction of ^3H-serotonin uptake in human blood platelets by the endogenous Na^+ pump inhibitor observed in whole plasma suggests that the inhibitor may be active in vivo.

The uptake of serotonin in blood platelets is a carrier-mediated, Na^+-dependent transport process.[19] Ouabain, which through the inhibition of the Na^+ pump decreases the transmembrane Na^+ gradient, is known to inhibit the serotonin uptake.[19] Our experiments showed that a similar inhibition could be achieved with the purified fractions of the endogenous inhibitor. It is thus possible that the endogenous Na^+ pump inhibitor plays a role in several cell processes depending on Na^+ gradient, such as cell excitability, cell volume and nutrition, and neurotransmitter uptake and release. The observed rise in blood pressure induced by central infusion could be one of these effects.

REFERENCES

1. Buckalew V.M., Nelson D.B.: Natriuretic and sodium transport inhibitory activity in plasma of volume expanded dogs. *Kidney Int.* 5:12, 1974.
2. Gonick H.C., Kramer H.J., Paul W., et al.: Circulating inhibitor of sodium-potassium activated adenosine triphosphatase after expansion of extracellular fluid volume in rats. *Clin. Sci. Mol. Med.* 53:329, 1977.
3. De Wardener H.E., MacGregor G.A., Clarkson E.M., et al.: Effect of sodium intake on ability of human plasma to inhibit Na^+,K^+-ATPase (adenosine triphosphatase) in vitro. *Lancet* 1:411, 1981.
4. Blaustein M.P.: Sodium ions, calcium ions, blood pressure regulation and hypertension: A reassessment and a hypothesis. *Am. J. Physiol.* 232:C165, 1977.
5. Blaustein M.P., Hamlyn J.M.: Role of a natriuretic factor in essential hypertension: A hypothesis. *Ann. Intern. Med.* 98:785, 1983.
6. De Wardener H.E., MacGregor G.A.: Dahl's hypothesis that a saliuretic substance may be responsible for a sustained rise in arterial pressure: Its possible role in essential hypertension. *Kidney Int.* 18:1, 1980.
7. Haddy F.J., Overbeck H.W.: The role of humoral agents in volume expanded hypertension. *Life Sci.* 19:935, 1976.
8. MacGregor G.A., Fenton S., Alghband-Zadeh J., et al.: Evidence of raised concentrations of a circulating sodium transport inhibitor in essential hypertension. *Br. Med. J.* 283:1355, 1981.
9. Edmondson R.P.S., Thomas R.D., Hilton P.J., et al.: Abnormal leukocyte composition and sodium transport in essential hypertension. *Lancet* 1:1003, 1975.
10. Poston L., Sewell R.B., Wilkinson S.P., et al.: Evidence for a circulating sodium transport inhibitor in essential hypertension. *Br. Med. J.* 282:847, 1981.
11. Edmondson R.P.S., MacGregor G.A.: Leukocyte cation transport in essential hypertension: Its relation to the renin angiotensin system. *Br. Med. J.* 282:1267, 1981.
12. Devynck M.A., Pernollet M.G., Rosenfeld J., et al.: Measurement of a digitalis-like compound in human plasma: Application to essential hypertension. *Br. Med. J.* 287(6393):631–634.
13. Hamlyn J.M., Ringel R., Shaeffer J., et al.: A circulating inhibitor of Na^+-K^+-ATPase associated with essential hypertension. *Nature* 300:650, 1982.
14. Cloix J.F., Devynck M.A., Elghozi J.L., et al.: Plasma endogenous sodium pump inhibitor in essential hypertension. *J. Hypertension,* to be published.
15. Cloix J.F., Miller E.D., Pernollet M.G., et al. Purification d'un inhibiteur endogène de la sodium-potassium-ATPase. *C. R. Seances Acad. Sci. III* 296:213, 1983.
16. De The H., Devynck M.A., Rosenfeld J., et al.: Plasma Na^+ pump inhibitor in

hypertension and hypertensive heredity. *J. Cardiovasc. Pharmacol.*, to be published.
17. Kamal L.K., Cloix J.F., Devynck M.A., et al.: Reduced ^{3}H-serotonin uptake in human blood platelets by ouabain and endogenous digitalis-like inhibitors of Na^+,K^+-ATPase. *Eur. J. Pharmacol.* 92:167, 1983.
18. Henning G., Cloix J.F.: Chromatographie d'affinité pour la détection d'un inhibiteur endogène humain de la Na^+,K^+-ATPase. *C. R. Seances Acad. Sci.*, to be published.
19. Sneddon J.M.: Sodium-dependent accumulation of 5-hydroxytryptamine by rat blood platelets. *Br. J. Pharmacol.* 37:680, 1969.
20. Kamal L.A., Le Quan-Bui K.H., Meyer P.: Decreased uptake of ^{3}H-serotonin and endogenous content of serotonin in blood platelets in hypertensive patients. *Hypertension,* to be published.
21. Whitmer K.R., Wallick E.T., Epps D.E.: Effects of extracts of rat brain on the digitalis receptor. *Life Sci.* 30:2261, 1982.
22. Gillis R.A., Quest J.A.: The role of the nervous system in the cardiovascular effects of digitalis. *Pharmacol. Rev.* 31:20, 1980.
23. Gruber K.A., Whitaker J.M., Buckalew V.M.: Endogeneous digitalis-like substance in plasma of volume expanded dogs. *Nature* 287:743, 1980.
24. Sealey J.E., Kirshman J.D., Laragh J.H.: Natriuretic activity in plasma and urine of salt-loaded man and sheep. *J. Clin. Invest.* 48:2210, 1969.
25. Brown P.R., Koutsaimanis K.G., De Wardener H.E.: Effect of urinary extracts from salt-loaded man on urinary sodium excretion by rat. *Kidney Int.* 2:1, 1972.
26. Buckalew V.M.: Variable factors affecting ultrafiltration of an humoral sodium transport inhibitor. *Nephron* 9:66, 1971.
27. Licht A., Stein S., MacGregor C.W., et al.: Progress in isolation and purification of an inhibitor of sodium transport obtained from dog urine. *Kidney Int.* 21:339, 1982.
28. Clarckson E.M., Young D.R., Raw S.M., et al.: Chemical properties, physiological action and further separation of low molecular weight natriuretic substance in the urine of the normal man, in *Hormonal Regulation of Sodium Excretion.* Amsterdam, North Holland Biochemical Press, 1980, pp. 333–340.
29. Ambrosioni E., Costa V., Montebugnoli L., et al.: Increased hypertension: An index of impaired Na^+ cellular metabolism. *Clin. Sci.* 61:181, 1981.
30. Garay R.P., Dagher G., Pernollet M.G., et al.: Inherited defect in a Na^+-K^+-cotransport system in erythrocytes of essential hypertensive patients. *Nature* 284:281, 1980.
31. Woods K.L., Beevers D.G., West M.: Familial abnormality of erythrocyte cation transport in essential hypertension. *Br. Med. J.* 282:1186, 1981.
32. Meyer P., Garay R.P., Nazaret C.: Inheritance of abnormal erythrocyte cation transport in essential hypertensives. *J. Lab. Clin. Med.* 94:764, 1979.
33. Heagerty A.M., Milner M., Bing R.F., et al.: Leucocyte membrane sodium transport in normotensive populations: Dissociation of abnormalities of sodium efflux from raised blood pressure. *Lancet* 2:894, 1982.
34. Costa F.V., Montebugnoli L., Giordani M.F., et al.: Evidence for a plasma factor affecting Na^+ cellular transport in genetic normotensive subjects and in borderline hypertensive subjects. *Clin. Sci.* 63:53s, 1982.
35. Grim C.E., Luft F.C., Miller I.Z., et al.: Effects of sodium loading and depletion in normotensive relatives of essential hypertensives. *J. Lab. Clin. Med.* 94:764, 1979.
36. Wiggins R.C., Basar I., Slater J.M.: Effect of arterial pressure and inheritance on the sodium excretory capacity of normal young men. *Clin. Sci. Mol. Med.* 54:639, 1978.
37. Araoye M.A., Khatri I.M., Yao L.L., et al.: Leucocytes intracellular cations in hypertension: Effect of antihypertensive drugs. *Am. Heart J.* 96:731, 1978.
38. Thomas R.D., Edmondson R.P.S., Hilton P.J., et al.: Abnormal sodium transport in leucocytes from patients with essential hypertension and the effect of treatment. *Clin. Sci. Mol. Med.* 48:169s, 1975.

Calcium Flux Regulation in Myocardial and Vascular Smooth Muscle

A.M. MOURA, M.D., G. HAMON, M.D., AND M. WORCEL, M.D.

Centre de Recherches Roussel-Uclaf, Romainville, 111 Route de Noisy, France

THE IMPORTANCE of Ca^{2+} ions in the cardiovascular system, from both the physiologic and the pharmacologic points of view, has been well established. The involvement of these ions in excitation-contraction coupling regulation has been known for a long time. In fact, it is generally admitted that the variation in intracellular concentration of free Ca^{2+} $(Ca^{2+})_i$ is the cause of modifications in the contractile force and basic tone of these cells. An increase in $(Ca^{2+})_i$ between $10^{-7}M$ and $10^{-6}M$ induces the formation of cross-bridges between myosin and action filaments.

Research carried out during the last decade has led to great progress in the understanding, at the molecular level, of the regulatory mechanism of cardiac and vascular contraction. This has opened the way for new privileged targets with important therapeutical repercussions.

Many reviews have been published on the role of Ca^{2+} in the excitation-contraction coupling of smooth muscles and cardiac cells.[9, 42, 52, 174] This chapter reviews the various regulatory mechanisms of transmembrane and intracytoplasmic Ca^{2+} movements and addresses the question of how pharmacologic

173

agents can modify these movements, and to what extent, therefore some of these mechanisms should be the object of top priority research.

Ca^{2+} Influx

In the resting state, the $(Ca^{2+})_i$ concentration is around $10^{-7}M$ and the extracellular concentration, $(Ca^{2+})_o$, is about $10^{-3}M$. An inward concentration gradient of about 10,000 through the cytoplasmic membrane is thus created. Moreover, the difference in the distribution of electrical charges on both sides of this membrane determines a resting potential of about -80 to -90 mV for cardiac cells and about -45 to -60 mV for vascular smooth muscle cells. This large membrane electrochemical gradient induces a passive influx of Ca^{2+} into the cell. However, these ions are not distributed in a homogeneous mannner in the intracellular medium. In fact, some intracellular organelles are able to store large amounts of Ca^{2+}. Thus, exchanges of Ca^{2+} between intracellular organelles and cytoplasm add to Ca^{2+} influxes through the plasmic membrane. During cell excitation, passive Ca^{2+} influxes are increased due to the opening of ionic channels admitting this cation selectively. These channels are activated by membrane depolarization, but a direct activation of a membrane receptor can also produce channel opening.

In Cardiac Muscle

In the resting state, cardiac cell membrane Ca^{2+} permeability is very low. Indeed, the passive Ca^{2+} influx is about 100 times less than the passive Na^+ influx.[102] Analysis of ^{45}Ca fluxes has showed that Ca^{2+} influx is sensitive to variations in the extracellular concentrations of Na^+, $(Na^+)_o$, and $(Ca^{2+})_o$.[101, 122] Moreover, experimental results show evidence of a competition between Na^+ and Ca^{2+} for a common carrier mechanism, according to a $(Ca^{2+})_o/(Na^+)_o^2$ ratio.[122] The intracellular concentration of Na^+ $(Na^+)_i$ also influences the entry of Ca^{2+}: increasing $(Na^+)_i$ by different means induces an increase in Ca^{2+} influx.[58, 103] To explain this influence of Na^+ on Ca^{2+} influx, many authors have suggested the intervention of an Na^+-Ca^{2+} countertransport mechanism. In the absence of clear experimental proofs, the existence of this pathway for the entry of extracellular Ca^{2+} has been much debated until recently.[42, 154] However, the existence of an Na^+-Ca^{2+} exchange mechanism has now been proved beyond doubt in the sarcolemma (see subsequent section on Ca^{2+} efflux). As its calculated reversal potential is between the diastolic resting potential and the mean polarization value of action potential (AP) plateau, this exchange mechanism must theoretically participate in Ca^{2+} entry (coupled with Na^+ efflux) during the AP plateau.[43, 105]

Nevertheless, the main pathway for Ca^{2+} entry is the slow Ca^{2+}-Na^+ channels activated during AP.

The contraction of cardiac tissue is physiologically triggered by a depolarization wave. Two main inward ionic currents contribute to the characteristic form of AP which triggers each heartbeat: a fast inward current, I_{Na}, responsible for the fast rising phase of AP, followed by a current activated by this depolarization, I_{si} (slow inward current), with a slower kinetic, and partly responsible for the AP plateau. The fast inward current results from the entry of Na^+ ions, whereas the slow current, which has a lower amplitude, mainly results from the influx of Ca^{2+} ions, but can also admit Na^+ and K^+ ions.[110, 137] It should be noted that the contribution of this Ca^{2+} current is most important for electrical activity of the sinus node[13, 125, 127] and atrioventricular node.[94, 126]

I_{si} is a fundamental current for the excitation-contraction coupling.[52, 103, 179] The passive Ca^{2+} influx during the opening of calcium channels triggered by membrane depolarization is, however, not sufficient by itself to fully activate the contractile apparatus in mammals.[194] However, this Ca^{2+} influx during the AP plateau is able to induce a Ca^{2+} release, mainly from the sarcoplasmic reticulum,[41, 42, 49] and probably also from the inner side of the sarcolemma. In some way, this process constitutes a mechanism of amplification that results in a sufficient rise in the level of $(Ca^{2+})_i$ for a full contraction.

The passive Ca^{2+} influx through the slow channel depends on $(Ca^{2+})_o$ and the duration and frequency of AP.[11]

Many authors have suggested that the opening mechanism of the calcium channels may be controlled by a metabolic process.[34] Based on biochemical data, a mechanism requiring the intervention of a Ca^{2+} dependent ATPase has been sug gested.[34] Recently, in light of more direct electrophysiologic results, it has been shown that the amplitude of I_{si} could be increased by a rise in $(ATP)_i$ and $(cAMP)_i$.[82] This seems to confirm the importance of the phosphorylation state of calcium channels as suggested by analysis of the mechanism of action of adrenaline on cardiac muscle. Other metabolic processes have been proposed in the regulation of Ca^{2+} transmembrane movements, but their role remains controversial.[34]

In Vascular Smooth Muscle

In quiescent smooth muscle cells as in cardiac cells, Ca^{2+} influx follows the transmembrane electrochemical gradient. This passive Ca^{2+} influx is sensitive to modifications of $(Na^+)_o$.[148, 150] In light of results obtained on visceral smooth muscles,[10, 174] it would seem that $(Na^+)_i$ could also influence Ca^{2+} influx. Some authors have suggested the presence of an Na^+-Ca^{2+} countertransport mechanism, identical to the one described for the heart.[8, 65, 130, 139] However, in the absence of experimental proofs, this pathway for Ca^{2+} entry remains controversial in the case of vascular smooth muscle as well as visceral smooth muscle.[23, 170, 191] The contraction of vascular smooth muscle cells is, in fact, triggered by a depolarization linked to a rise in the Ca^{2+}-Na^+ permeability.[8, 86, 89, 175] Ca^{2+} influx, following its own electrochemical gradient, takes place essentially through two types of channels whose opening is dependent on stimulus: channels sensitive to membrane potential, and channels linked to membrane receptors whose activation determines the opening.

Some vascular smooth muscles are able to generate AP, either spontaneously or during the action of nervous or humoral mediators (i.e., portal vein). A phasic contraction is linked to each AP. These AP essentially result from activation of a slow Ca^{2+}-Na^+, potential-dependent, inward current.[29, 68, 83, 86, 114]

Some smooth muscles do not generate AP (i.e., aorta). In the presence of some mediators (noradrenaline, angiotensin II) they generate a slow and sustained contraction. This tonic contraction is linked to a slow depolarization without AP. This depolarization is due to the opening of slow Ca^{2+}-Na^+ channels which do not depend on membrane potential.[9, 72] It has been shown that in these smooth muscles, the activation of the slow

Ca^{2+}-Na^+ conductance is counteracted by an excessively high membrane K^+ conductance, thus preventing the production of AP.[9]

Ca^{2+} can also enter the cells through channels directly activated by the occupation of membrane receptors which are linked to them (receptor-operated channels).[9] However, it seems, at least by analogy with the observations made on visceral smooth muscles, that the channels linked to receptors are also able to admit Na^+ ions. Thus, Hamon and Worcel[74] have shown that, in the rat uterus, depolarization induced by angiotensin II is due to a primary rise in Na^+ conductance. Due to this depolarization, AP are generated as the consequence of activation of potential-dependent Ca^{2+}-Na^+ channels.

Generally, the amount of Ca^{2+} entering through the different calcium channels does not seem sufficient to fully activate the contractile apparatus. As in cardiac muscle, Ca^{2+} influx would be amplified by a release of Ca^{2+} from intracellular binding sites.[9, 75] Two main mechanisms of mobilization of intracellular Ca^{2+} have been proposed: (1) a mechanism of release of Ca^{2+} bound to the sarcoplasmic reticulum, by Ca^{2+} influx during AP[9]; and (2) a direct release of Ca^{2+} from the superficial sarcoplasmic reticulum immediately underneath the plasmic membrane.[55] This could constitute a sort of electromechanical coupling.[86]

Release of Ca^{2+} from intracellular binding sites could also occur without any change in the resting membrane potential or pharmacomechanical coupling.[9, 149] In this case, it would be the release of Ca^{2+} linked to membrane receptors that would produce the release of Ca^{2+} from the sarcoplasmic reticulum. This mechanism could be responsible for the phasic component of contraction of large vessels devoid of electrical activity.[32, 33, 171, 172]

Ca^{2+} Efflux

In Cardiac Muscle

The increase in $(Ca^{2+})_i$ which takes place during each contraction has to be eliminated during diastole; in other words, a beat-to-beat regulation of $(Ca^{2+})_i$ is necessary for the normal activity of cardiac muscle. Two mechanisms have been proposed to explain the regulation of $(Ca^{2+})_i$ at a level lower than the threshold concentration required for the activation of contractile proteins: (1) an Na^+-Ca^{2+} exchange mechanism; and (2) an active pumping mechanism carried out by a calcium pump (see Fig 1,A).

Na^+-Ca^{2+} Exchange Mechanism

Some authors had observed, for a long time, that Na^+ ions had some effects on calcium metabolism in heart tissue,[105] when Reuter and Seitz[138] obtained clear experimental evidence enabling them to suggest the existence of an exchange mechanism between Na^+ and Ca^{2+}. In particular, Reuter and Seitz[138] have shown that Ca efflux is sensitive to Na^+ transmembrane gradient. In 1974, Reuter[136] developed this model and suggested an electrically neutral exchange of two extracellular Na^+ ions for one intracellular Ca^{2+} ion. According to this hypothesis, the energy required for the extrusion of Ca^{2+} is provided by the electrochemical transmembrane gradient of Na^+ in such a manner that the movement of Na following its gradient would ensure the supply of sufficient energy for the extrusion of Ca^{2+} against its own gradient. Ca^{2+} efflux through this pathway would only indirectly depend on ATP hydrolysis.

The energy provided by Na electrochemical gradient is, however, not sufficient to allow the transfer of one Ca^{2+} ion against two Na^+ ions.[105] If we accept that the Na^+-Ca^{2+} exchange system operates solely on the basis of Na^+ gradient, a coupling ratio higher than 2 is necessary.

Recent experimental results obtained from simultaneous measurements of intracellular Na^+ and Ca^{2+} activities have given a coupling ratio between 2.5 and 3.[5, 53] The analysis of ^{45}Ca efflux from sarcolemmal isolated vesicles has led Pitts[133] to calculate a coupling ratio of 3.

Since the transfer of electrical charges through the membrane is not equal, the system is not electroneutral and should be sensitive to variations in membrane potential.[118] The reversal potential of the exchange mechanism has a value which is between the resting membrane potential and the AP plateau.[105, 118] Thus, the Na^+-Ca^{2+} exchange mechanism seems to be able to contribute both to Ca^{2+} influx during AP plateau and to Ca^{2+} extrusion during diastole.

Ca^{2+} Pump

A Ca^{2+} extrusion mechanism directly dependent on ATP hydrolysis in cardiac cell membranes has been suggested by many authors and constitutes an alternative to the extrusion mechanism through Na^+-Ca^{2+} exchange. Indeed, studies carried out mainly on isolated cardiac sarcoplasmic membrane preparations reconstituted into vesicles have shown the existence of a Ca^{2+}-Mg^{2+}-ATPase which could be linked to a calcium pump. These vesicular preparations containing enriched sarcolemmal membranes are able to accumulate Ca^{2+} by an ATP- and Mg^{2+}-dependent process.[17, 19–21, 28, 98, 100, 116, 158] Ca^{2+} translocation rate, however, is slower through the calcium pump than through the Na^+-Ca^{2+} exchange mechanism.[19] Therefore, the Na^+-Ca^{2+} exchange mechanism, owing to its greater rate, could carry out the greater part of transmembrane Ca^{2+} extrusion during muscular activity, whereas the calcium pump would ensure transport when $(Ca^{2+})_i$ is below the micromolar concentration, during diastole.[19, 21]

Unlike the Na^+-Ca^{2+} exchange mechanism, the calcium pump is regulated by a phosphorylation-dephosphorylation mechanism dependent on cAMP, with phosphorylation increasing the activity of the enzyme rather than its affinity for Ca^{2+}.[20]

Calmodulin, a cytoplasmic calciprotein, also seems to be an important regulating factor in sarcolemmal calcium pump activity. It increases not only the V_{max} of the enzyme but also its affinity for Ca^{2+}.[19, 98, 158] Conversely, cyclic guanosine monophosphate decreases the rotation rate of the enzyme, and to a lesser extent, its affinity for Ca^{2+}.[28]

During relaxation, the membrane Ca^{2+} extrusion pathways play only a minor role in the elimination of $(Ca^{2+})_i$, which is increased during systole. Indeed, the reuptake by intracellular organelles, especially the sarcoplasmic reticulum, seems to be much more important.[2] The sarcoplasmic reticulum is able to accumulate Ca^{2+} against a large concentration gradient particularly because of a Ca^{2+}-ATPase which has a much higher capacity than the Ca^{2+}-ATPase of the sarcolemma.[22] This Ca^{2+}-ATPase of sarcoplasmic reticulum is stimulated by a protein kinase dependent on cAMP.[95, 157] The activity of the sarcoplasmic reticulum calcium pump can also be stimulated by calmodulin,[90] even though it seems to be involved only in case of an abnormal calcium overloading.[107]

In Vascular Smooth Muscle

Similarly, two Ca^{2+} extrusion mechanisms have been proposed for the vascular smooth muscle cells.

Na^+-Ca^{2+} Exchange Mechanism

In the absence of any external stimulation, some of these cells show a resting tone or myogenic tone,[168] probably resulting from the regulation of $(Ca^{2+})_i$ at a level higher than the contraction threshold. This vascular tone can show slow variations and could be modulated by an Na^+-Ca^{2+} exchange mechanism[8] identical to that described for cardiac cells. The Ca^{2+} electrochemical gradient would be maintained by the Na^+ electrochemical gradient. Thus, Na^+ and its concentration-regulating mechanisms could play an important role in controlling arterial contractility.[8, 65, 130, 139] However, in the absence of clear proofs, the participation of the Na^+-Ca^{2+} exchange mechanism in vascular smooth muscle relaxation remains controversial.[38]

Ca^{2+} Pump

Ca^{2+} can also be extruded from the cell by a mechanism directly dependent on ATP hydrolysis. A Ca^{2+}-Mg^{2+} ATPase has been identified in isolated membrane preparations from vascular smooth muscle cells reconstituted into vesicles. This Ca^{2+}-Mg^{2+}-ATPase could be linked to a calcium pump. Indeed, these vesicular preparations are able to accumulate Ca^{2+} by an ATP-dependent process.[48, 51, 65, 99, 195] These Ca^{2+} pumps are localized in plasmic membrane as well as in the sarcoplasmic reticulum membrane, at least as suggested by observations made on visceral smooth muscle.[193] According to some authors,[65] these two Ca^{2+} extrusion mechanisms could coexist. As in the heart, the Ca^{2+} pump could show a greater affinity for Ca^{2+} than does the Na^+-Ca^{2+} exchange mechanism. However, contrary to what has been observed in heart cells,[21] the Ca^{2+} pump could also have a larger capacity than the Na^+-Ca^{2+} exchange mechanism. Thus, the Na^+-Ca^{2+} exchange mechanism might modulate the slow variations of vascular tone, the Ca^{2+} pump being involved during a large increase in $(Ca^{2+})_i$.

As in the heart cell, calmodulin would regulate Ca^{2+} pump by increasing its affinity for Ca^{2+}.[117, 195] This calciprotein, which is a true Ca^{2+} receptor[26] and in itself inactive, probably also regulates intracytoplasmic Ca^{2+} movements. In particular, it would ensure the activation of myosine kinase by Ca^{2+}, thus allowing myosine phosphorylation, without which the interaction with actin cannot take place.[142] Furthermore, it appears that cAMP can modulate the effects of calmodulin[1] by interacting with dissociation of the calcium-calmodulin complex.

The reuptake of Ca^{2+} by intracellular organelles and particularly by the sarcoplasmic reticulum seems to largely participate, as in cardiac cells, in the normalization of $(Ca^{2+})_i$.[47, 50, 88, 115, 134, 152, 153]

Modulation of Calcium Movements by Endogenous Substances

Many endogenous substances can affect the heart and vessels, directly modifying their contractile force and their basic tone. Here we will consider only catecholamines, whose effects on calcium movements have been well documented.

In the Heart

Catecholamines induce a positive inotropic and chronotropic action. This double action, which mainly results from β-adrenergic receptor activation, is essentially due to an increase in I_{si} without any change in its kinetic.[137, 140, 141, 183] This cardiac β-adrenergic-stimulating effect seems to occur through an increase in intracellular cAMP concentration resulting from a stimulation of the membrane adenylate cyclase. Indeed, any treatment that increases the intracellular cAMP content mimics the increase in I_{si} induced by the stimulation of β-adrenergic receptors, including intracellular application of cAMP,[161, 163, 165, 184, 197] exposure to membrane-permeating cAMP analogues,[120, 164] phosphodiesterases inhibition,[16] and injection of cAMP-dependent protein kinase subunit.[129]

This regulating action of cAMP on I_{si} could be the result of a direct phosphorylation of the membrane calcium channels induced by a protein kinase activated by cAMP[140, 188] or by indirect action through local modifications in the cytoplasmic ionic concentrations following stimulation of the Ca^{2+} pumping mechanisms.[14, 43, 56]

In the Vessels

Catecholamines are also important vasoactive agents. By activating α-adrenergic and β-adrenergic receptors of vessels, they respectively produce a contraction and a relaxation.

Activation of α-Adrenergic Receptors

The activation of α-adrenergic receptors by catecholamines is linked to an increase in Ca^{2+} influx.[24, 59, 71, 91, 167, 185] The contraction thus produced is associated with a depolarization with or without an increase in electrical activity, depending on vessels.[32, 92, 132, 171]

In spontaneously active vessels, the membrane depolarization is accompanied by an acceleration of spontaneous AP.[81, 119, 149] This phenomenon is associated with an increase in Ca^{2+} conductance but also in Na^+ conductance.[111, 145]

In some vessels, this α-adrenergic stimulation seems to be associated with release of Ca^{2+} from intracellular stores.[32, 37, 69, 70, 79, 92, 152, 173] In vitro, noradrenaline can accelerate the dissociation of Ca^{2+} from rabbit aorta microsomes.[4] This release of Ca^{2+} from internal stores would be responsible for the noradrenaline-induced phasic component of contraction in large vessels devoid of any electrical activity, like aorta.[32, 33, 60, 69, 171, 172] It is very likely that the release of Ca^{2+} from internal stores is triggered by a release of Ca^{2+} linked to membrane receptors through a pharmacomechanical coupling.[9] Then the tension would be maintained by an influx of Ca^{2+}.[32, 33, 171, 172] Since the identification of α_1 and α_2 receptors in the plasmic membrane of vascular smooth muscles,[31, 35, 36, 160, 196] different hypotheses have been proposed as to the role of these receptor subclasses in the effect of catecholamines on Ca^{2+} movements. Some authors suggest[63, 64, 177] that the release of Ca^{2+} from internal stores is due to stimulation of α_1 receptors, the activation of α_2 receptors inducing the opening of membrane Ca^{2+} channels. The opposite hypothesis is suggested by Van Breemen et al.[176] and Vanhoutte et al.[182] These hypotheses are based on the differing sensitivity of α_1- and α_2-adrenergic receptors for Ca^{2+} antagonists. It is likely that the results are the consequence of a difference in the activation of calcium channels by α_1 and α_2 receptors.[25] Moreover, the heterogeneity of vascular smooth muscle cells on which these studies were carried out could contribute to the disparate findings.[182]

Activation of β-Adrenergic Receptors

The activation by catecholamines of β-adrenergic receptors of vessels induces a relaxation or a reduction in the amplitude of contractions produced by a stimulating agent.[92] This action is more pronounced in smaller vessels.[108] The activation of β-adrenergic receptors has two synergic effects: (1) a hyperpolarization or a rise in membrane potential, thus abolishing AP generation[84]; and (2) an increase in cAMP induced by the activation of adenylate cyclase.[7,44] Even though no cause-and-effect correlation has been established between phosphorylation stimulated by an increase in cAMP and relaxation,[80] these two actions ought to lead to a reduction in $(Ca^{2+})_i$ by different ways. Indeed, by increasing the cAMP-dependent Na^+-K^+-ATPase activity, cAMP could induce a relaxation by indirectly activating Na^+-Ca^{2+} exchange mechanism.[66,84,144]

A stimulation of the electrogenic Na^+ pump by cAMP is also able to induce a hyperpolarization.[189] It has been shown that cAMP and protein kinases activated by cAMP are able to increase Ca^{2+} sequestration in intracellular stores.[39,84,113] Moreover, due to competition between the cAMP-dependent protein kinase and calmodulin,[78,146,169] an increase in cAMP could bring about a dissociation of the Ca^{2+}-calmodulin complex.[1,112]

Pharmacologic Modulations

THE CARDIOTONIC GLYCOSIDES

The positive inotropic effects of cardiotonic glycosides are commonly explained by an interaction with the Na^+-K^+-AT-

Pase, a sarcolemmal enzyme that supplies energy to the Na^+ pump responsible for maintaining the Na^+ and K^+ transmembrane gradients. According to this hypothesis, inhibition of the Na^+ pump could result in an increase in $(Na^+)_i$, leading to an increase in Ca^{2+} influx or a decrease in Ca^{2+} extrusion through Na^+-Ca^{2+} exchange mechanism, especially in sarcolemmal membrane.[104] This mechanism is greatly debated, especially with regard to low therapeutic digitalis concentrations.[3, 6, 57, 61, 124, 128] Indeed, whereas the action of high concentrations (toxic concentrations) certainly seems to involve this Na^+-Ca^{2+} exchange mechanism,[2, 104] the intracellular ionic modifications produced by low concentrations of digitalis have been much more difficult to show. Only recently, owing to the use of Na^+-sensitive microelectrodes, has a close parallel been observed between an increase in intracellular Na^+ activity and the positive inotropic effect of digitalis.[53, 187] This observation favors the implication of an Na^+-Ca^{2+} exchange mechanism even at the lower digitalis concentrations. Moreover, it indicates that Na^+-K^+-ATPase activity may play a role in the modulation of $(Ca^{2+})_i$. The positive inotropic effect of glycosides seems also to result in part from their ability to stimulate I_{si}; an increase in the amplitude of this current by digitalis has been reported.[109, 166, 190]

Calcium Antagonists

Calcium homeostasis of contractile structures is closely linked to a fine adjustment of the various mechanisms controlling $(Ca^{2+})_i$. The upsetting of one of these mechanisms can lead to structural and functional alterations in cardiac and vascular cells, resulting in pathologic situations: angina and especially vasospastic angina, heart failure, arrhythmias, cardiomyopathy, etc. These alterations could also lead to some hypertensive states and cerebrovascular diseases. Indeed, calcium overloading not only can modify the contraction-relaxation cycle, it also can alter some metabolic steps, resulting in cell death. For example, in cardiac cells, ischemia or hypoxia induces a collapse in ATP stores, resulting in $(Ca^{2+})_i$ increase, which in turn produces a more severe depletion of energy reserves.[121] In preventing an excessive intracellular influx of Ca^{2+}, every substance able to selectively inhibit the penetration of these ions would have both a beneficial effect on energy metabolism of the cell and a protective effect.

Inorganic cations like Mn^{2+}, La^{3+}, Ba^{2+}, and Ni^+ behave as antagonists of several calcium-dependent processes.[9, 93, 135, 162] The calcium antagonist effects of these cations are probably the consequence of their interaction with Ca^{2+} binding sites. However, as a result of their lack of selectivity for a given function or a given tissue, these cations can only be used as pharmacologic tools. During the last decade, the development of substances that selectively block calcium channels has not only brought information on the role of Ca^{2+} transmembrane exchange in the heart and in vessels but also has opened the way to new therapeutical approaches. The selectivity of action of these substances can easily be observed at the level of both myocardiac and vascular smooth muscle cells.[46] Calcium antagonists do not constitute a homogeneous chemical class. At the present time, they are subdivided into four main groups: phenylalkylamines (verapamil-like), diphenylalkylamines (bepridil type), benzothiazapines (diltiazem type), and dihydropyridines (nifedipine type).

When administered in concentrations normally used in therapy, these substances seem to directly affect neither the Ca^{2+} sensitivity of myofibrils nor Ca^{2+} sarcoplasmic reticulum and mitochondria transport mechanisms.[121] Their action seems to be limited to the transmembrane flux of Ca^{2+} through the slow, potential-dependent, calcium-sodium channels; this justifies their common designation as slow calcium channel inhibitors.[121, 162]

In cardiac cells the application of verapamil or diltiazem or nifedipine results in a decrease in the amplitude of the slow I_{si} current without any change in activation kinetics.[106] The slow conducting intracardiac structures which show AP with a slow rising phase whose activation mainly depends on the development I_{si} would be highly sensitive to slow channel inhibitors. This is especially true for the sinus node pacemaker cells and atrioventricular nodal cells. However, such slow responses are also observed under various abnormal situations like ischemia, hypoxia, and during partial depolarization induced by catecholamines. Moreover, in isolated cardiac preparations, the slow calcium channel inhibitors greatly prolong the effective refractory period of slow response structures, especially in atrioven tricular nodal cells.[147] The blocking effect on cardiac calcium channels seems to be the result of a renal antagonism with Ca^{2+}, although this effect cannot be explained by a competition for the same binding site,[106] as opposed to the antagonism observed with inorganic cations.[73, 106] As suggested for D600,[77] the organic antagonist could bind to a site close to the internal side of the membrane.

The inhibiting effect of slow channel blockers depends on the frequency of APand membrane potentials. However, as for the blocking effect of local anesthetics on sodium channel, this action qualitatively depends on the chemical structures of molecules. Indeed, the antagonism increases with cell activity frequency, with a time constant of a few minutes for D600 and diltiazem but only a few seconds for nitrendipine.[106]

In AP-generating vessels it has been shown that Ca^{2+} antagonists reduce the amplitude and frequency of spontaneous contractions[67, 85, 178, 192] as well as the amplitude and frequency of the associated AP.[54, 67, 68, 70, 76, 85, 97, 156, 192] These electrical and contractile activities could even be abolished.[54, 70, 178] However, some authors have observed that nifedipine was able to suppress contractions induced by electrical stimulation in rat caudal artery without alteration of the associated AP.[155]

In vessels that do not readily generate AP, Ca^{2+} antagonists only inhibit calcium movements and the contractile phase associated with membrane depolarization. At therapeutic doses these substances do not affect Ca^{2+} movements resulting from the opening of channels linked to receptors. Therefore, as in the heart, Ca^{2+} antagonists preferentially inhibit Ca^{2+} movements through the ionic channels activated during membrane depolarization.[62, 65a, 174]

However, some Ca^{2+} antagonists, like verapamil and bepridil, accumulate in cardiac as well as in vascular smooth muscle cells, whereas nifedipine and diltiazem seem to equilibrate on both sides of cell membrane.[131] Many authors have suggested an additional intracellular effect in order to explain the mechanism of action of Ca^{2+} antagonists.[27, 87, 186] However, no experimental proof allows us to state that intracellular processes are brought into play by therapeutic concentrations.[30, 54, 96, 97, 143, 156] Nevertheless, an intracellular interaction has been reported with relatively high concentrations $(10^{-5}M)$ of antagonists, i.e., diltiazem[143] and verapamil.[159]

As in the case of cardiac cells, the inhibition of the influx of Ca^{2+} in vascular smooth muscle cells could well be related to the electrical activity frequency of the tissue. Indeed, results obtained by Bolton[9a] on a visceral smooth muscle support such a hypothesis. In vessels, it is possible to observe, for a given calcium antagonist molecule, some specificity of action, depending on the vascular bed and the vasoconstricting agent.[65a] In general, vascular arterial beds are more sensitive to Ca^{2+} antagonists than venous beds.[178] Moreover, their action seems to be more pronounced at the arterial level.[27, 40] It should also be noted that coronary and cerebral vessels are particularly sensitive to these agents.[46] The coronary excitation-contraction coupling is generally 3–10 times more sensitive to the action of Ca^{2+} antagonists than ordinary myocardiac fibers.[46]

On the other hand, it has been suggested that the activation of vessels by catecholamines could be differentially antagonized by Ca^{2+} antagonists, depending on the type of α-adrenergic receptor involved. Indeed, a higher sensitivity of α_2 compared to α_1 receptor stimulation has been reported.[177, 180] This selectivity is, however, debated.[181]

The overall cardiovascular effects of calcium antagonists in the animal and human being are quite different from those observed in isolated preparations. The outcome of the effects of these different substances at various levels of the circulatory apparatus largely depends on the degree of activation of the reflex regulation mechanisms. In particular, depending on the degree of the vasodilating and hypotensive effect of these molecules, their direct cardiac effect would be masked. In fact, it is by this mechanism that the various calcium antagonists can be differentiated one from another. This also conditions their therapeutic applications.[12, 147]

In conclusion, the modulation of intracellular Ca^{2+} concentration is the result of a close coordination of membrane and intracellular functions. By preventing an excessive influx of Ca^{2+}, Ca^{2+} antagonists exert a protective effect on vascular and cardiac cells as a result of a selective action on transmembrane Ca^{2+} transfers.

REFERENCES

1. Adelstein R.S., Eisenberg E.: Regulation and kinetics of the actin-myosin-ATP interaction. *Annu. Rev. Biochem,* 49;921, 1980.

2. Akera T., Brody T.M.: The role of Na-K-ATPase in the inotropic action of digitalis. *Pharmacol. Rev.* 29:187, 1978.

3. Akera T., Brody T.M.: Cardiotonic agents and the sodium transient. *TIPS* 2:191, 1981.

4. Baudouin-Legros M., Meyer P.: Effects of angiotensin, catecholamines and cyclic AMP on calcium storage in aortic microsomes. *Br. J. Pharmacol.* 47:377, 1973.

5. Bers D.M., Ellis D.: Intracellular calcium and sodium activity in sheep heart Purkinje fibers: Effects of changes of external sodium and internal pH. *Pflugers Arch.* 393:171, 1982.

6. Besch H.R., Watanabe A.M.: The positive inotropic effect of digitoxin: Independence from sodium accumulation. *J. Pharmacol. Exp. Ther.* 207:958, 1978.

7. Bhalla R.C., Webb R.C., Singh D., et al.: Role of cyclic AM in rat aortic microsomal phosphorylation and calcium uptake. *Am. J. Physiol.* 234:H508, 1978.

8. Blaustein M.P.: Sodium ions, calcium ions, blood pressure regulation and hypertension: A reassessment and a hypothesis. *Am. J. Physiol.* 232:C165, 1977.

9. Bolton T.B.: Mechanisms of action of transmitters and other substances on smooth muscle. *Physiol. Rev.* 59:607, 1979.

9a. Bolton T.B.: Use dependent effect of calcium entry blocking drugs on the electrical and mechanical activities on guinea-pig taenia coli. *Br. J. Pharmacol.* 78:174, 1983.

10. Brading A.F.: Calcium-induced increase in membrane permeability in the guinea pig taenia-coli: Evidence for involvement of a sodium-calcium exchange mechanism. *J. Physiol.* 275:65, 1978.

11. Braunwald E., Sonnenblick E.H., Ross J.: Contraction of the normal heart, Braunwald E. (ed.): in *Heart Disease.* Philadelphia, W.B. Saunders Co., 1980, pp. 413–451.

12. Braunwald E.: Mechanism of action of calcium-channel-blocking agents. *N. Engl. J. Med.* 307:1618, 1982.

13. Brown H.F., Giles W., Noble S.J.: Membrane currents underlying activity in frog sinus venosus. *J. Physiol.* 271:783, 1977.

14. Brown H.F., Kimura J., Noble S.J.: Calcium entry dependent inactivation of the slow inward current in the rabbit sinoatrial node. *J. Physiol.* 320:11P, 1981.

15. Carafoli E., Zurini M.: The Ca^{2+} pumping ATPase of plasma membranes: Purification, reconstitution and properties. *Biochim. Biophys. Acta* 683:279, 1982.

16. Carmeliet E., Vereecke J.: Adrenaline and the plateau phase of the cardiac action potential: Importance of Ca^{2+}, Na^+, and K^+ conductance. *Pflugers Arch.* 313:300, 1969.

17. Caroni P., Carafoli E.: An ATP-dependent Ca^{2+} pumping system in dog heart sarcolemma. *Nature* 283:765, 1980.

18. Caroni P., Reinlib L., Carafoli E.: Charge movements during the Na^+/Ca^{2+} exchange in heart sarcolemmal vesicles. *Proc. Natl. Acad. Sci. USA* 77:6354, 1980.

19. Caroni P., Carafoli E.: The Ca^{2+} pumping ATPase of heart sarcolemma: Characterization, calmodulin dependence, and partial purification. *J. Biol. Chem.* 256:3263, 1981.

20. Caroni P., Carafoli E.: Regulation of calcium in pumping ATPase of heart sarcolemma by a phosphorylation dephosphorylation process. *J. Biol. Chem.* 256:9371, 1981.

21. Caroni P., Zurini M., Clark A.: The calcium-pumping ATPase of heart sarcolemma, in *Transport ATPase. Ann. NY Acad. Sci.,* 402:402, 1982.

22. Caroni P. Zurini M., Clark A., et al.: Further characterization and reconstitution of the purified Ca^{2+} pumping ATPase of heart sarcolemma. *J. Biol. Chem.* 258:7305, 1983.

23. Casteels R.: Membrane potential in smooth muscle, Bülbring E., Brading A.F., Jones A.W., et al. (eds.): in *Smooth Muscle.* London, Arnold, 1981, pp.105–126.

24. Casteels R., Kitamura K., Kuriyama H., et al.: Excitation-contraction coupling in the smooth muscle cells of the rabbit main pulmonary artery. *J. Physiol.* 271:63, 1977.

25. Cauvin C., Loutzenhiser R., Hwang O., et al.: α-Adrenoreceptors induce Ca influx and intracellular Ca release in isolated rabbit aorta. *Eur. J. Pharmacol.* 84:233, 1982.

26. Cheung W.Y.: Calmodulin plays a pivotal role in cellular regulation. *Science* 207:19, 1980.

27. Church J., Zsoter T.T.: Calcium antagonistic drugs: Mechanism of action. *Can. J. Physiol. Pharmacol.* 58:254, 1980.

28. Church J.G., Sen A.K.: Regulation of canine heart sarcolemmal Ca^{2+}-pumping ATPase by cyclic GMP. *Biochim. Biophys. Acta* 728:191, 1983.

29. Daemers-Lambert C.: Voltage-clamp studies on rat portal vein, in Bülbring E., Shuba M.F. (eds.): *Physiology of Smooth Muscle.* New York, Raven Press, 1976, pp. 83–90.

30. Daly M.J., Perry S., Nayler W.G.: Calcium antagonists and calmodulin: Effects of verapamil, nifedipine and diltiazem. *Eur. J. Pharmacol.* 90:103, 1983.

31. De Mey J., Vanhoutte P.M.: Uneven distribution of postjunctional alpha$_1$ and alpha$_2$-like adrenoreceptors in canine arterial and venous smooth muscle. *Cir. Res.* 48:875, 1981.

32. Deth R., Van Breemen C.: Relative contributions of Ca^{2+} influx and cellular Ca^{2+} release during drug induced activation of the rabbit aorta. *Pflugers Arch.* 348:13, 1974.

33. Deth R., Van Breemen C.: Agonist-induced $^{45}Ca^{2+}$ release from smooth muscle cells of the rabbit aorta. *J. Membr. Biol.* 30:363, 1977.

34. Dhalla N.S., Pierce G.N., Panagia V., et al.: Calcium movements in relation to heart function. *Basic Res. Cardiol.* 77:117, 1982.

35. Diggs K.G., Summers R.J.: Characterization of postsynaptic alpha-adrenoreceptors in rat aortic strip and portal veins. *Br. J. Pharmacol.* 79:655, 1983.

36. Docherty J.R., McDonald A., McGrath J.C.: Further subclassification of α adron oceptors in the cardiovascular system, vas deferens and anococcygeus of the rat. *Br. J. Pharmacol.* 67:421P, 1979.

37. Droogmans G., Raeymaekers L., Casteels R.: Electro- and pharmaco-mechanical coupling in the smooth muscle cells of the rabbit ear artery. *J. Gen. Physiol.* 70:129, 1977.

38. Droogmans G., Casteels R.: Sodium and calcium interactions in vascular smooth muscle cells of the rabbit ear artery. *J. Gen. Physiol.* 74:57, 1979.

39. Ebashi S., Mikawa T., Hirata M., et al.: Regulatory proteins of smooth muscle, in Casteels R., Godfraind T., Rüegg J.C. (eds.): *Excitation-Contraction Coupling in Smooth Muscle.* Amsterdam, Elsevier/North Holland Biomedical Press, 1977, pp. 325–334.

40. Ekelund L.G.: Ca-blockers and peripheral circulation: Physiological viewpoints. *Acta Pharmacol. Toxicol.* 1(suppl. 33), 1978.

41. Fabiato A., Fabiato F.: Calcium release from the sarcoplasmic reticulum. *Circ. Res.* 40:119, 1977.

42. Fabiato A., Fabiato F.: Calcium and cardiac excitation-contraction coupling. *Annu. Rev. Physiol.* 41:473, 1979.

43. Fischmeister R., Vassort G.: The electrogenic Na-Ca exchange and the cardiac electrical activity: I. Simulation on Purkinje fibre action potential. *J. Physiol. (Paris)* 77:705, 1981.

44. Fitzpatrick D.F., Szentivanyi A.: Stimulation of calcium uptake into aortic microsomes by cyclic AMP and cyclic AMP-dependent protein kinase. *Naunyn-Schmiedebergs Arch. Pharmacol.* 298:255, 1977.

45. Fleckenstein A., Tritthart H., Fleckenstein B., et al.: A new group of competitive

Ca-antagonists (Iproveratril, D600, Prenylamine) with highly potent inhibitory effects on excitation-contraction coupling in mammalian myocardium. *Pflugers Arch.* 307:R25, 1969.

46. Fleckenstein A.: Specific pharmacology of calcium in myocardium cardiac pacemakers, and vascular smooth muscle. *Annu. Rev. Pharmacol. Toxicol.* 17:149, 1977.

47. Ford G.D.: Subcellular fractions of vascular smooth muscle exhibiting calcium transport properties. *Fed. Proc.* 35:1298, 1976.

48. Ford G.D.: Kinetic evidence that vascular smooth muscle sarcoplasmic reticulum possesses both a calcium stimulated and a basal magnesium ATPase. *Circulation* 62(3):111, 1980.

49. Ford L.E., Podolsky R.J.: Regenerative calcium release within muscle cells. *Science* 67:58, 1970.

50. Ford G.D., Hess M.L.: Calcium accumulating properties of subcellular fractions of bovine vascular smooth muscle. *Circ. Res.* 37:580, 1975.

51. Ford G.D., Hess M.L.: Influence of ATP on sarcoplasmic reticulum function of vascular smooth muscle. *Am. J. Physiol.* 242(3):C242, 1982.

52. Fozzard H.A.: Heart excitation-contraction coupling. *Annu. Rev. Physiol.* 39:201, 1977.

53. Fozzard H.A., Lado M.G., Sheu S.S.: Control of intracellular Na^+ and Ca^{2+} in cardiac muscle. *Jpn. Heart J.* 23(suppl.):26, 1982.

54. Fujiwara S., Ito Y., Itoh T., et al.: Diltiazem-induced vasodilatation of smooth muscle cells of the canine basilar artery. *Br. J. Pharmacol.* 75:455, 1982.

55. Gabella G.: Fine structure of smooth muscle. *Philos. Trans. R. Soc. Lond. (Biol.)* 265:7, 1973.

56. Garnier D., Nargeot J., Ojeda C., et al.: The action of acetylcholine on background conductance in frog atrial trabeculae. *J. Physiol.* 274:381, 1978.

57. Ghysel-Burton J., Godfraind T.: Stimulation and inhibition of the sodium pump by cardiotonic steroids in relation to their binding sites and their inotropic effect on guinea-pig isolated atria. *Br. J. Pharmacol.* 66:175, 1979.

58. Glitsch H.G., Reuter H., Scholz H.: The effect of the internal sodium concentration on calcium fluxes in isolated guinea-pig auricles. *J. Physiol.* 209:25, 1970.

59. Godfraind T.: Calcium exchange in vascular smooth muscle: Action of noradrenaline and lanthanum. *J. Physiol.* 260:21, 1976.

60. Godfraind T., Kaba A.: The role of calcium in the action of drugs on vascular smooth muscle. *Arch. Int. Pharmacodyn.* 196(suppl.):35, 1972.

61. Godfraind T., Ghysel-Burton J.: Binding sites related to ouabain-induced stimulation or inhibition of the sodium pump. *Nature* 265:165, 1977.

62. Godfraind T., Dieu D.: The inhibition of flunarizine of the norepinephrine-evoked contraction and calcium influx in rat aorta and mesenteric arteries. *J. Pharmacol. Exp. Ther.* 217:510, 1981.

63. Godfraind T., Miller R.C., Lima J.S.: Selective α_1 and α_2-adrenoreceptor agonist-induced contractions and ^{45}Ca-fluxes in the rat isolated aorta. *Br. J. Pharmacol.* 77:597, 1982.

64. Godfraind T., Miller R.C.: α_2-Adrenoreceptor stimulation and Ca fluxes in isolated rat aorta. *Arch. Int. Pharmacodyn. Ther.* 256:171, 1982.

65. Godfraind T., Morel N.: Na-Ca exchange in guinea-pig and rat smooth muscle. *J. Physiol.* 340:23P, 1983.

65a. Godfraind T., Miller R.C.: Specificity of action of Ca^{2+} entry blockers: A comparison of their actions in rat arteries and in human coronaries. *Circ. Res.* 52(suppl. 1):81, 1983.

66. Goldberg N.D., Haddox M.K., Nicol S.E., et al.: Biological regulation through opposing influence of cyclic AMP: The yin yang hypothesis. *Adv. Cyclic Nucleotide Res.* 5:307, 1975.

67. Golenhofen K., Lammel E.: Selective suppression of some components of spontaneous activity in various types of smooth muscle by iproveratril (verapamil). *Pflugers Arch.* 331:233, 1972.
68. Golenhofen K., Hermstein N., Lammel E.: Membrane potential and contraction of vascular smooth muscle (portal vein) during application of noradrenaline and high potassium and selective inhibitory effects of iproveratril (verapamil). *Microvasc. Res.* 5:73, 1973.
69. Golenhofen K., Hermstein N.: Spike-free activation mechanisms in vascular smooth muscle. *J. Physiol.* 231:14P, 1973.
70. Golenhofen K., Hermstein N.: Differentiation of calcium activation mechanisms in vascular muscle by selective suppression with verapamil and D600. *Blood Vessels* 12:21, 1975.
71. Greenberg S., Long J.P., Diecke F.P.J.: Differentiation of calcium pools utilized in the contractile response of canine arterial and venous smooth muscle to norepinephrine. *J. Pharmacol. Exp. Ther.* 183:493, 1973.
72. Haeusler G., Thorens S.: Effects of tetraethylammonium chloride on calcium fluxes in smooth muscle from rabbit main pulmonary artery. *J. Physiol.* 303:225, 1980.
73. Hagiwara S.: Calcium channel. *Annu. Rev. Neurosci.* 4:69, 1981.
74. Hamon G., Worcel M.: Electrophysiological study of the action of angiotensin II on the rat myometrium. *Circ. Res.* 45:234, 1979.
75. Hamon G., Worcel M.: Mechanism of action of angiotensin II on excitation-contraction coupling in the rat portal vein. *Br. J. Pharmacol.* 75:425, 1982.
76. Harder D.R., Sperelakis N.: Bepridil blockade of C^{2+}-dependent action potentials in vascular smooth muscle of dog coronary artery. *J. Cardiovasc. Pharmacol.* 3:906, 1982.
77. Hescheler J., Pelzer D., Trube G., et al.: Does the organic calcium channel blocker D600 act from inside or outside on the cardiac cell membrane? *Pflugers Arch.* 393:287, 1982.
78. Hidaka H., Yamaki T., Totsuka T., et al.: Selective inhibitors of Ca^{2+}-binding modulator of phosphodiesterase produce vascular relaxation and inhibit actin-myosin interaction. *Mol. Pharmacol.* 15:49, 1979.
79. Hinke J.A.M.: Calcium requirements for noradrenaline and high potassium ion concentration in arterial smooth muscle, in Paul W.M., Daniel E.E., Mary C.M., et al. (eds.): *Muscle.* New York, Pergamon Press, 1965, pp. 269–285.
80. Hirata M., Kuriyama H.: Does activation of cyclic AMP dependent phosphorylation induced by β-adrenergic agent control the tone of vascular muscle? *J. Physiol.* 307:143, 1980.
81. Holman M.E., Kasby C.B., Suthers M.B., et al.: Some properties of the smooth muscle of rabbit portal vein. *J. Physiol.* 196:111, 1968.
82. Irisawa H., Kokubun S.: Modulation by intracellular ATP and cyclic AMP of the slow inward current in isolated single ventricular cells of the guinea-pig. *J. Physiol.* 338:321, 1983.
83. Ito Y., Kuriyama H.: Membrane properties of the smooth muscle fibers of the guinea-pig portal vein. *J. Physiol.* 214:427, 1971.
84. Itoh T., Izumi H., Kuriyama H.: Mechanisms of relaxation induced by activation of β-adrenoreceptors in smooth muscle cells of the guinea-pig mesenteric artery. *J. Physiol.* 326:475, 1982.
85. Jetley M., Weston A.H.: Some effects of sodium nitroprusside, methoxyverapamil (D600) and nifedipine on rat portal vein. *Br. J. Pharmacol.* 68:311, 1980.
86. Johansson B., Somlyo A.P.: Electrophysiology and excitation-contraction coupling, in *Handbook of Physiology.* Vol. II: *The cardiovascular system,* ed. Bohr D.F., Somlyo A.P., Sparks H.V. Bethesda, Md., American Physiological Society, 1980, pp. 301–324.

87. Johnson J.D., Vaghy P.L., Crouch T.H., et al.: An hypothesis for the mechanism of action of some of the Ca^{2+} antagonist drugs: Calmodulin as a receptor. *Adv. Pharmacol. Ther.* 3:121, 1982.

88. Jonas Z., Zelck U.: The subcellular calcium distribution in the smooth muscle cells of the pig coronary artery. *Exp. Cell Res.* 89:352, 1974.

89. Jones A.W.: Content and fluxes of electrolytes, In *Handbook of Physiology*. vol. II: *The Cardiovascular System,* ed. Bohr D.F., Somlyo A.P., Sparks H.V. Jr., Bethesda, Md., American Physiological Society, 1980, pp. 253–299.

90. Katz S.: Mechanism of stimulation of calcium transport in cardiac sarcoplasmic reticulum preparations by calmodulin. *Ann. NY Acad. Sci.* 356:267, 1980.

91. Keene J.J., Seidel C.L., Bohr D.F.: Manganese on calcium flux and norepinephrine induced tension in arterial smooth muscle. *Proc. Soc. Exp. Biol. Med.* 139:1083, 1972.

92. Keatinge W.R.: Mechanical response with reversed electrical response to noradrenaline by Ca-deprived arterial smooth muscle. *J. Physiol.* 224:21, 1972.

93. Kohlardt M., Bauer B., Krause H., et al.: Selective inhibition of the transmembrane Ca conductivity of mammalian myocardial fibers by Ni, Co and Mn ions. *Pflugers Arch.* 338:115, 1973.

94. Kokubun S., Nishimura M., Noma A., et al.: Membrane currents in the rabbit atrioventricular node cell. *Pflugers Arch.* 393:15, 1982.

95. Kranias E.G., Mandel F., Wang T., et al.: Mechanism of the stimulation of calcium ion dependent ATPase of cardiac sarcoplasmic reticulum by cyclic AMP dependent protein kinase EC-2.7.1.37. *Biochemistry* 19:5434, 1980.

96. Kreye V.A.W., Ruegg J.C., Hofmann F.: Effect of calcium-antagonist and calmodulin-antagonist drugs on calmodulin-dependent contractions of chemically skinned vascular smooth muscle from rabbit renal arteries. *Naunyn-Schmiedebergs Arch. Pharmacol.* 323:85, 1983.

97. Kuriyama H., Ito Y., Suzuki K., et al.: Action of diltiazem on single smooth muscle cells and on neuromuscular transmission in vascular bed. *Circ. Res.* 52(suppl. 1):92, 1983.

98. Kuwayama H., Kanazawa T.: Purification of cardiac sarcolemmal vesicles: High sodium pump content and ATP dependent calmodulin activated calcium uptake. *J. Biochem.* 91:1419, 1982.

99. Kwan C.Y.: Magnesium or calcium activated ATPase activities of plasma membranes isolated from vascular smooth muscle. *Enzyme* 28(4):317, 1982.

100. Lamers J.M.J., Stinis J.T.: An electrogenic sodium-calcium antiporter in addition to the calcium pump in cardiac sarcolemma. *Biochim. Biophys. Acta* 640:521, 1981.

101. Langer G.A.: Kinetic studies of calcium distribution in ventricular muscle of the dog. *Circ. Res.* 15:393, 1964.

102. Langer G.A.: Ion fluxes in cardiac excitation and contraction and their relation to myocardial contractility. *Physiol. Rev.* 48:708, 1968.

103. Langer G.A.: Heart: Excitation-contraction coupling. *Annu. Rev. Physiol.* 35:55, 1973.

104. Langer G.A.: Relationship between myocardial contractility and the effects of digitalis on ionic exchange. *Fed. Proc.* 36:2231, 1977.

105. Langer G.A.: Sodium-calcium exchange in the heart. *Annu. Rev. Physiol.* 44:435, 1982.

106. Lee K.S., Tsien R.W.: Mechanism of calcium channel blockade by verapamil, D600, diltiazem and nitrendipine in single dialysed heart cells. *Nature* 302:790, 1983.

107. Louis C.F., Maffitt M.: Characterization of calmodulin mediated phosphorylation of cardiac muscle sarcoplasmic reticulum. *Arch. Biochem. Biophysiol.* 218:109, 1982.

108. Lundvall J., Hillman J., Gustafsson D.: Beta-adrenergic regulation of the capillary exchange and resistance functions, in Vanhoutte P.M., Leusen I. (eds.): *Vasodilatation*. New York, Raven Press, 1981, pp. 107–116.

109. Marban E., Tsien R.W.: Enhancement of the calcium current during digitalis inotropy in mammalian heart: Positive feedback regulation by intracellular calcium. *J. Physiol*. 329:589, 1982.

110. McDonald T.F.: The slow inward calcium current in the heart. *Annu. Rev. Physiol*. 44:425, 1982.

111. Mekata F., Niu H.: Biophysical effects of adrenaline on the smooth muscle of the rabbit common carotid artery. *J. Gen. Physiol*. 59:92, 1972.

112. Mueller R., Van Breemen C.: Role of intracellular Ca^{2+} sequestration in β-adrenergic relaxation of a smooth muscle. *Nature* 281:682, 1979.

113. Mikawa T., Nonomura Y., Hirata M., et al.: Involvement of an acidic protein in regulation of smooth muscle contraction by the tropomyosin-leiotonin system. *J. Biochem. Tokyo* 84: 1633, 1978.

114. Mironneau J., Gargouil Y.M.: Action of indapamide on excitation-contraction coupling in vascular smooth muscle. *Eur. J. Pharmacol*. 57:57, 1979.

115. Moore L., Hurwitz L., Davenport G.R., et al.: Energy dependent calcium uptake activity of microsomes from the aorta of normal and hypertensive rats. *Biochim. Biophys. Acta* 413:432, 1975.

116. Morcos N.C., Localization of calcium magnesium ATPase calcium pump and other ATPase activities in cardiac sarcolemma. *Biochim. Biophys. Acta* 668:747, 1982.

117. Morel N., Wibo M., Godfraind T.: A calmodulin stimulated Ca^{2+} pump in rat aorta plasma membranes. *Biochim. Biophys. Acta* 644:82, 1981.

118. Mullins L.J., The generation of electric currents in cardiac fibers by Na-Ca exchange. *Am. J. Physiol*. 236:C103, 1979.

119. Nakajima A., Horn L.: Electrical activity of single vascular smooth muscle fibers. *Am. J. Physiol*. 213:25, 1977.

120. Nargeot J., Nerbonne J.M., Engels J., et al.: Time-course of the increase in the myocardial slow inward current after a photochemically generated concentration jump of intracellular cAMP. *Proc. Natl. Acad. Sci. USA* 80:2395, 1983.

121. Nayler W.G., Grinwald P.: Calcium entry blockers and myocardial function. *Fed. Proc*. 40:2855, 1981.

122. Niedergerke R.: Movements of Ca in frog heart ventricles at rest and during contractions. *J. Physiol*. 167: 515, 1963.

123. Niedergerke R.: Movements of Ca in beating ventricles of the frog heart. *J. Physiol*. 167:551, 1963.

124. Noble D.: Mechanism of action of therapeutic levels of cardiac glycosides. *Cardiovasc. Res*. 14:495, 1980.

125. Noma A., Irisawa H.: Membrane currents in the rabbit sinoatrial node cell as studied by the double microelectrode method. *Pflugers Arch*. 364:45, 1976.

126. Noma A., Irisawa H., Kokobun S., et al.: Slow current systems in the AV node of the rabbit heart. *Nature* 285:228, 1980.

127. Noma A., Morad M., Irisawa H.: Does the "pacemaker current" generate the diastolic depolarization in the rabbit SA node cells? *Pflugers Arch*. 397:190, 1983.

128. Okita G.T.: Discussion of the Na^+-K^+ ATPase inhibition from digitalis inotropy. *Fed. Proc*. 36:2225, 1977.

129. Osterrieder W., Brum G., Hescheler J., et al.: Injection of subunits of cyclic AMP-dependent protein kinase into cardiac myocytes modulates Ca^{2+} current. *Nature* 298:576, 1982.

130. Ozaki H., Karaki H., Urakawa N.: Possible role of Na-Ca exchange mechanism in the contractions induced in guinea-pig aorta by potassium free solution and ouabain. *Naunyn Schmiedebergs Arch. Pharmacol*. 304:203, 1978.

131. Pang D.C., Sperelakis N.: Nifedipine, diltiazem, bepridil and verapamil uptakes into cardiac and smooth muscles. *Eur. J. Pharmacol.* 87:199, 1983.
132. Peiper U., Griebel I., Wende W.: Activation of vascular smooth muscle of rat aorta by noradrenaline and depolarization: Two different mechanisms. *Pflugers Arch.* 330:74, 1971.
133. Pitts B.J.R.: Stoichiometry of sodium-calcium exchange in cardiac sarcolemmal vesicles. *J. Biol. Chem.* 254:6232, 1979.
134. Popescu L.M., Diculescu I.: Calcium in smooth muscle sarcoplasmic reticulum in situ. *J. Cell. Biol.* 67:911, 1975.
135. Reuter H.: Divalent cations as charge carriers in excitable membranes. *Prog. Biophys. Mol. Biol.* 26:1, 1973.
136. Reuter H.: Exchange of calcium ions in the mammalian myocardium: Mechanisms and physiological significance. *Circ. Res.* 34:599, 1974.
137. Reuter H.: Properties of two inward membrane currents in the heart. *Annu. Rev. Physiol.* 41:413, 1979.
138. Reuter H., Seitz N.: The dependence of calcium efflux from cardiac muscle on temperature and external ion composition. *J. Physiol.* 195:45, 1968.
139. Reuter H., Blaustein M.P., Haeusler G.: Na-Ca exchange and tension development in arterial smooth muscle. *Philos. Trans. Soc. Lond. [Biol.]* 265:87, 1973.
140. Reuter H., Scholz H.: The regulation of the Ca conductance of cardiac muscle by adrenaline. *J. Physiol.* 264:49, 1977.
141. Reuter H., Stevens C.F., Tsien R.W., et al.: Properties of single calcium channels in cardiac cell culture. *Nature* 297:501, 1982.
142. Ruegg J.C., Paul R.J.: Vascular smooth muscle calmodulin and cyclic AMP-dependent protein kinase alter calcium sensitivity in porcine carotid skinned fibers. *Circ. Res.* 50:394, 1982.
143. Saida K., Van Breemen C.: Inhibiting effect of diltiazem on intracellular Ca^{2+} release in vascular smooth muscle. *Blood Vessels* 20:105, 1983.
144. Scheid C.R., Honeyman T.W., Fay F.S.: Mechanism of β-adrenergic relaxation of smooth muscle. *Nature* 277:32, 1979.
145. Shuba M.F., Gurkovskaya A.V., Klevetz N.J., et al.: Mechanism of the excitatory and inhibitory actions of catecholamines on the membrane of smooth muscle cells, in Bülbring E., Shuba M.F. (eds.): *Physiology and Pharmacology of Smooth Muscle*, New York, Raven Press, 1976, pp. 347–355.
146. Silver P., Disalvo J.: cAMP-dependent inhibition of myosin light chain phosphorylation in bovine aortic actinomyosin. *Fed. Proc.* 38:1243, 1979.
147. Singh B.N., Hecht H.S., Nademanee K., et al.: Electro-physiologic and hemodynamic effects of slow-channel blocking drugs. *Prog. Cardiovasc. Dis.* 25:103, 1982.
148. Sitrin M.D., Bohr D.F.: Ca and Na interaction in vascular smooth muscle contraction. *Am. J. Physiol.* 220:1124, 1971.
149. Somlyo A.P., Somlyo A.V.: Electromechanical and pharmacomechanical coupling in vascular smooth muscle. *J. Pharmacol. Exp. Ther.* 159:129, 1968.
150. Somlyo A.P., Somlyo A.V.: Electrophysiological correlates of the inequality of maximal vascular smooth muscle contration elicited by drugs, in Bevan J.A., Furchgott R.F., Maxwell R.A., et al. (eds.): *Physiology and Pharmacology of Vascular Neuroeffector Systems.* Basel, S. Karger, 1971, pp. 216–226.
151. Somlyo A.P., Devine C.E., Somlyo A.V., et al.: Sarcoplasmic reticulum and the temperature dependent contraction of smooth muscle in calcium-free solutions. *J. Cell Biol.* 51:722, 1971.
152. Somlyo A.V., Somlyo A.P.: Strontium accumulation by sarcoplasmic reticulum and mitochondria in vascular smooth muscle. *Science* 174:955, 1971.
153. Somlyo A.P., Somlyo A.V., Devine C.E., et al.: Electron microscopy and electron probe analysis of mitochondrial cation accumulation in smooth muscle. *J. Cell Biol.* 61:723, 1974.

154. Sulakhe P.V., St. Louis P.J.: Passive and active calcium fluxes across plasma membranes. *Prog. Biophys. Mol. Biol.* 35:135, 1980.
155. Surprenant A., Neild T.O., Holman M.E.: Effects of nifedipine on nerve-evoked action potentials and consequent contractions in rat tail artery. *Pflugers Arch.* 396:342, 1983.
156. Suzuki H., Itoh T., Kuriyama H.: Effects of diltiazem on smooth muscles and neuromuscular junction in the mesenteric artery. *Am. J. Physiol.* 242:H325, 1982.
157. Tada M., Yamamoto T., Tonomura Y.: Molecular mechanism of active calcium transport by sarcoplasmic reticulum. *Physiol. Rev.* 58:1, 1978.
158. Tuana B.S., Dzurba A., Panagia V., et al.: Stimulation of heart sarcolemmal calcium pump by calmodulin. *Biochem. Biophys. Res. Commun.* 100:1245, 1981.
159. Thorens S., Haeusler G.: Effects of some vasodilators on calcium translocation in intact and fractionated vascular smooth muscle. *Eur. J. Pharmacol.* 54:79, 1979.
160. Timmermans P.B.M.W.M., Kwa H.Y., Van Zieten P.A.: Possible subdivision of postsynaptic α-adrenoceptors mediating pressor responses in the pithed rat. *Naunyn Schmiedebergs Arch. Pharmacol.* 310:189, 1979.
161. Trautwein W., Taniguchi J., Noma A.: The effect of intracellular cyclic nucleotides and calcium on the action potentia and acetylcholine response of isolated cardiac cells. *Pflugers Arch.* 392:307, 1982.
162. Triggle D.J., Swamy V.C.: Pharmacology of agents that affect calcium. Agonists and antagonists. *Chest* 78(suppl.):1974, 1980.
163. Tsien R.W.: Adrenaline-like effects of intracellular iontophoresis of cyclic AMP in cardiac Purkinje fibers. *Nature New Biol.* 245:120, 1973.
164. Tsien R.W., Giles W., Greengard P.: Cyclic AMP mediates the effects of adrenaline on cardiac Purkinje fibers. *Nature New Biol.* 240:181, 1972.
165. Tsien R.W., Weingart R.: Inotropic effect of cyclic AMP in calf ventricular muscle studied by a cut end method. *J. Physiol.* 260:117, 1976.
166. Tsien R.W., Kass R.S., Weingart R.: Calcium ions and membrane current changes induced by digitalis in cardiac Purkinje fibers. *Ann. N.Y. Acad. Sci.* 307:483, 1978.
167. Turlapaty P.D.M.V., Hester R.K., Carrier O.: Role of calcium in different layers of vascular smooth muscle in norepinepharine contraction. *Blood Vessels* 13:193, 1976.
168. Uchida E., Bohr D.F.: Myogenic tone in isolated perfused resistance vessels: Occurrence among vascular beds and along vascular trees. *Circ. Res.* 25:549, 1979.
169. Vallet B., Molla A., DeMaille J.G.: Cyclic adenosine 3′, 5′-monophosphate-dependent regulation of purified bovine aortic calcium calmodulin-dependent myosin light chain kinase. *Biochem. Biophys. Acta* 674:256, 1981.
170. Van Breemen C.: Calcium requirement for activation of intact aortic smooth muscle. *J. Physiol.* 272:317, 1977.
171. Van Breemen C., Farinas B.R., Gerba P., et al.: Excitation-contraction coupling in rabbit aorta studied by the lanthanum method for measuring cellular calcium influx. *Circ. Res.* 30:44, 1972.
172. Van Breemen C., Farinas B.R., Casteels R., et al.: Factors controlling cytoplasmic Ca^{2+} concentration. *Philos. Trans. R. Soc. Lond. [Biol.]* 265:57, 1973.
173. Van Breemen C., Lasser P.: The absence of increased membrane calcium permeability during norepinephrine stimulation of arterial smooth muscle. *Microvasc. Res.* 3:113, 1974.
174. Van Breemen C., Aaronson P., Loutzenhiser R.: Sodium-calcium interactions in mammalian smooth muscle. *Pharmacol. Rev.* 30:167, 1978.
175. Van Breemen C., Aaronson P., Loutzenhiser R.: Ca^{2+} movements in smooth muscle. *Chest* 78(suppl.):157, 1980.
176. Van Breemen C., Hang O., Cauvin C.: Ca-antagonist inhibition of norepinephrine

stimulated Ca influx in vascular smooth muscle, in *International Symposium on Calcium Modulators*. Amsterdam, Elsevier/North Holland, 1982, p. 185.

177. Van Meel J.C.A., De Jonge A., Wilffert B., et al.: Vascular smooth muscle contraction initiated by post-synaptic α_2-adrenoceptor activation is induced by an influx of extracellular calcium. *Eur. J. Pharmacol.* 69:205, 1981.

178. Van Nueten J.M., Vanhoutte P.M.: Calcium entry blockers and vascular smooth muscle heterogeneity *Fed. Proc.* 40:2862, 1981.

179. Van Winkle W.B., Schwartz A.: Ions and inotropy. *Annu. Rev. Physiol.* 38:247, 1976.

180. Van Zwieten P.A., Van Meel J.C.A., Timmermans P.B.M.W.M.: Calcium antagonists and α_2-adrenoceptors: Possible role of extracellular calcium ions in α_2-adrenoceptor mediated vasoconstriction. *J. Cardiovasc. Pharmacol.* 4:5273, 1982.

181. Vanhoutte P.M.: Heterogeneity of postjunctional vascular α-adrenoceptors and handling of calcium. *J. Cardiovasc. Pharmacol.* 4:S91, 1982.

182. Vanhoutte P.M., Rimele T.J.: Calcium and α-adrenoceptors in activation of vascular smooth muscle. *J. Cardiovasc. Pharmacol.* 4:S280, 1982.

183. Vassort G., Rougier O., Garnier D., et al.: Effect of adrenaline on membrane inward currents during the cardiac action potential. *Pflugers Arch.* 309:70, 1969.

184. Vogel S., Sperelakis N.: Induction of slow action potentials by microiontophoresis of cyclic AMP into heart cells. *J. Mol. Cell. Cardiol.* 13:51, 1981.

185. Wahlstrom B.A.: A study on the action of noradrenaline on ionic content and sodium, potassium and choride effluxes in the rat portal vein. *Acta Physiol. Scand.* 89:522, 1973.

186. Walus K.M., Fondacaro J.D., Jacobson E.D.: Effect of calcium and its antagonists on the canine mesenteric circulation. *Circ. Res.* 48:692, 1981.

187. Wasserstrom J.A., Schwartz D.J., Fozzard H.A.: Relation between intracellular sodium and twitch tension in sheep cardiac Purkinje strands exposed to cardiac glycosides. *Circ. Res.* 52:697, 1983.

188. Watanabe A.M., Besch H.R. Jr.: Cyclic adenosine monophosphate modulation of slow calcium influx channels in guinea pig hearts. *Circ. Res.* 35:316, 1974.

189. Webb R.C., Bohr D.F.: Relaxation of vascular smooth muscle by isoproterenol, dibutyryl cyclic AMP and theophylline. *J. Pharmacol. Exp. Ther.* 217:26, 1981.

190. Weingart R., Kass R.S., Tsien R.W.: Is digitalis inotropy associated with enhanced slow inward calcium current? *Nature* 273:389, 1978.

191. Weiss G.B.: Calcium and contractility in vascular smooth muscle, in Narahashi T., Bianchi C.P. (eds.): *Advances in General and Cellular Pharmacology*. New York, 1977, pp. 71–154.

192. Weston A.H.: The effect of noradrenaline on electrical activity and calcium fluxes in rat portal vein, in Szabadi E., Brashaw C.M., Bevan D. (eds.): *Recent Advances in the Pharmacology of Adrenoceptors*. Amsterdam, Elsevier, 1978, pp. 15–22.

193. Wibo M., Morel N., Godfraind T.: Differentiation of Ca^{2+} pump linked to plasma membrane and endoplasmic reticulum in the microsomal fraction from intestinal smooth muscle. *Biochim. Biophys. Acta* 649:651, 1981.

194. Winegrad S.: Electromechanical coupling in heart muscle, in *Handbook of Physiology*. Vol. I: *The Cardiovascular System*, ed. Berne R.M., Sperelakis N. Bethesda, M., American Physiological Society, 1979, pp. 393–428.

195. Wuytack F., Casteels R.: Demonstration of a calcium magnesium ATPase activity probably related to calcium: II. Transport in the microsomal fraction of porcine coronary artery smooth muscle. *Biochim. Biophys. Acta* 595(2):257, 1980.

196. Yamaguchi I., Kopin I.J.: Differential inhibition of α_1 and α_2 adrenoceptor-mediated pressor responses in pithed rats. *J. Pharmacol. Exp. Ther.* 214:275, 1980.

197. Yamasaki Y., Fujiwara M., Toda N.: Effects of intracellularly applied cyclic 3′, 5′-adenosine monophosphate and dibutyryl cyclic 3′, 5′-adenosine monophosphate on the electrical activity of sinoatrial nodal cells of the rabbit. *J. Pharmacol. Exp. Ther.* 190:15, 1974.

Calcium Antagonists in the Treatment of Hypertension: A Critical Overview

P. WEIDMANN, A. GERBER, AND K. LAEDERACH

Medizinische Poliklinik, University of Berne, Switzerland

THE CENTRAL ROLE that calcium (Ca) plays in cardiovascular regulation is well apparent in several clinical situations. Chronic hypercalcemia due to hyperparathyroidism, vitamin D intoxication, or other etiologies is sometimes accompanied by hypertension,[14] and acute hypercalcemia induced by Ca infusion also may increase blood pressure, particularly in patients with impaired renal function.[87, 134] Conversely, acute severe hypocalcemia causes hypotension,[81] and the inhibition of transmembranous transport with Ca antagonists has more recently been noted to lower blood pressure in various forms of hypertension. The possible pressor action of Ca as well as the antihypertensive mechanisms and the potential value of Ca antagonists for practical antihypertensive pharmacotherapy have attracted great interest. Based on a comprehensive assessment of the available information, the following profile emerges.

Interaction Between Calcium and Some Blood Pressure–Regulating Factors

Clinical variations in Ca may modulate blood pressure through several mechanisms. The direct effect of changes in intracellular free Ca on vascular muscle tone is undoubtedly of prime importance[17, 18]; cardiac function also is regulated by

0084–5957/84/0014–0197–0232–$04.00

Ca.[45] Nevertheless, Ca may interact with other important pressor factors. In the sympathetic system, the role of Ca in the coupling between the electric signal and the release of noradrenaline from nerve terminals is well known. Moreover, studies in vitro have demonstrated that with increasing Ca concentrations in the incubation media, there is a parallel rise in the release of noradrenaline from sympathetic nerves and of adrenaline from adrenal medullary tissue[20, 25, 36, 50, 64, 72]; acute hypercalcemia in man was associated with an increase in the blood levels of both catecholamines.[16, 87] The latter observation suggested that in vivo, a modest hypercalcemia may induce mild activation of the sympathetic system which, in turn, may support the blood pressure–elevating influence of the excess Ca. Regarding renin and aldosterone, it has been shown that their production in vitro requires Ca.[28, 42, 43, 91, 117] On the other hand, a renin-inhibiting influence of increased Ca entry into the juxtaglomerular cells of the kidney has been proposed.[104] However, our studies in man did not reveal relevant changes in plasma renin activity and aldosterone levels during acute hypercalcemia[16, 87, 134] or in circulating renin levels during hypocalcemia[81]; therefore, we concluded that renin and aldosterone do not play an important role in the pathogenesis of acute hypercalcemic hypertension or hypocalcemic hypotension.[81] Yet another humoral factor, namely, parathormone (PTH), might also be involved in the pressor effect of hypercalcemia. Thus, PTH, which is thought to exert a vasodilating effect,[103] is inhibited during hypercalcemia of nonparathyroid origin. Finally, hypercalcemia promotes sodium diuresis and hypovolemia; the latter may possibly attenuate a blood pressure–elevating effect of increased serum Ca concentrations.

Effects of Calcium Antagonists on Blood Pressure–Regulating Factors

DIRECT EFFECT ON CARDIOVASCULAR FUNCTION

Ca antagonists exert a direct influence on the cardiovascular system. They inhibit the cellular transmembranous influx of Ca.[45] The level of intracellular free Ca is decisive for the initiation of contraction.[45] A reduction in Ca-dependent vascular

TABLE 1.—Potential Direct Effects of Therapeutic Doses of Calcium Antagonists on the Heart and Blood Vessels*

EFFECT	NIF	VER	DIL
Coronary arterial vasodilation	+ + + +	+ + +	+ + +
Peripheral arterial vasodilation	+ + + +	+ + +	+ + +
Inhibition of SA node automaticity	±	+ + +	+
Inhibition of AV conduction	±	+ + + +	+ + +
Inhibition of myocardial contractility	+ +	+ + +	+ +

*Nif, nifedipine; ver, verapamil; dil, diltiazem.

smooth muscle tone appears to be the major and common mechanism by which Ca antagonists influence blood pressure. Nifedipine, verapamil, and diltiazem are the most commonly used Ca antagonists. They have different chemical structures and also differ somewhat in their pharmacologic effects on the heart and blood vessels (Table 1).[45] Nifedipine induces a more pronounced arteriolar vasodilation and has only a minimal influence on the cardiac pacemakers. Verapamil is a somewhat weaker vasodilator but can have a distinct depressant effect on sinus node automaticity and atrioventricular conduction. Diltiazem resembles verapamil in its vasodilating potency, while its negative chronotropic and dromotropic effects seem to be somewhere between those of nifedipine and verapamil. The potential inhibition of myocardial contractility is perhaps slightly greater with verapamil than with nifedipine or diltiazem. Nevertheless, in vivo the potential negative chronotropic, dromotropic, and inotropic actions of these systemically administered Ca antagonists may be attenuated by sympathetic cardiovascular reflexes; these may also contribute to additional coronary vasodilation.[45]

Effect on Other Blood Pressure—Regulating Factors

The available data allow certain conclusions to be made on the effects of nifedipine and verapamil, while information on other Ca antagonists is still scarce.

Circulating Catecholamines and Renin

The influence of monotherapy with nifedipine or verapamil on plasma catecholamine and renin levels was recently assessed by a comprehensive analysis of published reports (see review by Laederach et al.[71]). In patients with benign essential hypertension, the administration of nifedipine, either as an acute single dose or as short-term monotherapy for up to 8 weeks, was often associated with modest increases in plasma renin and noradrenaline levels, averaging about 30%–70% (Fig 1). When verapamil was given in essential hypertension either as an acute single dose or as short-term monotherapy for up to 16 weeks, plasma renin levels were not consistently altered (Fig 2). Plasma noradrenaline levels also were not consistently altered in the two available single dose-studies, but tended to be increased mildly during short-term therapy with verapamil.

Differences between the humoral effects of nifedipine and verapamil are further corroborated by a comparative assessment of the average responses to these agents in the published reports on both patients with essential hypertension and normal subjects (Fig 3).[71] Nifedipine, given either acutely or as short-term therapy, increased plasma renin levels by an average of 60% in patients with essential hypertension, and at least as much in normal subjects. In contrast, following administration of verapamil, plasma renin levels were on the average unchanged or even slightly decreased. Plasma noradrenaline levels also increased by an average of 50% following an acute single dose of nifedipine but were largely unchanged after the acute administration of verapamil both in hypertensive and in normal subjects. During short-term therapy, plasma noradrenaline levels tended to increase slightly with both agents, although perhaps somewhat less with verapamil. Plasma adrenaline levels did not change during treatment with either nifedipine or verapamil (for a detailed review, see Laederach et al.[71]). The few data on renin or catecholamine responses to other Ca antagonists need further evaluation.

The mechanisms by which treatment with Ca antagonists may influence circulating renin and noradrenaline levels are not entirely clear. Nevertheless, the increases in plasma noradrenaline following administration of nifedipine resemble the

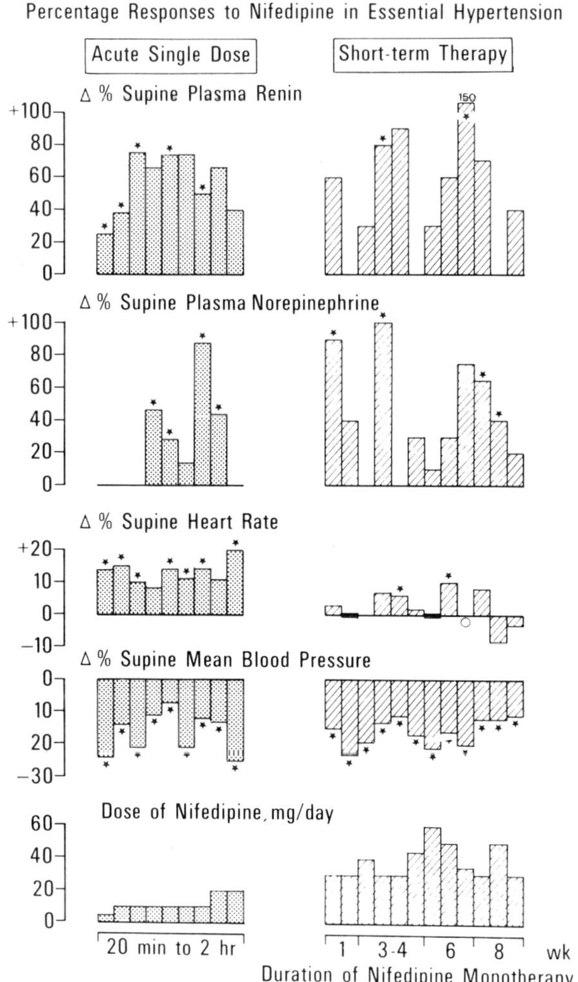

Fig 1.—Percentage responses, in supine subjects, of plasma renin, noradrenaline, heart rate, and mean blood pressure to acute single-dose or short-term monotherapy with nifedipine in essential hypertension. *Asterisks* indicate changes were reported as statistically significant. *Circle* indicates variations were reported as statistically significant but numerical data were not provided. In the acute single-dose studies, the duration of monotherapy *(bottom rank)* is given as the interval between drug administration and the time measurements were made.

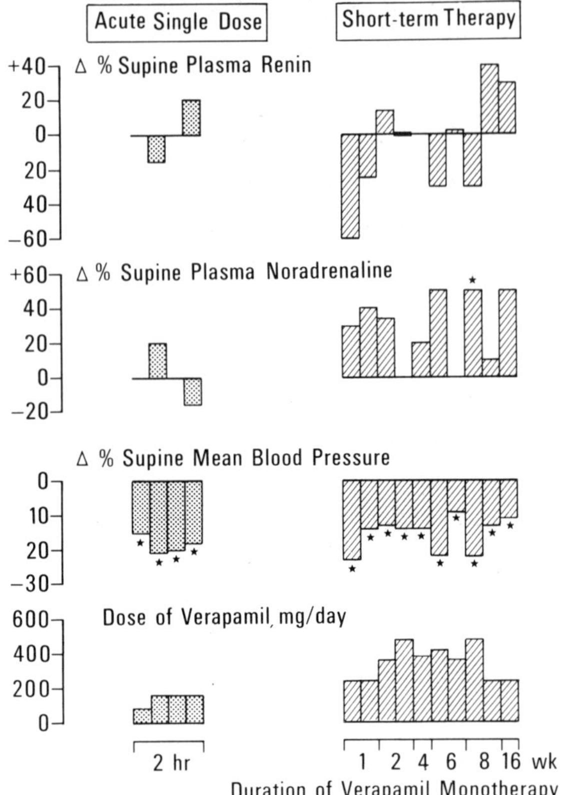

Fig 2.—Percentage responses, in supine subjects, of plasma renin, noradrenaline, heart rate, and mean blood pressure to acute single-dose or short-term monotherapy with verapamil in essential hypertension. *Asterisks* indicate changes were reported as statistically significant. In the acute single-dose studies, the duration of monotherapy *(bottom rank)* is given as the interval between drug administration and the time measurements were made.

mild changes induced by direct arteriolar vasodilators such as the hydralazines,[65] minoxidil,[15, 51] or carprazidil.[15] The degree of sympathetic stimulation by the latter agents appears to be determined largely by the degree of peripheral vasodilation and blood pressure reduction with consecutive activation of the baroreflex mechanism. Obviously, this does not apply in the case of verapamil, which caused a similar blood pressure reduc-

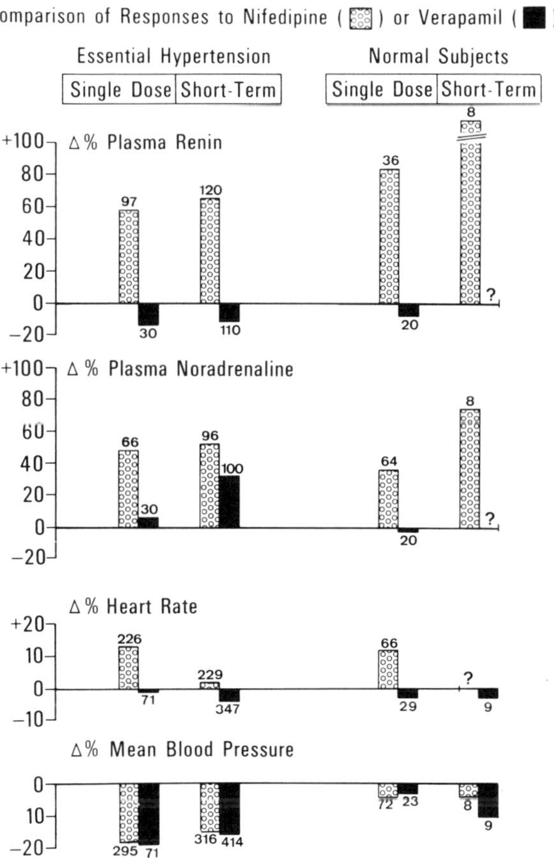

Fig 3.—Average percentage responses, in supine subjects, of plasma renin, nor-adrenaline, heart rate, and mean blood pressure to nifedipine or verapamil in essential hypertension or in normal subjects. All data shown in Figures 1, 2, 8, and 9 are incorporated in this analysis. Each bar represents the average response in the reported cases. The total number of subjects in whom measurements were made is given above or below the columns.

tion as nifedipine (see Fig 3). The relatively stable plasma nor-adrenaline levels, despite a distinct fall in blood pressure, following acute administration of verapamil in essential hypertension raises the possibility that verapamil per se may acutely inhibit the neural discharge of noradrenaline. Alternative explanations, such as different effects of nifedipine and verapamil on the baroreflex[67, 93] or the plasma clearance of nor-adrenaline, also deserve further consideration.

The potential of nifedipine to stimulate plasma renin also appears to be quite comparable to that of the direct arteriolar vasodilators. The increase in sympathetic activity and/or fall in systemic and renal arterial perfusion pressure induced by these vasodilators are known complementary factors that may activate renin secretion through renal β receptors, baroreceptors and perhaps also other mechanisms. Our analysis reveals no consistent relationship between variations in plasma renin levels and concomitant changes in mean blood pressure induced by the acute administration of nifedipine or verapamil in normal or hypertensive subjects (Fig 4). However, the finding of a significant correlation between the induced changes in circulating renin and noradrenaline levels suggests that renin variations following acute Ca antagonist therapy may closely reflect the individual effects of such drugs on sympathetic activity. Nevertheless, the relative importance of different degrees of renal vasodilation for the contrasting renin effects of nifedipine and verapamil cannot be assessed for this analysis, and a direct

Fig 4.—Relationship between percentage changes in supine plasma renin and plasma adrenaline levels or mean blood pressure after acute administration of a single dose of nifedipine or verapamil in supine normal or hypertensive subjects.

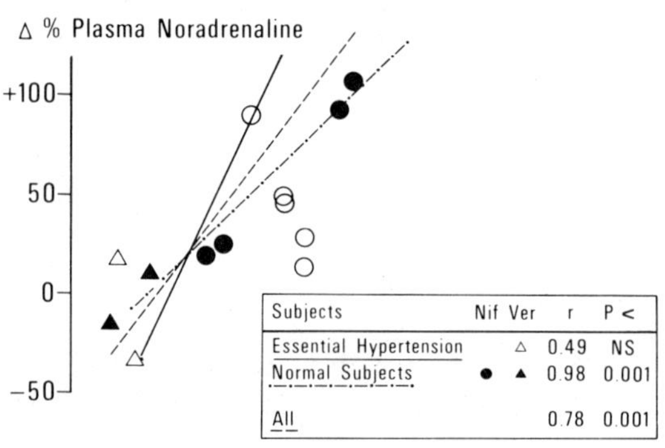

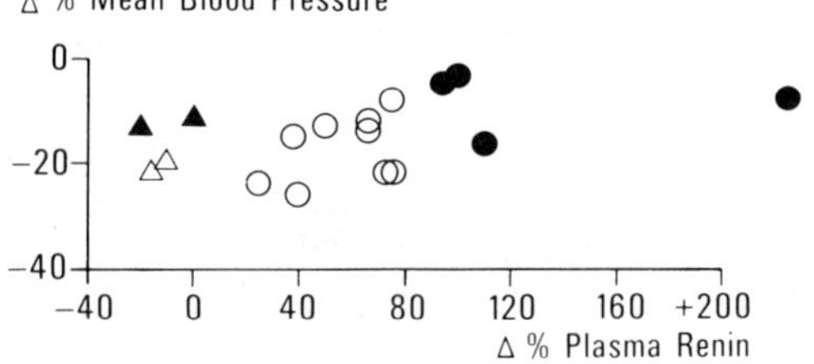

inhibitory effect of verapamil on renin release has not been excluded.

Relationship Between Heart Rate and Circulating Noradrenaline or Renin Levels Following Acute and Calcium Entry Blockade

The lack of an increase in heart rate following treatment with verapamil (see Figs 2 and 3) is generally attributed to a direct negative dromotropic and chronotropic action.[4] This well-established pharmacologic potential of verapamil[45] will not be disputed. However, our analysis revealed close correlations, in normal or hypertensive subjects, between variations in heart rate and concomitant changes in plasma noradrenaline or renin levels following acute Ca entry blockade (Fig 5). Circulating noradrenaline and renin levels may both be partial indices of sympathetic activity. Therefore, it appears possible that the different chronotropic effects of acutely administered nifedipine or verapamil may be determined, at least in part, by a different influence of these agents on the sympathetic system.

Fig 5.—Relationship between percentage changes in heart rate and plasma renin or noradrenaline levels after acute administration of a single dose of nifedipine or verapamil in normal or hypertensive subjects.

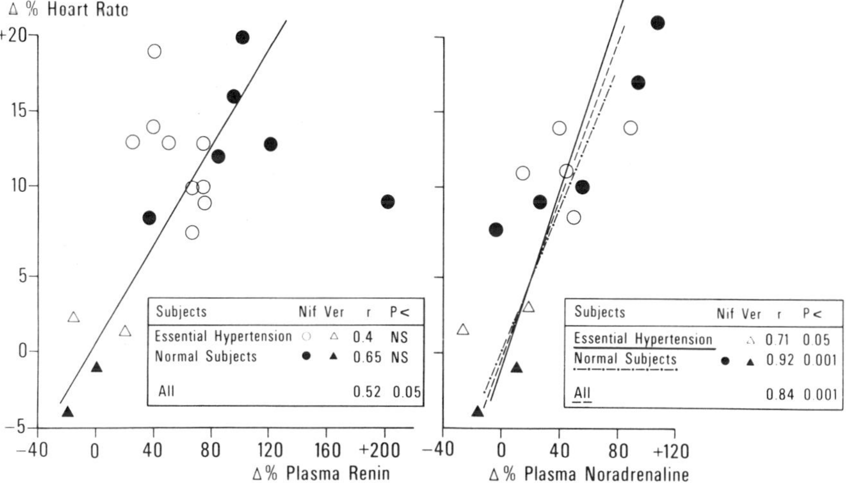

Effects on Plasma Aldosterone and Serum Electrolytes

Since aldosterone production in vitro requires Ca, the possibility of an inhibitory influence of Ca antagonists has been considered. Following acute administration of nifedipine, basal plasma aldosterone concentrations[31, 75, 118, 123] and aldosterone responsiveness to infused angiotensin II[92] tended on average to decrease slightly. However, both parameters were largely unchanged after short-term treatment with nifedipine (Fig 6).[14, 75, 95, 96] Short-term therapy with verapamil also did not consistently alter basal plasma aldosterone concentrations,[33, 95, 96] but the effect of such treatment on aldosterone responsiveness to adrenocortical stimuli and of acute single-dose verapamil on aldosterone metabolism remains to be clarified. Data with other Ca antagonists are largely lacking.

Fig 6.—Relationship between plasma aldosterone and plasma angiotensin II concentrations before and during angiotensin II infusion. *Open circles,* control values for angiotensin II infusion; *open triangles,* values for combined calcium-angiotensin II infusion; *closed triangles,* values for angiotensin II infusion during nifedipine treatment. Bars indicate SEM. (From Bianchetti et al.[14] Reproduced by permission.)

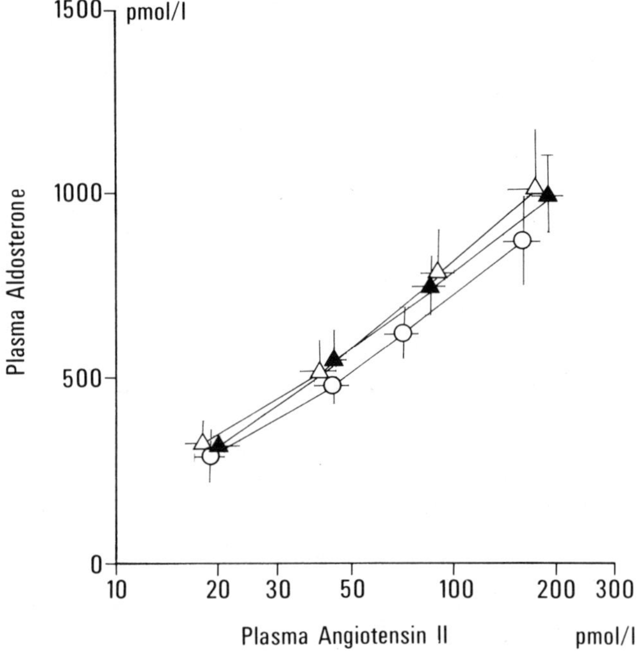

Plasma potassium, which may modulate aldosterone release and/or be changed as a consequence of slight variations in plasma aldosterone,[135, 136] was not consistently changed following short-term therapy with nifedipine, verapamil, or diltiazem in patients with essential hypertension.[4, 7, 49, 61, 71, 78, 83, 102, 112, 144] Plasma sodium and creatinine levels or creatinine clearance also were stable.

Effects on Cardiovascular Pressor Responsiveness

There is little doubt that clinical variations in Ca metabolism influence blood pressure, largely by their direct action on cardiovascular muscle cells. Nevertheless, hypercalcemia, acute hypocalcemia, and Ca entry blockade may modify not only the basal cardiovascular tone, but perhaps also the responsiveness to certain vasoactive hormones. Based on an inhibitory effect of calcium antagonists in vitro, it has been proposed that vasoconstriction due to α_2 receptor stimulation requires the influx of Ca from the extracellular space through the smooth muscle cell membrane.[129] This property is of particular interest with respect to certain human conditions with an exaggerated noradrenaline responsiveness. These include established essential hypertension, in which blood levels of noradrenaline and adrenaline are normal or sometimes even slightly increased,[105, 139, 140] normotension in children of hypertensive parents,[111] borderline hypertension,[90] nonazotemic diabetes mellitus,[10, 138] and mild renal functional impairment,[11] in which conditions circulating catecholamine levels generally are normal. It is possible that the noradrenaline hyperresponsiveness in some normotensive offspring of hypertensive parents may represent a familial predisposition for the development of essential hypertension. Cardiovascular hyperresponsiveness in patients with renal failure or diabetes mellitus might also contribute to the frequent development of high blood pressure. Therefore, agents that reduce the noradrenaline pressor responsiveness could possibly provide a rational antihypertensive therapy in these patients.

Previous studies in our laboratory indicated that treatment with certain diuretics tends to restore toward normal the exaggerated noradrenaline responsiveness in patients with essential hypertension or high blood pressure associated with mild renal impairment or diabetes mellitus.[52, 114, 137, 143] Moreover, based on preliminary observations, certain Ca antagonists may have a similar effect, at least when given acutely or for a few weeks. Following single-dose nifedipine administration to normal subjects, a reduction in the blood pressure responses to both noradrenaline and angiotensin II was reported.[131] In persons with normal or borderline increased blood pressure, nifedipine given for 2 weeks in a dose of 30–60 mg/day reduced blood pressure responsiveness to noradrenaline, as evidenced by a significant shift to the right of the relationship between increases in blood pressure and concomitant increases in plasma noradrenaline induced by a noradrenaline infusion; no influence on the pressor response to angiotensin II was noted.[16] In patients with established essential hypertension, a significant improvement of the previously exaggerated noradrenaline responsiveness was noted following 4 weeks of nifedipine therapy but not after a similar period of verapamil therapy.[116] Finally, the noradrenaline hyperresponsiveness was also improved in 10 patients with diabetes mellitus treated for 6 weeks with nitrendipine.[125] Clearly, more studies are necessary to clarify the time course and relative importance of modified cardiovascular responsiveness in the antihypertensive mechanism of single-dose or chronic treatment with different Ca antagonists in man.

Effects on Cardiac Output and Total Peripheral Resistance in Essential Hypertension

The antihypertensive effect of Ca antagonists in essential hypertension appears to be largely due to a decrease in total peripheral vascular resistance. This hemodynamic improvement is desirable, given the presence of vasoconstriction in most patients with untreated essential hypertension. Following an acute single dose, cardiac output was reported to be increased distinctly by nifedipine,[4, 5, 55, 63, 100] only slightly by verapamil,[80] and was largely unchanged by diltiazem.[5, 7, 102] Cardiac output was reported to be modestly increased after 3 weeks' monotherapy with nifedipine[100] but was unaltered after 6 weeks'[63] and 11 months'[82] therapy.

Do Calcium Antagonists Correct an Underlying Abnormality of Essential Hypertension?

Whether and to what extent abnormalities in Ca metabolism may play a primary pathogenic role in hypertensive states not associated with frank hypercalcemia is presently unclear. Disturbances in blood cell membrane cation metabolism have been described both in essential hypertension[17, 35, 48] and in normotensive offspring of hypertensive parents.[48] Moreover, the possibility of a more generalized tissue alteration, leading to an increased Ca content in cardiovascular muscle cells, has also been considered. Such a mechanism, although still speculative, could produce hypertension.[17]

Some observations with Ca antagonists have been interpreted in favor of a Ca-dependent dysregulation in essential hypertension. These include (1) the dependence of their blood pressure–lowering effect on the pretreatment blood pressure level (Fig 7) and the lack of influence in normotensive subjects (see Fig 3),[7, 31, 89] (2) the possibility that in essential hypertension the abnormally constricted brachial arteries may be dilated more completely by a Ca antagonist than by the potent direct vasodilator nitroprusside,[19, 57, 109, 124] and (3) the report of a close relationship between blood pressure and blood platelet Ca content before and after treatment with nifedipine or verapamil.[40] Nevertheless, blood pressure responses to other antihypertensive drugs, such as diuretics, β blockers, and sympatholytics, also tend to correlate with pretreatment blood pressure, and this as well as an altered platelet Ca content could theoretically represent unspecific phenomena associated with the hypertensive state.

Furthermore, the vasodilating, blood pressure–lowering, and platelet Ca–modifying effects of Ca antagonists in essential hypertension per se do not prove the pathogenic role of a primary disturbance of Ca metabolism in cardiovascular muscle cells. In fact, Ca is the common intracellular trigger for various pressor substances, and the potential of Ca antagonists to lower blood pressure at least acutely in different forms of hypertension is consistent with this.

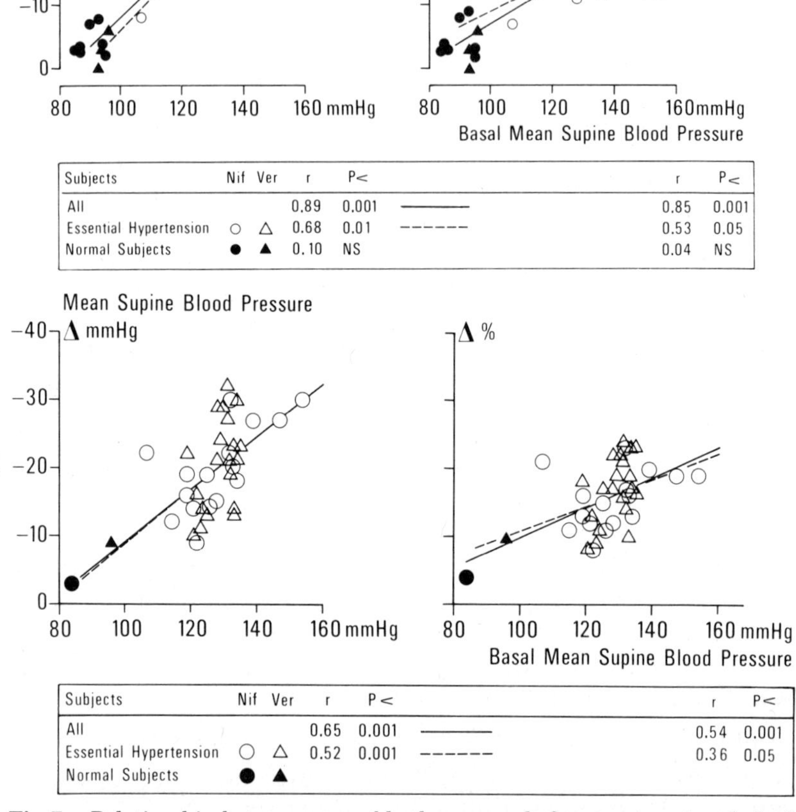

Subjects	Nif	Ver	r	P<		r	P<
All			0.89	0.001	————	0.85	0.001
Essential Hypertension	○	△	0.68	0.01	——————	0.53	0.05
Normal Subjects	●	▲	0.10	NS		0.04	NS

Subjects	Nif	Ver	r	P<		r	P<
All			0.65	0.001	————	0.54	0.001
Essential Hypertension	○	△	0.52	0.001	——————	0.36	0.05
Normal Subjects	●	▲					

Fig 7.—Relationship between mean blood pressure before treatment and absolute or percentage blood pressure responses to an acute single dose **(top)** or short-term monotherapy **(bottom)** with nifedipine or verapamil in patients with essential hypertension and normal subjects. Studies using the following drug dosages were analyzed: acute single-dose studies, nifedipine, 10–20 mg; verapamil, 80–160 mg. Short-term monotherapy, nifedipine, 30–60 mg/day; verapamil, 240–480 mg/day (in two to four daily doses).

Antihypertensive Efficacy

ESSENTIAL HYPERTENSION

Monotherapy

The influence of monotherapy with nifedipine or verapamil in essential hypertension was assessed by an analysis of published reports with a minimum of six subjects per study (see Laederach et al.[71]). It is evident that nifedipine (Fig 8) lowers supine mean blood pressure by about 10%–25% when given as an acute single dose (10–20 mg sublingually or 5–60 mg orally), and by about 10%–20% during short-term oral treatment of 1–22 weeks' duration (15–80 mg/day). Supine heart rate was increased acutely by an average of more than 10%, but this was distinctly less pronounced during short-term nifedipine therapy, despite a persistent blood pressure reduction. Nevertheless, the antihypertensive efficacy and associated chronotropic effects of nifedipine monotherapy beyond 6 months' duration remain to be clarified.

Verapamil (Fig 9), given either as an acute single dose (80–160 mg orally) or as short- to long-term therapy (240–480 mg/day), also reduced mean supine blood pressure by about 10%–23%. However, supine heart rate was not consistently changed and sometimes even was slightly decreased.

Various other Ca antagonists also exerted an antihypertensive effect when given as monotherapy to patients with essential hypertension. With respect to both blood pressure and heart rate, the effects of diltiazem and niludipine given either acutely or for a short term, resembled two effects of verapamil.[4, 6, 7, 49, 61, 62, 70, 78, 83, 102, 112, 144] Tiapamil may possibly also follow this tendency,[30] while a constellation of effects bearing a resemblance to those of nifedipine was noted following acute and/or short-term treatment with nitrendipine, nisoldipine given acutely, or nicardipine for a short term.*

The effects of Ca antagonists on blood pressure and heart rate in the upright subject generally resemble their effects in the supine subject.[6, 26, 71, 115, 130] Nevertheless, orthostatic hypo-

---

*References 2, 4, 20, 41, 47, 56, 60, 101, 115, 120, 121, 122, 130, 132

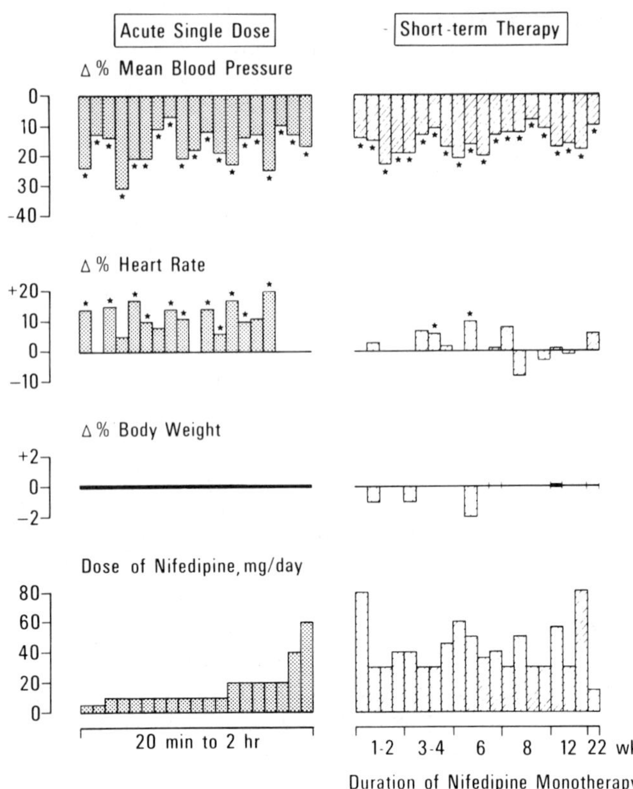

Fig 8.—Percentage responses of mean blood pressure, heart rate, and body weight to acute single-dose or short-term monotherapy with nifedipine in essential hypertension. Each column represents the average percent change in a series including at least six patients. *Asterisks* indicate changes reported as statistically significant. In the case of acute single-dose studies, the duration of monotherapy *(bottom rank)* is given as the interval between drug administration and the time measurements were made.

tension and/or dizziness may sometimes occur after emergency application, and we have sporadically encountered it following initiation of Ca antagonist therapy in elderly patients. Moreover, during short-term nifedipine monotherapy, heart rate tended to increase more distinctly in the standing than in the supine position.[38, 75, 95, 96]

Whenever body weight was reported, it was usually unchanged or even decreased slightly during short-term monotherapy with nifedipine, verapamil (see Figs 8 and 9), dilti-

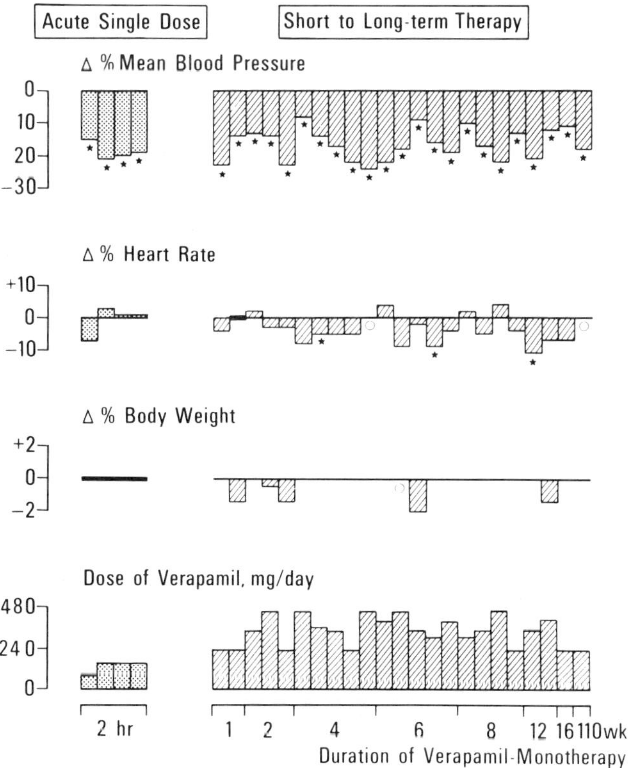

Fig 9.—Percentage responses of mean blood pressure, heart rate, and body weight to acute single-dose or short-term monotherapy with verapamil in essential hypertension. *Asterisks* indicate changes were reported as statistically significant. *Circle* indicates variations were reported as statistically significant but numerical data were not provided. In the acute single-dose studies *(bottom rank)*, the duration of monotherapy is given as the interval between drug administration and the time measurements were made.

azem, nitrendipine, or nicardipine.[60, 71, 130] This may be interpreted as indirect evidence that relevant body sodium fluid retention, which is a well-known side effect and may antagonize a long-term antihypertensive treatment of direct arteriolar vasodilators such as hydralazine, minoxidil, and the like, may often not occur with the Ca antagonists. In fact, natriuresis was unchanged or even slightly increased following a single dose of nifedipine[29] or verapamil,[118] while total plasma or blood volume was largely unchanged after short-term therapy with these agents.[33, 34, 63, 88, 95, 100] On the other hand, a tendency for slightly increased exchangeable body sodium has been noted following short-term therapy with nifedipine,[88] and mild sodium and water retention was reported in some patients on short- to long-term treatment.[58] The observation of a persistent antihypertensive with verapamil monotherapy of up to 2 years' duration (see Fig 9)[146] suggests that sodium fluid volume retention, if it occurred at all, was not a major antagonistic factor, at least in some patients.

The magnitude of blood pressure responses to a Ca antagonist monotherapy may depend on several factors. When we compared the various reported studies of patients with essential hypertension or normal subjects (see Fig 7)[71] who received nifedipine or verapamil acutely or for a short term, no close correlation of average percentage blood pressure reductions with the mean drug dosages was apparent. This does not exclude a certain dose-response in blood pressure in individual patients receiving stepwise increasing doses of Ca antagonists.[119, 122] Nifedipine was given acutely, either by the peroral or by the sublingual route. However, a further analysis of acute studies indicates that in patients with benign essential hypertension, the percentage responses of blood pressure and heart rate did not consistently differ between the two routes of administration, although drugs given by the sublingual route tended to act more rapidly.[71] The level of blood pressure before treatment seems to be an important determinant of the efficacy of Ca antagonists. In the published reports on patients with benign essential hypertension and normal subjects, a direct relationship between basal mean blood pressure and percentage or absolute blood pressure responses to nifedipine or verapamil is apparent under conditions of both acute single-dose or short-term therapy (see Fig 7). The existence of this relationship following acute single-dose or short-term therapy has already been noted by others[39, 63, 77, 86, 89, 145] and also applies to hypertensive emergencies.[12, 106] It follows that the blood pressure-lowering effect of Ca antagonists is minimal in normotensive subjects and tends to increase with the severity of essential hypertension. It is possible that patient age may be another important determinant. A positive relationship between age and the antihypertensive efficacy of verapamil has recently been reported,[39] suggesting that Ca antagonist therapy might be particularly useful in elderly patients. It is possible that additional factors, such as interactions with the sympathetic and renin–angiotensin systems and other blood pressure–regulating components, may also modulate the cardiovascular effects of Ca antagonists.

The potential value of monotherapy with Ca antagonists in essential hypertension requires further assessment of the efficacy and the benefit-risk ratio by long-term studies. At present, diuretics and β blockers are accepted step 1 drugs for the treatment of essential hypertension. With respect to antihypertensive efficacy, it is evident that on short-term administration, Ca antagonists may have a similar potency as thiazide-type diuretics or β blockers. Thus, drugs of all three classes given as a monotherapy may lower blood pressure by an average of about 15%,[24, 142] although β blockers may generally be more effective in younger[22] and diuretics and perhaps also Ca antagonists[24] more potent in elderly patients with essential hypertension.

Combination Therapy

Compared to a monotherapy, an additional blood pressure-lowering effect may be obtained in essential hypertension when Ca antagonists are combined with a thiazide-type diuretic, a β blocker, a sympatholytic such as α-methyldopa or reserpine, or a two-drug regime with a β blocker and diuretic. Table 2 summarizes some short-term and more prolonged studies. It is evident that the complementary potencies of various combinations deserve further clarification, particularly with respect to long-term administration. Nifedipine also induced a further blood pressure reduction acutely when administered as a single-dose treatment to some patients with essential hypertension pretreated with β blockers.[31, 29]

OTHER FORMS OF HYPERTENSION

A paucity of controlled data on the effect of Ca antagonist monotherapy in various secondary forms of hypertension prevents definite conclusions. Acute blood pressure reductions were noted following single doses of nifedipine in sporadic cases with pheochromocytoma, primary hyperaldosteronism, renal artery stenosis, and parenchymal disease, and in terminal

TABLE 2.—EFFECT OF COMBINED TREATMENT WITH CALCIUM ANTAGONISTS AND THIAZIDE-TYPE DIURETICS AND/OR β BLOCKERS AND OTHER SYMPATHOLYTICS ON SUPINE BLOOD PRESSURE AND HEART RATE IN PATIENTS WITH ESSENTIAL HYPERTENSION*

| | | PRECEDING TREATMENT | | COMBINED TREATMENT | | | |
STUDY, YEAR	N	Drug(s)	Duration (wk)	Drug added	Duration (wk)	Blood Pressure (% change)†	Heart Rate (% change)†
Ca antagonist added to thiazide type	D	D					
Anavekar et al., 1981[1]	17	D	2	VER	6	−9	−1
Maeda et al., 1981[83]	5	TCM‡	2–4	DIL	12–14	−27	
Thiazide-type D added to Ca antagonist							
Maeda et al., 1981[83]	5	DIL	2	TCM	12–14	−8	
Marone et al., 1984[88]	10	NIF	6–8	CHLOR	6–8	−6	NC
Ca antagonist added to thiazide type D or B							
Maeda et al., 1982[84]	22	TCM or PROP	?	NIF	12	−24	0
Maeda et al., 1982[84]	17	TCM or PROP	?	NIF	156	−10	0
Ca antagonist added to B							
Lederballe et al., 1980[76]	9	PROP, ATEN, TIM, or MET	≥ 4	NIF	4	−13	+6
Husted et al., 1982[58]	10	PROP, TIM, or MET	≥ 8	NIF	52–132	−21	0
Orö, 1982[101]	12	MET	3	NIT	4	−23	NC
Tammen et al., 1982[121]	8	MET or PROP	2–3	NIT	3	−14	+8

B added to Ca antagonist							
Corea et al., 1980[31]	15	NIF	4	MET	4	−12	−1
Imai et al., 1980[59]	6	NIF	1/2	PROP	1 1/2	−18	−20
Aoki & Sato, 1982[6]	7	NIL	8	PROP	8	0	−14
Eggertsen & Hansson, 1982[37]	26	NIF	12	MET	12	−4	
Ekelund et al., 1982[38]	12	NIF	4	MET	4	−7	−26
Ca antagonist added to D and B							
Brennan & Blake, 1982[21]	16	BFZ and MET	?	NIF	8–24	−18	
Dean & Kendall, 1982[22]	20	D + B	2	NIF	12	−10	−2
Murphy et al., 1983[98]	15	BFZ + ATEN	Chronic	NIF	2	−6 to −16	+3 to +5
						(dose dependent)	
Sympatholytics added to Ca antagonist							
Leary & Asmal, 1979[73]	40	VER	6	RES	6	−5	−14
Guazzi et al., 1980[54]	23	NIF	1 1/2	MD	1 1/2	−15	
Imai et al., 1980[59]	7	NIF	1/2	CLON	1 1/2	−15	−17
Ca antagonists added to sympatholytic							
Leary & Asmal, 1973[79]	40	RES	6	VER	6	−6	−4
Direct vasodilator added to Ca antagonist							
Ueda & Musakami, 1983[127]	16	NIF	2	HYDR	6	+2	−2
Ca antagonist added to direct vasodilator							
Ueda & Musakami, 1983[127]	68	HYDR	2	NIF	6	−19	−1

*ATEN, atenolol; B, β blocker, not specified or different types; BFZ, bendrofluazide; CHLOR, chlorthalidone; CLON, clonidine; D, diuretic, not specified or different types; DIL, diltiazem; HYDR, hydralazine; MD, α-methyldopa; MET, metoprolol; NC, no statistically significant change; NIL, niludipine; NIT, nitrendipine; PROP, propranolol; RES, reserpine; TCM, trichlormethiazide; NIF, nifedipine; TIM, timolol; VER, verapamil.

†Compared to values of preceding treatment.

‡Compared with sedative agent.

renal failure.[8, 66, 68, 133] A certain antihypertensive effect was obtained following short-term monotherapy with diltiazem in some patients with mild to moderate renal failure of various origin or chronic nephritis.[113, 144] Some combination studies with other agents are difficult to evaluate in terms of specificity of patient groups. An ongoing study in our institution suggests that monotherapy with nitrendipine is an effective and well-tolerated form of treatment of mild to moderate hypertension associated with diabetes mellitus type II.[125] A dose of 20–40 mg once daily provided satisfactory blood pressure control in all 10 patients observed for 6 weeks to 1 year. Moreover, there were no adverse effects of the Ca antagonist therapy on parameters of carbohydrate metabolism, such as blood HbA_1 and basal and stimulated levels of plasma glucose and insulin.

HYPERTENSIVE EMERGENCIES

Nifedipine is now established as an important alternative in the treatment of certain hypertensive emergencies. A single dose of 5–20 mg, administered sublingually or sometimes orally, acutely and effectively reduced blood pressure in many patients with life-threatening states complicating hypertension of various etiologies.[9, 12, 53, 69, 85, 106, 110] A typical series is shown in Figure 10.[12] In patients with severe hypertension and left ventricular failure, concomitant improvement of blood pressure and pulmonary congestion usually occurred.[9, 53, 106] Hypertensive encephalopathy was influenced favorably in some cases.[69] Blood pressure also responded in the few cases reported with pheochromocytoma.[12, 85]

An important consideration of any antihypertensive emergency therapy is its effect on cerebral circulation. With nifedipines, an unchanged or even increased cerebral blood flow in the setting of a concomitant marked fall in blood pressure has been reported.[12] However, perfusion may be compromised in certain cases.[3, 99] The relative efficacy and safety of nifedipine in different types of hypertensive emergencies need further clarification.

Following sublingual administration of nifedipine, the reduction in blood pressure is maximal at 15–30 minutes, and improvement may last for up to 4 hours. The response takes only slightly longer after oral administration.[71] Furthermore, the

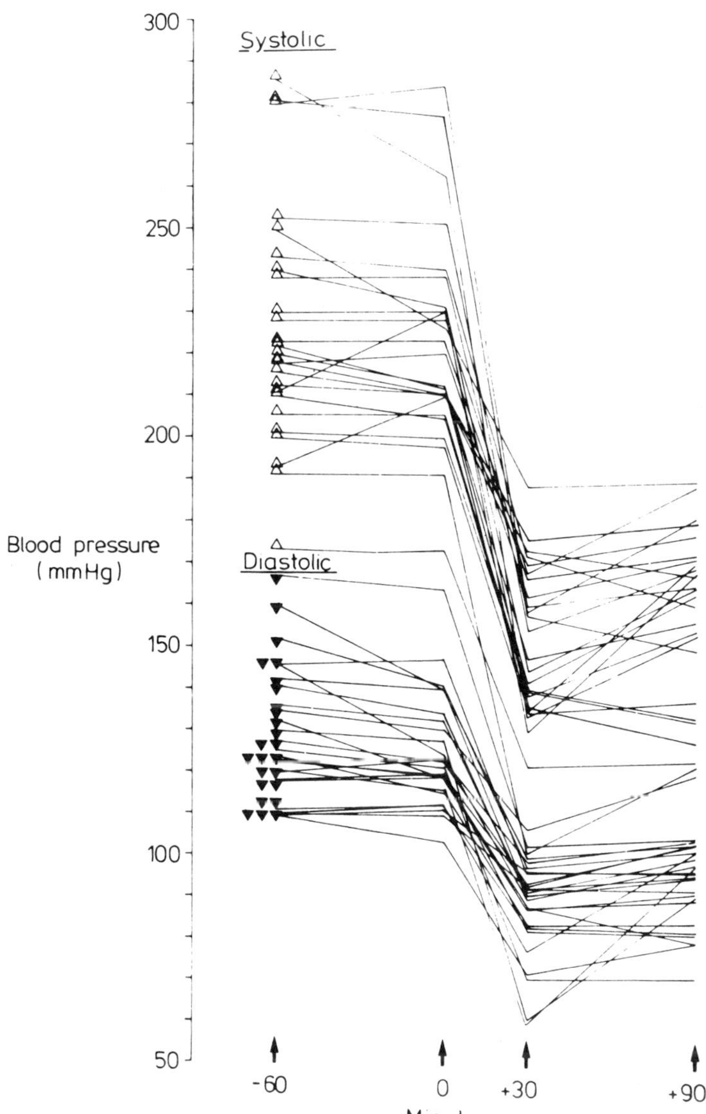

Fig 10.—Effect of nifedipine, 10–20 mg orally, in 25 patients with hypertensive emergencies of various types. Figure shows percentage responses of blood pressure and heart rate to an acute single dose of nifedipine taken perorally or sublingually. (From Bertel et al. Reproduced by permission.)

induced individual decreases in blood pressure correlate strongly with pretreatment blood pressure,[12, 106] as is also noted in benign essential hypertension. An exaggerated fall to hypotensive levels was not encountered with nifedipine monotherapy but sometimes may occur with the use of higher doses (15–20 mg) in patients already on diuretics or other potent antihypertensive therapy.

Other Ca antagonists, such as verapamil[13, 46] or diltiazem,[110] given intravenously, were found to be effective in some patients with hypertensive crises.

SIDE EFFECTS

Ca antagonist therapy is well tolerated by the majority of patients. Nevertheless, side effects may occur that are particularized to individual substances and sometimes lead to disruption of treatment. Table 3 lists only a few side effects reported in the literature, since the relative tolerance and frequency of

TABLE 3.—SIDE EFFECTS OF CALCIUM ANTAGONISTS IN SHORT- TO LONG-TERM ADMINISTRATION*

EFFECT	NIF	VER	DIL
Cardiovascular			
Headache	+ + + +	+ +	+ + + +
Facial flushing, burning of face or legs, palpitations	+ + +	+ +	+ +
Hypotension	+ + +	+ +	+ +
Bradycardia	—	+ + + +	+ +
AV blocks	—	+ +	(+)
Ankle edema	+ +	+	+
Gastrointestinal			
Anorexia, nausea	+ +	+	+ + +
Vomiting	+ +	—	+
Constipation or diarrhea	+	+ + +	+ +
Heartburn	+	—	(+)
Liver function disturbances			(+)
Skin rash	+ +	+	+ +
Neurologic			
Dizziness, vertigo	+ +	+ +	+ + +
Weakness, asthenia	+		+ +
Depression	(+)		

*Reported occurrence of side effects ranges from more common (+ + + +) to very rare (+). Nif, nifedipine; ver, verapamil; dil, diltiazem.

side effects of the various Ca antagonists, particularly when they are used for treatment of hypertension, have not been clarified by comparative assessment. Certain symptoms such as facial flushing, burning sensations, palpitations, and dizziness may be more pronounced in the initial stage and tend to diminish with progressive treatment. Intravenous administration of verapamil to patients with diseased hearts or already receiving another cardiodepressant such as β blockers or digitalis has occasionally provoked serious episodes of bradycardia, heart block, and/or hypotension. Therefore, intravenous administration of verapamil or diltiazem to such patients is contraindicated, and their oral administration in combination with other cardiodepressants warrants particular precaution. Pitting ankle edema, which appears following initiation of treatment and may improve with progressive Ca antagonist therapy, often reflects a local, harmless hemodynamic alteration rather than congestive heart failure or marked body sodium fluid volume retention.

Short-term Ca antagonist therapy has been remarkably free of relevant metabolic side effects. Thus, plasma potassium was generally unchanged except for a mild decrease with nifedipine in one study.[75] Serum total and high-density lipoprotein cholesterol, triglyceride, glucose, and insulin levels, when measured, usually were not affected adversely by nifedipine, verapamil, or diltiazem[7, 49, 71, 108, 115]; this was true for the use of nitrendipine in a group of patients with diabetes mellitus type II.[125] Nevertheless, the long-term situation still remains to be assessed.

Practical Antihypertensive Therapy

Based on the information presented, the following suggestions for practical therapy appear justified.

ESSENTIAL HYPERTENSION

Practical dosages, precautions, and contraindications to the use of nifedipine, verapamil, and diltiazem are summarized in Table 4. Ca antagonists may be useful step 2 or step 3 drugs when used in combination with a diuretic or/and a β blocker. Moreover, they can be tried as an alternative to diuretics or β

TABLE 4.—CALCIUM ANTAGONIST THERAPY IN ESSENTIAL HYPERTENSION

PRACTICAL USE:
 Possibly as a step 1 drug, particularly in the elderly.
 As a step 2 drug, combined with a diuretic or β blocker (see precautions).
 As a step 3 drug, combined with a diuretic and β blocker.
PRECAUTIONS:
 Avoid abrupt discontinuation in patients with coronary artery disease.
 Concerning verapamil and diltiazem:
  AV block I.
  Combined *oral* administration with β blocker or other cardiodepressant may tend
   to potentiate SA and AV nodal inhibition and/or a negative inotropic effect.
CONTRAINDICATIONS:
 Congestive heart failure.
 Pregnancy (except verapamil ?).
 Concerning verapamil and diltiazem:;
  Sick-sinus syndrome.
  AV block II or III.
  Bradycardia.
  Parenteral use in presence of β blocker or other cardiodepressant drugs.
  Digitalis toxicity.

	mg/day	doses/day
DOSAGE:		
Nifedipine or nif.-retard	30–80	2–3
Verapamil or ver.- retard	160–480	2–3
	(−720)	2–3
Diltiazem	90–360	3

blockers for step 1 pharmacotherapy. Young subjects may be initially treated with a β blocker, while in elderly subjects it may be best to start either with a diuretic or a Ca antagonist.[23] The subjective tolerance for all three drug types is quite acceptable. β Blockers and Ca antagonists are more expensive, but they, and Ca antagonists in particular, have less biochemical side effects than diuretics. Recently, some suspicion has arisen that thiazide-type diuretics may have an adverse influence on coronary heart disease in certain individuals with mild hypertension[97] and contribute to excess cardiac death in elderly hypertensive men.[94] Hypokalemia undoubtedly favors the appearance of cardiac arrhythmias in susceptible, usually elderly individuals. Therefore, the possibility of prescribing a Ca antagonist instead of a thiazide-type diuretic is of particular interest in those elderly patients in whom diuretic-induced symptomatic hypokalemia, associated cardiac arrhythmias, attacks of gout, or aggravation of a hyperglycemia have already devel-

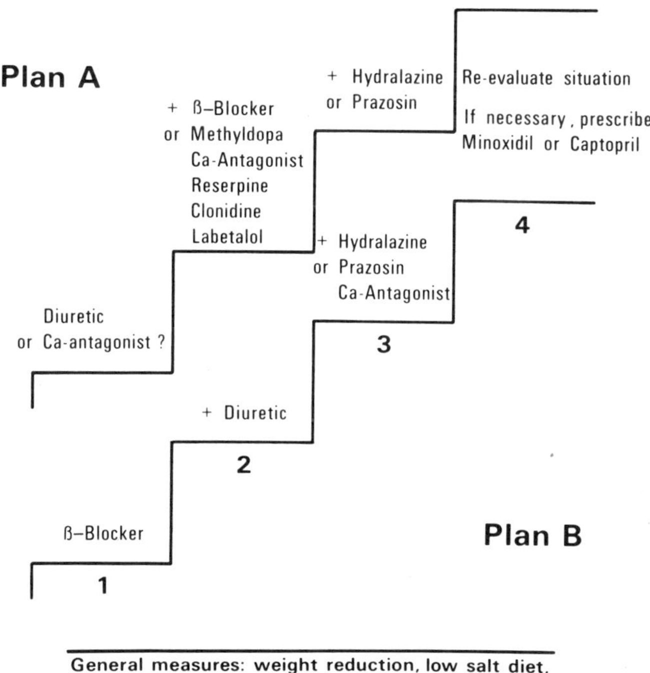

Fig 11.—Stepped-care therapeutic approach to patients with hypertension. Two alternative plans start with either a β blocker (preferred in younger patients) or a diuretic or antagonist (preferred in older patients).

oped or are to be avoided. Figure 11 shows our present steppedcare treatment plan, giving with the proposed place of Ca antagonists in relation to various well-established agents. A detailed description of this approach has been presented elsewhere.[142]

OTHER FORMS OF HYPERTENSION

The potential value of Ca antagonists remains to be clarified. Nevertheless, it may be particularly worthwhile to try these agents in hypertensive patients with diabetes mellitus in whom diuretics and β_2 blockers tend to have undesirable metabolic effects.

HYPERTENSIVE EMERGENCIES

The choice of Ca antagonists or other agents for initial drug therapy depends on the type of hypertensive emergency.

Malignant hypertension not accompanied by hypertensive encephalopathy, severe congestive heart failure, or dissecting aortic aneurysm is no longer an undisputed indication for rapidly acting drugs.[141] Very rapid blood pressure reduction carries a certain risk for the development of neurologic sequelae, which on rare occasions have been fatal or resulted in blindness. Even nifedipine is possibly not free of this risk.[3, 99] Therefore, the risks and benefits of rapid lowering of blood pressure versus a more gently acting therapy should be weighed carefully in such patients. Immediate initiation or intensification of the usual oral drug therapy (see Fig 11), together with in-hospital care, will often allow the blood pressure to fall satisfactorily and safely.

Severe or malignant hypertension complicated by severe congestive heart failure or simultaneous anticoagulant therapy, and hypertensive encephalopathy, and malignant hypertension without these complications but resistant to more gently acting drug therapy within the first 24 hours, are life-threatening conditions which require rapid lowering of blood pressure. Among the possible emergency drugs for this indication (Table 5), nifedipine taken sublingually is now considered to have particular value because of its easy and safe mode of administration as well as its possible lack of adverse effect on cerebral blood flow in many patients.

TABLE 5.—EMERGENCY TREATMENT OF SEVERE OR
MALIGNANT HYPERTENSION WITH ACUTE LEFT VENTRICULAR
FAILURE OR ENCEPHALOPATHY OR OF MALIGNANT
HYPERTENSION WITHOUT THESE COMPLICATIONS BUT
UNRESPONSIVE TO GENTLE DRUG THERAPY

Hospitalize and consider following alternative agents:	
Nifedipine, sublingually	5–20 mg*
Labetalol, IV bolus	60–100 mg*
or IV infusion	2 mg/min*
Clonidine, IV	0.15 mg over 5–10 min*
Nitroprusside, IV infusion and titration	0.5–10 mg/kg/minute
Diazoxide, IV bolus	(150)–300 mg*

*Repeat if necessary; complement with early buildup of usual oral drug combinations.

The potential value of a Ca antagonist in the other types of hypertensive emergencies, such as pheochromocytoma crisis or hypertension with stroke or dissecting aortic aneurysm, needs to be clarified.

Acknowledgment

Research was supported by the Swiss National Science Foundation.

REFERENCES

1. Anavekar S.N., Christophidis N., Louis W.J., et al.: Verapamil in the treatment of hypertension. *J. Cardiovasc. Pharmacol.* 3:287, 1981.
2. Andren L., Hansson L., Oroe L., et al.: Experience with nicardipine—a new calcium antagonist—in hypertension. *J. Cardiovasc. Pharmacol.* 4(suppl. 3):S387, 1982.
3. Anonymous: Calcium antagonists and aneurysmal subarachnoid haemorrhage. *Lancet* 1:141, 1983.
4. Antman E.M., Stone P.H., Mueller J.E., et al.: Calcium channel blocking agents in the treatment of cardiovascular disorders: Part I. Basic and clinical electrophysiologic effects. *Ann. Intern. Med.* 93:875, 1980.
5. Aoki K., Kawaguchi Y., Sato K., et al.: Clinical and pharmacological properties of calcium antagonists in essential hypertension in humans and spontaneously hypertensive rats. *J. Cardiovasc. Pharmacol.* 4(suppl. 3):S298, 1982.
6. Aoki K., Sato K.: Acute hypotensive, hemodynamic effects of long-term treatment with niludipine, a Ca^{2+}-antagonist, in patients with essential hypertension. *Drug Res.* 32:1141, 1982.
7. Aoki K., Sato K., Kondo S., et al.: Hypotensive effects of diltiazem on normals and essential hypertensives. *Eur. J. Clin. Pharmacol.* 25:475, 1983.
8. Aoki K., Yoshida T., Kato S., et al.: Hypotensive action and increased plasma renin activity by Ca^{2+}-antagonist (nifedipine) in hypertensive patients. *Jpn. Heart J.* 17:479, 1976.
9. Bartorelli C., Magrini F., Moruzzi P., et al.: Hemodynamic effect of a calcium-antagonistic agent (nifedipine) in hypertension: Therapeutic implications. *Clin. Sci. Mol. Med.* 55:291S, 1978.
10. Beretta-Piccoli C., Weidmann P.: Exaggerated pressor responsiveness to norepinephrine in non-azotemic diabetes mellitus. *Am. J. Med.* 71:829, 1981.
11. Beretta-Piccoli C., Weidmann P., Schiffl H., et al.: Enhanced cardiovascular pressor reactivity to norepinephrine in mild renal parenchymal disease. *Kidney Int.* 22:297, 1982.
12. Bertel O., Conen D., Radue E.W., et al.: Nifedipine in hypertensive emergencies. *Br. Med. J.* 286:19, 1983.
13. Bhat R.P., Wasir H.S.: Verapamil infusion in hypertension. *Indian Heart J.* 34:228, 1982.
14. Bianchetti M.G., Beretta-Piccoli C., Weidmann P., et al.: Studies on aldosterone responsiveness to angiotensin II during clinical variations in calcium metabolism in normal man. *Clin. Sci.* 63:325, 1982.
15. Bianchetti M.G., Weidmann P., Boehringer K., et al.: Comparative evaluation of the new vasodilator carprazidil and minoxidil in the treatment of moderate to severe hypertension. *Eur. J. Clin. Pharmacol.* 23:483, 1982.
10. Bianchetti M.G., Beretta-Piccoli C., Weidmann P., et al.: Calcium and blood pres-

sure regulation in normal and hypertensive subjects. *Hypertension* 5(suppl. II):57, 1983.

17. Blaustein M.P.: Sodium ions, calcium ions, blood pressure and hypertension: A reassessment and hypothesis. *Am. J. Physiol.* 132:C165, 1977.

18. Bohr D.F.: Vascular smooth muscle updated. *Circ. Res.* 32:665, 1973.

19. Bolli P., Hulthen L., Amann F.W., et al.: Verapamil-induced vasodilator response is enhanced in essential hypertension. *Gen. Pharmacol.* 14:185, 1983.

20. Boullin D.J.: The action of extracellular cations on the release of the sympathetic transmitter from peripheral nerves. *J. Physiol.* 189:85, 1967.

21. Brennan F.N., Blake S.: The use of nifedipine as a third-step agent in the treatment of refractory hypertension. *Ir. Med. J.* 75:29, 1982.

22. Buehler F.R., Burkhart F., Luetold B.E., et al.: Antihypertensive beta blocking action as related to renin and age: A pharmacologic tool to identify pathogenetic mechanisms in essential hypertension. *Am. J. Cardiol.* 36:653, 1975.

23. Buehler F.R., Hulthen U.L., Kiowski W., et al.: Greater antihypertensive efficacy of the calcium channel inhibitor verapamil in older and low renin patients. *Clin. Sci.* 63:S439, 1982.

24. Buehler F.R., Hulthen U.L., Kiowski W., et al.: The place of the calcium antagonist verapamil in antihypertensive therapy. *J. Cardiovasc. Pharmacol.* 4(suppl. 3):S350, 1982.

25. Burn J.H., Gibbons W.R.: The release of noradrenaline from sympathetic nerve fibers in relation to calcium concentration. *J. Physiol.* 181:214, 1965.

26. Burris J.F., Notargiacomo A.V., Papademetriou V., et al.: Acute and short-term effects of a new calcium-antagonist in hypertension. *Hypertension* 4:32, 1982.

27. Cauvin C., Saida K., Van Breemen C.: Effects of Ca-antagonists on Ca-fluxes in resistance vessels. *J. Cardiovasc. Pharmacol.* 4(suppl. 3):S287, 1982.

28. Chen D.S., Poisner A.M.: Direct stimulation of renin release by calcium. *Proc. Soc. Exp. Biol. Med.* 152:565, 1976.

29. Christensen C.K., Lederballe Pedersen O., Mikkelsen E.: Renal effects of acute calcium blockade with nifedipine in hypertensive patients receiving beta-adrenoceptor blocking drugs. *Clin. Pharmacol. Ther.* 32:572, 1982.

30. Chu D., De Gori D.: Antihypertensive effect of tiapamil, a calcium antagonist. *Cardiology* 69(suppl. I):99, 1982.

31. Corea L., Alunni G., Bentivoglio M., et al.: Acute and long-term effects of nifedipine on plasma renin activity and plasma catecholamines in controls and hypertensive patients before and after metoprolol. *Acta Ther.* 6:177, 1980.

32. Dean S., Kendall M.J.: Nifedipine in the treatment of difficult hypertensives. *Eur. J. Clin. Pharmacol.* 24:1, 1982.

33. De Leeuw P.W., Smout A.J.P.M., Willemse P.J., et al.: Effects of verapamil in hypertensive patients, in Zanchetti A., Krikler D. (eds.): *Proceedings of the International Symposium on Calcium Antagonism in Cardiovascular Therapy.* Amsterdam, Excerpta Medica, 1981, pp.233–37.

34. De Leeuw P.W., Van Soest G.A.W., Birkenhaeger W.H.: Aldosterone response to antihypertensive treatment. *Clin. Exp. Hypertens.* [A] 4:1913, 1982.

35. Dorst K.G., Zidek W., Losse H., et al.: Intrazelluläres Natrium und Calcium als genetische Marker der essentiellen Hypertonie. *Schweiz. Med. Wochenschr.* 111:1964, 1981.

36. Douglas W.W., Rubin R.P.: The role of calcium in the secretory response of the adrenal medulla to acetylcholine. *J. Physiol.* 159:40, 1961.

37. Eggertsen R., Hansson L.: Effects of treatment with nifedipine and metoprolol in essential hypertension. *Eur. J. Clin. Pharmacol.* 21:389, 1982.

38. Ekelund L.G., Ekelund C., Roessner S.: Antihypertensive effects at rest and during exercise of a calcium blocker, nifedipine, alone and in combination with metoprolol. *Acta Med. Scand.* 212:71–75, 1982.

39. Erne P., Bolli P., Bertel O., et al.: Factors influencing the hypotensive effects of calcium antagonists. *Hypertension* 5(Suppl. II):II–97, 1983.
40. Erne P., Buergisser E., Bolli P., et al.: Free calcium concentration in platelets closely relates to blood pressure in normal and essential hypertensive subjects. *Hypertension*, to be published.
41. Esper R.J., Esper R.C., Cassola D., et al.: Nitrendipine in treatment of essential hypertension: A multicenter trial. Read before the International Nitrendipin Workshop, Port Chester, New York, Oct. 13–15, 1982.
42. Fakunding J.L., Chow R., Catt R.J.: The role of calcium in the stimulation of aldosterone production by adrenocorticotropin, angiotensin II, and potassium in isolated glomerulosa cells. *Endocrinology* 105:327, 1979.
43. Farese R.V., Prudente W.J.: On the role of calcium in adrenocorticotropin-induced changes in mitochondrial pregnolone synthesis. *Endocrinology* 103:1264, 1978.
44. Fleckenstein-Gruen G., Fleckenstein A.: Calcium-antagonism, a basic principle in vasodilation, in Zanchetti A., Krikler D. (eds.): *Proceedings of the International Symposium on Calcium Antagonism in Cardiovascular Therapy.* Amsterdam, Excerpta Medica, 1981, pp. 30–48.
45. Fleckenstein A.: *Calcium Antagonism in Heart and Smooth Muscle: Experimental Facts and Therapeutic Prospects.* New York, John Wiley & Sons, 1983.
46. Freitas A.R.M.F., Francischetti E.A., Cardoso M.S., et al.: Uso do verapamil no controle da crise vascular hipertensiva e efeitos sobre as concentrações de sódio e potassio urinário e activitáde da renina plasmática. *Arq. Bras. Cardiol.* 31:101, 1978.
47. Fritschka E., Distler A., Gotzen R., et al.: Cross-over-Vergleich von Nitrendipin und Propranolol bei Patienten mit essentieller Hypertonie. *Therapiewoche* 33:45, 1983.
48. Garay R.P., Dagher G., Pernollet M.G., et al.: Inherited defect in Na^+, K^+-cotransport system in erythrocytes from essential hypertensive patients. *Nature* 284:281, 1980.
49. Giesecke H.J., Guckenbiehl W., Hagemann I.: Ergebnisse einer Multicenter-Studie mit Diltiazem bei Hypertonie, in *Calcium-Antagonisten zur Behandlung der Angina Pectoris, Hypertonie und Arrhythmie.* Amsterdam, Excerpta Medica, 1982, p. 220.
50. Greenberg R., Kolen C.A.: Effect of acetylcholine and calcium ions on the spontaneous release of epinephrine from catecholamine granules. *Proc. Soc. Exp. Biol. Med.* 121:1179, 1966.
51. Grim C.E., Luft F.C., Grim C.M., et al.: Rapid blood pressure control with minoxidil: Acute and chronic effects on blood pressure, sodium excretion, and renin-aldosterone system. *Arch. Intern. Med.* 139:529, 1979.
52. Grimm M., Weidmann P., Meier A., et al.: Correction of altered noradrenaline reactivity in essential hypertension by indapamide. *Br. Heart J.* 46:404, 1981.
53. Guazzi M., Olivari M.T., Polese A., et al.: Nifedipine: A new antihypertensive with rapid action. *Clin. Pharmacol. Ther.* 22:528, 1977.
54. Guazzi M.D., Fiorentini C., Olivari M.T., et al.: Short- and long-term efficacy of a calcium antagonistic agent (nifedipine) combined with methyldopa in the treatment of severe hypertension. *Circulation* 61:913, 1980.
55. Guazzi M.D., Polese A., Bartorelli A., et al.: Evidence of shared mechanisms of vasoconstriction in pulmonary and systemic circulation in hypertension: A possible role of intracellular calcium. *Circulation* 66:881, 1982.
56. Hansson L., Andren L., Oroe L., et al.: Pharmacokynetic and pharmacodynamic parameters in patients treated with nitrendipine. *Hypertension* 5(suppl. II):25, 1983.
57. Hulthen U.L., Bolli P., Amann F.W., et al.: Enhanced vasodilatation in essential hypertension by calcium channel blockade with verapamil. *Hypertension* 4(suppl. II):II–26, 1982.

58. Husted S.E., Nielsen H.K., Christensen C.K., et al.: Long-term therapy of arterial hypertension with nifedipine given alone or in combination with a beta-adrenoceptor blocking agent. *Eur. J. Clin. Pharmacol.* 22:101, 1982.

59. Imai Y., Abe K., Otsuka Y., et al.: Management of severe hypertension with nifedipine in combination with clonidine or propranolol. *Drug. Res.* 30(I):674, 1980.

60. Jones R.J., Hornung R.S., Sonecha T., et al.: The effect of a new calcium channel blocker nicardipine on 24-hour ambulatory blood pressure and the press or response to isometric and dynamic exercise. *J. Hypertension* 1:85, 1983.

61. Klein W.: Ergebnisse einer Vergleichsuntersuchung zwischen Nifedipin und Diltiazem bei essentieller arterieller Hypertonie, in *Calcium-Antagonisten zur Behandlung der Angina pectoris, Hypertonie und Arrhythmie*. Amsterdam, Excerpta Medica, 1982, p. 210.

62. Klein W., Brandt D., Vrecko K., et al.: Role of calcium antagonists in the treatment of essential hypertension. *Circ. Res.* 52(suppl. I):174, 1983.

63. Kiowski W., Bertel O., Erne P., et al.: Hemodynamics and reflex response to acute and chronic antihypertensive therapy with the calcium entry blocker nifedipine. *Hypertension* 5(suppl. I):I–70, 1983.

64. Kirpekar S.M., Misu Y.: Release of noradrenaline by splenic nerve stimulation and its dependence on calcium. *J. Physiol.* 188:219, 1967.

65. Koch-Weser J.: Hydralazine. *N. Engl. J. Med.* 295:320, 1967.

66. Kubo K., Shiraishi K., Muto H., et al.: Treatment of hypertension in hemodialysis patients with nifedipine. *Hypertension* 5(suppl. II):II–109, 1983.

67. Kunze D.L.: Calcium and magnesium sensitivity of the carotid baroreceptor reflex in cats. *Circ. Res.* 45:815, 1979.

68. Kusano E., Asano Y., Takeda K., et al.: Hypotensive effect of nifedipine in hypertensive patients with chronic renal failure. *Drug Res.* 32:1575, 1982.

69. Kuwajima I., Ueda K., Kamata C., et al.: A study on the effects of nifedipine in hypertensive crises and severe hypertension. *Jpn. Heart J.* 19:455, 1978.

70. Kuwajima I., Ueda K., Murakami M.: A study on the effects of niludipine in hypertensive patients. *Drug Res.* 32:398, 1982.

71. Laederach K., Gerber A., Weidmann P.: Effect of calcium antagonists on blood pressure, catecholamines, renin, aldosterone, and cardiovascular pressor responsiveness in normal and hypertensive man, in Althaus U., Burckhardt D., Vogt E. (eds.): *Proceedings of the International Symposium on Calcium Antagonism*. Frankfurt, PMI-Verlagsgesellschaft, 1984.

72. Lane J.D., Aprison M.H.: Calcium-dependent release of endogenous serotonin dopamine and norepinephrine from nerve endings. *Life Sci.* 20:665, 1979.

73. Leary W.P., Asmal A.C.: Treatment of hypertension with verapamil. *Curr. Ther. Res.* 25:747, 1979.

74. Lederballe Pedersen O.L., Mikkelsen E., Andersson K.E.: Effects of extracellular calcium on potassium and noradrenaline induced contractions in the aorta of spontaneously hypertensive rats: Increased sensitivity to nifedipine. *Acta Pharmacol. Toxicol.* 43:137, 1978.

75. Lederballe Pedersen O., Mikkelsen E., Christensen N.J., et al.: Effect of nifedipine on plasma renin, aldosterone and catecholamines in arterial hypertension. *Eur. J. Clin. Pharmacol.* 15:235, 1979.

76. Lederballe Pedersen O., Christensen C.K., Mikkelsen E., et al.: Relationship between the antihypertensive effect and steady state plasma concentration of nifedipine given alone or in combination with a beta adrenoceptor blocking agent. *Eur. J. Clin. Pharmacol.* 18:287, 1980.

77. Lederballe Pedersen O., Christensen N.J., Raemsch K.D.: Comparison of acute effects of nifedipine in normotensive and hypertensivae man. *J. Cardiovasc. Pharmacol.* 2:357, 1980.

78. Lenz K., Magometschnigg D.: Die hypotensive Wirkung von intravenös verabrei-

chtem Diltiazem, in *Calcium-Antagonisten zur Behandlung der Angina pectoris, Hypertonie und Arrhythmie.* Amsterdam, Excerpta Medica, 1982, p. 194.

79. Leonetti G., Cuspidi C., Sampieri L., et al.: Comparison of cardiovascular, renal, and humoral effects of acute administration of two calcium channel blockers in normotensive and hypertensive subjects. *J. Cardiovasc. Pharmacol.* 4(suppl. 3):S319, 1982.

80. Lewis G.R.J.: The long-term management of hypertension with verapamil. *Clin. Exp. Pharmacol. Physiol. Suppl.* 6, 1982, p. 107.

81. Llach F., Weidmann P., Reinhart R., et al.: Effect of acute and long-standing hypocalemia on blood pressure and plasma renin activity in man. *J. Clin. Endocrinol. Metab.* 38:841, 1974.

82. Lund-Johansen P., Omvik P.: Hemodynamic effects of nifedipine in essential hypertension at rest and during exercise. *J. Hypertension* 1:159, 1983.

83. Maeda K., Takasugi T., Tsukano Y., et al.: Clinical study on the hypotensive effects of diltiazem hydrochloride. *Int. J. Clin. Pharmacol. Ther. Toxicol.* 19:47–55, 1981.

84. Maeda K., Tanaka C., Minamikawa H., et al.: Antihypertensive effects of the calcium antagonistic agent nifedipine. *Drug Res.* 32:267, 1982.

85. Magometschnigg D.: Zur Therapie bei hypertonen Krisen: Nifedipin per os. *Dtsch. Med. Wochenschr.* 107:1423, 1982.

86. Magometschnigg D.: Acute hypotensive response to nifedipine. *Hypertension* 5(suppl. II):II 81, 1983.

87. Marone C., Beretta-Piccoli C., Weidmann P.: Acute hypercalcemic hypertension in man: Role of hemodynamics, catecholamines and renin. *Kidney Int.* 20:92, 1980.

88. Marone C., Luisoli S., Bomio F., et al.: Antihypertensive therapy with the calcium antagonist nifedipine alone or combined with a diuretic: Response of the body sodium-blood volume state and some other pressor factor. *Kidney Int.* to be published.

89. McGregor G.A., Rotellar C., Markandu N.D., et al.: Contrasting effects of nifedipine, captopril and propranolol in normotensive and hypertensive subjects. *J. Cardiovasc. Pharmacol.* 4(suppl. 3):S358, 1982.

90. Meier A., Weidmann P., Grimm H., et al.: Pressor factors and cardiovascular pressor responsiveness in borderline hypertension. *Hypertension* 3:367, 1981.

91. Michelakis A.: The effect of sodium and calcium on renin release in vitro. *Proc. Soc. Exp. Biol. Med.* 137:833, 1971.

92. Millar J.A., McLean K., Reid J.L.: Calcium antagonists decrease adrenal and vascular responsiveness to angiotensin II in normal man. *Clin. Sci.* 61:65s, 1982.

93. Millard R.W., Lathrop D.A., Grupp G., et al.: Different cardiovascular effects of calcium channel blocking agents: Potential mechanisms. *Am. J. Cardiol.* 49:499, 1982.

94. Morgan T.O., Adams W.R., Hodgson M., et al.: Failure of therapy to improve prognosis in elderly males with hypertension. *Med. J. Aust.* 2:27, 1980.

95. Muiesan G., Agabiti-Rosei E., Alicandri C., et al.: Influence of verapamil on catecholamines, renin, and aldosterone in essential hypertension patients, in Zanchetti A., Krikler D. (eds.): *Proceedings of the International Symposium on Calcium Antagonism in Cardiovascular Therapy.* Amsterdam, Excerpta Medica, 1980, p. 238.

96. Muiesan G., Agabiti-Rosei E., Castellano M., et al.: Antihypertensive and humoral effects of verapamil and nifedipine in essential hypertension. *J. Cardiovasc. Pharmacol.* 4(suppl. 3):S325, 1982.

97. Multiple Risk Factor Intervention Trial Research Group (MRFIT): Risk factor changes and mortality results. *JAMA* 248:1465, 1982.

98. Murphy M.B., Scriven A.J.I., Dollery C.T.: Efficacy of nifedipine as a step 3 antihypertensive drug. *Hypertension* 5(suppl. III)II–218, 1983.

99. Nobile-Orazio E., Sterzi R.: Cerebral ischemia after nifedipine treatment. *Br. Med. J.* 283:948, 1981.
100. Olivari M.T., Bartorelli C., Polese A., et al.: Treatment of hypertension with nifedipine, calcium antagonistic agent. *Circulation* 59:1056, 1979.
101. Oroe L.: Treatment of essential hypertension with the combination of nitrendipine and metoprolol. Read before the International Nitrendipine Workshop, Port Chester, New York, Oct. 13–15, 1982.
102. Oyama Y., Nakaya H., Kanda K.: Clinical application of diltiazem hydrochloride in hypertension. *J. Adult Dis.* 9:687, 1979.
103. Pang P.K.T.: Parathyroid hormone, a potent and specific vasodilator, in Jahn H. (ed.): *Contributions to Nephrology*. Basel, S. Karger, to be published.
104. Park C.S., Han D.S., Fray J.C.S.: Calcium in the control of renin secretion: Ca^{++} influx as an inhibitory signal. *Am. J. Physiol.* 240:F70, 1981.
105. Philip T.H., Distler A., Cordes U.: Sympathetic nervous system and blood pressure control in essential hypertension. *Lancet* 2:959, 1978.
106. Polese A., Fiorentini C., Olivari M.T., et al.: Clinical use of a calcium antagonistic agent (nifedipine) in acute pulmonary edema. *Am. J. Med.* 66:825, 1979.
107. Pozet N., Brazier J.L., Hadj Aïssa A., et al.: Pharmacokinetics of diltiazem in severe renal failure. *Eur. J. Clin. Pharmacol.* 24:635, 1983.
108. Riegger A.J.G., Kromer E., Junggerburth J., et al.: Wirkung des Calzium-Antagonisten Diltiazem auf Plasmareninkozentration, Plasmaaldosteron, antidiuretsiches Hormon, Plasmaosmolalität, freie Wasserclearance und Serum- Natrium- und Kaleiumkonzentration. *Therapiewoche* 33:6006, 1983.
109. Robinson B.F., Dobbs R.J., Bailey S.: Response of forearm resistance vessels to verapamil and sodium-nitroprusside in normotensive and hypertensive men: Evidence for a functional abnormality of vascular smooth muscle in primary hypertension. *Clin. Sci.* 63:33, 1982.
110. Rosenthal J.: Die Behandlung der hypertensiven Krisen mit Diltiazem, in Bender F., Greef K. (eds.): *1. Dilzem Symposium*. Amsterdam, Excerpta Medica, 1981, p. 227.
111. Rupp U., Beretta-Piccoli C., Weidmann P., et al.: Enhanced cardiovascular responsiveness to norepinephrine and angiotensin II in normotensive offspring of hypertensive families, in Rosenfeld J. (ed.): *Hypertension Control in the Community*. London Libbey Publishers, 1983.
112. Safar M.E., Simon A.C., Levenson J.A., et al.: Hemodynamic effects of diltiazem in hypertension. *Circ. Res.* 52:I169, 1983.
113. Sakurai T., Kurita T., Nagano S., et al.: Antihypertensive vasodilating and sodium diuretic actions of D-*cis*-isomer of benzothiazepine derivate (CRD-401). *Acta Urol. Jpn.* 18:695, 1972.
114. Schiffl H., Weidmann P., Beretta-Piccoli C., et al.: Antihypertensive mechanism of the diuretic muzolimine in mild renal failure: Roles of sodium and cardiovascular responsiveness to norepinephrine. *Eur. J. Clin. Pharmacol.* 23:215, 1982.
115. Schulte K.L., Meyer W.A., Distler A., et al.: Antihypertensive Langzeitbehandlung mit Diltiazem und Nifedipin bei essentieller Hypertonie. *Therapiewoche* 33:6011, 1983.
116. Schwietzer G., Distler A., Reeck S., et al.: Hypotensive action of calcium antagonists as related to plasma noradrenaline and reactivity to noradrenaline. *J. Hypertension,* to be published.
117. Shima S., Kawashima Y., Hirai M.: Studies on cyclic nucleotides in the adrenal gland: VIII. Effects of angiotensin on adenosine 3'5-monophosphate and steroid genesis in the adrenal cortex. *Endocrinology* 103:1361, 1978.
118. Soto M.E., Thibonnier M., Sire O., et al.: Antihypertensive and hormonal effects of single oral dose of captopril and nifedipine in essential hypertension. *Eur. J. Clin. Pharmacol.* 20:157, 1981.

119. Taburet A.M., Singlas E., Colin J.N., et al.: Pharmacokinetic studies on nifedipine tablet: Correlation of antihypertensive effects. *Hypertension* 5(part II):II–29, 1983.

120. Takabatake T., Ohta H., Yamamoto Q., et al.: Antihypertensive effect of nicardipine hydrochloride in essential hypertension. *Int. J. Clin. Pharmacol. Ther. Toxicol.* 20:346, 1982.

121. Tammen A.T., Stoepel K., Vollmer G., et al.: Efficacy and safety in patients with essential hypertension and coronary heart disease. Read before the International Nitrendipine Workshop, Port Chester, New York, Oct. 13–15, 1982.

122. Taylor S.H., Silke B., Ahuya C., et al.: Influence of nicardipine on the blood pressure at rest and on the pressor responses to cold, isometric exertion and dynamic exercise in hypertensive patients. *J. Cardiovasc. Pharmacol.* 4:803, 1982.

123. Thibonnier M., Bonnet F., Corvol P.: Antihypertensive effect of fractionated sublingual administration of nifedipine in moderate essential hypertension. *Eur. J. Clin. Pharmacol.* 17:161, 1980.

124. Thorens S., Haeusler G.: Effects of some vasodilators on calcium translocation in intact and fractionated vascular smooth muscle. *Eur. J. Pharmacol.* 54:79, 1983.

125. Trost B., Weidmann P.: Unpublished data.

126. Tsuyusaki T., Noro C., Yabata Y., et al.: Clinical study on long-term oral administratin of diltiazem hydrochloride (CRD-401). *Jpn. J. Clin. Exp. Med.* 53:247, 1976.

127. Ueda K., Musakami M.: A controlled, comparative multicenter study on the clinical efficacy of nifedipine in the treatment of severe hypertension, in Kaltenbach M., Neufeld H.N. (eds.): *5th International Adalat Symposium.* Amsterdam, Excerpta Medica, 1983, p. 146.

128. Valdes G., Soto M.E., Croxatto H.R., et al.: Effects of nifedipine during low, normal and high intakes of sodium in patients with essential hypertension. *Clin. Sci.* 63:S447, 1982.

129. Van Zwieten P.A., Van Meel J.C.A., Timmermanns P.: Calcium antagonists and alpha-2-adrenoceptors: Possible role of extracellular calcium ions in alpha-2-adrenoceptor-mediated vasoconstriction. *J. Cardiovasc. Pharmacol.* 4(suppl. 3):S273, 1982.

130. Ventura H.O., Messerli F.H., Oigman W., et al.: Immediate hemodynamic effects of a new calcium channel blocking agent (nitrendipine) in essential hypertension. *Am. J. Cardiol.* 51:783, 1983.

131. Vierhapper H., Waldhaeusl W.: Reduced pressor effect of angiotensin II and of noradrenaline in normal man following the oral administration of the calcium antagonist nifedipine. *Eur. J. Clin. Med.* 12:263, 1982.

132. Vogt A., Neuhaus K.L., Kreuzer H.: Hemodynamic effects of the new vasodilator drug Bay k 5552 in man. *Drug Res.* 38:2162, 1980.

133. Wasir H.S., Rao S.P.: Acute blood pressure lowering effect of sublingual nifedipine: A clinical study. *Clin. Sci.* 63:S471, 1982.

134. Weidmann P., Massry S.G., Coburn J.W., et al.: Blood pressure effects of acute hypercalcemia. Studies in patients with chronic renal failure. *Ann. Intern. Med.* 76:741, 1972.

135. Weidman P., Horton R., Maxwell M.H., et al.: Dynamic studies of aldosterone in anephric man. *Kidney Int.* 4:289, 1973.

136. Weidmann P., Maxwell M.H., Delima J., et al.: Control of aldosterone responsiveness in terminal renal failure. *Kidney Int.* 7:351, 1975.

137. Weidmann P., Keusch G., Meier A., et al.: Effects of indapamide on the body sodium-volume state, plasma renin, aldosterone and catecholamines, and cardiovascular pressor sensitivity in normal and borderline hypertensive man, *in Proceedings of the Second Int Symposium on Arterial Hypertension.* Amsterdam, Excerpta Medica, 1979, p. 169

138. Weidmann P., Beretta-Piccoli C., Keusch G., et al.: Sodium-volume factor, cardio-vascular reactivity and hypotensive mechanisms of diuretic therapy in hypertension associated with diabetes mellitus. *Am. J. Med.* 67:779, 1979.
139. Weidmann P., Keusch G., Flammer J., et al.: Increased ratio between changes in blood pressure and plasma norepinephrine in essential hypertension. *J. Clin. Endocrinol. Metab.* 48:727, 1979.
140. Weidmann P., Grimm M., Meier A., et al.: Pathogenic and therapeutic significance of cardiovascular pressor reactivity as related to plasma catecholamines in borderline and established essential hypertension. *Clin. Exp. Hypertension* 2:427, 1980.
141. Weidmann P.: Essential, renal and endocrine hypertension, in Massry S.G., Glassock R.J. (eds.): *Textbook of Nephrology.* Baltimore, Williams & Wilkins Co., 1983, vol. 2, p. 738.
142. Weidmann P.: Langzeitbehandlung der Hypertonie 1983. *Schweiz. Med. Wochenschr.* 113:984, 1983.
143. Weidmann P., Beretta-Piccoli C., Meier A., et al.: Antihypertensive mechanism of diuretic treatment with chlorthalidone: Complementary roles of sympathetic axis and sodium. *Kidney Int.* 23:320, 1983.
144. Yamakado M., Tagawa T.: Hypotensive effects of diltiazem HCl (Herbesser). *Mod. Clin. Med.* 20:1877, 1978.
145. Yoshimura M., Takashina R., Shikuma R., et al.: Antihypertensive effect of nifedipine and its relationship to severity of hypertension. *Drug Res.* 33:254, 1983.
146. Zawar P.B., Chawhan R.N. Gosavi S.V., et al.: Verapamil in hypertension: A long-term study. *Indian Heart J.* 34:38, 1982.

Synthesis of Prostaglandins by Vascular Endothelial Cells

FRANÇOISE RUSSO-MARIE,

Inserm U 90, Hôpital Necker, Université René Descartes, Paris

What are Prostanoids?

IN 1930 Kurzrok and Lieb,[11] two American gynecologists, reported that uterus strips, in contact with human sperm, either contract or relax. A few years later, Goldblatt[7] and Von Euler[24] confirmed these results and demonstrated similar effects on smooth muscle. Von Euler[24] showed that the substance involved is a lipid. He called this substance "prostaglandin," or hormone formed in the prostatic gland.

Thirty years passed before substantial progress was made in understanding these molecules. In 1962, Bergström and Samuelsson[2] identified the structure of the prostaglandins and successfully completed their first synthesis. Prostaglandins are unsaturated carboxylic acids with 20 carbons, including a pentane ring.

A few years later, it was reported that prostaglandins are derived from a polyunsaturated fatty acid, arachidonic acid (AA). Thereafter progress in elucidating the biochemical and pharmacologic nature of the prostaglandins was made rapidly. Initially only the prostaglandins of the E and F series were known, and their physiologic and pharmacologic properties were exhaustively studied.

In the 1970s, the discovery of new derivatives shed some

233

0084–5957/84/0014–0233–0240–$04.00

light on the importance of these compounds. In 1973, Hamberg and Samuelsson[9] and Nugteren and Hazelhof[18] reported the existence of endoperoxides, PGG_2 and PGH_2, peroxidation products of AA and precursors of all the prostaglandins.

In 1975 Hamberg, Svensson, and Samuelsson[10] reported for the first time the existence of the platelet metabolite, thromboxane A_2 (TXA_2), specifically formed by platelets and possessing the ability to aggregate platelets and to vasoconstrict smooth muscle. TXA_2 is very unstable and is rapidly metabolized into an inactive compound, TXB_2.

In 1976, Moncada, Gryglewski, Bunting, and Vane[16] reported that vascular endothelium and smooth muscle are able to synthesize from the same endoperoxides another molecule of the same prostaglandin family, prostacyclin. Prostacyclin possesses properties opposite to those of TXA_2. It is the most potent antiaggregatory agent described up to now, and it has vasodilatory effects on smooth muscle. Just as thromboxane is formed specifically in platelets, prostacyclin is formed specifically in the vascular wall. Prostacyclin is unstable and is rapidly metabolized into 6-keto $PGF_{1\alpha}$, which is stable but inactive.

Prostaglandin D_2 has been described and is also a potent antiaggregatory agent but its site of synthesis and other properties are not well known.

Prostanoids of the 2 series are all derived from the polyunsaturated fatty acid, AA, which possesses 20 carbons and four double bonds. AA is found in all membranes of all living cells. The cell type is responsible for the formation of one or more prostanoids. According to the cell type in which AA is liberated, five different prostanoids can be formed: PGE_2, $PGF_{2\alpha}$, PGD_2, PGI_2, or prostacyclin, and TXA_2. These prostanoids are called primary prostanoids. Their formation is due to the enzymic equipment present in the different cells, transforming endoperoxides into primary prostanoids.

Since 1976 the transformation of AA inside the cells has been widely studied. Indeed, all AA liberated inside the cell is not only metabolized into prostanoids, it then undergoes further changes, some of which take it along enzymic pathways. Once liberated in the cell under the action of one phospholipase, AA can be reincorporated into membrane phospholipids under the action of the enzymes known as acyltransferases, or trapped by extracellular albumin, in which case it crosses back over the membrane, or it enters enzymic pathways. One enzymic pathway is the cyclooxygenase, which we have just described. The second enzymic pathway is an oxidative pathway well known in plants, the lipoxygenase pathway. This pathway was initially believed to be a residual oxidative pathway, but since the discovery that the metabolites formed by lipoxygenases have biologic properties, the metabolic importance of this pathway has been reinforced.

It has been known for a long time that in platelets, in parallel to the products of the cyclooxygenase pathway, there appears a 12-peroxidative metabolite of AA; 12-hydroperoxyeicosatetraenoic acid, or 12-HPETE, an unstable compound, which is transformed into a stable product, 12-hydroxyeicosatetraenoic acid.[9] The biologic importance of this compound is not known. Chemotactic properties for neutrophils have been reported for this compound.[6]

In 1976 Borgeat et al.[3] described a 5-peroxidative pathway involving a 5-lipoxygenase in neutrophils.

In 1979 Borgeat and Samuelsson[4] described the intermediary metabolites and the end products of the 5-lipoxygenase pathway. Leukotrienes were then initially described. Leukotriene A_4 (LTA$_4$) is formed from AA through a 5-lipoxygenase pathway. LTA is the unstable precursor of all leukotrienes and can be compared with the endoperoxide PGH_2 of the parallel cyclooxygenase pathway. Leukotrienes B_4, C_4, D_4, and E_4 are then formed from LTA$_4$. LTC$_4$, LTD$_4$, and LTE$_4$ are formed from LTA$_4$ by addition of peptides on the lipid moiety, and have been described as being the active principle of slow-reacting substance of anaphylaxis (SRS-A), involved in anaphylactic reactions. LTB$_4$ is not a peptidolipid but is formed from LTA$_4$ under the action of a hydrolase. This compound is the most potent chemotactic agent for neutrophils described up to now.[5]

Another peroxydative pathway has been described in the vascular wall, involving a 15-lipoxygenase. This lipoxygenase would be specific for vascular cells. Its biologic role is not known.[12]

It can be concluded that three lipoxygenase enzymes, able to form biologically active compounds, exist for AA: a 5-lipoxygenase, mainly found in neutrophils, a 12-lipoxygenase, found in platelets, and a 15-lipoxygenase, found in the vascular wall.

What is Vascular Wall?

The vascular wall is formed by three cell layers. The monolayer endothelium faces the bloodstream. This cell layer is the link between the blood where all substances are carried and the living cells. The integrity of this layer is therefore fundamental.

Under this monocellular layer, and separated by the internal elastic lamina, is the multicellular layer of smooth muscle cells. This layer is perpendicular to the monocellular layer of endothelium. This smooth muscle layer is broader than the endothelial one. It is responsible for the tonus of the vessel, but it also possesses metabolic functions.

Under this smooth muscle layer is the adventitia, mainly formed of fibroblastic cells. The role of this layer is not known.

Each cell layer has a specific function. The endothelium has mainly a metabolic function; it is the first contact between the substances carried by the blood and the living cells. The smooth muscle cell layer controls the tonus of the vascular wall because of the ability of these cells to contract. The adventitia probably has a protective role for the other layers.

Differential Role of Each Vascular Layer in Prostanoid Formation

In 1976 the British group, together with Moncada and Vane, demonstrated the importance of endothelium for prostacyclin production. They found that in the mammals, there exists a gradient in the production of prostacyclin; the luminal part of the vessel is able to synthesize much more prostacyclin than the rest of the vessel wall, whereas the adventitial part of the vessel is almost unable to synthesize prostacyclin.[17]

Such a cell specificity was also reported by ourselves[19] and by other authors using cultured cells from the vascular wall.[14] Using cultured cells derived from piglet aorta, we showed that endothelium was only able to synthesize large amounts of prostacyclin. We could find neither thromboxane nor PGE_2 in this layer in culture. Nevertheless, it is noteworthy that fresh endothelial cells in culture almost exclusively formed prostacyclin,[12] whereas once in culture they are also able to form $PGF_{2\alpha}$, whose local role is negligible.

The smooth muscle layer is also able to form prostacyclin but its main products are PGE_2 and $PGF_{2\alpha}$. However, since smooth muscle cells are present in much greater amount, their secretion of prostacyclin might become more important than endothelial secretion. Nevertheless, the way prostacyclin crosses the endothelium in order to reach the vessel light is unknown, and the exact physiologic role of smooth muscle cells in the production of prostacyclin is not well known, although this production might become of primary importance when the endothelium is injured.

Adventitial cells in culture do not form prostacyclin but are able to synthesize TXA_2. Such results have also been reported in the human umbilical vein and calf aorta in culture.[1, 25] It seems that this scheme of secretion can be proposed as a general one.

In summary, in a physiologic and balanced situation, prostacyclin is mainly of endothelial origin, whereas in other situations, after endothelium has been injured, the smooth muscle may become the major source of prostacyclin.

Differential Function of Prostanoids

We will not describe recent results obtained with lipoxygenase derivatives in the vessel wall. The results are too preliminary to be reported in a review, and it is not possible to give a clear scheme of their functions.

On the other hand, the roles of the products of the cyclooxygenase pathway have been exhaustively studied. PGE_2 and $PGF_{2\alpha}$ do not seem to have important functions apart from those of relaxing or contracting smooth muscle. PGD_2 is a very potent antiaggregatory agent but is not synthesized in the vessel wall. It can be formed in platelets under certain circumstances. The importance of prostacyclin and thromboxane is fundamental. Briefly, TXA_2, formed mainly by platelets, is aggregatory and vasoconstricting for the smooth muscle, whereas prostacyclin is antiaggregatory and vasodilating.

Under normal physiologic circumstances, there exists a balance in the production of these two prostanoids. It is reasonable to posit that if this balance is shifted toward more thromboxane, aggregation will occur, whereas a shift of the balance toward more prostacyclin will favor bleeding. Many data have now been reported that support this theory.

Lipoxygenase derivatives formed in the vessel wall (15-lipoxygenase) and in the platelets (12-lipoxygenase) do not play a definite role in the balance between vascular wall and platelets.

Cellular Interactions

The function of these prostanoids in the vascular wall has been well defined. However, in vivo more complicated situations exist that involve cellular cooperation, rendering possible the formation of compounds derived from two different cells and linked to the enzymic equipment of each cell type.

There exists a platelet-endothelium cooperation. When platelet reaches the vicinity of the endothelium, platelet endoperoxides can be transferred to the endothelial cell and become a substrate for prostacyclin synthetase. In such conditions, proaggregatory substances can finally become powerful antiaggregatory substances. Such a cooperation is now well established, but the factors regulating this cooperation are not known.[3, 15]

Another cell cooperation has now been described[13] but its physiologic significance is not known. Leukocytes and platelets can make a product involving the 12-lipoxygenase and the 5-lipoxygenase enzymes. This product is formed in large amounts. Its biologic function is not known.

Pathology and Prostanoids

Although no defined pathology has been linked to an abnormal secretion of prostanoids, some diseases can be related to an abnormality in the balance between prostacyclin and thromboxane.

In atheroma, it has been suggested that during smooth muscle proliferation, the smooth muscle cells are loaded with peroxidated lipids, which are potent inhibitors of prostacyclin synthetase.[8] It is conceivable that after endothelium injury, if smooth muscle cells are no longer able to form prostacyclin, because of lipid loading, there is no possibility of increasing prostacylin secretion, and therefore thrombus formation can occur rapidly.

On the other hand, Remuzzi et al.[20] have demonstrated that in some chronic renal diseases associated with a bleeding tendency there is increased formation of prostacyclin and decreased formation of thromboxane owing to the presence of plasmatic proteins in the blood of these patients. Similarly, Remuzzi et al. have described another disease, thrombotic microangiopathy, in which they found a decreased synthesis of prostacyclin.[21]

In summary, it is difficult to determine whether a modification of the balance is the initial phenomenon or a secondary event following metabolic anomaly. But it is conceivable that a new therapeutic approach, modifying the prostacyclin-thromboxane balance, might open new investigations in pharmacology.

REFERENCES

1. Baenziger N.L., Dillender M.J., Majerus P.W.: Cultured human skin fibroblasts and arterial cells produce a labile platelet inhibitory prostaglandin. *Biochem. Biophys. Res. Commun.* 78:294, 1977.
2. Bergström S., Samuelsson B.: The prostaglandins. *Endeavour* 27:109, 1968.
3. Borgeat P., Hamberg M., Samuelsson B.: Transformation of arachidonic acid and homolinolenic acid by rabbit polymorphonuclear leukocytes to monohydroxy acids from novel lipoxygenase. *J. Biol. Chem.* 251:7816, 1976.
4. Borgeat P., Samuelsson B.: Metabolism in arachidonic acid in polymorphonuclear leukocytes. *J. Biol. Chem.* 254:7865, 1979.
5. Ford-Hutchinson A.W., Bray M.A., Doig M.V., et al.: Leukotriene B, a potent chemokinetic and aggregating substance released from polymorphonuclear leukocytes. *Nature* 286:264, 1980.
6. Goetzl E.J., Woods J.M., Gorman R.R.: Stimulation of human eosinophil and neutrophil polymorphonuclear leukocyte chemotaxis and random migration by 12-L-hydroxy-5,8,10,14-eicosatetraenoic acid. *J. Clin. Invest.* 59:179, 1977.
7. Goldblatt M.W.: Properties of human seminal fluid. *J. Physiol.* 84:208, 1935.
8. Gryglewski R.J., Dembinska-Kiec A., Zmuda A., et al.: Prostacyclin and thromboxane A_2 biosynthesis capacities of heart, arteries and platelets at various stages of experimental atherosclerosis in rabbits. *Atherosclerosis* 31:385, 1978.
9. Hamberg M., Samuelsson B.: Detection and isolation of an endoperoxide intermediate in prostaglandin biosynthesis. *Proc. Natl. Acad. Sci. USA* 70:899, 1973.
10. Hamberg M., Svensson J., Samuelsson B.: Thromboxane: A new group of biologically active compounds derived from prostaglandin endoperoxides. *Proc. Natl. Acad. Sci. USA* 72:2994, 1975.
11. Kurzrok R., Lieb C.C.: Biochemical studies of human semen: The action of semen on the human uterus. *Proc. Soc. Exp. Biol. Med.* 28:268, 1930.
12. Larrue J., Rigaud M., Razaka G., et al.: Formation of monohydroxyeicosatetraenoic acids from arachidonic acid by cultured rabbit aortic smooth muscle cells. *Biochem. Biophys. Res. Commun.* 112:242, 1983.
13. Maclouf J. Fruteau de Laclos B., Borgeat P.: Stimulation of leukotriene biosynthesis in human blood leukocytes by platelet derived 12-hydroperoxy-icosatetraenoic acid. *Proc. Natl. Acad. Sci. USA* 79:6042, 1982.
14. MacIntyre D.E., Pearson J.D., Gordon J.L.: Localisation and stimulation of PGI_2 production in vascular cells. *Nature* 271:549, 1978.
15. Marcus A.J., Weksler B.B., Jaffe A.E.: Enzymatic conversion of PGH_2 and arachidonic acid to PGI_2 by human endothelial cells. *J. Biol. Chem.* 253:7138, 1978.

16. Moncada S., Gryglewski R.J., Bunting S., et al.: An enzyme isolated from arteries transforms prostaglandin endoperoxides to an unstable substance that inhibits platelet aggregation. *Nature* 263:663, 1976.
17. Moncada S., Herman A.G., Higgs E.A., et al.: Differential formation of PGI_2 by layers of the arterial wall: An explanation for the antithrombotic properties of the vascular endothelium. *Thromb. Res.* 11:323, 1977.
18. Nugteren D.H., Hazelhof E.: Isolation and properties of intermediates in prostaglandin biosynthesis. *Biochim. Biophys. Acta* 326:448, 1973.
19. Ody C., Seillan C., Russo-Marie F.: 6-keto prostaglandin $F_{1\alpha}$, prostaglandin E_2, $F_{2\alpha}$ and thromboxane B_2 production by endothelial cells, smooth muscle cells and fibroblasts cultured from piglet aorta. *Biochim. Biophys. Acta* 712:103, 1982.
20. Remuzzi G., Bertani T., Livio M., et al.: Vascular factors in the pathogenesis of uraemic bleeding, in Robinson B.H.B., Hawkins J.B. (eds.): *Dialysis Transplantation Nephrology*, Turnbridge Wells, England, Pitman Medical, 1978, pp. 449–455.
21. Remuzzi G., Misiani R., Marchesi D., et al.: Haemolityc uraemic syndrome: Deficiency of plasma factors regulating prostacyclin activity. *Lancet* 2:871, 1978.
22. Siess W., Dray F., Seillan C., et al.: Prostanoid synthesis by vascular slices and cultured vascular cells of piglet aorta. *Biochem. Biophys. Res. Commun.* 99:608, 1981.
23. Tateson J.E., Moncada S., Vane J.R.: Effects of prostacyclin on cyclic AMP concentrations in human platelets. *Prostaglandins* 13:389, 1977.
24. Von Euler U.S.: On the specific vasodilating and plain muscle stimulating substance from accessory genital glands in man and certain animals (prostaglandin and vesiglandin). *J. Physiol.* 88:213, 1936.
25. Weksler B.B., Marcus A.J., Jaffe E.A.: Synthesis of prostaglandin I_2 (prostacyclin) by cultured human and bovine endothelial cells. *Proc. Natl. Acad. Sci. USA* 94:3922, 1977.

The Role of Prostaglandins in Arterial Hypertension: A Critical Review

HERMAN-JOSEF GROENE, M.D., AND
MICHAEL J. DUNN, M.D.

*Department of Medicine, Case Western Reserve University and Division of Nephrology,
University Hospitals of Cleveland, Cleveland, Ohio*

Introduction

PROSTAGLANDINS and thromboxane, also collectively called "prostanoids" or "eicosanoids," are oxygenated products of polyunsaturated fatty acids, especially arachidonic acid. Because prostaglandins have vasodilatory and natriurctic properties and thromboxane is a potent vasoconstrictor, many investigators have tried to elucidate the role of vasodilatory prostaglandins or vasoconstrictor thromboxane in different forms of experimental and human hypertension. Experimental and clinical data about the roles of prostaglandins and thromboxane in controlling blood pressure are sometimes contradictory. Hence, it is presently impossible to attribute pathophysiologic importance to these eicosanoids in hypertension. Nonetheless, this new and exciting field has provided both experimental and clinical insights that have enhanced our understanding of hypertension. This review is introductory, and additional information can be found in recently published works.[1, 2, 3]

241

0084–5957/84/0014–0241–0272–$04.00

Vascular and Renal Prostaglandins:
Synthesis and Degradation

Vascular and renal cells, like most mammalian cells, are capable of converting polyunsaturated fatty acids into prostaglandins (PG). Arachidonic acid (AA) is the polyunsaturated fatty acid that most often serves as the substrate for PG synthesis, but other polyunsaturated fatty acids may also be transformed into prostaglandins if tissue levels are high enough—e.g., through dietary supplementation. Dihoma-gamma-linolenic acid is the substrate for monoenoic prostaglandins with one double bond, arachidonic acid serves as precursor for dienoic prostaglandins with two double bonds, and trienoic prostaglandins with three double bonds are synthesized from eicosapentaenoic acid (EPA).

Monoenoic, dienoic, and trienoic eicosanoids may exert contrasting actions. For example, TxA_2 is a potent aggregatory and vasoconstrictive substance, while TxA_3 seems to be devoid of these characteristics and even increases platelet cyclic AMP levels like classical inhibitors of aggregation.[4] Whereas PGE_1 is a potent anti-aggregatory agent in platelets, PGE_2 has little effect or is pro-aggregatory.[5] Mammalian cells synthesize predominantly dienoic prostaglandins. AA and other polyunsaturated fatty acids are stored in membrane phospholipids and after a stimulus are deacylated by acylhydrolases primarily from phosphatidyl-choline and phosphatidylinositol (Fig 1). Phospholipase A_2 directly releases AA, bound to the phosphoglyceryl structure of the phospholipid in the C_2 position. A second possible release reaction consists of phospholipase C splitting the phospholipid into a diglyceride and the phosphorylated base, and diglyceride lipase then frees AA from the diglyceride. Both phospholipases are calcium-dependent enzymes with varying dependence on calmodulin. Miscellaneous stimuli (Table 1) may cause an increase of intracellular calcium (Ca) and an activation of phospholipases.

During basal or nonhormonal stimulation of prostaglandin synthesis, only about 5–10% of the released AA is actually converted to PG; the remainder is reincorporated into phospholipid pools or is lipoxygenated to leukotrienes and hydroxy fatty acids. After hormonal stimulation—for example, bradykinin or angiotensin—greater amounts of AA are converted to prosta-

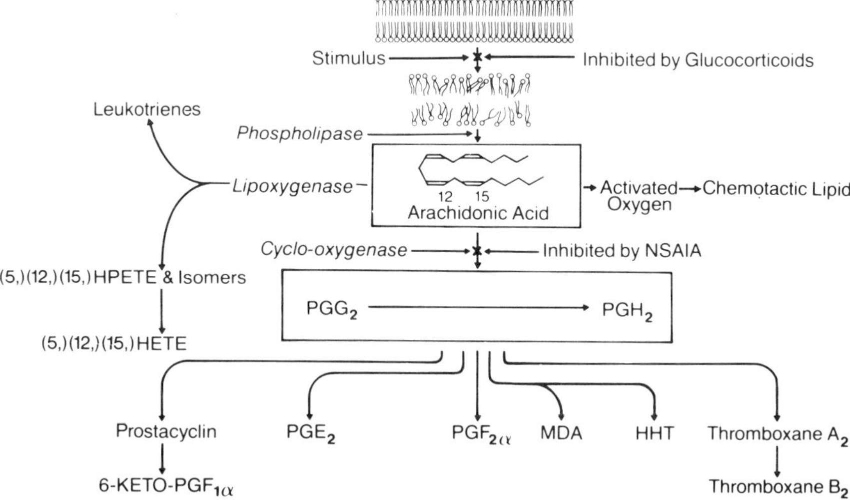

Fig 1.—Outline of arachidonic acid's conversion to oxygenated products via the lipoxygenase and cyclo-oxygenase pathways. Abbreviations: NSAID = nonsteroidal antiinflammatory agents; HPETE = hydroperoxyeicosatetraenoic acid; HETE = hydroxyeicosatetraenoic acid; MDA = malondialdehyde; HHT = hydroxyheptadecatrienoic acid. (Reproduced with permission of the Upjohn Company, Kalamazoo, Mich.)

glandins, probably through a hormone-sensitive phospholipid pool tightly coupled to the prostaglandin-synthesizing enzyme cyclooxygenase.[6, 7]

Endogenous inhibitors of phospholipase activity have been described—macrocortin isolated from lung, lipomodulin in rabbit peritoneal neutrophils.[8, 9] Adrenal steroids stimulate the synthesis of these phospholipase-inhibitory proteins. Intracellular cAMP, which is stimulated by different prostaglandins in different cells, inhibits phospholipase activity, establishing a

TABLE 1:—STIMULI OF RENAL PG SYNTHESIS

PEPTIDES	DISEASES
Angiotensin II, III	Bartter's syndrome
Bradykinin	Hypertension (SHR)
Vasopressin	Ischemia
MISCELLANEOUS	Ureteral or renal venous obstruction
Arachidonic acid	Glomerulonephritis
Calcium	
Catecholamines	
Loop diuretics	

negative feedback loop for prostaglandins and cAMP synthesis.[10]

Free AA is metabolized by an enzyme complex called "cyclo-oxygenase," which is located primarily in the endoplasmic reticulum. A co-oxidase converts AA to PGG_2 which is subsequently metabolized by a hydroperoxidase to PGH_2. PGG_2 and PHG_2 are known as endoperoxides. Cyclo-oxygenase is deactivated during the generation of PGH_2 by oxygen radicals released during the conversion of PGG_2 to PGH_2. Specific enzymes then act on PGH_2 to form prostacyclin (PGI_2), thromboxane (TxA_2), PGE_2 or $PGF_{2\alpha}$ (Fig 1). Thromboxane synthetase can also catalyze the conversion of PGH_2 into 12 L-hydroxy-5,8,10, heptadecanoic acid (HHT) and malondialdehyde (MDH). MDA has been measured as an index of TxA_2 generation. The lipoxygenase enzymes synthesize monohydroxy fatty acids and leukotrienes. Since the cardiovascular and renal actions of these compounds are still incompletely understood, we will focus on eicosanoids derived from the cyclo-oxygenase pathway.

Prostaglandin-degrading enzymes are located in the cytosol. There, 15-hydroxy prostaglandin dehydrogenase forms inactive 15-keto-Pg, and these are then reduced to 13,14-dihydro-15 keto prostaglandins. TxA_2 and PGI_2, which possess a half-life of 0.5 and 3 minutes, respectively, decay spontaneously to their hydrolysis products, TxB_2 and 6-keto-$PGF_{1\alpha}$. Kidney cells possess additional degradative PG enzymes such as prostaglandin 9-keto-prostaglandin reductase and 9-hydroxy-prostaglandin dehydrogenase, which convert PGE_2 to $PGF_{2\alpha}$ or $PGF_{2\alpha}$ to PGE_2. The physiological importance of these enzymes is unknown. Most of the prostaglandins synthesized in the kidney are metabolized either within the same cell or by contiguous cells and only a limited amount is released into renal venous blood. The lung inactivates most of the prostanoids delivered to the pulmonary circulation with the notable exception of PGI_2. The liver and kidney constitute major degradative sites for PGI_2.

Qualitative and quantitative differences of prostaglandin synthesis exist for different cells in one organ as exemplified by the vascualr wall and the kidney (Table 2). Whereas prostaglandin synthetic capacity is greatest in the renal medulla, the degradative enzymes are greater in renal cortex (tubules).[11]

TABLE 2:—RENAL AND VASCULAR CELLULAR SITES OF
PROSTAGLANDIN SYNTHESIS

Glomeruli (whole)	$PGF_{2\alpha} \gtrless PGE_2 > TxA_2 > PGI_2$
Glomerular epithelial cells	$PGE_2 >> TxA_2 > PGF_{2\alpha} > PGI_2$
Glomerular mesangial cells	$PGE_2 >> PGF_{2\alpha} > PGI_2 > TxA_2$
Cortical tubules (mixed)	Negligible
Collecting tubule:	
Cortical	PGE_2
Papillary	$PGE_2 >> PGF_{2\alpha} > TxA_2, PGI_2$
Medullary thick ascending limb	$PGE_2 >> PGF_{2\alpha}$
Medullary interstitial cells	$PGE_2 >> PGF_{2\alpha}$
Arteries, arterioles	$PGI_2 > PGE_2 > PGE_{2\alpha} > TxA_2$
Endothelial cells	$PGI_2 > PGF_{2\alpha} > PGE_2 (> TxA_2)$
Vascular smooth Muscle cells	$PGI_2 > PGF_{2\alpha} > PGE_2$

Data are based on microdissection and cell culture studies of rats
and rabbits.

Degradative prostaglandin enzymes can also be found in the
cells of the vascular wall.[12]

Measuring Prostaglandins

Because prostaglandins are rapidly metabolized and are not
stored, most investigators have studied in vitro prostaglandin
synthesis, or measured stable prostaglandin or prostaglandin
metabolites in urine or plasma. The first approach is to remove
the kidneys or a portion of vasculature and measure its capacity to synthesize prostanoids in vitro. The alternative approach,
for in vivo experiments, is to measure prostaglandins or prostaglandin metabolites in peripheral or renal venous plasma or
in urine. The in vitro techniques with isolated renal or vascular tissue allow one to assess prostaglandin synthesis in a single organ, but obviously they can only be applied to experimental animals. Human experimentation has emphasized in vivo
measurements of prostaglandins, especially in urine.

Urinary excretion of prostaglandins and prostaglandin metabolites has been studied extensively in animals and humans
because it is a noninvasive way of assessing systemic and renal
prostaglandin synthesis. Since intrarenal stimuli (AA and AN-
GII), which increase renal PGE_2 and $PGF_{2\alpha}$ synthesis, also el-

evate urinary PGE_2 and $PGF_{2\alpha}$ excretion, it is generally accepted that urinary PGE_2 and $PGF_{2\alpha}$ are of renal origin.[13] Urinary 2,3 dinor 6-keto-$PGF_{1\alpha}$ and 2,3 dinor TxB_2 are measured as metabolites and indices of systemic PGI_2 and TxA_2 synthesis. Controversy continues about the origin of urinary 6-keto-$PGF_{1\alpha}$ and TxB_2. It seems that under normal conditions urinary 6-keto-$PGF_{1\alpha}$ and TxB_2 are solely derived from the kidney. However, in pathophysiological states with increased synthesis of TxA_2 and PGI_2, TxB_2 and 6K-$PGF_{1\alpha}$ in the urine may partially reflect extrarenal TxB_2 or PGI_2.[14]

Male urine can be contaminated by prostaglandin-rich seminal fluid, so it is advisable to collect urine for prostaglandin measurements from females.[15] Urinary prostanoid determinations require extraction and chromatography of the sample before radioimmunoassay. Measuring urinary prostanoids does not indicate the specific intrarenal origin of the measured prostanoid—i.e., glomerular, tubular, vascular, etc.

Prostaglandin Action on Blood Vessels and Kidneys

Infusion of AA into the renal artery increases the renal blood flow as well as sodium and water diuresis, which can be blocked by cyclo-oxygenase inhibitors, thereby showing that these physiologic responses are secondary to enhanced synthesis of PGE_2 and PGI_2.[16, 17] Infused prostaglandins (PGA_1, PGD_2, PGE_2 and PGI_2) vasodilates the renal vascular bed of the rabbit, dog, and human being.[18, 19] PGE_2 increased renal vascular resistance in the rat kidney in vivo and in isolated perfused kidneys.[3] This PGE_2 vasoconstrictive action can be reversed by competitive blockade of ANG II.[20] Low doses of PGE_2 seem to directly vasodilate the renal vascular bed, and the final effect of PGE_2 on the renal vasculature depends on the pre-existing renal vascular resistance as well as the amount of renin stimulation in response to PGE_2.[21] The effects of exogenous prostaglandins may not reflect the physiological actions of renal prostaglandins. The influence of inhibitors of prostaglandin synthesis on renal vascular resistance has been investigated under different situations to assess the contribution of prostaglandins to the effective tone of renal arteries. Nonsteroidal anti-inflammatory drugs (NSAID), used to inhibit the synthesis of prostaglandins, inhibit irreversibly (e.g., acetylsalicyclic acid) or reversibly (e.g., indomethacin) the cyclo-oxygenase.[22] Renal vascular resistance in dogs increased during NSAID therapy, in states in which the activities of the renin-angiotensin and the sympatho-adrenal systems were increased (e.g., anesthesia, hypovolemia, and abdominal operations). Autoregulation of renal blood flow was preserved.[23, 24]

Contradictory results have been reported in anesthetized rats. In one study, renal blood flow was decreased by 25% by indomethacin, while others could not detect any increase of vascular resistance after indomethacin or meclofenamate.[3, 25] Conscious awake animals, with the exception of the rabbit, showed no decrease in renal blood flow or glomerular filtration rate in most studies during NSAID therapy.[24, 26–28] In man, inhibition of systemic vascular and renal prostaglandins causes significant elevations of systemic and renal vascular resistance and decrements of the glomerular filtration rate if blood pressure or plasma volume are lowered.[29] In this situation, prostaglandins are necessary to counteract activated vasoconstrictive systems like the renin-angiotensin system.

Renal medullary prostaglandins alter water and electrolyte excretion in different ways. Micropuncture experiments provide evidence that prostaglandins inhibit NaCl transport distal to the proximal tubule. PGE_2 seems to inhibit sodium chloride reabsorption in the medullary thick ascending loop of Henle and in the cortical and medullary collecting tubule.[39] In the collecting tubule, urea reabsorption is decreased by PGE_2.[30] Medullary blood flow is increased by prostaglandins, because cyclo-oxygenase inhibition reduces medullary blood flow.[31, 32] In the isolated perfused collecting tubule, PGE_2 can reduce the osmotic water permeability induced by vasopressin. The results of these medullary effects of prostaglandins are decreased medullary tonicity, and increased NaCl excretion.[39]

Interactions Among Prostaglandins, the Renin-Angiotensin and Kallikrein Systems

Vasoconstrictor stimuli like angiotensin II, vasopressin, norepinephrine, and sympathetic nerve stimulation provoke increased renal prostanoid synthesis.[33–35] When ANGII and ANGIII are infused into the dog, rabbit, or human kidneys, PGE_2 and PGI_2 increase in the venous effluent and urine.[36] Norepinephrine or renal nerve stimulation releases renal PGE_2 and PGI_2. In studies in human volunteers, intravenous norepinephrine infusion led to elevated PGE_2 and 6-keto-$PGF_{1\alpha}$ excretion in the urine.[37] The kidney cells responding to ANGII include arterioles, glomeruli, and medullary interstitial cells. PGE_2 synthesis by isolated glomeruli, as well as cultured rat mesangial and epithelial glomerular cells, is stimulated by ANGII.[1,38] The renomedullary interstitial cell also responds to ANGII and vasopressin with increments of PGE_2 synthesis.[40] PGI_2 synthesis by perfused arteries or by vascular endothelial and smooth muscle cells in culture is increased by ANGII and vasopressin.[41] The stimulatory effect of vasoconstrictive agents on the synthesis of vasodilatory prostaglandins can be interpreted as a counter-regulatory process. Prostaglandins attenuate the effects of sympathetic nerve stimulation by pre- and postsynaptic mechanisms. PGE_2, in addition to antagonizing the vasoconstrictive action of norepinephrine by its direct effect on the vascular smooth muscle, inhibits norepinephrine release presynaptically. PGI_2 does not inhibit norepinephrine release presynaptically, but it interferes with its action on the postsynaptic receptor site.[1,42,43]

Many in vitro and in vivo studies have unequivocally established that certain prostaglandins most notably PGE_1, PGE_2, and PGI_2 as well as AA are capable of stimulating renin release.[44–47] Studies on kidney slices, isolated glomeruli, and denervated nonfiltering kidneys have shown a direct stimulatory effect of AA on renin release. This response could be blocked by cyclo-oxygenase inhibitors, which suggests that AA releases renin after its conversion to prostaglandins. In experiments in which renal baroreceptors and renin release were activated by different means—for example, hemorrhagic hypotension or suprarenal aortic clamping—cyclo-oxygenase inhibitors attenuated, but never abolished, renin release.[48] β-adrenergic stimulation of renin secretion is not predictably reduced by inhibiting prostaglandin synthesis with indomethacin.[49–60] If ANGII stimulates vasodilatory prostaglandin and if these prostaglandins can increase renin release and ANGII formation, one is left with a positive feedback system. ANGII inhibition of renin release may constitute the necessary negative input to avoid continual re-enforcement of renin secretion (Fig 1).

Kinins activate phospholipase and the synthesis of prostaglandins in vascular and kidney cells. Bradykinin stimulates PGE_2 synthesis in glomerular epithelial and mesangial cells, in renal medullary interstitial cells, and in tubular cells of the medulla. The vasodilatory effect of kinins seems to be largely independent of prostaglandins, while their natriuretic effect apparently depends on prostaglandin synthesis in the renal medulla.[1, 51] Because urinary kallikrein, the enzyme catalyzing the formation of kinins from kininogen, has been reported to be decreased in essential hypertension, the interaction between the kallikrein-kinin system and prostaglandins may be important in regulating arterial hypertension (Fig 2).[51, 52]

Prostaglandins and Experimental Hypertension

Many investigators have examined the biosynthetic capacity of vascular and renal structures to produce and degrade prostanoids. Others have measured the tissue levels of prostanoids and the urinary excretion of prostaglandins and their metabolites. Probably because of the different methods used and the various stages of hypertension studied, divergent and contrasting results have been reported, even for the same hypertensive animal model.

In the spontaneously hypertensive rat (SHR) of the Kyoto strain, we have demonstrated increased PGE_2 synthetase activity in renal medullary microsomes with the differences between the normotensive Wistar Kyoto control rat (WKy) and

Fig 2.—Interrelationships of prostaglandins with the renal kallikrein, kinin, and renin-angiotensin-aldosterone systems. ACE = angiotensin converting enzyme; LBK = lysol bradykinin; BK = bradykinin. Solid arrows depict stimulation and the broken arrows show inhibition or degradation. (Reprinted with permission from Smith M.C., Dunn M.J.: Renal kallikrein, kinins, and prostaglandins in hypertension. Brenner B.M., Stein J.H. (eds.): In *Hypertension*. (New York: Churchill Livingstone, pp. 168-202, 1981).

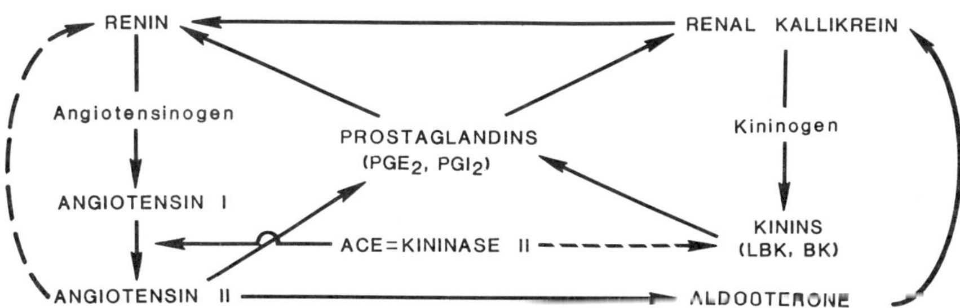

SHR becoming more pronounced with age.[53] This suggested an adaptive process in the kidney in response to rising blood pressure. However, in our studies the SHR's medullary PGE_2 content, renal venous concentrations of PGE_2 and $PGF_{2\alpha}$ and urinary excretion of PGE_2 and $PGF_{2\alpha}$ did not differ from those of normotensive WKy.[53, 54] In other investigations, urinary PGE_2 excretion was either increased or decreased.[55, 56]

The in vitro experiments may have indicated a greater synthetic capacity for prostaglandins in kidney medulla of SHR incubated with AA while AA availability in vitro may have been rate-limiting. Experiments in isolated perfused kidneys indirectly confirmed the data obtained in microsomal preparations of the kidney. Isolated, ex vivo perfused kidneys of young SHR released more TxA_2 than WKy kidneys after stimulation with either ANGII or AA and showed a rise in perfusion pressure. The renal venous perfusate of old SHR contained more vasodilatory prostaglandins of the E-series and 6-keto-$PGF_{1\alpha}$ rather than TxA_2.[57, 58] In congruence with these in vitro results, urinary excretion of TxB_2 was increased in young, 6-weeks-old, volume- and salt-loaded SHR while $6KPGF_{1\alpha}$ and PGE_2 urinary excretion were elevated in older, 18-weeks-old SHR in comparison to age-matched WKy rats.[59]

The increased renal TxA_2 synthesis in young SHR, in the developmental phase of hypertension, provokes the following hypothesis. Because TxA_2 is a potent, though admittedly very short-lived, vasoconstrictor and because young SHR have greater renal vascular resistance with a decreased renal plasma flow and glomerular filtration rate, TxA_2 may directly contribute to the pathogenesis of the hypertension. In an effort to locate the renal structure producing more TxA_2 in the SHR, we found that isolated SHR glomeruli, even after prolonged blood pressure reduction, produce significantly more TxA_2, as well as other prostaglandins, than age-matched WKy rats.[60] In addition, SHR thrombocytes synthesize large amounts of TxA_2 during aggregation in vitro. As the thrombocyte survival time is shortened in the SHR, TxA_2 release from activated thrombocytes in vivo has been postulated to aggravate the hypertension.[61]

The physiological relevance of these biochemical observations has been partially tested. In saline-expanded anesthetized SHR, acute selective inhibition of the action of TxA_2 with pinane thromboxane, a TxA_2 receptor antagonist and partial TxA_2 synthetase inhibitor, caused an increase in renal plasma flow and the glomerular filtration rate in the young, but not in older SHR and in young WKy.[62, 63]

In our laboratory, we have used a selective thromboxane synthetase inhibitor, UK38485, animidazole derivative. Infusion of UK38485 acutely increased the renal plasma flow and the glomerular filtration rate in young, anesthetized, euvolemic SHR, this effect could not be demonstrated but after chronic therapy.[64] The increase of blood pressure was not attenuated with prolonged inhibition of TxA_2 synthesis. This latter finding is in contrast to another report that demonstrated a decrease in arterial pressure in SHR by chronic treatment with another TxA_2 synthetase inhibitor.[65] We believe that renal and platelet TxA_2 exert minor and transient effects on renal function and no direct effects on blood pressure in the SHR. The increase in arterial pressure in the young SHR, although temporally linked to increased renal TxA_2 synthesis, cannot be prevented by TxA_2 inhibition.

Other recent investigations have focused on the excretion of vasodilatory prostaglandins in the SHR. Falardeau and Martineau have reported recently that SHR did not increase the excretion of the PGI_2 metabolite, 2,3 dinor 6-keto-$PGF_{1\alpha}$, after salt loading, but this metabolite increased in WKy.[66] Thus, SHR seem to lack appropriate responses of the vascular and renal prostaglandins to down regulate vasoconstrictive stimuli. This finding agrees with data obtained in the Dahl salt-sensitive hypertensive rat, but is contrary not only to the increased prostaglandin synthesis in renal microsomes but also to the repeatedly documented increased synthesis of PGI_2 in SHR vascular rings. In vitro, the arterial wall of SHR increases the synthesis of PGI_2 in parallel with the rise in arterial pressure due to increased phospholipase and cyclo-oxygenase activity.[67–71] If one postulates an inhibitor of prostaglandin synthesis in SHR that causes an adaptive increase in the activity of prostaglandin-synthesizing enzymes, the in vivo and in vitro results may be reconciled.

In vivo and in vitro findings on prostaglandin synthesis correlate more closely in the Dahl salt-sensitive rat. Female Dahl salt-sensitive rats excreted less PGE_2 than Dahl salt-resistant rats at a stage when arterial pressure did not differ between the two strains, as well as at stages when arterial pressure was elevated in the Dahl salt-sensitive rat.[72] The PGE_2 content of papillary slices was decreased in Dahl salt-sensitive rats.[73] Investigations of the prostaglandin metabolism in medullary microsomes in salt-sensitive and salt-resistant rats and normotensive Sprague-Dawley rats revealed a reduced PGE_2, $PGF_{2\alpha}$ and PGD synthesis in salt-sensitive rats under low NaCl intake. Synthesis of these prostaglandins did not increase to the same degree as prostaglandin synthesis in the other two control groups on a high NaCl diet.[74] It appears that the net synthetic rate of medullary prostaglandins is significantly reduced in Dahl salt-sensitive rats.

A recent report also revealed a decreased in vivo capacity in the Dahl salt-sensitive rat's systemic vasculature to synthesize vasodilatory prostaglandins in response to a high salt intake; Dahl salt-resistant rats significantly elevated the 2,3 dinor $6KPGF_1$-metabolite of prostacyclin-excretion during a salt diet, while Dahl salt-sensitive rats did not show this response.[56] In summary, one may assume that the SHR and Dahl salt-sensitive rats lack the ability to synthesize appropriate amounts of vasodilatory and natriuretic prostaglandins in response to hypertensive stimuli and the young SHR produce significant amounts of vasoconstrictor TxA_2.

In the Lyon strain of hypertensive rats, urinary excretion of PGE_2 and $PGF_{2\alpha}$ only decreased significantly as compared to the normotensive control rats after hypertension had developed. This makes it unlikely that renal prostaglandins are important factors in the development of high arterial pressure in Lyon hypertensive rats.[75]

In the New Zealand hypertensive rat, a reduced renal prostaglandin 15-hydroxy-dehydrogenase (PGDH) activity was described that was associated with increased vascular reactivity to noradrenaline.[76] The authors, Wong et al., hypothesized that reduced activity of the degrading enzyme for renal PGE_2 may aggravate the hypertension because they considered PGE_2 to be vasoconstrictor in the rat. In a recent investigation, the PGDH differences could only be demonstrated in male rats; female hypertensive and normotensive rats of the New Zealand strain had a similar renal PGDH. Only female rats differed with regard to PGE_2 excretion in the urine.[77] In addition, PGE_2

vasodilated the renal vascular bed of the New Zealand hypertensive rat in another study.[78] The pathogenesis of the hypertension in the New Zealand hypertensive rat may thus be independent of changes in prostaglandin synthesis.

Prostaglandins and Human Hypertension

In vitro assessment of human prostaglandin production is not feasible. Since urinary PGE_2 and $PGF_{2\alpha}$ originate in the kidney, the analysis of urinary prostaglandins may serve to elucidate the role of renal prostaglandins in essential hypertension. A reduced excretion of PGE_2, measured by bio- and radioimmunoassay, has been reported in essential hypertensives. Furosemide did not adequately stimulate the urinary PGE_2 excretion in patients with essential hypertension.[52, 79–83] The ratio of urinary PGE_2 to $PGF_{2\alpha}$ was decreased in hypertensive groups, which agrees with the finding of a diminished $PGE_2/PGF_{2\alpha}$ ratio in renal venous blood of essential hypertensives.[81, 83] Patients with low renin hypertension tended to have especially low urinary PGE_2 excretion rates.[80] However, recently published investigations, in which urine prostaglandin excretion was measured in defined states of sodium chloride intake, could not detect differences in PGE_2 urine values among patients with high, normal, or low renin hypertension and no differences between normotensives and hypertensives with regard to PGE_2 and $PGF_{2\alpha}$ excretion.[84, 85] Campbell et al. studied PGE_2, $PGF_{2\alpha}$, $6KPGF_{1\alpha}$, and TxB_2 excretion under high, normal, and low Na intake in black and white female patients with high, normal, and low renin hypertension and could detect no significant alterations in prostanoid excretion patterns.[86] The contradictory results do not allow any definite conclusion about the role of renal prostaglandins in essential hypertension. Nevertheless, it seems that some essential hypertensives display a significantly reduced synthesis of renal prostaglandins (PGE_2).[84] In this group of patients, a repressed renal PGE_2 synthesis may aggravate the arterial hypertension. There are few studies on renal prostanoid synthesis in human renovascular hypertension. Renal venous PGE_2 ratios tend to correlate with the renal venous renin activity ratios.[87] The increased synthesis of prostaglandins in the stenosed kidney is probably due to increased ANGII levels and may be part of a delicate balance between vasoconstrictive and vasodilatory influences in the clipped kidney to maintain its excretory function.

CYCLO-OXYGENASE INHIBITORS

Inhibition of the synthesis of PGE_2 and PGI_2 in the kidney and blood vessels should enhance the vasoconstrictive response to vasopressors. It has been demonstrated that normotensive subjects show an enhanced pressor response to ANGII during indomethacin therapy.[88, 89] Cyclo-oxygenase inhibition with NSAID increased arterial pressure in most hypertensive animal models (Table 3). As can be seen, NSAID caused a decrease in blood pressure in some experiments. The renin angiotensin system and prostaglandins are interdependent and NSAID, like indomethacin, can effectively lower plasma renin activity (PRA). In renovascular hypertension with a pronounced stimulation of the renin angiotensin system, the depression of the renin angiotensin system by indomethacin may outweigh the concomitant reduction in vasodilatory prostaglandins. The si-

TABLE 3:—RENAL PROSTAGLANDINS AND HUMAN ESSENTIAL HYPERTENSION

AUTHOR	NUMBER OF CASES (Male; Female)	OBSERVATION
Papanicolaou et al.[145]	15 M; 6 F	Urine PGE inversely proportional to BP
Abe et al.[52]	15 M; 4 F	↓ Urine PGE and ↓ furosemide - stimulated urine PGE
Abe et al.[135]	26 M and F	↓ Urine PGE; normal $PGF_{2\alpha}$
Tan et al.[82]	22 M; 28 F	↓ Urine PGE_2, especially low renin hypertension
Tan et al.[146]	32 M; 53 F	↓ Urine PGE_2, ↓ furosemide-stimulated
Weber et al.[83]	14 M; 21 F	↓ Urine PGE_2, ↓ furosemide-stimulated
Scherer et al.[81]		urine PGE_2, normal $PGF_{2\alpha}$
Grose et al.[147]	6 M; 7 F	↓ Urine 6-keto-$PGF_{1\alpha}$
Campbell et al.[86]	16 F	Normal PGE_2, $PGF_{2\alpha}$, TxB_2 on 120 μequ Na
Lebel et al.[84]	33 M; 25 F	PGE_2 $PGF_{2\alpha}$ no significant Δ
Ruilope et al.[148]	16 M; 10 F	↑ PGE_2 NRH; ↓ PGE_2 LRH
Sato et al.[85]	48 M; 18 F	No Δ in basal and stimulated PGE_2 between HRH, NRH, LRH
Rathaus et al.[80]	28 M; 7 F	↓ PGE_2 in LRH ↑ $PGF_{2\alpha}$ in NRH

M: Male
F: Female
LRH: Low renin hypertension
NRH: Normal renin hypertension
HRH: High renin hypertension
Δ: Change

TABLE 4:—The Effects of Indomethacin on Blood Pressure

AUTHORS	SPECIES AND MODEL	DOSE AND DURATION OF INDOMETHACIN	OBSERVATIONS
Terragno et al.[24]	dog, normal	10 mg/kg i.v.	No Δ BP
Zambraski, Dunn[28]	dog, normal	2 mg/kg i.v.	No Δ BP
Larsson, Anggard[149]	rabbit, normal	15 mg/kg i.v.	↑ BP
Collina-Chourio et al.[27]	rabbit, normal	15 mg/kg, 14 d	↑ BP
Romero, Strong[150]	rabbit, normal	3 mg/kg, 10 d	No Δ BP
Murihead et al.[151]	rabbit, normal	10 mg/kg, i.m., 10 d	No Δ BP
Romero, Strong[150]	rabbit, 1C1KH and 1C2KH	3 mg/kg 10 d	↑ BP
Scholkens and Steinbach[152]	rat, 2C2KH	2.5 mg/kg. 10 d	↑ BP
Cangiano et al.[153]	rat, 1C2KH	5 mg/kg, 14 d	↑ BP
McQueen, Bell[154]	rat, 2C2KH	meclofenamate, 5 mg/kg, 30 d	No Δ or ↓ BP
Levy[31]	rat, SHR	5 inhibitors i.v.	↑ BP
Chrysant et al.[155]	rat, SHR and NaC1	meclofenamate 10 mg/kg, 3 mo	↑ BP
Quirion et al.[156]	rat, SHR	50 mg/kg, i.v.	No Δ BP
Pugsley et al.[157]	rat, DOCA-salt	2 mg/kg for 30 d	↑ BP
Paulson, Eversole[158]	rat, adrenal regeneration	0.2 and 2 mg/kg, 3, 5, and 7 w	variable ↑ BP
Schölkens et al.[159]	rat, cerebroventricular injection of renin	5 mg/kg, 10 d	↑ BP
Donker et al.[160]	man, normal	2–3 mg/kg, 3 d	No Δ BP
Nowak & Wennmalm[90]	man, normal	0.3 mg/kg, i.v.	↑ BP
Patak et al.[91]	man, normal & EH	200 mg/d, 4 d	↑ BP (slight)
Ylitalo et al.[92]	man, EH	75 mg/d, 1 w	↑ BP (slight)
Lopez-Overjero et al.[143]	man, EH	200 mg/d, 7 d	No Δ BP

All intravenous (i.v.) administration of indomethacin was acute.
SHR = spontaneously hypertensive rat
1C2KH = 1 clip, 2 kidney hypertension
2C2KH = 2 clip, 2 kidney hypertension
EH = Essential hypertension

multaneous blockade of vasodilatory and natriuretic prostaglandins and vasoconstrictive TxA_2 during NSAID therapy may result in no discernible change of arterial blood pressure. In this regard, a report showing no influence of indomethacin on arterial pressure rise in young SHR, which have a high glomerular TxA_2 synthesis, is interesting (Table 4).

The effects of NSAID therapy on arterial pressure in normotensive and hypertensive man are not dramatic. In normotensive subjects, a mean blood pressure increase of 10 mm Hg occurred after acute intravenous infusion of indomethacin.[90] Indomethacin (200 mg/d for 4 days) caused a slight increase of blood pressure in normotensive and hypertensive subjects.[91] Therapy with indomethacin, 75 mg/kg, for a week, likewise elevated arterial pressure in another group of essential hypertensives,[92] but other investigators could not demonstrate an effect on arterial pressure in hypertensives during NSAID therapy.[39]

DIETARY CHANGES OF POLYUNSATURATED FATTY ACIDS

Recent experimental and human studies demonstrate that diets containing different amounts of polyunsaturated fatty acids, such as linoleic acid, linolenic acid, and eicosapentaenoic acid, change cardiovascular, renal, and hemostatic functions. As already stated, linoleic acid is converted to AA and hence to dienoic prostaglandins; linolenic acid is metabolized to eicosapentaenoic acid, which in turn is converted to trienoic prostaglandins. Diet-induced changes in prostaglandin synthesis may assume an important role in future antihypertensive therapy regimens.

ESSENTIAL FATTY ACID DEFICIENCY

Animal Studies

The animal with essential fatty acid deficiency can be regarded as similar to the animal treated with NSAID without incurring the problems of non-specific, prostaglandin-independent effects of NSAID. Studies in essential fatty acid-deficient rats clearly demonstrate the importance of prostaglandins in water, electrolyte excretion, and arterial pressure regulation. Hoffmann et al. demonstrated that the isolated perfused kid-

TABLE 5:—THE EFFECTS OF POLYUNSATURATED FATTY ACIDS ON BLOOD PRESSURE

AUTHOR	SPECIES AND MODEL	FATTY ACID	OBSERVATIONS
Laborit et al.[161]	Rat DOCA-salt	AA	↑ BP
Bayorh et al.[105]	Rat SHR	AA	↓ BP
Hoffmann et al.[93]	Rat Wistar high salt	Sunflower Seed Oil	↓ BP
Ten Hoor et al.[99]	Rat Wistar high salt	Linoleic Acid	↓ BP
Feinberg et al.[162]	Rat SHR	Linolenic Acid	No Δ BP
Schoene et al.[103]	Rat SHR	Corn Oil	↓ BP Urine PGE$_2$ increased
MacDonald et al.[96]	Rat Wistar	Linoleic Acid	↓ BP
Smith-Barbaro et al.[98]	Rat Sprague Dawley high salt	Corn Oil	↓ BP
Box et al.[101]	Rat SHR	Corn Oil	↑ BP
Hoffmann et al.[102]	Rat SHR	Linoleic Acid	↓ BP
		Linoleic Acid	during pregnancy
Comberg et al.[109]	Man EH	Sunflower Oil	↓ BP
Vergroesen et al.[113]	Man EH		↓ BP
Fleischman et al.[163]	Man EH	Linoleic Acid	↓ BP
Oster et al.[110]	Man Normal	Linoleic Acid	↓ BP
Stern et al.[117]	Man (Adolescents) EH	Linoleic Acid	↓ BP
Vergroesen et al.[114]	Man	Linoleic Acid	↓ BP
Brussard et al.[108]	Man Normal	Linoleic Acid	↓ BP
Rao et al.[164]	Man EH		↓ BP
Ianoco et al.[107]	Man Normal EH	P/S 0.95	↓ BP
Roux et al.[112]	Man Normal	P/S 0.8	↓ BP
Puska et al.[111]	Man EH	P/S 1.0	↓ BP
Sanders et al.[87]	Man Normal	Cod Liver Oil	↓ BP
Mortensen et al.[115]	Man Normal	Eicosapentaeonoioc acid	↓ BP
Lorenz et al.[118]	Man Normal	Cod Liver Oil	↓ BP
Singer et al.[116]	Man	Mackerel	↓ BP

SHR: Spontaneously hypertensive rat
EH: Essential hypertension
Changes in systolic arterial pressure are 5–20 mm/Hg
ΔBP: Change in blood pressure
P/S: Ratio of polyunsaturated to saturated fatty acids. (Polyunsaturated fatty acid mostly linoleic acid)
DOCA: Deoxycorticosterone acetate

neys of salt-loaded rats on a four-week essential fatty acid-deficient diet released significantly smaller amounts of PGE$_2$ than control rats.[93] Cox et al. found urinary PGE$_2$ excretion in fatty acid-deficient rats to be about five times lower than in control rats. The arachidonic acid content of deficient rats' kidneys decreased.[94] Prostacyclin synthesis in aortic vascular rings was significantly lower in fatty acid deficient rats than in rats with a higher linoleic acid intake; conversely, TxB$_2$, released during platelet aggregation in whole blood, and plasma thromboxane B$_2$ concentrations rose in essential fatty acid-deficient rats over the values in control rats.[95]

Normotensive or spontaneously hypertensive rats fed an essential fatty acid-deficient diet showed increased systolic blood pressure in contrast to rats with an essential fatty acid supplemented diet.[93–100] Blood pressure decreased after returning linoleic acid to the diet. While an essential fatty acid-deficient diet did not alter renal blood flow and glomerular filtration rate, the ability to excrete an acute salt or water load was decreased.[95]

These studies suggest that essential fatty acid deficiency decreases the renal medullary PGE_2 synthesis, with a concomitant increase in sodium chloride and water reabsorption. Arterial pressure may ultimately increase to compensate for the disturbed renal medullary function in order to enhance the excretion of water and sodium chloride. Because urinary sodium and potassium excretion were reported to be the same in essential fatty acid-deficient and essential fatty acid-supplemented rats, the increase in arterial pressure found in another study was thought to be due solely to an imbalance of the vasodilator prostacyclin to the vasoconstrictor thromboxane B_2 in the vascular system, not a renal medullary excretory defect.[95] We favor the former explanation.

Supplementation of Polyunsaturated Fatty Acids

Experimental Hypertension

In the Dahl salt-sensitive and salt-resistant rats, Tobian et al., showed that treatment with 15% linoleic acid in the diet significantly increased the renal papillary PGE_2 content in both strains, compared to control groups that had only 1.5% linoleic acid in their diet. Nevertheless, the PGE_2 medullary content was still significantly lower in the linoleic acid-supplemented salt-sensitive strain than in the salt-resistant strain. The expected increments of blood pressure were prevented in the linoleic acid-treated, salt-sensitive rat until the 12th week of a high 5% sodium chloride diet, and subsequent blood pressure increases were markedly attenuated.[73] It seems likely that a higher renal medullary PGE_2 synthesis improved the sodium chloride and water renal excretory capacity in the linoleic acid groups, preventing the retention of sodium chloride and water that would elevate arterial pressure. Contradictory results have been obtained in SHR treated with high fat diets. Box et al. found that young SHR fed a diet with a low linoleic acid content had lower arterial pressures than SHR with a higher linoleic acid content in their diet.[101] The authors concluded that all increased synthesis of "vasoconstrictor prostaglandins" aggravated the hypertension in SHR with a high diet content of linoleic acid. Hoffmann et al. observed that a diet rich in linoleic acid or α linolenic acid, the precursor of eicosapentaenoic acid, attenuated the pressure rise in SHR. The blood pressure decrease could be shown only when the mothers already received the diets during pregnancy.[102] Other studies demonstrated reduced blood pressure in SHR with linoleic acid and with high fat diets.[103, 104] Chronic subcutaneous administration of arachidonic acid dose-dependently attenuated the arterial pressure rise in SHR; simultaneous indomethacin treatment prevented a blood pressure decrease. Arachidonic acid-treated SHR rats gained less body weight and prostaglandin synthesis was not assessed in any organ, so the relative effects of weight loss and vasodilatory prostaglandins on the reduction in blood pressure cannot be evaluated.[105]

Human Hypertension

Intravenous infusion of linoleic acid into human volunteers increased the urinary excretion of 6-keto-PGF$_{1\alpha}$ and, to a lesser degree, PGE$_2$.[106] Several investigators have explored the hypothesis that an increased intake of linoleic acid, and thereby a higher synthesis of prostaglandins, can induce a reduction in arterial pressure and greater urinary sodium chloride excretion in human beings.[109] In most of these studies, though, no data on prostaglandin synthesis in the vascular system or the kidney are reported that indicate a causal relationship between the described hemodynamic and renal effects and the prostaglandins. When normotensive subjects consumed a diet enriched with linoleic acid, arterial pressure (the systolic more than the diastolic) fell significantly. Blood pressure can also be reduced in hypertensive subjects by a diet high in linoleic acid.[70, 108–114] An increased excretion of sodium and potassium in the urine was documented in two of these studies.[110] It is worth noting that the decreases in systolic arterial pressure achieved by diets supplemented with polyunsaturated fatty acid vary between 5 and 20 mm Hg.

Because Greenland Eskimos, who have a low incidence of heart disease and an increased bleeding time, consume large amounts of polyunsaturated fatty acids, which are the precursor of arienoic prostaglandins, several trials have been performed on the hemostatic and hemodynamic effects of diets high in α-linolenic acid or eicosapentaenoic acid. Open and double blind cross-over studies documented a reduction in systolic and, to a lesser extent, diastolic pressure during a diet high in eicosapentaenoic acid.[87, 115–117] The effect of this diet on prostanoids was assessed by Lorenz et al. in an investigation in which a polyunsaturated fatty acid diet with eicosapentaenoic acid led to a reduction in upright arterial pressure and a decreased pressure response to ANGII or norepinephrine administered intravenously.[118] After about three weeks of this diet— 10 ml of cod liver oil added to an otherwise unaltered diet in men 22 to 42 years of age—the eicosapentaenoic acid content of platelet phospholipids increased and the linoleic and arachidonic acid contents decreased. Platelet aggregability and the release of TxB_2 were inhibited, especially at low concentrations of ADP and collagen. Plasma immunoreactive TxB_2 was lowered. Urinary PGE_2 and $PGF_{2\alpha}$ excretions were reduced, probably because of lower renal linoleic and arachidonic acid stores in the men. Lorenz et al. found that urinary sodium excretion increased, perhaps because of greater synthesis of natriuretic trienoic prostaglandins (which were not measured).[28] Only scanty information exists about the kidney's ability to convert eicosapentaenoic acid into prostaglandins of the 3-series. In rats fed a high α-linolenic acid diet, renal eicosapentaenoic acid content increased, but higher PGE_3 excretion could not be documented.[119] In contrast, another report affirmed that the kidney can synthesize trienoic prostanoids.[120] Because the umbilical artery can effectively synthesize prostanoids of the three series when exposed to eicosapentaenoic acid, vascular effects of PGI_3 and PGD_3 may have been important for the renal and systemic hemodynamic effects described in the study. On the other hand, the diet may have changed membrane fluidity and receptor affinity for vasoactive agents, thereby causing the hemodynamic alterations.

Prostaglandins as Antihypertensive Agents

Prostaglandins A_2, E_1, E_2, I_2, and synthetic analogues of PGI_2 lower arterial pressure after systemic administration in the SHR.[121–125] As is true for other blood pressure-lowering agents, the extent of arterial pressure reduction seems to correlate positively with the height of the pressure, although Dusting states that PGI_2 prostacyclin has a stronger antihypertensive effect in SHR.[122] Normotensive animals may not show any reduction of arterial pressure or a lesser decrement. Administration of PGE_2, prostacyclin, or its analogues to normotensive conscious animals can significantly stimulate the renin-angiotensin-aldosterone system.[123] In conscious rats, an analogue of prostacyclin lowered blood pressure only after the ANGII-antagonist saralasin was administered simultaneously.[124]

Anesthetized one-kidney, one-clip, hypertensive rats demonstrated a fall in arterial pressure after being injected with prostacyclin.[122] When conscious rats received a continuous infusion of prostacyclin at a dose of 100 ng/kg/min from the time of nephrectomy and clipping of the contralateral renal artery, the rise in arterial pressure occurring in the PGI_2-treated group was totally prevented for the six days of the study. After four weeks of established one-kidney, one-clip hypertension, prostacyclin infusion into conscious rats only temporarily lowered arterial pressure slightly. Cessation of prostacyclin infusion, though, caused the arterial pressure to rise above control levels for five days.[72] The animal studies establish that certain prostaglandins have significant antihypertensive effects, although part of their capacity to lower blood pressure is attenuated in the conscious animal by activating the vasoconstrictive systems.

Lee and his coworkers were the first to report that intravenous PGA_1 dose-dependently decreased arterial pressure in patients with essential hypertension.[126, 127] Prostacyclin decreased arterial pressure in normotensive subjects.[128, 129] These vasodilatory prostanoids and their analogues have the disadvantage that they must be given intravenously and tend to produce headache and gastrointestinal side effects, in addition to stimulating the vasoconstrictive systems. Orally active PGI_2 analogues, which already have been shown to reduce arterial pressure chronically in dogs with renal hypertension, may make antihypertensive therapy with prostaglandins clinically feasible.[130]

The Interaction of Prostaglandins with Antihypertensive Agents

In the last few years, several investigations have tried to establish a causal relationship between the vasodilatory action of antihypertensive drugs and their effects on prostaglandins. A minimum requirement for the argument that prostaglandins are significantly involved in the action of antihypertensive drugs would be to document the stimulation of prostaglandin production, preferably in vivo, by a specific antihypertensive agent.

DRUGS THAT INHIBIT ANGIOTENSIN CONVERTING ENZYME (ACE).—The relationship between ACE inhibitors and prostaglandin synthesis is complex.[131] ACE inhibition blocks ANGII generation, and ANGII stimulates prostaglandin synthesis. Thus, ACE inhibition may actually decrease prostaglandin production.[131] On the other hand, ACE inhibition is accompanied by reduced kinase activity, and therefore can increase the kinins in plasma and urine, which may increase prostaglandin synthesis.

We believe that the effect of ACE inhibition in states of high renin activity and high ANGII concentration are not mediated by prostaglandins. Plasma PGE_2 concentrations actually fell in captopril-treated patients with high renin activity.[131] ACE inhibitors also lower arterial pressure in forms of hypertension that are not characterized by elevated activity of the renin angiotensin system, so it has been postulated that ACE inhibition significantly stimulates vasodepressor systems like the kinins and prostaglandins and by that measure lowers arterial pressure. In patients with essential hypertension, ACE inhibition was followed by an increase in urinary kinins and a rise in plasma PGE, which correlated with the fall in blood pressure.[132] Increased plasma levels of the PGE_2 metabolite, 13,14 dihydro-15 keto PGE_2 were also measured in normo- and hypertensive subjects during captopril therapy.[133, 134] Captopril may also directly stimulate prostaglandin formation; it increases the release of PGI_2 from aortic rings, whole glomeruli and cultured endothelial cells.[131] Cyclo-oxygenase inhibitors, such as indomethacin and, to a lesser extent, sulindac, have been reported to decrease the antihypertensive effect of captopril in essential hypertension.[135–137] However, elevated urinary PGE_2 could not be demonstrated after administration of the ACE inhibitor. In summary, the hypothesis that ACE inhibition reduces blood pressure partly by augmenting prostaglandin synthesis seems unsubstantiated for forms of arterial hypertension that clearly depend on ANGII, and is not proved to be important in the long-term effect of ACE inhibition in other forms of high blood pressure.

DIURETICS β BLOCKERS.—Loop diuretics, such as furosemide and ethacrynic acid administered intravenously, induce an increase in urinary PGE_2 simultaneously with a rise in sodium and potassium excretion. Furosemide increases free arachidonic acid in human beings and inhibits PG degradative enzymes.[39, 138] These observations suggest an interaction between prostaglandins and the renal action of some diuretics, and thereby a role for prostaglandins in the antihypertensive action of diuretics. Prostaglandin synthetase inhibitors, such as aspirin and indomethacin, antagonize the diuretic and blood pressure-lowering effect of such diuretics as furosemide, hydrochlorothiazide, and chlorthalidone.[1, 139] The antihypertensive effect of β blockers, such as pindolol, propranolol, and atenolol, can be attenuated by NSAID.[140, 141] Therefore, it was stated that β blocker partly exert their blood pressure-lowering activity by stimulating vasodilatory prostaglandins.[142] Propranolol has been reported to increase the excretion of urinary prostaglandins during antihypertensive treatment and to stimulate PGI_2 synthesis in aortic strips. Others could not confirm elevated PGE_2 and $PGF_{2\alpha}$ excretion in the urine of hypertensive patients treated with propranolol or atenolol.[39, 143] The evidence that β blockers increase prostaglandins synthesis in human beings is thus not conclusive.

Although there is no proof that diuretics or β blockers act via an elevation of systemic or renal prostaglandins synthesis, it is evident that an inhibition of prostaglandin synthesis by NSAID antagonizes the antihypertensive action of these drugs.[39, 144] Doses of 100–150 mg indomethacin/day will lessen the antihypertensive action of these drugs by about 10 mm Hg. The adverse effect of NSAID on the antihypertensive potency of diuretics may be overcome in most cases by increasing the dose of the diuretic. Nevertheless, cyclo-oxygenase inhibitors are to be avoided in hypertensives.

Acknowledgments

We are indebted to Linda Goldberg and Cheryl Inman for secretarial assistance.

The work was partially supported by the National Institutes of Health (HL 22563).

REFERENCES

1. Dunn M. J.: Renal Prostaglandins, in Dunn, M.J. (ed.): Renal Endocrinology, Baltimore, Williams & Wilkins Co., 1983, pp. 1–74.

2. Romero J.C., Beierwaltes W.H.: Renal prostaglandins in hypertension. *Mineral Electrolyte Metab.* 6:90, 1981.

3. Spokas E.G., Quilley J., McGiff J.G.: Prostaglandins in hypertension. Genest J., Kuchel D., Hamet P., Cantin M. (eds.): *Hypertension* (2nd ed.). (New York: McGraw Hill Co., pp. 373–393, 1983.)

4. Needleman P., Raz A., Minkes M.S., et al.: Triene prostaglandins: Prostacyclin and thromboxane biosynthesis and unique biological properties. *Proc. Natl. Acad. Sci. USA* 76:944, 1979.

5. Kloeze J.: Relationship between chemical structure and platelet aggregation activity of prostaglandins. *Biochim. Biophys. Acta* 187:285, 1969.

6. Israkson P.G., Raz A., Denny S.E.: Hormonal stimulation of arachidonate release from isolated perfused organs. Relationship to prostaglandin biosynthesis. *Prostaglandins* 14:853, 1977.

7. Raz A., Schwartzman M.: Distinct acylhydrolase and PG synthetase systems in the perfused rabbit kidney. Selective activation by vasoactive peptide hormones and by adenine nucleotides. Dunn M.J., Patrono C., Cinotti G.A. (eds.): *In Prostaglandins and the Kidney.* (New York: Plenum Medical Book Company, pp. 67–73, 1982.)

8. Flower R.J., Blackwell G.J.: Anti-inflammatory steroids induce biosynthesis of phospholipase A_2 inhibitor which prevents prostaglandin generation. *Nature* 278:450, 1979.

9. Hirata F., Schiffman E., Venkatasubramanian K., et al.: A phospholipase A_2 inhibitory protein in rabbit neutrophils induced by glucocorticoids. *Proc. Natl. Acad. Sci. USA* 77:2533, 1980.

10. Hassid A.H.: Regulation of prostaglandin biosynthesis in cultured cells. *Am. J. Physiol.* 243:C205, 1982.

11. Bohman S.O., Larsson G.: Prostaglandin synthesis in membrane fractions from the rabbit renal medulla. *Acta Physiol. Scand.* 94:244, 1975.

12. Pace-Asciak C.R., Rangaraj G.: Prostaglandin biosynthesis and catabolism in the lamb ductus arteriosus, aorta and pulmonary artery. *Biochim. Biophys. Acta* 529:13, 1978.

13. Froelich J.C., Wilson T.W., Sweetman B.J., et al.: Urinary prostaglandins: Identification and origin. *J. Clin. Invest.* 55:763, 1975.

14. Pugliese F., Ciabattoni G.: Investigations of renal arachidonic acid metabolites by radioimmunoassay. Dunn M.J., Patrono C., Cinotti G.A. (eds.): In *Prostaglandins and the Kidney.* (New York: Plenum Medical Book Company, pp. 83–98, 1982.)

15. Patrono C., Wennmalm A., Ciabattoni G., et al.: Evidence for an extrarenal origin of urinary prostaglandin E_2 in healthy men. *Prostaglandins* 78:623, 1979.

16. Feigen L.P., Chapnick B.M., Flemming J.E., et al.: Renal vascular effects of endoperoxide analogs, prostaglandins and arachidonic acid. *Am. J. Physiol.* 233:H573, 1977.

17. Gerber J.G., Data J.L., Nies A.S.: Enhanced renal prostaglandin production in the dog. The effect of sodium arachidonate in nonfiltering kidney. *Circ. Res.* 42:43, 1978.

18. Fuelgraff G., Bradenbusch G.: Comparison of the effects of the prostaglandins A_1, E_1, $F_{2\alpha}$ on kidney function in dogs. *Pflugers Arch.* 349:9, 1974.

19. Sustarsic D.L., McPartland R.P., Rapp J.P.: Developmental patterns of blood pressure and urinary protein, kallikrein, and prostaglandin E_2 in Dahl salt-hypertension-susceptible rats. *J. Lab. Clin. Med.* 98:599, 1981.
20. Schor N., Ichikawa I., Brnner B.M.: Mechanisms of action of various hormones and vasoactive substances on glomcrular ultrafiltration in the rat. *Kidney Int.* 20:442, 1981.
21. Haylor J.: Vasodilation, the major vascular response to PGE_2 in the rat kidney. *Br. J. Pharmacol.* 75:9P, 1982.
22. Dunn M.J., Zambraski E.J.: Renal effects of drugs that inhibit prostaglandin synthesis. *Kidney Int.* 18:609, 1980.
23. Chrysant S.G.: Renal functional changes induced by prostaglandin E_1 and indomethacin in the anesthetized dog. *Arch. Int. Pharmacodyn. Ther.* 234:156, 1978.
24. Terragno N.A., Terragno D.A., McGiff J.C.: Contribution of prostaglandins to the renal circulation in conscious, anesthetized and laparotomized dogs. *Circ. Res.* 40:590, 1977.
25. Mimran A., Casellas D., DuPont M., et al.: Effect of a competitive angiotensin antagonist on the renal haemodynamic changes induced by inhibition of prostaglandin synthesis in rats. *Clin. Sci. Mol. Med.* 48:299s, 1975.
26. Beilin L.J., Bhattacharya J.: The effect of prostaglandin synthesis inhibitors on renal blood flow distribution in conscious rabbits. *J. Physiol (London)* 269:395, 1977.
27. Collina-Chourio J., McGiff J.C., Nasjleti A.: Effect of indomethacin on blood pressure in the normotensive unanesthetized rabbit; possible relation to prostaglandin synthesis inhibition. *Clin. Sci.* 57:359, 1979.
28. Zambraski E.J., Dunn M.J.: Renal prostaglandin E_2 secretion and excretion in conscious dogs. *Am. J. Physiol.* 236:F552, 1979.
29. Muther R.S., Bennett W.M.: Effects of aspirin on glomerular filtration rate in normal humans. *Ann. Intern. Med.* 92:386, 1980.
30. Roman R.J., Lechene C.: Prostaglandin E_2 and $F_{2\alpha}$ reduces urea reabsorption from the rat collecting duct. *Am. J. Physiol.* 241:F53, 1981.
31. Levy J.V.: Changes in systolic arterial blood pressure in normal and spontaneously hypertensive rats produced by acute administration of inhibitors of prostaglandin biosynthesis. *Prostaglandins* 13:153, 1977.
32. Solez K., Fox J.A., Miller M., et al.: Effects of indomethacin on renal inner medullary plasma flow. *Prostaglandins* 7:91, 1974.
33. DesJardins-Giasson L., Gutkowska J., Garcia R., et al.: Effect of angiotensin II and norepinephrine on release of prostaglandins E_2 and I_2 by the perfused rat mesentery artery. *Prostaglandins* 24:105, 1982.
34. McGiff J.C., Crowshaw K., Terragno N.A., et al.: Release of prostaglandin-like substance into renal venous blood in response to angiotensin II. *Circ. Res.* 26–27:I121, 1970.
35. McGiff J.C., Crowshaw K., Terragno N.A., et al.: Differential effect of noradrenaline and renal nerve stimulation on vascular resistance in the dog kidney and the release of a prostaglandin E-like substance. *Clin. Sci.* 42:223, 1972.
36. Dunn M.J., Liard J.F., Dray F.: Basal and stimulated rates of renal secretion and excretion of prostaglandins E_2, $F_{2\alpha}$, and 13,14-dihydro-15-keto F_α in the dog. *Kidney Int.* 13:136, 1978.
37. Nadles J., Zipser R.D., Coleman R., et al.: Stimulation of renal prostaglandins by pressor hormones in man: Comparison of prostaglandin E_2 and prostacyclin (6 keto prostaglandin $F_{1\alpha}$). *J. Clin. Endocrinol. Metab.* 56:1260, 1983.
38. Beierwaltes W.H., Schryver S., Olson P.S., et al.: Interaction of the prostaglandin and renin-angiotensin systems in isolated rat glomeruli. *Am. J. Physiol.* 239:F602, 1980.
39. Stokes J.G.: Tubular actions of arachidonic acid motabolites. Effects on NaCl and water transport. Dunn M.J., Patrono C., Cinotti G.A. (eds.): In *Prostaglandins*

and the Kidney. (New York: Plenum Medical Book Company, pp. 133–149, 1982.)

40. Larsson C., Weber P., Anggard E.: Arachidonic acid increases and indomethacin decreases plasma renin activity in the rabbit. *Eur. J. Pharmacol.* 28:391, 1974.
41. Hassid A., Williams C.: Vasoconstrictor-evoked prostaglandin synthesis in cultured vascular smooth muscle. *Am. J. Physiol.* 245:C278, 1983.
42. Hedquist P.: Further evidence that prostaglandins inhibit the release of noradrenaline from adrenergic nerve terminal by restriction of availability of calcium. *Br. J. Pharmacol.* 58:599, 1976.
43. Malik K.U., McGiff J.C.: Modulation by prostaglandins of adrenergic transmission in the isolated perfused rabbit and rat kidney. *Circ. Res.* 36:599, 1975.
44. Gerkens J.F., Williams A., Branch R.A.: Effect of precursors of the 1,2, and 3 series prostaglandins on renin release and renal blood flow in the dog. *Prostaglandins* 22:513, 1981.
45. Patrono C., Wennmalm A., Ciabattoni G., et al.: Evidence for an extrarenal origin of urinary prostaglandin E_2 in healthy men. *Prostaglandins* 78:623, 1979.
46. Seymour A.A., Zehr J.E.: Influence of renal prostaglandin synthesis on renin control mechanisms in the dog. *Circ. Res.* 45:13, 1979.
47. Whorton A.R., Lazar J.D., Smigel M.D., et al.: Prostaglandins and renin release. III. Effects of PGE_1, E_2, $F_{2\alpha}$ and D_2 on renin release from rabbit renal cortical slices. *Prostaglandins* 22:455, 1981.
48. Data J.L., Gerber J.G., Crump W.J., et al.: The prostaglandin system. A role in canine baroreceptor control of renin release. *Circ. Res.* 42:454, 1978.
49. Henrich W.L., Anderson R.J., Berns A.S., et al.: The role of renal nerves and prostaglandins in control of renal hemodynamics and plasma renin activity during hypotensive hemorrhage in the dog. *J. Clin. Invest.* 61:744, 1978.
50. Zahajsky T., Fejes-Toth G.: Effect of alpha-receptor and adrenergic neuron blockade on indomethacin-induced changes of renal haemodynamics. *Acta Physiol. Acad. Sci. Hung.* 55:97, 1980.
51. Smith M.C., Dunn M.J.: Renal kallikrein, kinins, and prostaglandins in hypertension. Brenner B.M., Stein J.H. (eds.): In *Hypertension.* (New York: Churchill Livingstone, pp. 168–202, 1981.)
52. Abe K., Seino M., Uasujima M., et al.: Studies on renomedullary prostaglandin and renal kallikrein-kinin system in hypertension. *Jpn. Circ. J.* 41:873, 1977.
53. Dunn M.J.: Renal prostaglandin synthesis in the spontaneously hypertensive rat. *J. Clin. Invest.* 58:862, 1976.
54. Dunn M.J.: Renal prostaglandin production in the Japanese (Kyoto) spontaneously hypertensive rat. *Clin. Sci. Mol. Med.* 55:191s, 1978.
55. Herlitz H., Lundin L., Henning U., et al.: Hormonal pattern during development of hypertension in spontaneously hypertensive rat SHR. *Clin. Exp. Hypertens.* A4:915, 1982.
56. Martineau A., Robillard M., Falardeau P.: Defective synthesis of vasodilator prostaglandins in spontaneously hypertensive rats in vivo. *Hypertension* 1984 (in press).
57. Shibouta Y., Inada Y., Terashita Z., et al.: Angiotensin-II-stimulated release of thromboxane A_2 and prostacyclin (PGI_2) in isolated, perfused kidneys of spontaneously hypertensive rats. *Biochem. Pharmacol.* 28:3607, 1979.
58. Shibouta Y., Terashita Z.I., Inada Y., et al.: Enhanced thromboxane A_2 biosynthesis in the kidney of spontaneously hypertensive rats during development of hypertension. *Eur. J. Pharmacol.* 70:247, 1981.
59. Campbell W.B., Graham R.M., Jackson E.K.: Role of renal prostaglandins in sympathetically mediated renin release in the rat. *J. Clin. Invest.* 64:448, 1979.
60. Konieczkowski M., Dunn M.J., Stork J.E., et al.: Glomerular synthesis of prostaglandins and thromboxane in spontaneously hypertensive rats. *Hypertension* 5:446, 1983.
61. De Cerck F., Van Gorp L., Xhonneux B., et al.: Enhanced platelet turnover and

prostaglandin production in spontaneously hypertensive rats. *Thromb. Res.* 27:243, 1982.

62. Nicolaou K.C., Magolda R.L., Smith J.B., et al.: Synthesis and biological properties of pinane-thromboxane A_2, a selective inhibitor of coronary artery constriction, platelet aggregation and thromboxane formation. *Proc. Natl. Acad. Sci.* 76:2566, 1979.

63. Shibouta Y., Terashita Z.I., Inada Y., et al.: Renal effects of pinanethromboxane A_2 and indomethacin in saline volume-expanded spontaneously hypertensive rats. *Eur. J. Pharmacol.* 85:51, 1982.

64. Groene H.J., Dunn M.J.: The role of thromboxane (TxB_2) in the control of renal function and blood pressure (BP) in young spontaneously hypertensive rats (SHR). *Clin. Res.* 31:749A, 1983.

65. Underman H.D., Workman R.J., Jackson E.K.: Attenuation of the development of hypertension in spontaneously hypertensive rats by the thromboxane synthetase inhibitor 4'-(Imidazole-1-YL) acetophenone. *Prostaglandins* 24:237, 1982.

66. Falardeau P., Martineau A.: In vivo production of prostaglandin I_2 in Dahl salt-sensitive and salt-resistant rats. *Hypertension* 5:701, 1983.

67. Limas C., Goldman P., Limas C.: Age-dependency of vascular phospholipid deacylation-regulation in spontaneously hypertensive rats. *Biochim. Biophys. Acta* 713:446, 1982.

68. Ozawa Y., Kan K., Kouishi K., et al.: Renal and vascular wall prostaglandins in spontaneously hypertensive rats. *Clin. Sci.* 63:253s, 1982.

69. Pace-Asciak C.R., Carrara M.C.: Ontogeny of aortic PGI_2 formation in the developing spontaneously hypertensive rat - correlation with elevations in blood pressure. *Adv. Prostaglandin Thromboxane Res.* 7:797, 1980.

70. Quirion R., Rioux F., Regoli D.: Effects of arachidonic acid and indomethacin on the *in vitro* release of prostaglandins by aortic strips of spontaneously hypertensive rats. *Can. J. Physiol. Pharmacol.* 56:509, 1978.

71. Rioux F., Quiron R., Regoli D.: The role of prostaglandins in hypertension. I. The release of prostaglandins by aorta strips of renal, DOCA salt and spontaneously hypertensive rats. *Can. J. Physiol. Pharmacol.* 55:1330, 1977.

72. Sutter D.M., Weeks J.: An antihypertensive effect of prostacyclin. *Adv. Prostaglandin Thromboxane Res.* 8:789, 1980.

73. Tobian L.: Prostaglandin E_2 (PGE_2) in renal papilla in NaCl hypertension. Dunn M.J., Patrono C., Cinotti G.A. (eds.): In *Prostaglandins and the Kidney.* (New York: Plenum Medical Book Company, pp. 197–204, 1983.)

74. Limas C., Goldman P., Limas C.J., et al.: Effect of salt on prostaglandin metabolism in hypertension prone and resistant Dahl rats. *Hypertension.* 3:219, 1981.

75. Benzoni D., Vincent M., Sassard J.: Urinary prostaglandins in the Lyon strains of hypertensive, normotensive and low blood pressure rats. *Hypertension* 4:325, 1982.

76. Wong P.Y.-K., Baer P.G., McGiff J.C.: Evidence for an endogenous inhibition of 15-hydroxyprostaglandin dehydrogenase in New Zealand genetically hypertensive rat kidneys. *Jpn. Heart J.* 20(Suppl 1): 186, 1979.

77. Baer P.G., Cagen L.M.: Renal prostaglandin excretion and metabolism in male and female New Zealand normotensive and genetically hypertensive rats. *Hypertension* 3:257, 1981.

78. Haylor J.: PGE_2-induced renal vasodilation in the genetically hypertensive New Zealand rat. *Br. J. Pharmacol.* 80:441P, 1983.

79. Abe K., Yasujima M., Chiba S., et al.: Effect of furosemide on urinary excretion of prostaglandin E in normal volunteers and patients with essential hypertension. *Prostaglandins* 14:513, 1977.

80. Rathaus M., Korzets Z., Bernheim J.: The urinary excretion of prostaglandins E_2 and $F_{2\alpha}$ in essential hypertension. *Eur. J. Clin. Inv* 13:13, 1983.

81. Scherer E., Held E., Lange H-H., et al.: Erniedrigte renale Prostaglandin E_2-Aus-

scheidung und verminderte Stimulierbarkeit der Plasmaren inaktivität bei Patienten mit essentieller Hypertonie. *Klin. Wochenschr.* 57:567, 1979.

82. Tan S.Y., Sweet P., Mulrow P.J.: Impaired renal production of prostaglandin E_2: A newly identified lesion in human essential hypertension. *Prostaglandins* 15:139, 1978.

83. Weber P.C., Scherer B., Held E., et al.: Urinary prostaglandins and kallikrein in essential hypertension. *Clin. Sci.* 57:259s, 1979.

84. Lebel M., Grose J.H.: Renal prostaglandins in borderline and sustained essential hypertension. *Prostaglandins Leukotrienes and Medicine* 8:409, 1982.

85. Sato K., Abe K., Sato M., et al.: Prostaglandin E synthesis in the kidney in renin subgroups of essential hypertension. *Prostaglandins, Leukotrienes and Medicine* 9:577, 1982.

86. Campbell W.B., Holland O.B., Adams B.V., et al.: Urinary excretion of prostaglandin E_2, prostaglandin $F_{2\alpha}$ and thromboxane B_2 in normotensive and hypertensive subjects of varying sodium intakes. *Hypertension* 4:735, 1982.

87. Sanders T.A.B., Vickers M., Haines A.P.: Effect on blood lipids and haemostasis of a supplement of cod liver oil, rich in eicosapentaenoic and docosahexaenoic acids in healthy young men. *Clin. Sci.* 67:317, 1981.

88. Negus P., Tannen R.L., Dunn M.J.: Indomethacin potentiates the vasoconstrictor actions of angiotensin II in normal man. *Prostaglandins* 12:175, 1976.

89. Vierhapper H., Waldhausl W., Nowotny P.: Effect of indomethacin upon angiotensin-induced changes in blood pressure and plasma aldosterone in normal man. *Eur. J. Clin. Invest.* 11:85, 1981.

90. Nowak J., Wennmalm A.: Influences of indomethacin and of prostaglandin E_1 on total regional blood flow in man. *Acta Physiol. Scand.* 102:484, 1978.

91. Patak R.V., Mookerjee B.K., Bentzel C.J., et al.: Antagonism of the effects of furosemide by indomethacin in normal and hypertensive man. *Prostaglandins* 10:649, 1975.

92. Ylitalo P., Pitkajarvi T., Metsa-Ketela T., et al.: The effect of inhibition of prostaglandin synthesis on plasma renin activity and blood pressure in essential hypertension. *Prostaglandins Med.* 1:479, 1978.

93. Hoffmann P., Foerster W.: Influence of dietary linoleic acid content on blood pressure regulation in salt-loaded rats (with special reference to the prostaglandin system). *Adv. Lipid Res.* 18:203, 1981.

94. Cox J.W., Rutecki G.W., Francisco L., et al.: Studies of the effects of essential fatty acid deficiency in the rat. *Circ. Res.* 51:694, 1982.

95. Duesing R., Scherhag R., Glaenzer K.: Dietary linoleic acid deprivation: effects on blood pressure and PGI_2 synthesis. *Am. J. Physiol.* 244:H228, 1983.

96. Mac Donald M.C., Kline R.L., Morgenson G.J.: Dietary linoleic acid and salt-induced hypertension. *Can. J. Physiol. Pharmacol.* 59:872, 1981.

97. Rosenthal J., Simone P.G., Silbergast A.: Effect of PG deficiency on natriuresis, diuresis, and blood pressure. *Prostaglandins* 5:435, 1974.

98. Smith-Barbaro P.A., Puchak G.J.: Dietary fat and blood pressure. *Ann. Intern. Med.* 92(2):828, 1983.

99. Ten Hoor F., Van De Graaf M.M.: The influence of a linolenic acid rich diet and of acetyl salicylic acid on NaCl induced hypertension, Na and H_2O balance and urinary prostaglandin secretion in rats. *Acta Biol. Med. Ger.* 37:875, 1978.

100. Triebe G., Block H.-N., Foerster W.: On the blood pressure response of salt-loaded rats under different content of linoleic acid in the food. *Acta Biol. Med. Ger.* 35:1223, 1976.

101. Box B.M., Mogenson G.J.: Blood pressure differences in spontaneously hypertensive rats produced by varying the source of dietary fats. *Nutrition Research* 2:619, 1982.

102. Hoffmann P., Foerster W., Markov Ch.M.: Attenuation of blood pressure increase

in spontaneously hypertensive rats by diets enriched with polyunsaturated fatty acids. *Prostaglandins, Leukotrienes and Medicine* 8:151, 1982.

103. Schoene N.W., Reeves V.B., Jerretti A.: Effects of dietary linoleic acid on the biosynthesis of PGE_2 and $PGF_{2\alpha}$ in kidney medullae in spontaneously hypertensive rats. *Adv. Prostaglandin Thromboxanc Res.* 8:1791, 1980.

104. Wexeler B.C.: Inhibition of the pathogenesis of spontaneous hypertension in spontaneously hypertensive rats by feeding a high fat diet. *Endocrinology* 108:981, 1981.

105. Bayorh M.A., Zukowska-Grojec Z., Ezra D., et al.: Cardiovascular and sympathetic responses to chronic arachidonate in SHR and WKy rats. *Hypertension* 5:172, 1983.

106. Epstein M., Lifshitz M., Rapport K.: Augmentation of prostaglandin production by linoleic acid. *Clin. Sci.* 63:565, 1982.

107. Ianoco J.M., Dongherty R.M., Puska P.: Reduction of blood pressure associated with dietary polyunsaturated fat. *Hypertension.* 4(Supp. III):34, 1982.

108. Brussard J.H., Van Raaj J.M.A., Stasse-Wolthuis M., et al.: Blood pressure and diet in normotensive volunteers, absence of an effect of dietary fiber, protein or fat. *Am. J. Clin. Nutr.* 34:2023, 1981.

109. Comberg H.U., Heyden L., Hames C.G., et al.: Hypotensive effect of dietary prostaglandin precursor in hypertensive man. *Prostaglandins* 15:193, 1978.

110. Oster P., Arab L., Schellenberg B., et al.: Linoleic acid and blood pressure. *Prog. Food Nutr. Sci.* 4:39, 1980.

111. Puska P., Nissinen A., Vartiainen E., et al.: Controlled, randomised trial of the effect of dietary fat on blood pressure. *Lancet* 1:1, 1983.

112. Roux J.L., Armstrong B.K., Beilin L.J., et al.: Blood-pressure-lowering effect of a vegetarian diet: Controlled trial in normotensive subjects. *Lancet* 1:5, 1983.

113. Vergoesen A.J., Fleischman A.J., Comberg H.U., et al.: The influence of dietary linoleate on essential hypertension in man. *Acta Biol. Med. Ger.* 37:1879, 1978.

114. Vergroesen A.J., Dedeckere E.A.M., Ten Hoor F., et al.: Cardiovascular effects of linoleic acid. *Prog. Food Nutr. Sci.* 4·13, 1980.

115. Mortensen J.Z., Schmidt E.B., Nielsen A.H., et al.: The effect of w-6 and n-3 polyunsaturated fatty acids on hemostasis, blood lipids and blood pressure. *Thromb. Hacmost.* 50:543, 1983.

116. Singer P., Jaeger W., Wirth M., et al.: Lipid and blood pressure-lowering effect of mackerel diet in man. *Atherosclerosis* 49:99, 1983.

117. Stern B., Heyden L., Miller D., et al.: Intervention study in high school students with elevated blood pressures. Dietary experiment with polyunsaturated fatty acids. *Nutr. Metab.* 24:137, 1980.

118. Lorenz R., Spengler U., Fischer S., et al.: Platelet function, thromboxane formation and blood pressure control during supplementation of the Western Diet with cod liver oil. *Circulation* 67:504, 1983.

119. Hansen H.J., Jensen B.: Urinary prostaglandin E_2 and vasopressin excretion in essential fatty-acid deficient rats: Effect of linoleic acid supplementation. *Lipids* 18:682, 1983.

120. Schoene N.W., Feretti A., Fiore D.: Production of prostaglandins in homogenates of kidney medullae and cortices of spontaneously hypertensive rats fed menhaden oil. *Lipids* 16:866, 1981.

121. Armstrong J.M., Boura A.L.A., Hamberg M., et al.: A comparison of the vasodepressor effects of cyclic endoperoxides PGG_2 PGH_2 with those of PGD_2 and PGE_2 in hypertensive and normotensive rats. *Eur. J. Pharmacol.* 38:251, 1976.

122. Dusting G.J., DiNicolantonio R., Drysdale T., et al.: Vasodepressor effects of arachionic acid and prostacyclin (PGI_2) in hypertensive rats. *Clin. Sci.* 61:315s, 1981.

123. Hockel G.M., Cowley A.W.: Role of the renin-angiotensin system in prostaglandin E_2-induced hypertension. *Hypertension* 2:529, 1980.

123a. Leach B.E., Armstromg F.B., Germain G.S., et al.: Vasodepressor action of prostaglandins A_2 and E_2 in the spontaneously hypertensive rat (SH rat): Evidence for an action mediated by the vagus. *J. Pharm. Exp. Ther.* 185:479, 1973.

124. Mueller B., Schneider J., Wilsmann K., et al.: Role of renin release in the hemodynamic renal and dipsogenic actions of the prostacyclin analogue CG4203 in conscious rats. *Prostaglandins, Leukotrienes and Medicine* 11:361, 1983.

124a. Pace-Asciak C.R., Carrara M.C., Nicolaou K.G.: Prostaglandin I_2 has more potent hypotensive properties than prostaglandin E_2 in the normal and spontaneously hypertensive rat. *Prostaglandins* 15:999, 1978.

125. Simpson L.L.: The effect of prostaglandin E_2 on the arterial blood pressure of normotensive and spontaneously hypertensive rats. *Br. J. Pharm.* 51:559, 1974.

126. Lee J., Kannegiesser H., O'Toole J., et al.: Hypertension and the renomedullary prostaglandins: A human study of the antihypertensive effects of PGA_1. *Ann. NY Acad. Sci.* 180:218, 1971.

127. Okada F., Nukada T., Yamauchi Y., et al.: The hypotensive effect of prostaglandin E_1 on hypertensive cases of various types. *Prostaglandins* 7:99, 1974.

128. O'Grady J., Warrington S., Motti M.J.: Effects of intravenous infusion of prostacyclin (PGI_2) in man. *Prostaglandins* 19:319, 1980.

129. Patrono C., Pugliese F., Ciabattoni G., et al.: Evidence for a direct stimulatory effect on renin in man. *J. Clin. Invest.* 69:231, 1982.

130. Scholkens B.A., Gehring D., Jung W.: The orally active thia-immunoprostacyclin HOE892: Antiaggregatory and cardiovascular activities. *Prostaglandins, Leukotrienes and Medicine* 10:231, 1983.

131. Mullane K., Moncada L., Vane J.R.: Does prostaglandin release contribute to the hypotension induced by inhibitors of angiotensin converting enzyme? Dunn M.J., Patrono C., Cinotti G.A., (eds.): In *Prostaglandins and the Kidney. (New York: Plenum Medical Book Company,* pp. 213–233, 1983.)

132. Vinci J.M., Horwik D., Zusman R.M.: The effect of converting enzyme inhibition with SQ 20881 on plasma and urinary kinins, prostaglandin E and angiotensin II in hypertensive man. *Hypertension* 1:416, 1979.

133. Moore T.J., Crantz F.R., Hollenberg N.K.: Contribution of prostaglandins to the antihypertensive action of captopril in essential hypertension. *Hypertension* 3(2):168, 1981.

134. Swartz S.L., Williams G.H., Hollenberg N.K.: Converting enzyme inhibition in essential hypertension. The hypotensive response does not reflect only reduced angiotensin II formation. *Hypertension* 1:106, 1979.

135. Abe K., Itoh T., Imai Y., et al.: Implication of endogenous prostaglandin system in the anti-hypertensive effect of captopril SQ14,225 in low renin hypertension. *Jpn. Circ. J.* 44:422, 1980.

136. Salvetti A., Pedrinelli R., Magagna A., et al.: Differential effects of selective and nonselective prostaglandin synthesis inhibition on the pharmacological responses to captopril in patients with essential hypertension. *Clin. Sci.* 63:267s, 1982.

137. Witzgall H., Sherer B., Weber P.C.: Involvement of prostaglandins in the actions of captopril. *Clin. Sci.* 63:265s, 1982.

138. Stone K.J., Hart M.: Inhibition of renal PGE_2-9-heteroreductase by diuretics. *Prostaglandins* 12:197, 1976.

139. Susic D., Sparks J.C.: Effects of aspirin on renal sodium excretion, blood pressure, and plasma and extracellular fluid volume in salt-loaded rats. *Prostaglandins* 10:875, 1975.

140. Durao V., Ria J.M., Giao T.: Modification by indomethacin of the blood pressure lowering effect of pindolol and propranolol in conscious rabbits. *Eur. J. Pharmacol.* 43:377, 1977.

141. Durao V., Prato M.U., Goncalves L.M.P.: Modification of antihypertensive effect of beta-adrenoceptor-blocking agents by inhibition of endogenous prostaglandin synthesis. *Lancet* 2:1005, 1977.

142. Salvetti A., Pedrinelli R., Magagna A., et al.: The influence of indomethacin on some pharmacologic actions of atenolol. Dunn M.J., Patrono C., Cinotti G.A. (eds.): In *Prostaglandin and the Kidney* (New York: Plenum Medical Book Company, pp. 287–295, 1983).

143. Lopez-Ovejero J.A., Weber M.A., Drayer J.I., et al.: Effects of indomethacin alone and during diuretic or β-adrenoreceptor-blockade therapy on blood pressure and the renin system in essential hypertension. *Clin. Sci. Mol. Med.* 55:203s, 1978.

144. Watkins J., Abbott E.C., Hensby C.N., et al.: Attenuation of hypotensive effect of propranolol and thiazide diuretics by indomethacin. *Br. Med. J.* 281:702, 1980.

145. Papaicolaou N., Mountokalikis T., Safar M., et al.: Deficiency in renomedullary prostaglandin synthesis related to the evolution of essential hypertension. *Experientia* 32:1015, 1976.

146. Tan S.Y., Bravo E., Mulrow P.: Impaired renal prostaglandin E_2 biosynthesis in human hypertensive states. *Prostaglandins Med.* 1:76, 1978.

147. Grose J.H., Lebel M., Gbeassor F.M.: Diminished urinary prostacyclin metabolite in essential hypertension. *Clin. Sci.* 59:127s, 1980.

148. Ruilope L., Robles R.G., Barrentos A., et al.: The role of urinary PGE_2 and renin-angiotensin aldosterone system in the pathogenesis of essential hypertension. *Clin. Exp. Hypertens.* A4:989, 1982.

149. Larrson C., Anggard E.: Arachidonic acid lowers and indomethacin increases the blood pressure of the rabbit. *J. Pharm. Pharmacol.* 25:653, 1973.

150. Romero J.C., Strong C.G.: The effect of indomethacin blockade of prostaglandin synthesis on blood pressure of normal rabbits and rabbits with renovascular hypertension. *Circ. Res.* 40:35, 1977.

151. Muirhead E.E., Brooks B., Brosius W.L.: Indomethacin and blood pressure control. *J. Lab. Clin. Med.* 88:578, 1976.

152. Scholkens B.A., Steinbach R.: Increase of experimental hypertension following inhibition of prostaglandin biosynthesis. *Arch. Int. Pharmacodyn. Ther.* 214:328, 1975.

153. Cangiano J.L., Rodriquez-Sargent C., Martinez-Maldonado M.: Modification of experimental renal hypertension in the rat by indomethacin and hydralazine. *J. Lab. Clin. Med.* 92:516, 1978.

154. McQueen D., Bell K.: The effects of prostaglandin E_1 and sodium meclofenamate on blood pressure in renal hypertensive rats. *Eur. J. Pharmacol.* 37:223, 1976.

155. Chrysant S.G., Townsend S.M., Morgan P.R.: The effects of salt and meclofenamate administration on the hypertension of spontaneously hypertensive rats. *Clin. Exp. Hypertens.* 1:381, 1978.

156. Quirion R., Rioux F., Regoli D.: The effect of an acute or chronic treatment with indomethacin on the blood pressure of DOCA/salt and spontaneously hypertensive rats. *Clin. Exp. Hypertens.* 1:286, 1978.

157. Pugsley D.J., Mullins R., Beilin L.J.: Renal prostaglandin synthesis in hypertension induced by deoxycorticosterone and sodium chloride in the rat. *Clin. Sci. Mol. Med.* 51:253s, 1976.

158. Paulson D.J., Eversole W.J.: Effects of prostaglandin E_2 and prostaglandin inhibitors on adrenal regeneration hypertension. *Am. J. Physiol.* 232:E95, 1977.

159. Scholkens B.A., Steinbach R., Ganten D.: Blood pressure effects of endogenous brain angiotensin in rats are increased by inhibition of prostaglandin biosynthesis. *Clin. Sci.* 57:271s, 1979.

160. Donker A.J.M., Arisz L., Brentjens J.R.H., et al.: The effect of indomethacin on kidney function and plasma renin activity in man. *Nephron.* 17:288, 1976.

161. Laborit H., Valette N.: The action of arachidonic acid on experimental hypertension in the rat. *Chem. Biol. Interact.* 10:239, 1975.

162. Feinberg G., Trachte G.J., Curtis M., et al.: Dietary modification of the vascular effect of prostacyclin in hypertensive rats. *Prostaglandins Med.* 5:235, 1980.
163. Fleischman A.J., Bierenbaum M.L., Steir A., et al.: Hypotensive effect of increased dietary linoleic acid in mildly hypertensive humans. *J. Med. Soc. NJ* 76:181, 1979.
164. Rao R.H., Rao U.B., Srikantia S.G.: Effect of polyunsaturated-rich vegetable oils on blood pressure in essential hypertension. *Clin. Exp. Hypertens.* 3:27, 1981.

Effects of Nonsteroidal Anti-Inflammatory Drugs on Blood Pressure and Renal Function in Man

M. B. VALLOTTON AND L. FAVRE

Division of Endocrinology, Department of Medicine, University Cantonal Hospital, CH-1211 Geneva 4 - Switzerland

The Kidney at the Center of an Endocrine Crossroad

THE KIDNEY plays a crucial role among the pathophysiologic processes leading to the onset and maintenance of hypertension. This is a consequence of its major function in both the qualitative and quantitative regulation of intravascular and extravascular spaces. Such a vital role calls for an ability to adapt to ever-changing external conditions to which the organism is being exposed. The kidney receives and sends regulatory signals[29]: it is both a source of hormones and a target organ for hormones and for neurotransmitters liberated at sympathetic nerve endings; it is also the site of interplay between these hormones and eicosanoids that are synthesized in situ and modulate their actions. The synthesis of these local factors is in turn dependent on a series of hormones (Fig 1). Thus angiotensin II, generated by the serial action of renin and then converting enzyme (in the general circulation and in situ), directly stimulates the production of prostaglandins, mainly PGE_2. The synthesis of renal prostaglandins is also fostered indirectly: the angiotensin-dependent synthesis and release of aldosterone set up the liberation of kallikrein and thereby of kinins, such as

0084-5957/84/0014-0273-0284-$04.00

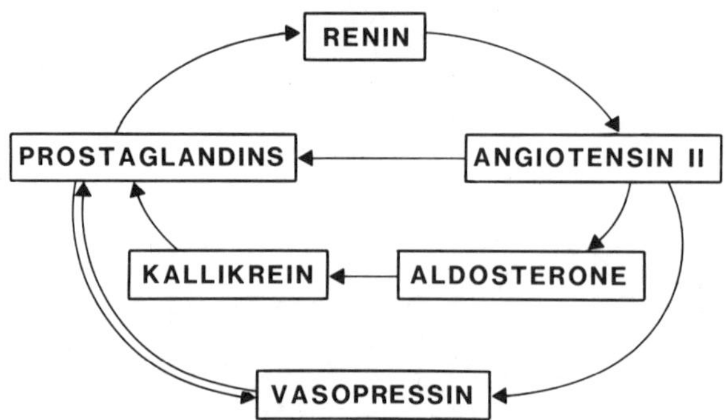

Fig 1.—Relationships between renal prostaglandins, the renin-angiotensin-aldosterone system, kallikrein, and vasopressin. (From Favre and Vallotton.[8] Reproduced by permission.)

bradykinin, that stimulate the synthesis of renal prostaglandins. The loop closes back on renin, since PGE_2 and prostacyclin are potent stimuli of renin release; furthermore, kallikrein might act as a maturating enzyme, converting inactive prorenin into active renin. It should be noted that this circle represents a positive feedback type of regulation. The same is true for the antidiuretic hormone arginine-vasopressin (AVP), which stimulates the synthesis of PGE_2 in renomedullary cells.

In order to understand the homeostatic control of kidney function exerted by these intricate positive feedback loops, one should understand the antagonistic actions that eicosanoids exert on angiotensin and AVP. The maintenance of blood pressure through the vasoconstrictive action of angiotensin II (and possibly also AVP, in some circumstances) is opposed by the vasodilation induced by PGE_2 and prostacyclin. The maintenance of body volumes through retention of saline by the renin-angiotensin-aldosterone system is opposed by the natriuretic effect of the kallikrein-kinin-prostaglandin system.[10, 28] Finally, the antidiuretic action of AVP is challenged by the diuretic action of PGE_2, which inhibits AVP-induced adenylate cyclase activation.[11, 27] To these roles of global importance for the whole organism one should add a local role in the kidney, maintaining its proper function. The compartmentalization of the biosynthesis of arachidonic acid metabolites within renal parenchyma[19, 21] is crucial for the continuing appropriate distribution of intrarenal blood flow.[3] Renal prostaglandins exert a local protecting function when the kidney is exposed to an excess of vasoconstrictive factors, sometimes required for maintaining blood pressure and body volumes, but at the same time potentially harmful for renal hemodynamics (Fig 2).

With this knowledge, we can now approach the study of the nonsteroidal anti-inflammatory drug (NSAID) effects on blood pressure and renal function.

Effects of NSAIDs on Blood Pressure

Before considering these effects of NSAIDs, we should examine whether an abnormal production of prostaglandins is observed in hypertensive subjects. An imbalance between pressor and depressor agents might indeed be involved in the genesis of high blood pressure (see Fig 2). The role of prostaglandins in the regulation of blood pressure in experimental animals[16, 20] and in clinical settings[8] was recently reviewed. Because the kidney is the source of antihypertensive factors,[14, 20] two possibilities should be considered: either essential hypertension results from a prostaglandin deficiency, or, in order to counteract

Fig 2.—Influence of the sympathetic nervous system, the renin-angiotensin system, and renal prostaglandins E_2 and I_2 on the balance between vasoconstriction and vasodilation.

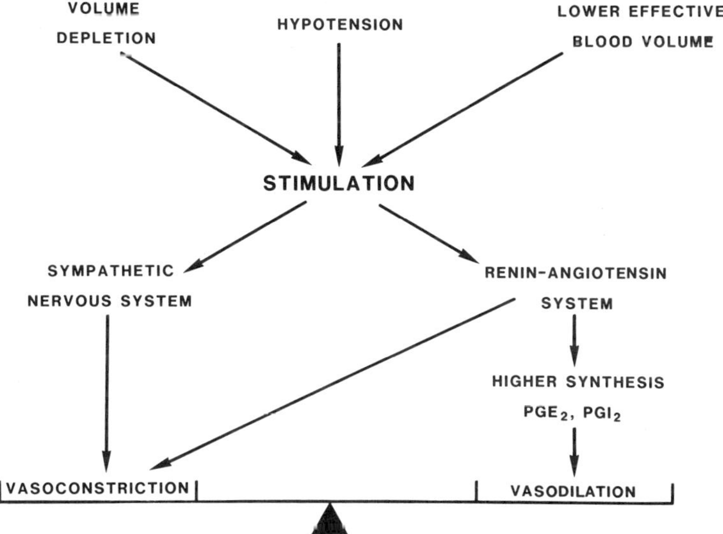

the action of an excess of vasopressors, the kidney synthesizes prostaglandins in larger amount.

A lowered urinary excretion of prostaglandins has been reported.[1, 17, 23] Yet other authors were unable to observe a difference in prostaglandin excretions between normotensive and hypertensive subjects.[13] Our own observations are in agreement with the latter. Among 53 patients with essential hypertension, matched for sex and age with normotensive subjects, we found no significant differences in the excretion of PGE_2, $PGF_{2\alpha}$ and 6-keto-$PGF_{1\alpha}$ (one stable metabolite of prostacyclin) (Table 1).

Another approach consists of modifying prostaglandin synthesis,[8] either through stimulation by furosemide or loading with prostaglandin precursors, or through reduction by restriction of prostaglandin precursors or by administration of NSAIDs. We will consider here only the latter maneuver. While administration of indomethacin tends to elevate blood pressure in some experimental animal models,[16] this is not the case in normotensive human subjects. According to our experience, indomethacin administered orally, whether acutely or chronically, does not modify blood pressure (Table 2).

It is well known that NSAIDs induce salt retention. Yet, as is the case with mineralocorticoids, the kidney escapes this action within 3–6 days.[5] On the other hand, if basal pressure is not modified, the pressure response to vasopressors such as angiotensin II and norepinephrine is potentiated.[25, 32] This indicates that under such circumstances the organism defense against pressor agents is lessened. In hypertension, the response to hypotensive drugs such as diuretics,[2] β-blocking

TABLE 1.—URINARY EXCRETION RATE OF PROSTAGLANDINS E_2, $F_{2\alpha}$ AND 6-KETO-$F_{1\alpha}$ IN NORMOTENSIVE SUBJECTS AND UNTREATED PATIENTS WITH ESSENTIAL HYPERTENSION*

	NORMOTENSIVES	HYPERTENSIVES	
PGE_2 (ng/24 hr)	259 ± 21 ($n = 84$)	213 ± 22 ($n = 53$)	NS
$PGF_{2\alpha}$ (ng/24 hr)	774 ± 51 ($n = 84$)	693 ± 74 ($n = 53$)	NS
6-keto-$PGF_{1\alpha}$ (ng/24 hr)	397 ± 38 ($n = 19$)	326 ± 31 ($n = 18$)	NS

*Values are in means $\pm$ SEM.

TABLE 2.—EFFECTS OF INDOMETHACIN AND FLUOROHYDROCORTISONE IN HEALTHY SUBJECTS*

PARAMETER	CONTROL	INDOMETHACIN	FLUOROHYDROCORTISONE
Weight gain (kg)	0.5 ± 0.2	0.9 ± 0.1 NS	1.9 ± 0.3 $P < .001$
Blood pressure (mm Hg)	$128 \pm 2/82 \pm 2$	$123 \pm 4/84 \pm 2$ NS	$120 \pm 4/83 \pm 2$ NS
Urinary sodium (mmoles/24 hr)	215 ± 35	215 ± 37 NS	145 ± 17 NS
Plasma sodium (mmoles/L)	143 ± 1.4	140 ± 1.4 NS	141 ± 0.6 NS
Plasma potassium (mmoles/L)	4.3 ± 0.1	4.2 ± 0.1 NS	3.8 ± 0.1 $P < .05$
Creatinine clearance (ml/min)	109 ± 6	107 ± 7 NS	116 ± 7 NS
Plasma renin activity (ng/ml/hr)	2.0 ± 0.5 $P < .02$	0.4 ± 0.1 $P < .02$	0.2 ± 0.1 $P < .005$
Urinary aldosterone (μg/24 hr)	6.5 ± 1.0	2.4 ± 0.4 $P < .005$	1.6 ± 0.3 $P < .005$
Urinary PGE_2 (ng/24 hr)	125 ± 25	74 ± 12 $P < .001$	230 ± 40 NS
Urinary $PGF_{2\alpha}$ (ng/24 hr)	593 ± 132	257 ± 49 $P < .005$	799 ± 50 NS

*Values are in means ± SEM. P values of comparisons with control values (two-tailed unpaired t test) are indicated (NS, not significant). The values were determined on the fifth day of daily administration of indomethacin, 150 mg, or fluorohydrocortisone, 0.6 mg. (Modified from Bonhomme M., Favre L., Vallotton M.B.: Influence of a prostaglandin inhibitor and a mineralocorticoid on the antidiuretic and hormonal response to an osmolar load. *Acta Endocrinol.* 103:331, 1983. Reproduced by permission).

agents[33] and the converting-enzyme inhibitor, captopril,[15, 22, 34] is also lowered when prostaglandin synthesis is inhibited.

In summary, if a pathogenic role of prostaglandins in the initiation or maintenance of arterial hypertension has not yet been conclusively demonstrated, inhibition of their synthesis by NSAIDs deprives the organism of their useful depressor effect, placing the hypertensive subject in an unfavorable situation of imbalance between pressor and depressor components.

Effects of NSAIDs on Renal Function

First, we must distinguish renal effects of NSAIDs[4] from nephropathies induced by analgesic agents, especially those containing phenacetin.[10] Analgesic agents constitute another class of drugs having different renal effects related to reduction of glutathion, their co-oxidation, or their protein binding.[35]

Since their introduction in the 1950s, pyrazole derivatives with anti-inflammatory properties were noted to induce salt retention with formation of edema, accompanied by a reduction in renal blood flow.[30] This saline retention is reminiscent of that induced by mineralocorticoids and is also followed by the renal escape phenomenon. This escape mechanism occurs later with pyrazole compounds (around the tenth day) than with more recently introduced NSAIDs, such as indomethacin (around the third day), which produces less salt retention and rarely edema formation (Fig 3). As with mineralocorticoids, this saline retention inhibits plasma renin activity and urinary excretion of aldosterone, despite renal escape (Figs 3 and 4; see also Table 2).[5] Yet other effects of NSAIDs and mineralocorti-

Fig 3.—Effects of an inhibitor of prostaglandin synthesis (indomethacin) and a mineralocorticoid (9α-fluorohydrocortisone) on the weight and the sodium and potassium balance in normal subjects. **A,** 5 subjects were given indomethacin (150 mg/day) for 3 days with a constant daily intake of sodium (230 mmoles) and potassium (110 mmoles). **B,** 10 subjects given the same sodium and potassium intake were treated with fluorohydrocortisone (0.6 mg/day) for 12 days, and with indomethacin (150 mg/day) for 3 days. Note the sodium retention followed by an escape during the three phases of treatment, and the kaliuretic action specific for fluorohydrocortisone.

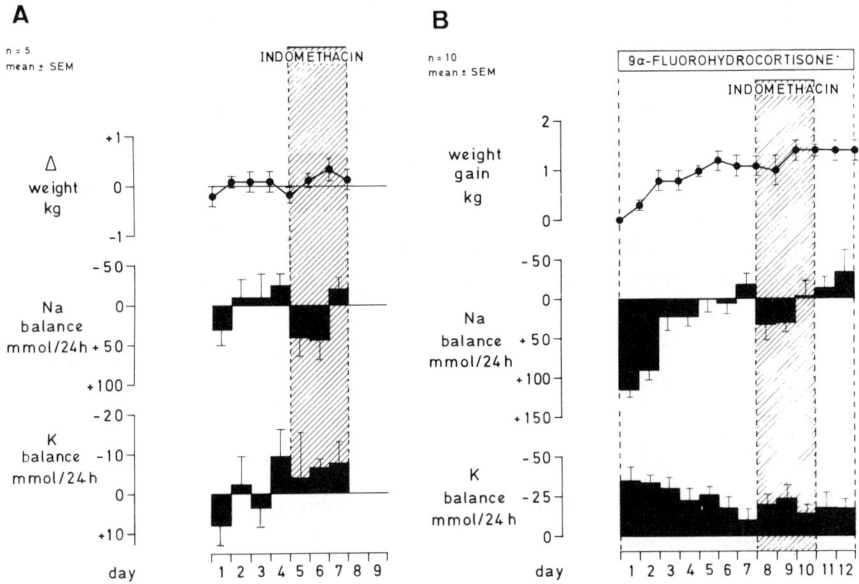

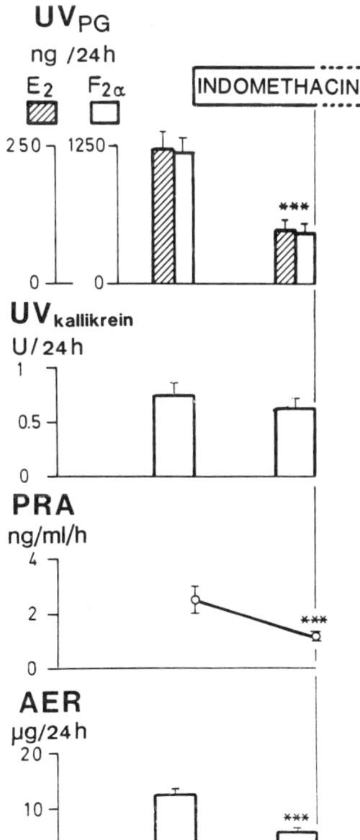

Fig 4.—Influence of indomethacin (150 mg/day for 3 days) on 24-hour urinary excretion of prostaglandins E_2 and $F_{2\alpha}$, kallikrein, and aldosterone, and on plasma renin activity.

coids are opposed. Following mineralocorticoid administration, renal prostaglandin excretion tends to rise (see Table 2),[5] whereas following NSAID administration it is obviously reduced. The administration of a mineralocorticoid is followed by a reduction in kalemia, whereas when indomethacin is administered for more than 5 days, a slight increase in kalemia is observed.[10, 24]

One can make use of this latter effect to correct the severe hyperkalemia of various syndromes, associated or not with excessive production of renal prostaglandins, such as Bartter's syndrome and other renal tubulopathies. When renal function is severely compromised, a frank hyperkalemia can occur when NSAIDs are given.[24] It has been proposed that the proximal cause of Bartter's syndrome is defective resorption of chloride along the thick ascending loop of Henle. We have examined whether a relation obtains between prostaglandins E_2 and $F_{2\alpha}$ and the fractional distal resorption of chloride, sodium, and magnesium in eight healthy subjects and nine patients with hypokalemia of various causes, including four patients with Bartter's syndrome.[9] The distal load as well as the fractional distal resorption were determined under conditions of maximal volume expansion, before and after indomethacin administration. The distal resorption of chloride, sodium, and magnesium, although reduced in Bartter's syndrome, was not modified by inhibition of prostaglandin production. Similarly, the transtubular transport of these electrolytes was not affected by indomethacin in the other hypokalemic patients and the controls. No correlation was seen between electrolyte transport and prostaglandin excretion in this condition of volume expansion.

What happens when sodium chloride resorption is inhibited by diuretics? Theoretically, two questions should be raised (Fig 5):

1. Does diuretic administration induce an increased production of renal prostaglandins, which then mediate natriuresis?

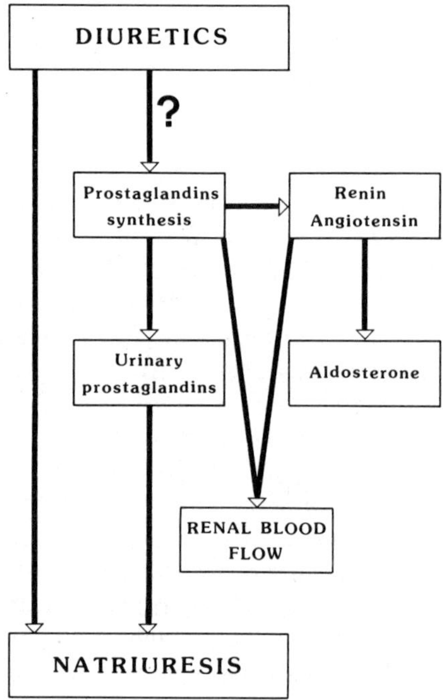

Fig 5.—Humoral hypothesis of renal prostaglandin involvement in the mechanism of action of diuretics.

2. Does concomitant administration of NSAIDs and a diuretic interfere with natriuresis?

No conclusive answer can be given to the first question. Some authors have reported elevated renal prostaglandin excretion after administration of loop diuretics, such as furosemide given IV,[2] as after administration of spironolactone and hydrochlorothiazide.[12] We have observed elevated urinary prostaglandin excretion after triamterene[6, 7] acetazolamide[9] administration but not after furosemide (PO), hydrochlorothiazide, spironolactone,[7] or amiloride administration.[9] There is more agreement on an answer to the second question: aspirin or indomethacin administration abolishes the natriuretic effect of spironolactone and furosemide,[7, 12] whereas various effects have been reported with hydrochlorothiazide.[7, 12] In all cases, the counter-regulation of the renin-angiotensin-aldosterone system was blunted or suppressed.[7, 10, 12] Triamterene was special in that, given alone, it induced an increased excretion of PGE_2 and $PGF_{2\alpha}$, but when given with indomethacin, a dramatic reduction in glomerular filtration without oliguria supervened in two healthy subjects.[6] This unexpected interaction suggests that the increased production of renal prostaglandins was playing a protective role by maintaining adequate renal hemodynamics against a harmful action of triamterene. Such a protective role has been attributed to renal prostaglandins when the renal function is threatened by exogenous or endogenous agents, causing a reduction in renal blood flow.[3] In fact, in numerous clinical reports the occurrence of acute (usually of the nonoliguric vasomotor type) renal failure has been described following NSAID administration to patients with preexisting nephropathy.[25, 26, 30] In view of the absence of oliguria or anuria, it is likely that this type of functional and reversible renal failure often goes undetected, rendering difficult an accurate evaluation of its true incidence.

Conclusion

NSAIDs are often given to alleviate pain in patients with arthritic problems. Nevertheless, practitioners should not prescribe NSAIDs indiscriminately without understanding the risks involved in case of preexisting nephropathy, of reduction of effective blood volume, of salt restriction, or of antihypertensive treatment, particularly involving diuretics.

REFERENCES

1. Abe K.: The kinins and prostaglandins in hypertension. *Clin. Endocrinol. Metab.* 10:577, 1981.
2. Attallah A.A.: Interaction of prostaglandins with diuretics. *Prostaglandins* 18:369, 1979.
3. Baer Ph.G., McGiff J.C.: Hormonal systems and renal hemodynamics. *Annu. Rev. Physiol.* 42:589, 1980.
4. Dunn M.J., Zambraski E.J.: Renal effects of drugs that inhibit prostaglandin synthesis. *Kidney Int.* 18:609, 1980.
5. Dürr J., Favre L., Gaillard R., et al.: Mineralocorticoid escape in man: Role of renal prostaglandins. *Acta Endocrinol.* 99:474, 1982.
6. Favre L., Glasson P., Vallotton M.B.: Reversible acute renal failure from combined triamterene and indomethacin: A study in healthy subjects. *Ann. Intern. Med.* 96:317, 1982.
7. Favre L., Glasson Ph., Riondel A., et al.: Interaction of diuretics and non-steroidal anti-inflammatory drugs in man. *Clin. Sci.* 64:407, 1983.
8. Favre L., Vallotton M.B.: Prostaglandines et pression artérielle. *J. Suisse Med.* 113:1042, 1983.
9. Favre L., Wicht Ch., Vallotton M.B.: Effects of triamterene, amiloride and acetazolamide on urinary prostaglandins, vasopressin and aldosterone. *J. Hypertension,* to be published.
10. Glasson P., Gaillard R., Riondel A., et al.: Role of renal prostaglandins and relationship to renin, aldosterone and antidiuretic hormone during salt depletion in man. *J. Clin. Endocrinol. Metab.* 49:176, 1979.
11. Glasson Ph., Vallotton M.B.: Inhibition of prostaglandin biosynthesis lowers antidiuretic hormone excretion in man. *Adv. Prostaglandin Thromboxane Res.* 7:1115, 1980.
12. Kramer H.J., Düsing R., Stinnesbeck B., et al.: Interaction of conventional and antikaliuretic diuretics with the renal prostaglandin system. *Clin. Sci.* 59:67, 1980.
13. Lebel M., Grose J.H.: Renal prostaglandins in borderline and sustained essential hypertension. *Prostaglandins Leukotrienes Med.* 8:409, 1982.
14. Margolius H.S.: Vasodepressor systems, in Genest J., Kuchel O., Hamet P., et al. (eds.): *Hypertension: Physiopathology and Treatment.* New York, McGraw-Hill Book Co., 1983, pp. 360–373.
15. Mullane K., Moncada S., Vane J.R.: Does prostaglandin release contribute to the hypotension induced by inhibitors of angiotensin converting enzyme? in Dunn M.J., Patrono C., Cinotti G.A. (eds.): *Prostaglandins and the Kidney.* New York, Plenum Publishing Corp., 1983, pp. 213–233.
16. Nasjletti A., Malik K.U.: Interrelations between prostaglandins and vasoconstrictor hormones: Contribution to blood pressure regulation. *Fed. Proc.* 41:2394, 1982.
17. Sato K., Abe K., Seino M., et al.: Reduced urinary excretion of prostaglandin E in essential hypertension. *Prostaglandins Leukotrienes Med.* 11:189, 1983.
18. Prescott L.F.: Analgesic nephropathy: A reassessment of the role of phenacetin and other analgesics. *Drugs* 23:75, 1982.
19. Smith W.L., Grenier F.C., DeWitt D.L., et al.: Cellular compartmentalization of the biosynthesis and function of PGE2 and PGI2 in the renal medulla, in Dunn M.B., Patrono C., Cinotti G.A., (eds.): *Prostaglandins and the Kidney.* New York, Plenum Publishing Corp., 1983, pp. 27–39.
20. Spokas E.G., Quilley J., McGiff J.C.: Prostaglandins in hypertension, in Genest J., Kuchel O., Hamet P., et al.(eds.): *Hypertension—Physiopathology and Treatment.* New York, McGraw-Hill Book Co., 1983, pp. 373–393.
21. Sraer J., Siess W., Dray F., et al.: Regional differences in in vitro prostaglandin synthesis by the rat kidney, in Dunn M.J., Patrono C., Cinotti G.A. (eds.): *Prostaglandins and the Kidney.* New York, Plenum Publishing Corp., 1983, pp. 41–52.

22. Swartz S.L., Willliams G.H., Hollenberg N.K., et al.: Captopril-induced changes in prostaglandin production: Relationship to vascular responses in normal man. *J. Clin. Invest.* 65:1257, 1980.
23. Tan S.Y., Sweet P., Mulrow P.J.: Impaired renal production of prostaglandin E_2: A newly identified lesion in human essential hypertension. *Prostaglandins* 15:139, 1978.
24. Tan S.Y., Shapiro R., Franco R., et al.: Indomethacin-induced prostaglandin inhibition with hyperkalemia: A reversible cause of hyporeninemic hypoaldosteronism. *Ann. Intern. Med.* 90:783, 1979.
25. De Torrente A.: Anti-inflammatoires non stéroïdiens et insuffisance rénale iguë vasomotrice. *Rev. Suisse Med.* 22:944, 1982.
26. De Torrente A.: Effets secondaires des anti-inflammatoires nonstéroïdiens sur la fonction rénale. *J. Suisse Med.* 113:1019, 1983.
27. Vallotton M.B.: Relationship between renal prostaglandins and antidiuretic hormone, in Mantero F., Biglieri E.G., Edwards C.R.W. (ed.): *Endocrinology of Hypertension*. New York, Academic Press, 1982, pp. 217–222.
28. Vallotton M.B., Favre L., Glasson P., et al.: Renal prostaglandin in human adaptation to modifications of sodium balance, in Dunn M.B., Patrono C., Cinotti G.A. (eds.): *Prostaglandins and the Kidney*. New York, Plenum Publishing Corp., 1983, pp. 167–175.
29. Vallotton M.B.: Le rein, carrefour endocrinien. *J. Suisse Med.* 112:1775, 1982.
30. Vallotton M.B., Favre L., Glasson P.: Agents anti-inflammatoires non-stéroïdiens, diurétiques et fonction rénale: Une mise en garde. *J. Suisse Med.* 113:1198, 1983.
31. Vierhapper H., Waldhäusl W., Nowotny P.: Effect of indomethacin upon angiotensin-induced changes in blood pressure and plasma aldosterone in normal man. *Eur. J. Clin. Invest.* 11:112, 1981.
32. Vierhapper H., Grubeck-Loebenstein B., Korn A., et al.: Release and vasoactive actions of catecholamines during inhibition of prostaglandin synthesis in normal man. *Hypertension* 4:112, 1982.
33. Watkins J., Abbott E.C., Hensby C.N., et al.: Attenuation of hypotensive effect of propranolol and thiazide diuretics by indomethacin. *Br. Med. J.* 281:702, 1980.
34. Witzgall H., Hirsch F., Scherer B., et al.: Acute haemodynamic and hormonal effects of captopril are diminished by indomethacin. *Clin. Sci.* 62:611, 1982.
35. Zenser T.V., Mattammal M.B., Rapp N.S., et al.: Effect of aspirin on metabolism of acetaminophen and benzidine by renal inner medulla prostaglandin hydroperoxidase. *J. Lab. Clin. Med.* 101:58, 1983.

New Approaches to the Diagnosis of Renovascular Hypertension

*MORTON H. MAXWELL, M.D. **MICHAEL R. RUDNICK, M.D. *ABRAHAM U. WAKS, M.D.

*UCLA School of Medicine, Los Angeles, California. **The Graduate Hospital, Philadelphia, Pennsylvania

ALTHOUGH renovascular hypertension (RVH) is the most common type of potentially curable hypertension, there is no agreement on which hypertensive patients should be screened for this disorder, or on the sensitivity and specificity of the various diagnostic tests available. Clinically, the decision matrix is usually based on suspicion of renovascular disease from the history and physical examination, or from the chance finding of inappropriately elevated plasma renin activity (PRA), or from disparity of kidney function as demonstrated by radionuclide or roentgenographic tests, if these tests are performed (Table 1).

The availability of newer antihypertensive drugs that are usually successful in lowering the blood pressure in patients with RVH, and the development of percutaneous transluminal angioplasty (PTA) as an alternative to operative treatment, drastically change the decision matrix, particularly with regard to risk-benefit and cost-benefit considerations.

This chapter reviews the diagnostic accuracy of the available tests and assesses their role in the evaluation of patients with suspected RVH. We conclude that most of the tests purported to diagnose renal artery stenosis or renovascular hypertension

285

0084-5957/84/0014-0285-0304-$04.00

© 1984, Year Book Medical Publishers, Inc.

TABLE 1.—Screening Methods, Diagnosis, and Significance of Renovascular Disease

SCREENING METHODS
    History
        Inappropriate age at onset
        Sudden worsening of hypertension
        Young white female, negative family history
        Diffuse atherosclerosis
    Physical examination
        Abdominal bruit
        Grade III–IV retinopathy
    Laboratory tests
        High plasma renin activity
        Abnormal radioisotope renogram/scan
        Abnormal rapid intravenous urogram
        Disparity on kidney function tests
        Positive saralasin test
DIAGNOSIS
    Renal arteriography
    Digital subtraction angiography
SIGNIFICANCE
    Saralasin test
    Renal vein renin level
    Renal arteriogram
    Response to percutaneous transluminal angiography

are nonspecific and have low predictive value. It is our belief (1) that hypertensive patients who are at high risk of a cardiovascular incident or in whom there is clinical suspicion of RVH should be screened, (2) that renal arteriography is the only procedure that can accurately diagnose renal artery stenosis, and (3) that the immediate blood pressure response to PTA diagnoses RVH. PTA thus can be utilized as a diagnostic test as well as a therapeutic procedure.

Dilemmas in the Diagnosis of Renovascular Hypertension

Renovascular Hypertension Responds to Antihypertensive Drug Therapy

There have been no published prospective, randomized trials of medical versus operative treatment of RVH. Furthermore, available reports vary widely with regard to selection of patients, definition of RVH, types of medications used, and length of follow-up.

Two of the earliest reports indicated that standard antihypertensive drugs were effective in lowering the blood pressure of some patients with RVH,[16, 55] which suggested an alternative mode of therapy for patients who were poor operative risks or who had inoperable renal arterial lesions. The largest comparative study showed much better long-term results in operatively treated patients.[32]

The better results achieved with medical therapy in more recent reports have been attributed to the use of new antihypertensive drugs, particularly β blockers and captopril.[7]

In the Cooperative Study of Renovascular Hypertension, 79% of patients with unilateral renovascular disease derived benefit from operative treatment, and the operative mortality was 5.9%.[20] More recent large operative series have reported better results than those of the Cooperative Study.[3, 36, 50, 54, 56, 57, 65–67, 72] with about 90%–95% of patients usually deriving benefit. The operative mortality has been lower than that reported in the Cooperative Study, ranging from 0%[13, 54, 65, 67] to 5%.[36]

The use of PTA to dilate renal arteries offers a potentially more cost-effective alternate to operative treatment. There are few long-term follow-up studies, however, so the precise indications for PTA cannot yet be delineated.

Successful initial dilation is possible in about 80% of cases.[23, 39, 61, 63, 70] There has been no patient deaths reported, and the immediate morbidity ranges from 5% to 15%.

Deaths associated with operative revascularization are seen almost exclusively in elderly patients with atherosclerotic renal artery stenosis and evidence of coronary and/or peripheral atherosclerosis.[3, 21, 64] Therefore, it was initially hoped that the safer procedure of PTA could replace surgery in this group of patients. Unfortunately, several investigators have noted frequent and early restenoses of atherosclerotic renal artery stenosis following PTA.[26, 34, 70] Successful redilation by PTA, however, has been repeated up to four times in some patients.[26]

If the hypertension can be controlled with antihypertensive drug therapy in most patients with RVH, two legitimate questions remain. Why bother to do any diagnostic tests? Why not treat all hypertensive patients with drugs, and test only those whose blood pressure cannot be controlled?

The answers to these questions are complex and depend on one's ethical viewpoint and clinical experience. Persons diagnosed as having high blood pressure are committed to a lifetime of antihypertensive drug therapy and physician visits, so that the costs for the diagnosis and correction of renovascular hypertension even in a small proportion of patients may be comparable to those of long-term drug therapy.[28] In our opinion physicians should be more concerned with risk-benefit than with cost-benefit ratios.

All antihypertensive drugs have undesirable (and sometimes dangerous) side effects that interfere with the quality of life. Furthermore, a large proportion of drug-treated hypertensive patients are noncompliant and have poor long-term blood pressure control. Better long-term results have been reported in operatively treated than in medically treated patients with renal artery stenoses.[32]

Another consideration is preservation of renal function. Although the situation in an individual patient is unpredictable, renal arterial stenotic lesions are often progressive,[52] sometimes to total arterial occlusion. An apparently stable serum creatinine value may be misleading, representing hypertrophy of the contralateral kidney during loss of renal mass on the stenotic side. Renal function improves following successful revascularization.[1, 63]

In summary, we believe that treatment by diagnosis and cure of significant renal artery stenosis is superior to long-term medical therapy. With careful selection of patients and appropriate tests, the costs and risks will be far lower than was the case when it was assumed that all hypertensive patients would be screened indiscriminately.[51]

RENOVASCULAR HYPERTENSION IS A RETROSPECTIVE DIAGNOSIS

A technically acceptable renal arteriogram can establish the diagnosis and usually the etiology of renal artery stenosis, and may also suggest whether the arterial lesion is hemodynamically significant (according to estimated degree of stenosis, poststenotic dilation, presence of collateral vessels, relative size of the kidneys).[6] The arteriogram, however, does not establish the diagnosis of RVH. If the elevated blood pressure decreases substantially after corrective surgery or PTA, then the diagnosis of RVH is made retrospectively.

All of the other diagnostic tests, whether intended for diagnosing renovascular disease (isotope renogram/scan, urography, PRA, kidney function tests, saralasin test) or for judging the significance of known renal artery stenosis, i.e., the probability of RVH (renal vein renin ratios, saralasin test) are nonspecific and may be positive in conditions other than renovascular disease. An abdominal bruit does not necessarily indicate renal artery stenosis but may be caused by turbulent blood flow in any large abdominal artery or by hyperdynamic circulation in young individuals. Radionuclide studies[1] and intravenous urography[5, 43] are not diagnostic, but merely show disparity in kidney function between the two kidneys. Lateralization of renal vein renin levels may occur in conditions other than significant renal artery stenosis, for example in patients with renin-secreting tumor of the kidney, and there is little agreement on a critical renal vein renin ratio (RVRR) in renovascular hypertension.[44] A positive saralasin test (decreased blood pressure) suggests renin-mediated hypertension, either renovascular or from another cause (essential, glomerulonephritis).[22] Thus, there is no single test or combination of tests that reliably diagnose RVH.

RENOVASCULAR HYPERTENSION IS A "RARE" DISORDER

The true prevalence of renovascular disease and RVH in the hypertensive population is unknown, but estimates based on selected referral populations range from 4% to 10%.[1, 45] Compared with essential hypertension, therefore, RVH is a relatively "rare" disorder, which greatly influences cost-benefit and risk-benefit ratios of the tests used in its diagnosis.[51]

The sensitivity of a given test is calculated by determining the percentage of positive tests in a group of patients with a specific disease. The specificity is the percentage of negative tests in subjects without the disease. The predictive value of a positive test is the percentage of subjects with a positive test who have the disease. Since none of the tests for RVH is truly diagnostic, a positive test result usually leads to other more costly and possibly more dangerous procedures. Since the proportion of patients with essential hypertension is at least 20 times greater than the proportion of patients with RVH, even a test of high sensitivity and specificity may have a low predictive value and result in a large number of patients with essential hypertension being subjected to unnecessary procedures.

As an example, let us assume that the prevalence of RVH is 5% and the prevalence of essential hypertension 95%. Test A for RVH is positive in 95% of patients with RVH (test sensitivity, 95%). Test A yields false positive results in only 5% of patients with essential hypertension (test specificity, 95%). Then, in 1,000 unselected hypertensive patients, test A will be positive in 47.5 (95%) of 50 patients with RVH but will also yield false positive results in another 47.5 (5%) of the 950 patients with essential hypertension. The predictive value of test A is thus only 50%, i.e., in random testing of patients with hypertension, if test A is positive, a patient has an equal chance of having essential hypertension or RVH.

Although persons with RVH represent only a small proportion of the total hypertensive population, the prevalence of hypertension in the general population is so high that renovascular hypertension is not a rare disorder in absolute numbers.

Clinical Characteristics of RVH

In the Cooperative Study of Renovascular Hypertension, in which 502 patients with renovascular disease were compared with 1,128 subjects judged to have primary (essential) hypertension, the question was asked: Do patients with RVH have clinical characteristics which differentiate them from patients with essential hypertension?[62] The differences in clinical characteristics between patients with RVH and those with essential hypertension were quantitative rather than qualitative. Truly distinctive features of RVH, suggested by a number of investigators, were not found. RVH may occur in either sex at any age and may range in severity from mild to severe. RVH is less frequent in blacks than whites.[45]

The presence of a bruit in the upper abdomen in patients with RVH was the finding that most sharply differentiated the two groups of patients. Body habitus is an important consideration in the prevalence of abdominal bruits, since vascular murmurs are transmitted poorly through body fat. The frequency of bruits in the upper abdomen in patients with renal artery stenosis was related to body habitus, being more frequent in thin and less frequent in obese individuals. Regardless of body habitus, upper abdominal bruits were 6–8 times more frequent in RVH than in essential hypertension.[62]

In a more recent prospective study, Grim et al.[24] excluded abdominal bruits heard exclusively during systole, reasoning that only systolic-diastolic bruits indicate the presence of a stenosis sufficient to produce a pressure gradient during diastole.[53] Systolic-diastolic bruits were detected in 39% of patients with RVH (sensitivity, 39%) but in only two of 379 patients with essential hypertension (specificity, 99%). Even assuming a prevalence of RVH of only 5%, the presence of an abdominal systolic-diastolic bruit had a predictive value of 67%.[24]

An abdominal bruit is thus a clear indication to perform additonal diagnostic tests for RVH. Other clinical characteristics that may influence our decision to search further for RVH are listed in Table 1 and include inappropriate age at onset of hypertension (< 20 or > 50 years); sudden worsening of severity of hypertension; a young or middle-aged woman with an abdominal bruit (possible fibrous dysplasia); and evidence of diffuse atherosclerosis (coronary, cerebral, peripheral) in hypertensive patients older than 40. Although RVH is often mild or moderate in degree, its prevalence in unselected patients with accelerated and malignant hypertension (grade III and IV hypertensive retinopathy) has been reported to be 31%.[12]

Comparative Risks of Diagnostic Tests

There is essentially no risk in PRA determination or in obtaining a radioisotope renogram/scan. Potential complications of RVRR determinations include groin hematoma, venous thrombosis, and venous perforation; we could find no published reports of morbidity or of deaths and therefore conclude that the risk of major complications is very low. Serious complications from intravenous urography are uncommon. In a large series (33,000 procedures), 1.7% of patients had adverse side effects, which were major in only 5%; there was one death (0.003%).[74] Major complications of transfemoral renal arteriography were seen in 1.2% of patients and mostly consisted of hemorrhage, thrombosis, or renal injury; the mortality in the

Cooperative Study was 0.1%.[59] If digital subtraction techniques, smaller catheters, and much smaller amounts of contrast material are used, the complication rate of renal arteriography may be considerably decreased.[2] Adverse reactions to the saralasin test consist solely of transient hypotensive or hypertensive responses in a small number of patients; no serious side effects or deaths have been reported in over 6,000 procedures.[22] The safety of digital subtraction angiography (DSA) is unknown. The dose of contrast medium used is often 2–3 times greater than that used for a urogram, theoretically increasing the risk of acute renal failure in susceptible patients. Furthermore, the technique of catheter insertion to the vena cava and bolus injection of contrast material suggests such possible complications as ruptured vessel wall, chemical thrombophlebitis, or pericardial injection.

Comparative Costs of Diagnostic Tests

The costs of diagnostic tests leading to the diagnosis and cure of RVH must be compared with the costs and inconveniences of chronic antihypertensive drug therapy.[28] In certain groups of patients, cost-effectiveness is relatively unimportant. These include patients with severe or accelerated hypertension and patients with moderate hypertension whose blood pressure cannot be controlled by means of medication or who are intolerant of medication. Cost should not be an important consideration in patients with a high probability of RVH, such as patients with a systolic-diastolic abdominal bruit, young children, patients with a sudden worsening of benign hypertension, and patients of inappropriate age at onset of hypertension. Cost may be a consideration in patients with mild hypertension and in young adults with moderate hypertension who are not particularly likely to have RVH.

CHARACTERISTICS OF DIAGNOSTIC TESTS

There is considerable disagreement on the sensitivity, specificity, and predictive value of the various diagnostic tests, alone or in combination. Our views are summarized in the following sections.

Screening Tests for the Possible Diagnosis of Renovascular Disease

Renovascular disease (renal artery stenosis) may occur in patients with essential hypertension and therefore may be an incidental finding.[15, 17, 31] Nevertheless, the disparity in renal function caused by significant renal artery stenosis results in abnormalities on radionuclide and roentgenographic tests. These tests have no predictive value as to the success or failure of operative repair.[5, 45]

Radioisotope Renogram/Scan

Renography is less accurate than hypertensive urography in screening for renovascular disease.[1, 4, 45] Renal scans, however, are safe, rapid, and relatively inexpensive. We use renal scans instead of urography only in patients who may be sensitive to radiographic contrast media or who may be in greater jeopardy when exposed to them, such as diabetics, and patients with azotemia.

Rapid-Sequence Intravenous Urography

The urogram is positive in about 80% of patients with significant renovascular disease,[5, 24, 45, 68] with false positive results ranging from 1.5%[24] to 12%[5] in patients with essential hypertension. A negative urogram in a patient without an abdominal bruit has a high exclusion ratio, making the likelihood of RVH less than 2%.[24, 25] A urogram may also reveal other unsuspected causes of hypertension, such as ureteropelvic obstruction, pyelonephritis, or renal calculi.

Tests for the Diagnosis of Renovascular Disease

DSA

The technology of DSA is changing rapidly. In a comparison with conventional catheter angiography, DSA was sufficient for diagnostic purposes in only 19 of 30 cases (63%),[8] although better results have been reported by others.[29] It is a curious semantic aberration that DSA has been called "noninvasive" because the catheter is in the venous rather than in the arterial vasculature; morbidity and mortality have not yet been reported. In our experience, visualization of the main renal arteries is not comparable to that of standard arteriography, and the renal arterial branches are seldom visualized at all. Practically, even with a positive DSA, surgeons seldom operate on a patient with renal artery stenosis without first requesting a renal arteriogram.

Renal Arteriography

Conventional renal arteriography remains the best method for delineating, diagnosing the etiology, and judging the operability and severity of renal arterial lesions.[6] It offers the further advantage of permitting possible dilation of a stenotic lesion by PTA during the same procedure.[47, 48] Its main limitations compared to DSA are cost and possible safety.

TESTS FOR RVH

The high morbidity and large percentage of uninterpretable test results have virtually eliminated the use of individual kidney function tests for judging the significance of renal artery stenosis.

There is convincing evidence that the hypertension secondary to renovascular disease, both experimental and occurring naturally in humans, is mediated by increased secretion of renin angiotensin and/or increased vascular responsiveness to angiotensin.[42] For this reason, diagnostic tests involving the renin-angiotensin system have been utilized to diagnose RVH. These tests include determination of peripheral PRA, RVRR, and the vasodepressor response to saralasin.

We recently reviewed the published literature on each test in terms of test accuracy (i.e., sensitivity and specificity), both in the basal state and after a variety of stimulatory maneuvers.[60] Only those series describing the blood pressure responses following technically successful surgery were included in these analyses. The following comments reflect our conclusions (Table 2).[60]

TABLE 2.—ACCURACY OF PRA, RVRR, AND SARALASIN TEST IN PATIENTS WITH RENOVASCULAR HYPERTENSION*

TEST[†]	SENSITIVITY[‡]	SPECIFICITY[§]	SURGICAL IMPROVEMENT	
			Neg. PRA	*Pos. PKA*
PRA	310/540	96/146	230/326	310/360
	(57%)	(66%)	(71%)	(86%)
			Neg. RVRR	*Pos. RVRR*
RVRR	896/1123	125/203	227/352	896/974
	(80%)	(62%)	(64%)	(92%)
Saralasin	126/170	273/324		
	(74%)	(84%)		

*Based on a review of the literature, from Rudnick and Maxwell.[60] PRA, plasma renin activity; RVRR, renal vein renin ratio.

†Criteria for positive test results were defined by authors of each study reviewed.

‡Sensitivity: percentage of positive tests in patients with RVH

§Specificity: percentage of negative tests in patients who do not have RVH.

PRA

The sensitivity and specificity of elevated PRA in the diagnosis of RVH were 57% and 66%, respectively. Thus, the false negative and false positive rates for this test are 43% and 34%, respectively. In a total of 540 patients (24 publications), 71% of patients with normal PRA and 86% of patients with elevated PRA benefited from surgery. About 15% of patients with essential hypertension had elevated PRA.[33, 37]

It appears that PRA is of very limited value in predicting which patients with renal artery stenosis and hypertension have RVH.

RVRR

In our analysis of published articles reporting on 1,097 patients, the RVRR had a sensitivity of 80% and a false negative rate of 20%. The specificity was 62%, with a false positive rate of 38%. Various stimulatory maneuvers (sodium depletion, upright posture, stimulatory drugs) did not improve the predictive value of RVRR.[60]

These data confirm earlier, smaller studies which indicated that corrective surgery would benefit more than 90% of patients with lateralizing RVRR.[44] Our analysis also confirmed that when surgery is performed in patients with renal artery stenosis and nonlateralizing RVRR, more than 50% will still benefit from the procedure.[40, 44]

Saralasin Test

We and others have found that in the presence of renal artery stenosis, the saralasin test is more predictive than the RVRR, particularly when both changes in blood pressure and changes in PRA are used in judging saralasin test results.[9, 46]

In our literature review, 126 of 170 patients with proved RVH had a positive saralasin test, for a sensitivity of 74%.[60] The specificity in essential hypertension (324 patients) was 84%. The false positive rate of 16% in essential hypertension probably identified those with high renin levels.[33, 37] In patients with suspected RVH but a nonlateralizing RVRR, a positive saralasin test would be highly suggestive of a favorable surgical outcome.[41, 58, 73]

Diagnostic Approaches to RVH

The suggested strategy detailed below is based on several premises:

1. Most patients with RVH do *not* present with the history of sudden onset of severe hypertension at an inappropriate age, but are clinically indistinguishable from patients with essential hypertension.[62] Nonetheless, in hypertensive patients with unusual clinical features (abdominal bruit, inappropriate age at onset, sudden worsening of hypertension), the physician's estimate of the disease probability *before* ordering diagnostic tests greatly enhances predictive accuracy.[27]

2. Because RVH is a rare disorder, its low prior probability precludes any valid estimate of posterior probability based on the usual type of formal decision analysis.[14] Decision-making, therefore, reverts back to clinical acumen and the physician's perception of risk-benefit ratio for a particular patient.

3. PTA is simple to perform, has no appreciable mortality, and has a low complication rate,[11, 19, 25, 35, 38, 39, 63, 69, 71] in contrast to operative treatment. *Initial* dilation of main renal artery lesions is successful in 90% of patients with fibrous dysplasia and in more than 75% of patients with nonostial

atherosclerotic lesions.[11, 19, 35, 38, 39, 63, 71] Initial dilation is less successful in lesions at the ostium which arise from aortic plaques extending into the renal artery, and these lesions are likely to recur.[10]

4. A short-term (hours, day, weeks) significant reduction of blood pressure following successful initial dilation of renal artery stenosis by PTA is per se evidence of RVH, even if restenosis subsequently occurs and the blood pressure increases.

5. Renal arteriography is diagnostic of the type, degree, and operability of renal artery stenosis. At present, DSA is not as dependable as standard arteriography in visualizing main renal artery lesions,[8] and the renal arterial branches are seldom adequately visualized.

The following classification of patients and selection of diagnostic tests is not meant to be rigid, and there is overlapping of patient groups.

Patients in Whom Intervention With Possible Cure or Improvement of Hypertension Is Preferable to Long-Term Drug Therapy

This group includes children, patients with severe and accelerated hypertension, and patients with hypertension uncontrollable (poor blood pressure response, adverse side effects, lack of compliance) with antihypertensive drug therapy (Fig 1). Patients in this category constitute about 10% of the hypertensive population[18] and should be also tested for other types of secondary hypertension.

The usual type of diagnostic workup for RVH—PRA, radionuclide studies, intravenous urography, DSA, RVRR, testing with angiotensin analogues or converting enzyme inhibitors—is complicated, costly, nondiagnostic, and aimed at determining the need for renal arteriography. In clinical practice, because the need for intervention is so great in this type of patient, a negative or questionably positive screening test is often ignored and the next, more complicated study is ordered. Renal arteriography is usually eventually performed, regardless of prior test results. Therefore, why not proceed directly to renal arteriography? With further technological improvement, DSA may replace arteriography as the initial examination in this patient group

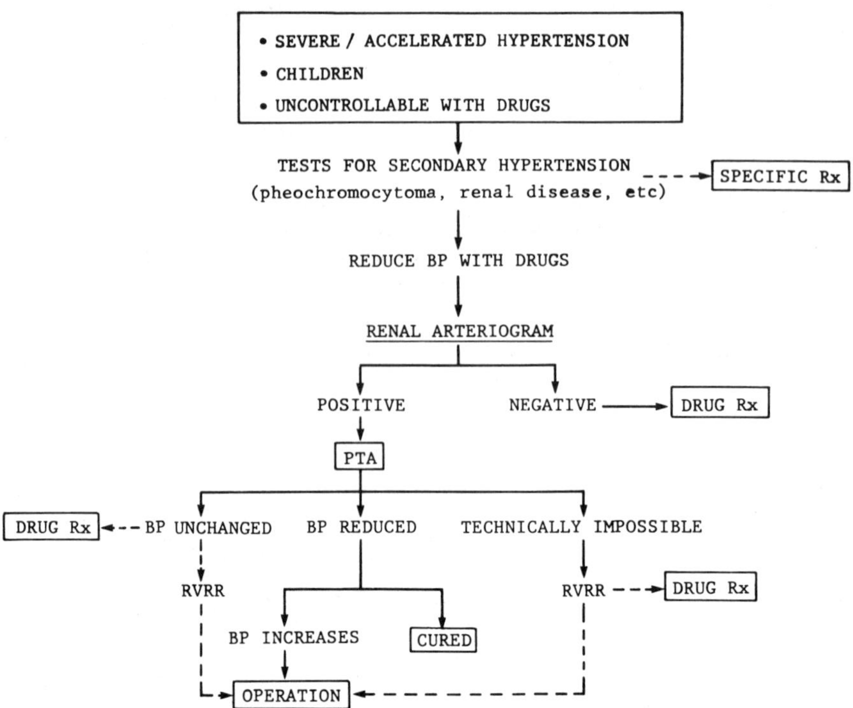

Fig 1.—Decision matrix for patients in whom intervention with possible cure or improvement of hypertension is preferable to long-term drug therapy. This group includes children and patients at high risk of cardiovascular incidents.

Regardless of the type or degree of stenosis demonstrated arteriographically, PTA is attempted during the same procedure. If initial dilation is successful, as judged by the radiologic appearance and confirmed by a decreased pressure gradient, then the short-term blood pressure response offers the most accurate and practical diagnosis of RVH: if the blood pressure falls significantly, the diagnosis of RVH is established, even if the blood pressure should subsequently increase because of restenosis. Thus, PTA is used as a diagnostic test as well as a therapeutic modality. When PTA is not technically feasible or is initially unsuccessful in dilating a stenotic lesion, then the usual diagnostic tests to ascertain its significance (renal vein renin levels, saralasin test) are employed.

This approach permits diagnosis and therapy to be undertaken during a brief hospital admission and reduces the costs and risks of the traditional approach.

PATIENTS SUSPECTED OF HAVING RVH

Clinical correlates of RVH include inappropriate age at onset, sudden onset or abrupt worsening of preexisting hypertension, and systolic-diastolic epigastric bruits (Fig 2). The degree of blood pressure elevation in patients in this group is irrelevant. Duration of hypertension has an inverse relationship to the operative cure rate in renovascular disease, and the possibility of cure should be offered before the long-term cardiovascular sequelae of high blood pressure develop. These patients should be screened for RVH with DSA or with rapid-sequence intravenous urography, with renal arteriography performed only if the screening test is positive. A negative rapid-sequence urogram has a high exclusion value.[24] Radionuclide studies and saralasin testing (utilizing both blood pressure and renin responses for interpretation) are useful if administration of radiocontrast material is contraindicated.

Fig 2.—Decision matrix for patients who have a high likelihood of renovascular disease. The degree of blood pressure elevation and cardiovascular risk are secondary.

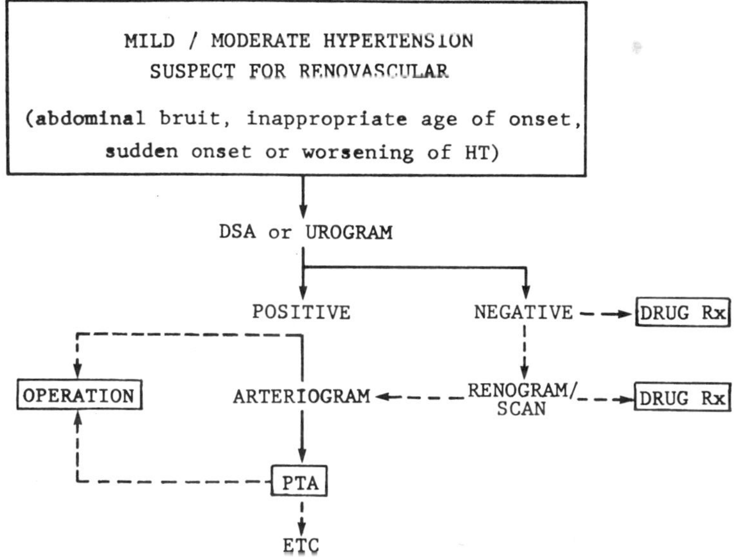

Patients With Moderate Hypertension and Not Suspected of Having RVH

Diagnostic workup in this category of patients, which represents over 75% of the hypertensive population, is most controversial. Most patients with renovascular disease do not have distinctive clinical features and resemble patients with essential hypertension. The decision as to further testing is based on clinical judgment (patient compliance, target organ damage, family history, drug side effects) and the desire of the individual patient.

We use the blood pressure response to diuretics as a gross screening test (Fig 3). Over 60% of these patients will have a

Fig 3.—Decision matrix for patients with mild or moderate hypertension and no clinical features suggestive of renovascular hypertension. The extent of testing in these patients is based on clinical circumstances and is arrived at jointly by physician and patient.

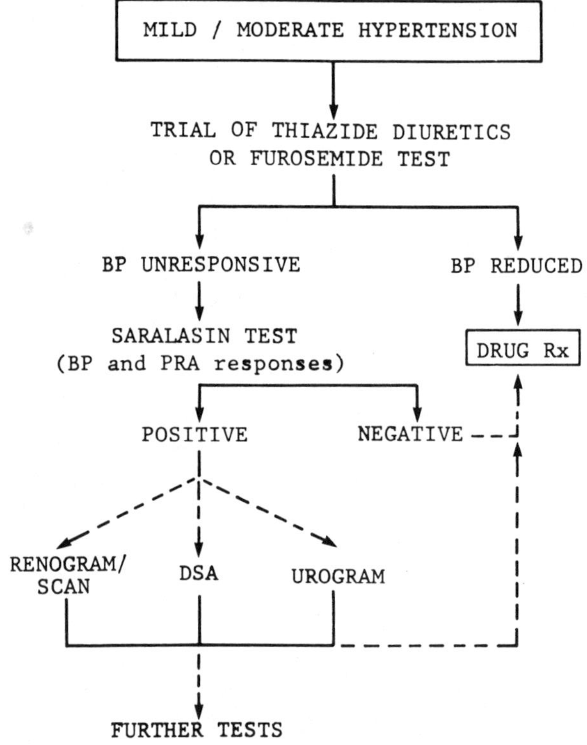

significant reduction of blood pressure following a brief period of thiazide therapy or the morning after a single oral dose of furosemide (1 mg/kg of body weight) administered the evening before.[30, 49] This responsive group is not studied further for RVH (volume-mediated hypertension?). Patients whose blood pressure fails to respond to a diuretic are more likely to have renin-dependent hypertension. Moderate sodium depletion following thiazide or furosemide administration improves the predictive value of the saralasin test, especially when PRA following saralasin administration as well as blood pressure response are used to evaluate test results.[9, 46] Thus, when there is no vasodepressor response to diuretic administration, the natriuresis will have served to prepare the patient for a saralasin bolus test.[30] Only those with a positive saralasin test result are considered for further studies for RVH. This sequence is cost-effective and avoids unnecessary invasive procedures.

The strategies described in this chapter are not intended to be exclusive or categorical. The decisions are based on particular clinical circumstances and risks as well as the likelihood of renovascular disease rather than on a fixed sequence of diagnostic tests for all patients. When the patient is at high cardiovascular risk and/or the likelihood of renovascular disease is great, then renal arteriography is used to rule out this disorder or to delineate the renal artery lesion, and the early blood pressure response to PTA determines its significance. When the likelihood of renovascular disease is lower, then standard tests are used. Obviously, further technical improvements in DSA could change these strategies.

REFERENCES

1. Arlart I., Rosenthal J., Adam W.E., et al.: Predictive value of radionuclide methods in the diagnosis of unilateral renovascular hypertension. *Cardiovasc. Radiol.* 2:115, 1979.
2. Barbaric Z., Kaufman J.J., Maxwell M.H.: Unpublished data, 1982.
3. Bergentz S.E., Ericsson B.F., Husberg B.: Technique and complications in the surgical treatment of renovascular hypertension. *Acta Chir. Scand.* 145:143, 1979.
4. Bianchi C., Donadio C., Tramonti G., et al.: Assessment of sequential scintigraphic rapid sequence pyelography and renography in the screening for renovascular hypertension. *J. Nucl. Med. Allied Sci.* 23:31, 1979.
5. Bookstein J.J., Abrams H.L., Buenger R.E., et al.: Cooperative study of renovascular hypertension: 2. The role of urography in unilateral renovascular disease. *JAMA* 220:1225, 1972.
6. Bookstein J.J. Abrams H.L., Buenger R.E., et al.: Cooperative study of renovascular hypertension: 3. Appraisal of arteriography. *JAMA* 221:368, 1979.

7. Brunner H.R., Gavras H.: Medical therapy of renovascular hypertension, in *Proceedings of the 8th International Congress of Nephrology*. Athens, 1981, p. 1135.

8. Buonocore E., Meany T.F., Borkowski G.P., et al.: Digital subtraction angiography of the abdominal aorta and renal arteries. *Radiology* 139:281, 1981.

9. Case D.B., Atlas S.A., Laragh J.H.: Reactive hyperreninaemia to angiotensin blockade identifies renovascular hypertension. *Clin. Sci.* 57:313s, 1979.

10. Cicuto K.P., McClean G.K., Oleaga J.A., et al.: Renal artery stenosis: Anatomic classification for percutaneous transluminal angioplasty. *AJR* 139:727, 1982.

11. Collapinto R.F., Stronell R.D., Harries-Jones E.P., et al.: Percutaneous transluminal dilatation of the renal artery: Follow-up studies on renovascular hypertension. *AJR* 139:727, 1982.

12. Davis B.A., Crook S.E., Vestal R.E., et al.: Prevalence of renovascular hypertension in patients with grade III or IV hypertensive retinopathy. *N. Engl. J. Med.* 301:1273, 1979.

13. Dean R.H., Lawson J.D., Hollified J.W., et al.: Revascularization of the poorly functioning kidney. *Surgery* 85:44, 1979.

14. Diamond G.A., Forrester J.S.: Clinical trials and statistical verdicts: Probable grounds for appeal. *Ann. Intern. Med.* 98:385, 1982.

15. Dustan H.P., Humphries A.W., deWolfe V.G., et al.: Normal arterial pressure in patients with renal arterial stenosis. *JAMA* 187:138, 1964.

16. Dustan H.P., Page I.H., Poutasse E.F., et al.: An evaluation of treatment of hypertension associated with occlusive renal arterial disease. *Circulation* 27:1018, 1963.

17. Eyler W.R., Clark M.D., Garman J.E., et al.: Angiography of the renal areas including a comparative study of renal arterial stenoses in patients with and without hypertension. *Radiology* 78:879, 1962.

18. Hypertension Detection and Follow-up Program Cooperative Group: Five-year findings of the Hypertension Detection and Follow-up Program: I. Reduction in mortality of persons with high blood pressure, including mild hypertension. *JAMA* 242:2562, 1979.

19. Flechner S., Novick A.C., Vidt D., et al.: The use of percutaneous transluminal angioplasty for renal artery stenosis in patients with generalized atherosclerosis. *J. Urol.* 127:1072, 1982.

20. Foster J.H., Maxwell M.H., Franklin, S.A., et al.: Renovascular occlusive disease: Results of operative treatment. *JAMA* 231:1043, 1975.

21. Franklin S.S., Young J.D. Jr., Maxwell M.H., et al.: Cooperative study of renovascular hypertension: Operative morbidity and mortality in renovascular disease. *JAMA* 231:1148, 1975.

22. Frohlich E., Maxwell M.H.: Use of saralasin as a diagnostic test in hypertension: Report of a consensus committee. *Arch. Intern. Med.* 142:1437, 1982.

23. Geyskes G.G., Puylaert C.B., Oei H.Y., et al.: Intraluminal dilatation of renal artery stenosis. *Clin. Sci.* 57(suppl. 5):441s, 1979.

24. Grim C.E., Luft F.C., Weinberger M.H., et al.: Sensitivity and specificity of screening tests for renal vascular hypertension. *Ann. Intern. Med.* 91:617, 1979.

25. Grim C.E., Luft F.C., Yune H.Y., et al.: Percutaneous transluminal dilatation in the treatment of renal vascular hypertension. *Ann. Intern. Med.* 95:439, 1981.

26. Grim C.E., Luft F.C., Yune H.Y., et al.: Balloon dilatation of renal artery stenosis causing hypertension: Contrasting cure rate by lesion type, in *Proceedings of the 8th International Congress of Nephrology*. Athens, 1981, p. 1154.

27. Griner P.F., Mayewski R.J., Mushlin A.I., et al.; Selection and interpretation of diagnostic tests and procedures. Principles and applications: Part 2. *Ann. Intern. Med.* 94:557, 1981.

28. Hillman B.J., Ovitt T.W., Capp W.P., et al.: The potential impact of digital video subtraction angiography on screening for renovascular hypertension. *Diagn. Radiol.* 142:577, 1982.

29. Hillman B.J., Ovitt T.W., Nudelman S., et al.: Digital video subtraction angiography of renovascular abnormalities. *Radiology* 139:277, 1981.

30. Hollenberg N.K., Williams G.H., Adams D.F., et al.: Response to saralasin and angiotensin's role in essential and renal hypertension. *Medicine* 58:115, 1979.
31. Holley K.E., Hunt J.C., Brown A.L. Jr., et al.: Renal artery stenosis: A clinical-pathologic study in normotensive and hypertensive patients. *Am. J. Med.* 37:14, 1964.
32. Hunt J.C., Strong C.G.: Renovascular hypertension: Mechanisms, natural history and treatment. *Am. J. Cardiol.* 32:562, 1973.
33. Kaplan N.M.: Renin profiles: The unfulfilled promises. *JAMA* 238:611, 1977.
34. Kuhlmann U., Vetter W., Furrer J., et al.: Renovascular hypertension: Treatment by percutaneous transluminal dilatation. *Ann. Intern. Med.* 92:1, 1980.
35. Kuhlmann U., Vetter W., Grüntzig A., et al.: Percutaneous transluminal dilatation of renal artery stenosis: 2 years' experience. *Clin. Sci.* 61:481S, 1981.
36. Lankford N.S., Donohue J.P., Grim C.E., et al.: Results of surgical treatment of renovascular hypertension. *J. Urol.* 122:439, 1979.
37. Laragh J.H., Baer L., Brunner H.R., et al.: Renin, angiotensin and aldosterone in pathogenesis and management of hypertensive vascular diseases. *Am. J. Med.* 52:633, 1972.
38. Madias N.E., Ball J.T., Millan V.G.: Percutaneous transluminal renal angioplasty in the treatment of unilateral atherosclerotic renovascular hypertension. *Am. J. Med.* 70:1078, 1981.
39. Mahler F., Probst P., Haertel M., et al.; Lasting improvement of renovascular hypertension by transluminal dilatation of atherosclerotic and nonatherosclerotic renal artery stenosis: A follow-up study. *Circulation* 65:611, 1982.
40. Marks L.S., Maxwell M.H.: Renal vein renin: Value and limitations in the prediction of operative results. *Urol. Clin. North Am.* 2:311, 1975.
41. Marks L.S., Maxwell M.H., Kaufman J.J.: Renin, sodium and vasodepressor response to saralasin in renovascular and essential hypertension. *Ann. Intern. Med.* 87:176, 1977.
42. Maxwell M.H.: Use of angiotensin antagonists in experimental and human renovascular hypertension, in Hamburger J., Crosnier J., Grünfeld J.P., ct al. (eds.): *Advances in Nephrology.* Chicago, Year Book Medical Publishers, 1979, pp. 297–319.
43. Maxwell M.H., Gonick H.C., Wiita R., et al.: Use of the rapid sequence intravenous pyelogram in the diagnosis of renovascular hypertension. *N Engl. J. Mcd.* 270:213, 1964.
44. Maxwell M.H., Marks L.S., Lupu A.N., et al.: Predictive value of renin determinations in renal artery stenosis. *JAMA* 238:2617, 1977.
45. Maxwell M.H., Varady P.D.: Cooperative study of renovascular hypertension, in Berlyne G.M., Giovanetti S. (eds.): *Contributions to Nephrology.* Basel, S. Karger, 1976, pp. 1–19.
46. Maxwell M.H., Varady P.D., Zawada E.T., et al.: Maximal discrimination of renovascular from essential hypertension by the saralasin test. *Clin. Sci.* 55:297s, 1978.
47. Maxwell M.H., Waks A.U.: Application of diagnostic procedures in patient management, in van Schilfgaarde R., Stanley J.C., van Brummelen P., et al. (eds.): *Clinical Aspects of Renovascular Hypertension.* Boston, Martinus Nijhoff, 1983, pp. 74–95.
48. Maxwell M.H., Waks A.U.: Strategies in renovascular hypertension: The real world. *Hypertension,* to be published.
49. Maxwell M.H., Waks A.U., Burkhalter J.F.: Blood pressure response to furosemide: Initial screening test for renovascular hypertension, in *Abstracts of the Fifth Scientific Meeting of the International Society of Hypertension.* Paris, 1978, p. 174.
50. McNair A., Neilsen M.D., Gammelgaard P.A., et al.: A follow-up study of hypertensive patients after operative treatment of unilateral renovascular or renal disease. *Acta Med. Scand.* 205:569, 1979.
51. McNeil, B.J., Varady P.D., Burrows B.A., et al.: Measures of clinical efficacy. *N. Engl. J. Med.* 293:216, 1975.

52. Meaney T.F., Dustan H.P., McCormach L.J.: Natural history of renal arterial disease. *Radiology* 91:881, 1968.
53. Meyers J.D., Murdaugh H.V., McIntosh H.D.: Observations on continuous murmurs over partially occluded arteries. *Arch. Intern. Med.* 97:726, 1956.
54. Nordhus O., Ekeström S., Liljeqvist L., et al.: Renal artery reconstruction in renovascular hypertension. *Scand. J. Thorac. Cardiovasc. Surg.* 12:111, 1978.
55. Pinedo H.M., DeGraeff J., Struyvenberg A.: Prognosis in arteriosclerotic renovascular hypertension. *Clin. Sci.* 45(suppl. 2):309s, 1973.
56. Pinkerton J.A. Jr., Crouch T.T., Sharma J.N.: Surgical treatment of renovascular hypertension. *Am. J. Surg.* 138:759, 1979.
57. Polterauer P., Dean R.H., Hollifield J.W.: Surgical treatment of renovascular hypertension: Results of operation in 400 patients with renal artery stenosis. *Wien. Klin. Wochenschr.* 92:433, 1980.
58. Poutasse E.F., Dustan H.P.: Arteriosclerosis and renal hypertension: Indications for aortography in hypertensive patients and results of surgical treatment of obstructive lesions of the renal artery. *JAMA* 165:1521, 1957.
59. Reiss M.D., Bookstein J.J., Bleifer K.H.: Radiologic aspects of renovascular hypertension: Part 4. Arteriographic complications. *JAMA* 221:374, 1972.
60. Rudnick M.R., Maxwell M.H.: Diagnosis of renovascular hypertension: Limitations of renin assays, in Narins R. (ed.): *Controversies in Nephrology and Hypertension.* New York, Churchill Livingstone, to be published.
61. Schwarten D.E., Yune H.Y., Latte E.C., et al.: Clinical experience with percutaneous transluminal angioplasty (PTA) of stenotic renal arteries. *Radiology* 135:601, 1980.
62. Simon N., Franklin S.A., Bleifer K.H., et al.: Cooperative study of renovascular hypertension: Clinical characteristics of renovascular hypertension. *JAMA* 220:1209, 1972.
63. Sos T.A., Pickering T.G., Sniderman K., et al.: Percutaneous transluminal renal angioplasty in renovascualr hypertension due to atheroma or fibromuscular dysplasia. *N. Engl. J. Med.* 309:274, 1983.
64. Stanley J.C., Fry W.V.: Surgical treatment of renovascular hypertension. *Arch. Surg.* 112:1291, 1977.
65. Starr D.S., Lawrie G.M., Morris G.C. Jr.: Surgical treatment of renovascular hypertension: Long-term follow-up of 216 patients up to 20 years. *Arch. Surg.* 115:494, 1980.
66. Stefanini P., Benedetti-Valentini F. Jr., Fiorani P.: Selection for surgery and long-term results in renovascular hypertension. *Int. Surg.* 63:73, 1978.
67. Stoney R.J., Silane M., Salvatiera O. Jr.: Ex vivo renal artery reconstruction. *Arch. Surg.* 113:1272, 1978.
68. Streeten D.H.P., Anderson G.A., Sunderlin F.S. Jr., et al.: Identifying renin participation in hypertensive patients, in Laragh J.H., Buhler F.R., Seldin D.W. (eds.): *Frontiers in Hypertension Research.* New York, Springer-Verlag, 1981, pp. 204–211.
69. Tegtmeyer C.J.: Percutaneous transluminal renal angioplasty. The evolution of a procedure, editorial. *Arch. Intern. Med.* 142:1085, 1982.
70. Tegtmeyer C.J., Dyer R., Teates C.D., et al.: Percutaneous transluminal dilatation of the renal arteries: Techniques and results. *Radiology* 135:589, 1980.
71. Tegtmeyer C.J. Elson J., Glass T.A., et al.: Percutaneous transluminal angioplasty: The treatment of choice for renovascular hypertension due to fibromuscular dysplasia. *Radiology* 143:631, 1982.
72. Vetter W., Wetter H., Tenschert W., et al.: Renovascular hypertension: Prognostic value of renal venous renin determinations. *Klin. Wochenschr.* 57:863, 1979.
73. Wilson H.M., Wilson J.P., Slaton P.E., et al.: Saralasin infusion in the recognition of renovascular hypertension. *Ann. Intern. Med.* 87:36, 1977.
74. Witten D.M.: Reactions to urographic contrast media. *JAMA* 231:974, 1975.

Recent Advances on the Mechanisms and Genetic Aspects of Lupus Erythematosus

ALFRED D. STEINBERG, M.D.

*Chief, Section on Cellular Immunology, ARB, NIADDK, National Institutes of Health;
Medical Director, U.S. Public Health Service, Bethesda, Md.*

SYSTEMIC LUPUS ERYTHEMATOSUS (SLE) appears to be a disorder in which multiple factors combine to determine whether or not disease will be expressed, and to what extent. In some individuals, the genetic predisposition may be so strong that trivial environmental factors or no environmental factors may be necessary for the disease to be expressed. In other individuals, the genetic predisposition may be modest and moderately strong environmental factors may be required for disease expression. Additional factors, such as sex hormone metabolism and the state of the immune system, may be sufficient to allow or prevent disease expression. Clues to the multifactorial nature of SLE in a given individual and to the differing factors in different individuals come from studies of mice that spontaneously develop SLE.

Murine Systemic Lupus

The genetic basis for illness may be different in different mice with lupus (Table 1). The most commonly studied mice have been the New Zealand black (NZB), (NZB × NZW) F₁,

0084-5957/84/0014-0305-0332-$04.00

TABLE 1.—HETEROGENEITY OF MURINE LUPUS

FEATURE	NZB	(NZB × NZW)F$_1$	MRL-MP/lpr/lpr	BXSB
Genetic	At least 6 autosomal genes	Multiple genes, some from NZW	Multiple background genes, lpr major accelerator	Multple background genes, Y chromosome gene major accelerator
Major histocompatibility	d/d	d/z	k/k	b/b
Sex	Little effect Recessive gene for androgen insensitivity	Marked effect Androgens protect Estrogens worsen	Androgens protect slightly	Marked acceleration in males, not hormonal
Immunoglobulins	↑ IgM	↑ IgM, ↑ IgG$_2$	↑ IgG$_1$, ↑ IgG2a	↑ IgG$_1$, ↑ IgG2b
Lymphoid organs	Lymphoid hyperplasia	Lymphoid hyperplasia	Marked ↑ T cells	Moderate ↑ B cells
Effects of *xid*	Prevents disease	Prevents disease	Retards disease	Prevents disease
Disease manifestations	Anti-T cell antibodies Coombs-positive hemolytic anemia Late-life renal disease Splenic hyperdiploidy Death occurs after 1 year	Anti-DNA, LE cells Membranoproliferative glomerulonephritis Sjögren's syndrome Females die in first year of life	Marked lymphadenopathy Anti-DNA, anti-Sm Arthritis and anti-Ig Membranoproliferative glomerulonephritis Vasculitis Males and females die in first year of life	Immune complex glomerulonephritis Degenerative coronary artery disease Serologically less abnormal than others Moderate adenopathy Males die in first year of life

MRL-lpr/lpr, and BXSB strains.[59, 87, 96, 105] These mice have differences in pace of illness and sex hormone effects. The BXSB mice have a male-oriented illness; the males have accelerated disease relative to the females. Some factor associated with the Y chromosome of the BXSB mouse appears to be responsible. Sex hormones are not able to reverse this male disease.[17] However, whereas the BXSB Y chromosome leads to disease in BXSB mice and in male offspring of BXSB males and autoimmune-prone females, BXSB Y chromosome does not lead to accelerated disease in offspring of BXSB males and non-autoimmune-prone females.[18, 96] Therefore, the BXSB Y chromosome factor is an accelerating factor rather than a lupus-inducing factor. Another accelerating factor is the lpr gene. Originally described on the MRL background, this gene has now been bred onto many backgrounds.[59] In homozygous form, this gene leads to lymphoproliferation. The proliferating cell is a dull Ly 1^+ T cell (helper phenotype).[55] Eventually, massive lymphadenopathy and splenomegaly result. Female sex hormones are an accelerating factor and androgens a retarding factor in (NZB × NBW) F_1 mice.[77, 98] Females experience a much more rapid onset of disease and earlier death than their brothers; however, that difference can be reversed by opposite sex hormone treatment. NZB mice tend to have late-onset "middle-age" lupus, with only a small difference between males and females. Some of these features are summarized in Table 2.

Of considerable interest are mice about which little has been written. (NZB × normal) F_1 mice have milder disease than either parent. This stands in contrast to the (NZB × NZW) F_1 female, which has more severe disease than either parent. Thus, gene interactions may give rise to either accelerated or retarded disease in offspring. These results have particular importance for human family and population studies. In addition, it is clear that high titers of autoantibodies may be associated with a normal life span without therapy in mice.

A careful analysis of the genetic basis for disease in NZB mice by use of F_1 and backcross mice has indicated that genes for anti-DNA and anti-T cell antibodies are unlinked and coded for by single dominant or codominant genes.[73] Additional genes from the NZW mouse contribute to disease in the (NZB × NZW) F_1. More recently, studies of recombinant inbred lines of mice derived originally from NZD and normals have indicated

TABLE 2.—GENETICS OF MURINE AUTOIMMUNITY: RELATIONSHIP TO HUMAN SLE

MOUSE STRAIN	MURINE SYSTEM	HUMAN SLE
NZB	Inherited autoimmune traits with a lack of sex differences[96]	Familial incidence of SLE[5] Concordance in identical twins[7]
F_1 hybrids with NZB	Androgens suppress and mask genetic mechanisms[73, 98]	Female predominance in SLE[5, 7]
BXSB	Male-linked inheritance[87, 96, 105]	Inheritance of male-predominant SLE[44]
Recombinant inbred lines of NZB × Normal	Independent inheritance of many autoimmune traits[71]	Familial members of SLE patients develop some autoimmune features without clinical SLE[52, 58, 75]
F_1 and backcross analysis	Dominant and recessive inheritance of autoimmune traits with additional modifying genes; many genes show gene dosage effects[73]	Dominant inheritance of ANA and anti-ssDNA[48]; two genes may give greater abnormality than one[75]
Modifying factors *xid* gene retards	Prediposing factors[87, 96, 105] Retarding factors[87, 100–102, 104]	B cell hyperactivity in SLE[6, 9, 25, 38]

that multiple genes are responsible for the full disease of NZB mice. At least six genes contribute to the disease of NZB mice.[71] A similar analysis of background genes in MRL and BXSB mice would be helpful. In addition to the above, congenital factors other than mammalian genes may be critical to the expression of disease. An oncornavirus may cause accelerated disease by virtue of increasing the load of pathogenic immune complexes.[16, 50] Thus, such a virus in an animal with a defect in tolerance could induce antiviral antibodies and exacerbate immune complex–mediated disease. Although such a virus is not necessary for disease,[110] it could be a factor, similar to what is seen in other viral infections.[107] Another factor is a maternally transmitted antigen that is present in some, but not all, mice. This antigen may result from cytoplasmic genetic material that is passed on from the mother's egg. Mice with the antigen may be protected from the full expression of autoimmune disease.

A detailed analysis of the cellular basis for illness in the different strains of mice that develop lupus is beyond the scope of this chapter. Nevertheless, it is helpful to point out some of the findings. The role of the thymus in retarding or preventing disease in the different strains may be very different. Neonatal thymectomy of MRL-lpr/lpr mice has a profoundly ameliorating effect on disease. These mice, which ordinarily die at about age 6 months, are essentially cured by neonatal thymectomy.[99] In contrast, neonatal thymectomy causes accelerated disease in BXSB males.[88] In our studies, neonatal thymectomy had a less dramatic retarding effect in NZB mice and an accelerating effect in (NZB × NZW) F_1 mice. Thus, the mouse strains must differ in terms of the cellular basis for illness if neonatal thymectomy can have such dramatically different effects in the different strains. These differences are explainable. The proliferation observed in MRL-lpr/lpr mice is primarily one of T cells. These T cells cannot proliferate without a thymus; therefore, neonatal thymectomy prevents disease. A corollary is that the autoantibody production is T cell dependent. In contrast, most proliferation in BXSB mice is of B cells. The thymus ordinarily holds in check the proliferation of these B cells, albeit not completely. Neonatal thymectomy allows the B cells to proliferate in an uninhibited fashion, giving rise to massive lymphoproliferation and markedly increased autoantibody production.

Immune Abnormalities that Lead to Disease Versus Those that Result From Disease

It is relatively easy to study individual mice prior to the onset of clinical illness and then after illness occurs. Such studies clearly indicate that there are many immune abnormalities. However, those that are found at the time of clinical illness may not be those that set off the process. This concept is especially important because patients with SLE are rarely studied prior to the onset of symptoms, and therefore abnormalities observed at the time of active disease are given great importance with regard to pathogenesis of the disorder. Some of these may in fact serve to perpetuate the disease process but may not have been important in its initiation. For example, antigen nonspecific suppressor function falls prematurely early in the life of the (NZB $\times$ NZW) F_1 mouse but rises abnormally after the onset of disease.[70] It is possible that the abnormality observed at the time of illness—increased suppression—is important in perpetuating the process; however, it has nothing to do with its initiation. In fact, the increased suppressor function probably results from the markedly increased immune reactivity which is observed as autoimmune disease. The marked hyperactivity is, however, not adequately controlled by the reactive suppressor factors.

What can be said of the early abnormalities of mice with murine lupus? In general, it appears that all have a stem cell disorder. That is, they have defects which may be expressed in mature cells of the immune system but which are encoded in the stem cells and can be transferred with stem cells.[3, 15, 18, 56, 57] The precise defects may be different in the different mice. For example, a defect associated with T cell proliferation is associated with MRL-lpr/lpr stem cells.[69, 85] Similarly, a defect for interference with normal tolerance is characteristic of NZB pre-T cell stem cells.[46] In both cases, the stem cells must be acted on by a thymus for the defect to be expressed. In contrast, non-T cells appear to be critical to the failure of normal tolerance and disease expression in the BXSB male.[28] Thus, the defects in the mature lymphoid cells may differ even though the information for the defects may be present in the stem cells in all of the mice.

Many abnormalities are observed late in the course of disease. These include autoantibody production, immune complex–mediated renal disease, impaired responsiveness to T cell mitogens, impaired IL2 production, and impaired immune responsiveness to exogenous stimulation, found in association with vigorous immune activity during the course of the autoimmune process. In other words, at the same time that there is vigorous B cell activity and production of autoantibodies, immune responsiveness to stimulation with nonspecific mitogens or foreign antigens may be markedly impaired. This paradox may be viewed teleologically as follows: the body is preoccupied making autoantibodies and autoimmune responses and cannot be bothered with the new stimuli. At a more mechanistic level, two explanations are available. First, the autoimmune process leads to the production of vigorous immunosuppressive signals that impair the responses to foreign antigens and mitogens. Second, the pre-B cell stem cell pool is preempted by the maturation into autoantibody-producing cells and the T cells are functionally inactivated by suppressor factors, many secreted by nonlymphoid mononuclear cells. These two explanations are not mutually exclusive. Additional factors occur in some but not all individuals: anti-T cell antibodies interfere with T cell regulation. These various defects may be partly overcome by treatment with immunosuppressive regimens (including corticosteroids and cyclophosphamide) to restore more normal immune system function. Therefore, the problem is not just a deficiency of adequate numbers of particular lymphocytes but active interference with normal cellular function.

Human SLE: An Approach Based on Murine Studies

In the next several sections, information regarding human SLE lymphocytes will be put forth. An attempt will be made to consider the data from the perspective derived from the murine studies. This perspective includes the idea that different individuals with SLE may have different genetic and cellular bases for illness, that immune abnormalities observed during the course of active disease may not be those that induced the disease, and that many immune abnormalities may actually result from the disease process. Finally, it must be appreciated throughout that most studies of humans have been limited to sampling of peripheral blood, whereas in animals lymphoid organs such as spleen and lymph nodes have been studied and sophisticated transfer experiments between animals have been conducted.

LYMPHOID CELLS IN PATIENTS WITH SLE

Patients with active SLE often have leukopenia.[72] Although this leukopenia is accounted for on an absolute basis primarily by a reduction in granulocytes, there is also an absolute reduction in lymphocytes. Thus, there is the paradox of an increased percentage of lymphocytes in the differential but a decreased absolute number of lymphocytes per cubic millimeter of peripheral blood. Individuals vary greatly. Some patients have leukocytosis, even without steroid therapy. Others have profound leukopenia that may actually improve with immunosuppressive drug therapy.

Peripheral blood lymphocyte counts may be greatly depressed, in the normal range, or increased. In active disease, the average lymphocyte count is reduced approximately 70%, with approximately equal reductions in B and T cells.[25, 72] This leads to a relative increase in the numbers of cells of the monocyte-macrophage series. In other words, patients with SLE have a relative decrease in lymphocytes among their peripheral blood mononuclear cells (Table 3). Therefore, if studies are performed on peripheral blood mononuclear cells (without further cell separation), there will be a relatively stronger influence of the nonlymphoid cells. This is especially important because such cells may exert profound suppressive influences.[37, 93] A variety of in vitro tests may record impaired immune function solely because of this relative increase in monocyte-macrophages.

B CELL FUNCTIONS IN SLE

Patients with active SLE are characterized by hypergammaglobulinemia and the production of large amounts of various autoantibodies. Such patients have circulating cells, resembling activated lymphocytes,[12, 13, 40, 51] which are able to produce immunoglobulin after removal from the blood.[34] Such antibody-forming cells have been studied by a reverse hemolytic plaque technique that allows enumeration of immunoglobulin-

TABLE 3.—IMMUNE ABNORMALITIES IN SLE PATIENTS*

IMMUNE MEASURES	ACTIVE DISEASE	INACTIVE DISEASE
Lymphopenia	+ + + + ↓	+ ↓
Absolute numbers of T cells	+ + + + ↓	+ ↓
Absolute numbers of B cells	+ + + ↓	0
Percentage of T cells	+ + ↓	± ↓
Percentage of B cells	+ + ↑	+ ↑
Percentage of TG cells	+ + + ↓	± ↓
Skin tests	+ + + + ↓	+ ↓
Responses to ConA (proliferation; other)	+ + + + ↓	+ + ↓
Responses to phytohemagglutinin	+ + + ↓	+ ↓
Responses to pokeweed mitogen	+ + + ↓	+ ↓
Suppressor function (T cell)	+ + + + ↓	+ ↓
Monocyte-macrophage suppression	+ + ↑	+ ↑
Helper T cell function	+ + + + ↓	+ ↓
B cell proliferation (spontaneous)	+ + + ↑	+ + ↑
B cell differentiation (Ig production)	+ + + + ↑	+ ↑
Marrow proliferation	+ + + ↑	+ ↑
Natural killer cell activity	+ + + ↓	+ ↓

*Since human SLE is very heterogeneous and patients differ markedly, these generalizations apply to the majority of patients; exceptions are found. ↑ = increase; ↓ = decrease; 0 = no change; + = small; + + = moderate; + + + = large; + + + + = very large. All comparisons are with normals.

secreting cells of different classes. These studies have demonstrated a marked increase in immunoglobulin-secreting cells in patients with active SLE.[6, 23, 103] Of interest, IgG and IgA antibody-forming cells were markedly increased, whereas IgM antibody-forming cells often were not.[6, 23] Moreover, the degree of increase in antibody-secreting cells was highly correlated with disease activity.[6] Of interest, numbers of IgG-secreting cells correlated better with disease activity than did levels of anti-DNA, C3, and other classic serologic measures.[100] Moreover, the immunoglobulin-secreting cells correlated in that study with multisystem disease activity, but not with major organ involvement. In other words, arthritis and serositis were as likely to be associated with large numbers of IgG-secreting cells as renal or CNS disease (the latter were associated only if the disease was recently reactivated).

It might be anticipated from the preceding comments that all of the immunoglobulin-secreting cells were secreting autoantibodies. Although this is possible, it has been found that patients with active SLE have immunoglobulin-secreting cells of many different specificities,[9, 19, 53] many of them being chemical haptens to which the patients might not be expected to have been exposed.[9, 53] These results suggest that the patients are polyclonally activated and that not all the antibodies are directed at autoantigens (see Table 3). One caveat remains: it is possible that unexpected cross-reactivities between the chemical haptens mask the true hyperproduction of only autoantibodies. Although I believe this is not a likely explanation, recent studies on the cross-reactivity of monoclonal antibodies leaves open the possibility.[2, 42, 86]

Thus, we find that patients with active SLE manifest large amounts of antibody production, much of which is autoantibody. The exact amount of autoantibody is difficult to quantify in many patients. As much as 4 mg/ml anti-DNA has been found in the serum of a patient with active SLE.[97] It is possible that some patients have enormous amounts of autoantibody, which could account for the majority of their excessive immunoglobulin production.

Despite the known hypergammaglobulinemia and increase in spontaneous antibody-forming cells, the greater the disease activity, the poorer the response of SLE mononuclear cells to stimulation with the B cell mitogen, pokeweed mitogen.[8, 103] In fact, patients with active SLE frequently have impaired B cell responses relative to normals. The basis for the impairment is complex; however, the phenomenon is only superficially paradoxical. It is clear that patients with active SLE have in vivo activation of cells. It is not really a great surprise that such cells cannot be activated in vitro. If many cells have already proliferated and differentiated in vivo, they will be unable to provide much of a contribution following in vitro stimulation. Moreover, macrophages can suppress the responses in SLE or in T cell populations in vitro.

Some authors have emphasized the known requirement for helper T cells in the pokeweed response of B cells and the defective helper T cell function of patients with SLE,[14, 103] which will be discussed below. Stimulation with a T cell–independent B cell mitogen elicited a relatively normal response in a few patients.[103] Therefore, it is possible that multiple mechanisms may be responsible for the impaired B cell responses in vitro. Drs. Jane Grayson, R. Michael Blaese, and I followed a few such patients with active SLE and impaired responsiveness to pokeweed mitogen. We found that in a given patient, different mechanisms of impaired responsiveness predominated at different times, despite no change in either disease activity or treatment.

Like many of the in vitro studies, in vivo studies of patients' B cell functions are affected by changes in other cell populations. This may explain the lack of uniform results. Patients have had normal or decreased antibody titers following immunization with influenza vaccine.[109] The primary responses were much more blunted than the secondary responses. Similar results were obtained following immunization with *Brucella* and with KLH antigens. In these studies, IgG responses were normal, but IgM responses were subnormal. This is consistent with an impaired primary response and a normal secondary response; however, it could represent a defect specifically in IgM responses. A number of publications have emphasized the elevated titers of antibody reactive with a variety of viral antigens; however, not all of these elevations may be real, as some of the assays allow SLE autoantibodies to react with cellular materials in the viral antigen preparations so as to yield a false positive test.[66] Moreover, since SLE patients have preferential decreases in IgM responses, any assay that is especially sensitive to IgM antibody (e.g., hemagglutination or hemolysis) might show a decreased titer due to the particular class of antibody produced.

The in vivo studies suggest that patients with active SLE have impaired primary and IgM antibody responses to immunization but normal or even elevated secondary and IgG responses. A similar impairment of primary responses with normal secondary responses have been observed in the NZB mouse model of SLE[22, 96, 105] with regard to both antibody production and skin graft survival. It appears that for both mice and humans, two explanations are available. One is that the ongoing autoimmune response leads to production of nonspecific suppressor factors, as in antigenic competition.[1] This phenomenon is mediated by suppressor cells and can be eliminated with low doses of cyclophosphamide. The second explanation involves the known defects in helper T cell functions, functions which may be necessary to a much greater extent in primary than in secondary responses (e.g., growth factor production). Moreover, primary responses are much more easily suppressed than secondary responses. Therefore, multiple immunizations may be necessary to achieve the desired antibody response.

Studies of B cell proliferation, as opposed to immunoglobulin secretion, have also provided important information regarding the B cell functions in SLE. Patients with active SLE often have B cells with impaired proliferative responses to pokeweed mitogen in vitro, a defect that may relate to impaired T cell help. Much more interesting are studies of spontaneous proliferation, since such studies might provide a clue to the in vivo situation.

A much greater degree of spontaneous proliferation of SLE B cell–enriched fractions was observed when cells were studied right out of the body than after 3 days in culture.[25, 26] Of interest in that study, patients with inactive SLE demonstrated as much proliferation as patients with active SLE. Therefore, the difference between inactive SLE and active SLE appears to be a signal that induces the B cells to start to differentiate into immunoglobulin-secreting cells. However, such a signal takes place in the context of already proliferating B cells. Therefore, activation does not require a signal for proliferation, only one for differentiation. It is possible that SLE B cells are more susceptible to such a trigger because of altered membrane potential or because of an increase in the number of receptors for T cell factors.

Patients who go into prolonged remission may revert toward normal and then require signals for both proliferation and differentiation in order for B cell hyperactivity to develop.

Recent studies of stem cells in SLE suggest that the B cell hyperactivity has a basis in increased stem cell activity. Patients with SLE were found to have increased numbers of B cell colony-forming cells.[38] This increase was independent of T cell function; in fact, the ability of SLE T cells to support colonies was impaired. More recent studies by Dr. Carl Laskin (unpublished data) have indicated that marrow stem cells from patients with active SLE show a fivefold increase in number at the end of 1 week in Dexter cultures in vitro.

T CELL FUNCTIONS IN SLE

A very large number of studies have evaluated T cells and T cell functions. The first question is whether or not the amazing B cell hyperproliferation and hypersecretion are related to abnormally active T cell help. Many years ago we attempted to answer this question in collaboration with Dr. T. Waldmann and found that patients with active SLE had markedly impaired help for polyclonal immunoglobulin production (unpublished studies). More recently, similar observations have been published.[14] It therefore appears that in the majority of patients, excess T cell help is not present at the time of B cell hyperactivity. Whether or not such decreased T cell help precedes the B cell hyperactivity is unknown; however, it does not appear to be likely. Therefore, on the basis of in vitro studies, one would have to attribute the B cell hyperactivity more to abnormal responsiveness of the B cells than to excessive help from the T cells (see Table 3).

In addition to helper T cell function, suppressor T cell function could be abnormal and fail to hold in check the excessive B cell activity. A number of studies have attempted to demonstrate impaired suppressor T cell function. Many papers have been written demonstrating that patients with SLE have impaired concanavalin (ConA)-induced T suppressor function.[72] However, even when such has been reported, the individual patients differ among themselves with regard to this type of defect; moreover, some patients have a defect in one function and not another.[82] As a result, there appears to be substantial functional heterogeneity. Others have claimed that there is no such defect, largely by calling into question the ConA-induced suppressor system.[60] This may be a premature negation, since defects in suppressor function in SLE may be observed in the absence of ConA.[40] In addition, the immune system is more complex than a simple accumulation of helper and suppressor cells. It appears that inducer cells are necessary for suppressor cells to become functional. Thus, T4$^+$ inducer cells are necessary to activate T8$^+$ suppressor cell precursors to become suppressor effector cells.[76, 106] As a result, a patient with SLE could have a defect in T8$^+$ cells (at the precursor or effector stage) and impaired function. Alternatively, a patient may have impaired inducer cells. In the absence of adequate T4$^+$ suppressor inducer function, suppressor function would be impaired even with an intact T8$^+$ suppressor system. In fact, recent studies suggest that patients with SLE may be quite heterogeneous in terms of the T cell defects they manifest. Some of these defects may not represent a primary problem but may be secondary to the anti-T cell antibodies produced by patients with SLE (see below).

Consistent with the possibility that SLE patients may have different functional abnormalities is the observation that some patients with SLE may have high, low, or normal ratios of T4[+] to T8[+] cells.[90] Those with high ratios appear to have clinical disease features different from those with low ratios. Thus, SLE may not be a single illness in which we can hope to find a single mechanism of cellular dysfunction. Rather, it may be a syndrome with different cellular bases. Therefore, different individuals may have different T cell dysfunctions.

Another type of T cell subdivision is division into T cells that bind autologous erythrocytes (Tar) and those that do not. The ability to bind autologous RBCs appears not to relate to any kind of self-recognition, since heterologous RBCs are bound as well as autologous RBCs.[94] Nevertheless, the cells that bind human RBCs do seem to have special functional properties. These Tar cells are highly enriched in a suppressor function.[40, 63] Moreover, anti-T cell antibodies from patients with active SLE may preferentially eliminate such cells and their function.[39, 40] As a result, it appears that anti-T cell antibodies may be important in many of the functional abnormalities in SLE T cell populations (see below).

In addition to impaired helper and suppressor functions, SLE T cells appear to be inadequate in other areas.[65, 72] Patients with active SLE have markedly impaired dermal responses to recall antigens[27] and have impaired sensitization.[32, 45] Since SLE patients have circulating T cell lymphopenia, it is possible that these deficiencies merely reflect reduced numbers of T cells. We and others have observed restoration of many skin test responses following low-dose oral immunosuppressive drug treatment, suggesting that part of the impairment is due to suppressor efforts which are counteracted by the drugs. However, the dermal response to tuberculin is impaired even in relatively inactive patients with reasonable lymphocyte numbers, suggesting a more severe abnormality.[72] In fact, studies have demonstrated a specific defect in responsiveness to mycobacteria.[108]

Recent advances in cellular immunology have demonstrated that many of the cell interactions observed over the past 15 years or more do not arise from cells touching each other, but rather from the first cell elaborating a soluble factor that is able to bind to a receptor on the second cell so as to trigger it.

The factors produced by lymphocytes are called lymphokines, and those produced by monocytes are called monokines. These factors appear to be abnormally produced by the cells in many SLE patients. Thus, SLE patients have abnormally increased production of interferon[31] and impaired production of the monokine IL1 and the lymphokine IL2.[4, 33] Since these latter factors are necessary for normal T cell activation and function, it is likely that some of the defects ascribed to the T cells of SLE patients may have a biochemical basis in a deficiency of adequate stimulatory signals. Since antibodies to interferon have been described in SLE,[64] it is possible that some of these deficiencies result from, rather than cause, that autoimmune problem.

ANTI-T CELL ANTIBODIES

Initially viewed as a curiosity, anti-T cell antibodies were subsequently held responsible for many abnormalities of SLE T cells, were again exonerated, and more recently were again held accountable. Patients with SLE produce a great variety of autoantibodies, some of which react with leukocytes. Some of these are specific for T lymphocytes or their subsets. The most easily demonstrated anti-T cell antibodies are cold-reactive IgM antibodies. These have been shown to be capable of specifically eliminating T cells necessary for suppressor function.[79, 83] However, it has been argued that at body temperature, such antibodies would not be able to have any effect. This argument is specious. Although the IgM antibodies may not induce complement-mediated lysis at body temperature, they could certainly alter T cell recirculation patterns and cause the T cells to be eliminated by the reticuloendothelial system. This problem has been largely resolved by the discovery of IgG anti-T cell antibodies capable of eliminating suppressor function by the mechanism of antibody-dependent direct cellular cytotoxicity (ADCC).[39, 62] Since this is a likely mechanism for tissue injury in many immune system—mediated diseases, such antibodies could plausibly be capable of eliminating T cell in vivo.

In addition to the initial studies demonstrating that SLE anti-T cell antibodies are capable of eliminating suppressor T cell function, it has been found that such antibodies may preferentially kill Tar cells and eliminate their suppressor function[39, 40] and that an SLE antibody may eliminate T cell suppressor inducer (T4) cells or suppressor effector (T8) cells, with resulting impaired suppressor function for immunoglobulin synthesis.[54] This finding suggests two mechanisms by which anti-T cell antibodies could interfere with suppressor function and allow unhindered immunoglobulin synthesis, as well as resolving the problem of some of the antibodies reacting with T4 cells. Since Ia^+ T cells tend to include $T8^+$ cells preferentially,[35] it is possible that anti-Ia antibodies found in patients with SLE may contribute to a selective loss of T cell subsets. In addition, anti-Ia antibodies could prevent T cell activation in vivo, which would help to explain impaired T cell functions in general.

Natural Killer Cells

Natural killer (NK) cells are cells that are related to T cells by virtue of surface membrane characteristics and the ability to kill target cells. Unlike cytotoxic T cells, NK cells do not require prior sensitization to the target cell determinants in order to kill it. Unlike cells mediating ADCC, the NK cell does not require the target cell to be coated by antibody. Nevertheless, the exact interrelationships among NK activity, ADCC, and cytotoxic T cells remain to be worked out. Of special note, NK cells appear to be unusual in having a positive feedback loop in which pre-NK cells are induced to become NK cells in the presence of interferon and the resulting cells produce interferon so as to recruit more NK cells from precursors. This phenomenon is of special interest in SLE, since many patients spontaneously produce large amounts of interferon during the course of active disease.

Patients with SLE have been reported to be deficient in NK activity. This is somewhat surprising, in view of the increase in interferon produced by many patients with SLE. However, a careful analysis by Katz et al.[36] has demonstrated that patients with SLE have a defect in NK activity which is secondary to a deficiency in the NK cell's capacity to kill bound target cells. Since interferon is known to make target cells more resistant to such NK killing, increased interferon production by SLE cells could be one explanation. Effects of antilymphocyte antibodies, previously reported to interfere with NK cell activity in

SLE, were not found in that study to interfere. Of interest, only the patients with active disease were found to be defective; those with inactive disease had normal NK cell activity.

NK cells are known to be well endowed with Fc receptors, which are capable of binding immune complexes. The association of increased disease activity and decreased NK function could reflect the binding of immune complexes by NK cells and the resultant decreased function. Nevertheless, studies specifically investigated this possibility and excluded it.[36] Not appreciated is the possibility that the most efficient NK cells were already inactivated and eliminated in vivo. This point was raised, however, by another group, who reported that patients with SLE had a decrease in NK activity that correlated with disease activity and also impaired augmentation of NK activity by interferon and virus-induced interferon.[61] Moreover, patients sometimes showed a dissociation among these functions, suggesting that the NK cells might have one or more defects in different patients. The failure of SLE NK cells to be stimulated by interferon[20, 61] is reminiscent of the failure of SLE T cells and B cells to be easily stimulated in vitro (see above). A recent study has confirmed the impaired NK activity in patients with active SLE as well as in patients followed serially.[87] In addition, the NK cells failed to respond well to interferon inducers, even if the baseline NK activity was in the normal range. The investigators found a normal ability of SLE cells to form effector target conjugates; however, the SLE NK cells failed adequately to produce a soluble cytotoxic factor necessary for lysis of the target. Whatever the mechanism of decreased NK activity in patients with active SLE, this deficiency could provide another reason for increased susceptibility to certain types of infections in patients with active disease.

The Autologous Mixed Lymphocyte Reaction

T lymphocytes from normal people are capable of mounting a vigorous proliferative response when cocultured with allogeneic non-T cells (cells from unrelated individuals). This reaction is called the mixed lymphocyte reaction and is conveniently studied by treating the stimulatory population in such a manner that it cannot contribute to the reaction being observed. Patients with SLE often manifest a defect in this reaction, especially when the disease is active.[72]

A somewhat related reaction is the responsiveness of T cells to stimulation by autologous non-T cells, called the autologous mixed lymphocyte reaction (AMLR). The AMLR has been demonstrated in both experimental animal and human cell systems; however, it has often been regarded as a curious reaction. Moreover, substantial controversy has existed regarding its existence in view of the presence of foreign materials (xenogeneic erythrocytes or fetal bovine serum or antibodies) used in cell separations or to support the culture growth. Most workers in the field not only believe that the AMLR is real, but that it provides an important insight into normal cell-cell interactions. Moreover, this reaction is defective in murine lupus and in many immune system–mediated diseases.[24, 30, 89]

In the AMLR, T cells proliferate in response to autologous non-T cells.[29, 41] The proliferating T cells are of the T4[+] and the T8[+] phenotype; however, the T8[+] cells require help from the T4[+] cells.[10, 92] This help can be replaced by IL2.[91, 92] The proliferating cells ultimately can provide help or suppression for immunoglobulin synthesis and can mount cytotoxic reactions.[21] Thus, the reaction represents a mirror of normal cell-cell interactions that might be operative in vivo. These interactions are known to be defective in patients with active SLE. Indeed, so is the AMLR.[80] Patients with very active disease were found to be uniformly defective.[80, 81] Moreover, the defect in the AMLR correlated with a defect in suppressor T cell function.[80] Advances have been made in analyses of the AMLR, several of which are important to the SLE story: (1) different non-T cells vary in their stimulatory capacity[78, 93]; (2) the magnitude of the AMLR is itself regulated by T cells and macrophages, either of which can suppress the reaction, but both together suppress best.[91] As a result, the AMLR in SLE recently has been re-examined.

It has been found that patients with active SLE have cells which in vitro have reduced IL2 production and reduced IL2 receptors on T4 cells (but with normal retention of IL2 receptors on T8 cells). Therefore, the T4 cells do not make IL2 and do not proliferate. IL2 addition corrects the T4–T8 interactions because there are normal receptors on the T8 cells; however, exogenous IL2 does not correct T4–T4 interactions because of the defect in IL2 receptors on the T4 cells.[103] In addition, patients with different defects have different responses to different stimuli, suggesting that the cellular basis for immune defects in different patients with SLE may be different.[95]

GENETIC FEATURES OF HUMAN SLE

Human SLE does not appear to be inherited as a single dominant trait. Far less than one half of offspring of affected individuals ultimately develop SLE. Nevertheless, it is clear that a predisposition to develop SLE can be inherited.[5, 7] The concordance of disease in identical twins is greater than 67% (more than seven unpublished observations), whereas dizygotic twins are at no greater risk than other first-degree relatives.[7] Family studies indicate that relatives of patients with SLE have a much greater chance of developing the disease than people in the general population.[5] Certain North American Indian tribes have a marked increase in SLE,[58] and in the United States, blacks develop the disease more readily than caucasians. These larger populations augment the family studies in pointing to a genetic mechanism, although environmental factors could conceivably explain such clustering. The latter worry is illustrated by the lack of concordance for SLE in more than 30% of identical twins with the disease.[7]

Recent family studies have helped to clarify the genetic patterns.[44, 48, 75] These studies have provided evidence for aspects of the genetic basis for SLE already appreciated in studies of murine lupus: a single dominant or codominant gene can predispose to anti-DNA antibodies,[48, 71, 73] disease is inherited in a multigenic fashion,[71, 75] and a subset of patients with SLE inherit an accelerating factor on the Y chromosome from the father.[44, 59, 87, 105] Thus, it is possible that different patterns of inheritance may be associated with disease in the two sexes. Moreover, as in mice, it is likely that early in life disease may be inherited differently from later in life (middle-age lupus). The former may require requisite "background" genes but may be mediated primarily by a single gene. This is probably the explanation for the Y chromosome–linked inheritance as well as the occurrence of disease in some females in those families (see Table 1).

What could the genes for predisposition to lupus be? No answer is currently available; nevertheless, it is worth considering some of the possibilities. If antinuclear antibodies represent an important aspect of disease, an immune response gene for anti-DNA might be inherited as a single dominant or codominant gene. Alternatively, if DNA metabolic abnormalities are largely responsible for anti-DNA production by virtue of the release of especially immunogenic DNA,[84] genes which code for an enzyme or other defect in this pathway (e.g., in DNA repair) could appear to act as genes for anti-DNA. In addition, abnormal estrogen metabolism reported in patients with SLE[43] might be inherited as a single gene; such a gene would be one of the background genes that would augment immune responses, decrease immune regulation, and predispose to heightened autoantibody responses. A defect in normal suppressor cell function could be inherited as one of many background genes that predispose to SLE. Evidence for such a process has been put forth in families of SLE patients.[52] Since not all of those affected by the defect have autoimmune disease, it appears that additional genes (or a critical environmental influence) is necessary. Thus, a defect in immune regulation leading to excessive B cell activation might come about by any of several abnormalities in the immune system; the genes coding for any of these defects could serve as "background" genes that predispose to SLE.

So far nothing has been mentioned of the major histocompatibility types in patients with SLE. Although much has been made of disease associations with HLA types, the relative risks associated with SLE and HLA-D3 and HLA-D2 are models.[74] It is likely that a gene association with HLA-D3 predisposes to increased antibody responses and decreased antigen clearance and thereby predisposes to immune complex- and antibody-mediated diseases.[47] A most interesting association is that of SLE and decreased numbers of C3b receptors on erythrocytes.[110] Rather than representing an immune response gene, this form of inheritance probably decreases the clearance of injurious antibodies and antigen-antibody complexes and thereby predisposes to disease. Thus, a great variety of "background" genes can predispose to SLE. The more of these genes that are found in a given individual, the more likely it is that disease will be expressed. On the other hand, a single gene in mice can entirely or largely prevent the expression of autoimmunity and the development of lupus.[87, 101, 102, 104] Whether or not such protective genes are present in humans is unknown. The presence of such genes could help to explain some of the incomplete penetrance observed in family studies. In addition, knowledge of such genes could help family planning and also approaches to therapy.

Synthesis

Is it possible to put the above information together so as to shed light on pathogenetic events in SLE? A complete picture cannot be drawn; however, some of the outlines fall into place. Since SLE may be genetically and clinically heterogeneous, it is probably a syndrome rather than a single disease. This is in some measure a semantic matter; however, if we recognize that the basis for disease might be different in different individuals, it allows us to deal better with diversity of biologic abnormalities as well as diversity in clinical manifestations.

The central aspect of SLE is a predisposition of B cells to proliferate and differentiate into immunoglobulin-secreting cells. Therefore, patients must have abnormalities leading to excessive B cell proliferation and differentiation. This abnormality might be an inherited defect. The precise defect might be different in different individuals, some having excess stimulation of the B cells, some having impaired regulation of the B cells, and some having excessively activatable B cells. In some individuals, excessive production of B cells from stem cells might be an underlying problem. Finally, some patients may have no major inherited predisposition to B cell hyperactivity but might be stimulated sufficiently by exogenous sources to yield disease.

The second major abnormality in patients with SLE is the production of particular kinds of autoantibodies. Although patients may produce a great variety of autoantibodies, antibodies reactive with DNA and other nuclear antigens are especially characteristic. Of interest, nucleic acids are capable of acting as immune adjuvants. Therefore, it is possible for a nucleic acid to act both as an immunogen and as a polyclonal immune activator in patients. However, it may require the appropriate second kind of gene, one that leads to a biochemical abnormality of nucleic acid metabolism or one that allows a vigorous immune response to nucleic acid antigens or some antigen that induces antibodies that crossreact with DNA. In this regard, we should recognize that the antibodies produced to self-antigens could actually be induced by cross-reactive immunogens that bear only a modest relationship to the self-antigens.

The process of polyclonal immune activation leads to a great variety of secondary phenomena. These are most of the phenomena we measure when we study cells from patients with active SLE. They include (1) spontaneous B cell hyperactivity but impaired B cell responses to in vitro stimuli, and (2) impaired in vivo and in vitro T cell functions of many kinds, many related to a decrease in necessary growth factor production as well as suppression as a result of the in vivo immune activation and a form of endogenous antigenic competition. Finally, antilymphocyte antibodies, immune complexes, etc. act to further interfere with normal immunoregulatory processes. The activated immune system leads to in vivo interferon production and further resistance to interferon-mediated phenomena, including NK cell activity, in vitro.

How is this process triggered? It should be clear that studying the full-blown process provides one with many abnormalities, some of which are very important in disease production and many of which are important in perpetuating the defective state, but very few of which initiate the process. Possible triggers are endogenous metabolic abnormalities and exogenous stimuli. Among the latter, viral infections that induce interferon production could initiate the process. Bacterial infections that induce Ia expression by macrophages also could initiate the process. Additional agents that mimic the various growth factors also are capable of pushing the immune system toward increased activity. Ultraviolet light acts as a trigger in some individuals. Two explanations readily present themselves: DNA alteration, and interference with macrophage functions. Ultraviolet light is capable of altering the structure of DNA; such an alteration might make it especially good at inducing either polyclonal immune activation or anti-DNA production. This is especially so in the face of impaired DNA repair in SLE. Less well appreciated is the profound suppressive effect of ultraviolet light on the ability of macrophages to handle antigens. This effect could have an adverse affect remote from the skin. A critical feature is failure of the system to turn itself off once the process is initiated. Thus, a perpetual anti-self immune reaction is possible. Only by interfering with the immune circuitry can we bring the entire process to an end. From a therapeutic point of view, it might be possible to allow the immune defects to continue and merely eliminate the final common pathway—autoantibody production or its consequences. Thus, it might be possible to eliminate the subpopulation of B cells which makes autoantibodies or reduces the impact of mediator release[67, 68] and thereby bring about a useful end result without altering the fundamental processes. With the advent of modern immunotechnology, novel approaches to the treatment of SLE and other immune complex–mediated diseases are moving from the realm of possibility.

REFERENCES

1. Adler F.L.: Competition of antigens. *Prog. Allergy* 8:41, 1964.
2. Agnello V., Arbetter A., Ibanez de Kaspep G., et al.: J. Exp. Med. 151:1514, 1981.
3. Akizuki M., Reeves J.P., Steinberg A.D.: Expression of autoimmunity by NZB/NZW marrow. *Clin. Immunol. Immunopathol.* 10:247, 1978.
4. Aloccer-Varela J., Alarcon-Segovia D.: Decreased production of and response to interleukin 2 by cultured lymphocytes from patients with systemic lupus erythematosus. *J. Clin. Invest.* 69:1388, 1982.
5. Arnett F.C., Shulman L.E.: Studies in familial systemic lupus erythematosis. *Medicine* 55:313, 1976.
6. Blaese R.M., Grayson J., Steinberg A.D.: Elevated immunoglobulin secreting cells in the blood of patients with active systemic lupus erythcmatosus. Correlation of laboratory and clinical assessment of disease activity. *Am. J. Med.* 69:345, 1980.
7. Block S.R., Lockshin M.D., Winfield J.B., et al.: Immunological observations on 9 sets of twins either concordant or discordant for SLE. *Arthritis Rheum.* 19:454, 1976.
8. Bobrove A.M., Miller P.: Depressed in vitro B-lymphocyte differentiation in systemic lupus erythematosus. *Arthritis Rheum.* 20:1326, 1977.
9. Budman D.R., Merchant E.B., Steinberg A.D., et al.: Increased spontaneous activity of antibody-forming cells in the peripheral blood of patients with active SLE. *Arthritis Rheum.* 20:829, 1977.
10. Damle N.K., Gupta S.: Autologous mixed lymphocyte reaction in man: V. Functionally and phenotypically distinct human T-cell subpopulations respond to non-T and activated T cells in AMLR. *Scand. J. Immunol.* 16:269, 1982.
11. Datta S.D., Owne F.L., Womack J.E., et al.: Analysis of recombinant inbred lines derived from "autoimmune" (NZB) and "high leukemia" (C58) strains: Independent multigenic systems control B cell hyperactivity, retrovirus expression, and autoimmunity. *J. Immunol.* 129:1539, 1982.
12. Delbarre F., Go L.A., Kahan A.: Hyperbasophilic immunoblasts in the circulating blood in chronic inflammatory rheumatoid and collagen diseases. *Ann. Rheum. Dis.* 34:422, 1975.
13. Delbarre F., Pompidou A., Kahan A., et al.: Study of blood lymphocytes during systemic lupus erythematosus. *Pathol. Biol.* 19:379, 1971.
14. Delfraissy J.F., Segond P, Galanaud P., et al.: Depressed primary *in vitro* anti-

body response in untreated systemic lupus erythematosus: T helper cell defect and lack of defective suppressor cell function. *J. Clin. Invest.* 66:141, 1980.

15. Denman A.M., Russell A.S., Denman E.J.: Adoptive transfer of the disease of NZB mice to normal mouse strains. *Clin. Exp. Immunol.* 5:677, 1969.

16. Dixon F.J., Oltstone M.B.A., Tonietti G.: Pathogenesis of immune complex glomerulonephritis of New Zealand mice. *J. Exp. Med.* 134:65s, 1971.

17. Eisenberg R.A., Dixon F.J.: Effect of castration on male-determined acceleration of autoimmune disease in BXSB mice. *J. Immunol.* 125:1959, 1980.

18. Eisenberg R.A., Izui S., McConahey P.F., et al.: Male determined accelerated autoimmune disease in BXSB mice: Transfer by bone marrow and spleen cells. *J. Immunol.* 125:1032, 1980.

19. Fauci A.S., Steinberg A.D., Haynes B.F., et al.: Immunoregulatory aberrations in systemic lupus erythematosus. *J. Immunol.* 121:1473, 1978.

20. Fitzharris et al.: *Clin. Exp. Immunol.* 47:110, 1982.

21. Gatenby P.A., Kotzin B.L., Kansas C.S., et al.: Immunoglobulin secretion in the human autologous mixed leucocyte reaction: Definition of a suppressor-amplifier circuit using monoclonal antibodies. *J. Exp. Med.* 156, 1982.

22. Gelfand M.C., Parker L.M., Steinberg A.D.: Mechanism of allograft rejection in New Zealand mice: II. Role of a serum factor. *J. Immunol.* 113:1, 1974.

23. Ginsburg W.W., Finkelman F.D., Lipsky P.E.: Circulating and pokeweed mitogen-induced immunoglobulin-secreting cells in systemic lupus erythematosus. *Clin. Exp. Immunol.* 35:76, 1979.

24. Glimcher L.H., Steinberg A.D., House S.B., et al.: The autologous mixed lymphocyte reaction in strains of mice with autoimmune disease. *J. Immunol.* 125:1832, 1980.

25. Glinski W., Gershwin M.E., Budman D.R., et al.: Study of lymphocyte subpopulations in normal humans and patients with systemic lupus erythematosus by fractionation of peripheral blood lymphocytes on a discontinuous Ficoll gradient. *Clin. Exp. Immunol.* 26:228, 1976.

26. Glinski W., Gershwin M.E., Steinberg A.D.: Fractionation of cells on a discontinuous Ficoll gradient: Study of subpopulations of human T cells using anti-T cell antibodies from patients with systemic lupus erythematosus. *J. Clin. Invest.* 57:604, 1976.

27. Gottlieb A.B., Lahita R.G., Chiorazzi N., et al.: Immune function in systemic lupus erythematosus: Impairment of *in vitro* T-cell proliferation and *in vivo* antibody response to exogenous antigen. *J. Clin. Invest.* 63:885, 1979.

28. Hang L., Izui S., Slack J.H., et al.: The cellular basis for resistance to induction of tolerance in BXSB systemic lupus erythematosus male mice. *J. Immunol.* 129:787, 1982.

29. Hausmann P.B., Stobo J.D.: Specificity and function of human autologous reaction T cell. *J. Exp. Med.* 149:1537, 1979.

30. Hom J.T., Talal N.: Decreased syngeneic mixed lymphocyte response in autoimmune susceptible mice. *Scand. J. Immunol.* 15:195, 1982.

31. Hooks J.J., Moutsopoulos H.M., Geis S.A., et al.: Immune interferon in the circulation of patients with autoimmune disease. *N. Engl. J. Med.* 301:5, 1979.

32. Horwitz D.A., Garrett M.A.: Lymphocyte reactivity to mitogens in subjects with systemic lupus erythematosus, rheumatoid arthritis and scleroderma. *Clin. Exp. Immunol.* 27:92, 1977.

33. Horwitz D.A., Linker-Israeli M., Bakke A.C., et al.: Characterization of the mechanisms responsible for interleukin 1 and 2 deficiencies in patients with systemic lupus erythematosus. *Arthritis Rheum.* 26:28s, 1983.

34. Jasin H.E., Ziff M.: Immunoglobulin synthesis by peripheral blood cells in systemic lupus erythematosus. *Arthritis Rheum.* 18:219, 1975.

35. Kaszuhowski S.A., Goodwin J.S., Williams R.C.: Ia antigen on the surface of a subfraction of T cells that bear Fc receptors for IgG. *J. Immunol.* 124:1075, 1980.

36. Katz: *J. Immunol.* 129:1966, 1982.
37. Kirchner H., Fernbach B.R., Herberman R.B.: Macrophages suppressing T and B cell mitogen responses and the mixed leukocyte reaction, in Oppenheim J.J., Rosenstreich D.L. (eds.): *Mitogens in Immunology.* New York, Academic Press, 1976, p. 495.
38. Kumagai S., Sredni B., House S., et al.: Defective regulation of B lymphocyte colony formation in patients with systemic lupus erythematosus. *J. Immunol.* 128:258, 1981.
39. Kumagai S., Steinberg A.D., Green I.: Antibodies to T cells in patients with systemic lupus erythematosis mediated ADCC against human T cell. *J. Clin. Invest.* 67:604, 1981.
40. Kumagai S., Steinberg A.D., Green I.: Immune responses to hapten-modified self and their regulation in normal individuals and patients with SLE. *J. Immunol.* 127:1643, 1981.
41. Kuntz-Crow M., Kunkel H.G.: Human dendritic cells: Major stimulators of the autologous and allogeneic mixed lymphocyte reactions. *Clin. Exp. Immunol.* 49:338, 1982.
42. Lafter E.M., Rauch J., Andrzejewski C., et al.: *J. Exp. Med.* 153:897, 1981.
43. Lahita R.G., Bradlow L., Fishman J., et al.: Estrogen metabolism in systemic lupus erythematosus: Patients and family members. *Arthritis Rheum.* 25:843, 1982.
44. Lahita R.G., Chiorazzi N., Gibofsky A., et al.: Familial systemic lupus erythematosus in males. *Arthritis Rheum.* 26:39, 1983.
45. Landry M.: Phagocyte function and cell-mediated immunity in systemic lupus erythematosus. *Arch. Dermatol.* 113:147, 1977.
46. Laskin C.A., Smathers P.A., Reeves J.P., et al.: Studies of defective tolerance induction in NZB mice: Evidence for a marrow pre-T cell defect. *J. Exp. Med.* 155:1025, 1982.
47. Lawley T.J., Hall R.P., Fauci A.S., et al.: Defective Fc-receptor functions associated with HLA-B8/DR3 haplotype. *N. Engl. J. Med.* 304·185, 1982.
48. Lippman S.M., Arnett F.C., Conley C.L., et al.: Genetic factors predisposing to autoimmune disease. *Am. J. Med.* 73:827, 1982.
49. Marmont A.M., Damasio E.: Circulating hyperbasophilic mononuclear cells in systemic lupus erythematosus, in Linder J., Ruttner J., Miescher P., et al. (eds.): *Arthritis-Arthrose.* Stuttgart, Verlag Hans Huber, 1971, pp. 287–303.
50. Mellors R.C., Shiari T., Aoki T.: Wildtype gross leukemia virus and the pathogenesis of the glomerulonephritis of New Zealand mice. *J. Exp. Med.* 133:113, 1971.
51. Michael S.R., Yural I.L., Basson V.A., et al.: The hematologic aspects of disseminated (systemic) lupus erythematosus patients. *Blood* 6:1059, 1951.
52. Miller K.B., Schwartz R.S.: Familial abnormalities of suppressor-cell function in systemic lupus erythematosus. *N. Engl. J. Med.* 301:803, 1979.
53. Morimoto C., Abe T., Hara M., et al.: *In vitro* TNP-specific antibody formation by peripheral lymphocytes from patients with systemic lupus erythematosus. *Scand. J. Immunol.* 6:575, 1977.
54. Morimoto C., Reinherz E.L., Steinberg A.D., et al.: Relationship between SLE T cell subsets, anti-T cell antibodies, and T cell functions. *Arthritis Rheum.* 26:s27, 1983.
55. Morse H.C. III, Davidson W.F., Yetter R.A., et al.: Abnormalities induced by the mutual gene *lpr:* Expansion of a unique lymphocyte subset. *J. Immunol.* 129:2612, 1982.
56. Morton J.I., Siegel B.V.: Transplantation of autoimmune potential: I. Development of antinuclear antibodies in H-2 histocompatible recipients of bone marrow from New Zealand black mice. *Proc. Natl. Acad. Sci. USA* 71:2162, 1974.
57. Morton J.I., Siegel B.V.: Transplantation of autoimmune potential: III. Immunological hyper-responsiveness and elevated endogenous spleen colony formation in

lethally irradiated recipients of NZB bone marrow cells. *Immunology* 34:863, 1978.

58. Morton R.O., Gershwin M.E., Brady C., et al.: Incidence of systemic lupus erythematosus (SLE) in North American Indians. *J. Rheum.* 3:186, 1976.

59. Murphy E.D.: Lymphoproliferation (LPR) and other single-locus models for murine lupus, in Gershwin M.E., Merchant B. (eds.): *Immunologic Defects in Laboratory Animals.* New York, Plenum, 1981, vol. 2, p. 143.

60. Nakamura Z., Asano T., Yano K., et al.: Reevaluation of suppressor cell function in systemic lupus erythematosus. *Clin. Immunol. Immunopathol.* 24:72, 1982.

61. Neighbor J., et al.: *Clin. Exp. Immunol.* 49:11, 1982.

62. Okudaira K., Searles R.P., Tanimoto K., et al.: T lymphocyte interaction with immunoglobulin G antibody in systemic lupus erythematosus. *J. Clin. Invest.* 69:1026, 1982.

63. Palacios R., Alarcon-Segovia D., Llorente L., et al.: Human post-thymic precursor cells in health and disease. *Immunology* 42:127, 1981.

64. Panem S., Check I.J., Henriksen D., et al.: Antibodies to α-interferon in a patient with systemic lupus erythematosus. *J. Immunol.* 129:1, 1982.

65. Paty J.G., Sienknecht C.W., Tomnes A.S., et al.: Impaired cell-mediated immunity in systemic lupus erythematosus. *Am. J. Med.* 59:769, 1975.

66. Pincus T., Steinberg A.D., Blacklow N., et al.: Reactivities of systemic lupus erythematosus sera with cellular and virus antigen preparations. *Arthritis Rheum.* 21:873, 1978.

67. Prickett J.D., Robinson D.R., Steinberg A.D.: Dietary enrichment with the polyunsaturated fatty acid eicosapentaenoic acid prevents proteinuria and prolongs survival in NZB NZW F_1 mice. *J. Clin. Invest.* 68:556, 1981.

68. Prickett J.D., Robinson D.R., Steinberg A.D.: Effects of dietary enrichment with eicosapentaenoic acid upon autoimmune nephritis in female (NZB × NZW) F_1 mice. *Arthritis Rheum.* 26:133, 1983.

69. Prud'homme G.J., et al.: *J. Exp. Med.* 157:730, 1983.

70. Ranney D.F., Steinberg A.D.: Differences in the age-dependent release of a low molecular weight suppressor (LMWS) and stimulators by normal and NZB/W lymphoid organs. *J. Immunol.* 117:1219, 1976.

71. Raveche E.S., Novotny E.A., Hansen C.T., et al.: Genetic studies in NZB mice: V. Recombinant inbred lines demonstrate that separate genes control autoimmune phenotype. *J. Exp. Med.* 153:1187, 1981.

72. Raveche E.S., Steinberg A.D.: Lymphocytes and lymphocyte functions in systemic lupus erythematosus. *Clin. Haematol.* 15:344, 1979.

73. Raveche E.S., Steinberg A.D., Klassen L.W., et al.: Genetic studies in NZB mice: I. Spontaneous autoantibody production. *J. Exp. Med.* 147:1487, 1978.

74. Reinertsen J.L., Klippel J.H., Johnson A.H., et al.: B lymphocyte alloantigens associated with systemic lupus erythematosus. *N. Engl. J. Med.* 299:515, 1978.

75. Reinertsen J.L., Klippel J.H., Johnson A.H., et al.: Family studies of B lymphocyte alloantigens in systemic lupus erythematosus. *J. Rheumatol.* 9:253, 1982.

76. Reinherz E.L., Morimoto C., Fitzgerald K.A., et al.: Heterogeneity of human T4[+] inducer T cells defined by a monoclonal antibody that delineates two function subpopulations. *J. Immunol.* 128:463, 1982.

77. Roubinian J.R., Talal N., Greenspan J.S., et al.: Effect of castration and sex hormone treatment on survival, antinucleic acid antibodies, and glomerulonephritis in NZB/NZW F_1 mice. *J. Exp. Med.* 147:1568, 1978.

78. Sakane T., Steinberg A.D., Arnett F.C., et al.: Studies of immune functions of patients with systemic lupus erythematosus: III. Characterization of lymphocyte subpopulations responsible for defective autologous mixed lymphocyte reactions. *Arthritis Rheum.* 22:770, 1979.

79. Sakane T., Reeves J.P., Steinberg A.D., et al.: Studies of immune functions of patients with systemic lupus erythematosus: Complement dependent immuno-

globulin M anti-thymus-derived cell antibodies preferentially inactive suppressor cells. *J. Clin. Invest.* 63:954, 1979.
80. Sakane T., Steinberg A.D., Green I.: Failure of autologous mixed lymphocyte reactions between T and non-T cells in patients with systemic lupus erythematosus. *Proc. Natl. Acad. Sci.* 75:3464, 1978.
81. Sakane T., Steinberg A.D., Green I.: Studies of immune functions of patients with systemic lupus erythematosus: V. T-cell suppressor function and autologous MLR during active and inactive phases of disease. *Arthritis Rheum.* 23:225, 1980.
82. Sakane T., Steinberg A.D., Green I.: Studies of immune functions of patients with systemic lupus erythematosus: I. Failure of suppressor T cell activity related to impaired generation of, rather than response to, suppressor cells. *Arthritis Rheum.* 21:657, 1978.
83. Sakane T., Steinberg A.D., Reeves J.P., et al.: Studies of immune functions of patients with systemic lupus erythematosus: T cell subsets and antibodies to T cell subsets. *J. Clin. Invest.* 64:1260, 1979.
84. Sano H., Imokawa M., Steinberg A.D., et al.: Accumulation of guanine-cytosine enriched low M.W. DNA fragments in lymphocytes of patients with systemic lupus erythematosus. *J. Immunol.* 130:187, 1983.
85. Santoro T.J., Benjamin W.R., Oppenheim J.J., et al.: The cellular basis for immune interferon production in autoimmune MRL-*lpr/lpr* mice. *J. Immunol.* 131:265, 1983.
86. Shoenfeld Y., Rauch J., Massicotte H., et al.: *N. Engl. J. Med.* 308:414, 1983.
87. Sibbitt, et al.: *J. Clin. Invest.* 71:1230, 1983.
87. Smith H.R., Steinberg A.D.: Autoimmunity: A perspective. *Annu. Rev. Immunol.* 1:175, 1983.
88. Smith H.R., Chused T.M., Smathers P.A., et al.: Evidence for thymic regulation of autoimmunity in BXSB mice: Acceleration of disease by neonatal thymectomy. *J. Immunol.* 130:1200, 1983.
89. Smith J.B., Pasternak R.D.: Syngenic mixed leukocyte reaction in mice; strain distribution, kinetics, participating cells, and absence in NZB mice. *J. Immunol.* 122:1889, 1978.
90. Smolen J.S., Chused T.M., Leiserson W.M., et al.: Heterogeneity of immunoregulatory T cell subsets in systemic lupus erythematosus: Correlation with clinical features. *Am. J. Med.* 72:783, 1982.
91. Smolen J.S., Chused T.M., Novotny E.A., et al.: The human autologous mixed lymphocyte reaction: III. Immune circuits. *J. Immunol.* 129:1050, 1982.
92. Smolen J.S., Luger T.A., Chused T.M., et al.: Responder cells in the human autologous mixed lymphocyte reaction. *J. Clin. Invest.* 68:1601, 1981.
93. Smolen J.S., Sharrow S.O., Reeves J.P., et al.: The human autologous mixed lymphocyte reaction: Suppression by macrophages and T cells. *J. Immunol.* 127:1987, 1981.
94. Smolen J.S., Sharrow S.O., Steinberg A.D.: Characterization of autologous rosette forming cells: A non-restricted phenomenon. *J. Immunol.* 127:737, 1981.
95. Smolen J.S., Siminovitch K., Luger T.A., et al.: Responder cells in the human autologous mixed lymphocyte reaction (AMLR): II. Characterization and interactions in healthy individuals and patients with systemic lupus erythematosus, in *Proceedings of the First International Symposium on the AMLR*. Behring Institute, 1983, p. 72.
96. Steinberg A.D., Huston D.P., Taurog J.D., et al.: The cellular and genetic basis for murine lupus. *Immunol. Rev.* 55:121, 1981.
97. Steinberg A.D., Kaltreider H.B., Staples P.J., et al.: Cyclophosphamide in lupus nephritis: A controlled trial. *Ann. Intern. Med.* 75:165, 1971.
98. Steinberg A.D., Melez K.A., Raveche E.S., et al.: Approach to the study of the role of sex hormones in autoimmunity. *Arthritis Rheum.* 22:1170, 1979.
99. Steinberg A.D., Roths J.B., Murphy E.D., et al.: Effects of thymectomy or andro-

gen administration upon the autoimmune disease of MRL/MP-*lpr/lpr* mice. *J. Immunol.* 125:871, 1980.

100. Steinberg A.D., Smolen J.S., Sakane T., et al.: Immune regulatory abnormalities in systemic lupus erythematosus, in Cummings N., Michael A., Wilson C. (eds.): *Immune Mechanisms of Renal Disease*. New York, Plenum Press, 1983, pp. 529–548.

101. Steinberg B.J., Smathers P.A., Frederiksen K., et al.: Ability of the *xid* gene to prevent autoimmunity in (NZB × NZW) F_1 mice during the course of their natural history, after polyclonal stimulation, following immunization with DNA. *J. Clin. Invest.* 70:587, 1982.

102. Steinberg E.B., Santoro T.J., Chused T.M., et al.: Studies of congenic MRL-*lpr/lpr xid* mice. *J. Immunol.* Vol. 131, 1983.

103. Takada S., Murakawa Y., Ueda Y., et al.: Abnormalities in autologous mixed lymphocyte reaction-activated immune circuits in systemic lupus erythematosus and their possible correction by interleukin 2. *J. Immunol.*, to be published.

104. Taurog J.D., Raveche E.S., Smathers P.A., et al.: T cell abnormalities in NZB mice occur independently of autoantibody production. *J. Exp. Med.* 153:221, 1981.

105. Theofilopolous A.N., Dixon F.J.: Etiopathogenesis of murine systemic lupus erythematosus. *Immunol. Rev.* 55:179, 1981.

106. Thomas Y., Rogozinski L., Irigoyen O.H., et al.: Functional analysis of human T cell subsets defined by monoclonal antibodies: V. Suppressor cells within the activated OKT4$^+$ population belong to a distinct subset. *J. Immunol.* 128:1386, 1982.

107. Tonietti G., Oldstone M.B., Dixon F.J.: The effect of induced chronic viral infections on the immunologic diseases of New Zealand mice. *J. Exp. Med.* 132:89, 1970.

108. Wades A.A., Gear A.J., Rabson A.R.: Production of a suppressor factor by human adherent cells treated with *Mycobacterium tuberculosis:* Absence in systemic lupus erythematosus. *Clin. Exp. Immunol.* 46:82, 1981.

109. Williams G.W., Steinberg A.D., Reinertsen J.L., et al.: Influenza immunization in systemic lupus erythematosus: A double-blind trial. *Ann. Intern. Med.* 88:729, 1978.

110. Wilson J.G., Wong W.W., Schur P.H., et al.: Mode of inheritance of decreased C3b receptors on erythrocyte of patients with systemic lupus erythematosus. *N. Engl. J. Med.* 307:981, 1982.

Atypical Lupus With Special Reference to ANA Negative Lupus and Lupus Subsets

G.R.V. HUGHES, M.D., F.R.C.P., AND
R.A. ASHERSON, M.B., Ch.B., F.C.P. (SA)

Department of Rheumatology, The Royal Postgraduate Medical School, Hammersmith Hospital, London, England

Introduction

The most prominent serologic abnormality in systemic lupus erythematosus (SLE) is the presence of autoantibodies that react against self-antigens. These antigens exist both in cell nuclei and in cytoplasm. They include double-stranded DNA, single-stranded DNA, soluble and insoluble nucleo-proteins, saline-extractable nuclear antigens (ENA), especially Sm and ribonucleoprotein. The antinuclear antibody test is positive in over 90% of patients with SLE, and in recent years the significance of these antinuclear as well as anticytoplasmic autoantibodies in defining different subsets and "overlap" syndromes in the various connective tissue diseases has become increasingly defined.

The discovery of the lupus erythematosus (LE) cell phenomenon in the 1940s first led to the recognition of the extent of the immunological disturbance in this disease. The phenomenon results from the presence in blood of an IgG antibody to DNA-histone complex (antinucleoprotein).[1] The wide variety of antinuclear and anticytoplasmic antibodies existing in SLE are

333

detectable by the usual immunofluorescent tests,[2] using tissue, such as rat liver cells. Proliferating cells in tissue culture monolayers are larger and richer in nuclear and cytoplasmic antigens than the resting cells of frozen organ sections and, although used in some centers, inevitably provide differences in the spectrum of autoantibodies detected.

Counterimmunoelectrophoresis and Immuno Diffusion

Twenty or more antibodies that react with soluble cellular components extracted for tissues (Table 1) have so far been identified and there are probably dozens more that are as yet not characterized. These are detected by precipitation reaction in gels using immuno diffusion or counter immunoelectrophoresis, which is a quick and sensitive method of detecting antibodies reacting with negatively-charged (acidic) antigens. Precipitin lines are identified by comparison with reference sera[3] (Figs 1 and 2).

"ANA-ve Lupus"

The frequency of ANA-ve SLE is by definition unknown, though it has been estimated that some 5% of the SLE population fall into this category (Table 2). The clinical character-

TABLE 1.—Non-histone Extractable
Cellular Antigens

ANTIGENS	
Sm	SLE
MA	Severe SLE
PM-I	Polymyositis
Mi(Mi-I)	Myositis
Jo-I	Myositis
	Pul. fibrosis
ScI-70	PSS
TM	SLE; CTD
r-RNP(MU)	SLE; CTD
PCNA	SLE
SS-A(Ro)	SLE; SS
SS-B(La,Ha)	SLE; SS
SS-C(RANA,RAP)	RA
RNP(Mo)	MCTD
SL	SLE, CTD
Ku	Polymyositis/Scleroderma

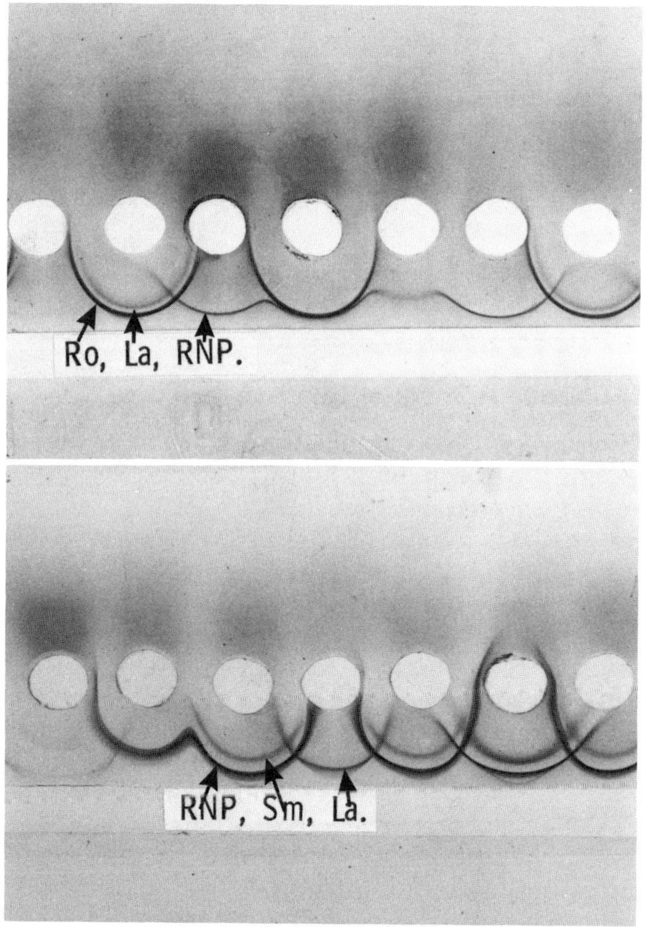

Fig 1 (top).—Counterimmunoelectrophoresis showing anti-ENA precipitin lines from human spleen extract.

Fig 2 (bottom).—Counterimmunoelectrophoresis showing anti-ENA precipitin lines from a rabbit thymus extract.

istics of this group are a high incidence of photo-sensitive dermatitis and a low incidence of nephritis and CNS disease.

The "ANA negative" group may be further characterized on the basis of the presence of anti-Ro antibody systems and the absence of complement. The clinical features of all the subsets associated with ANA negativity show strong "overlap" features, and these will be discussed in this article.

TABLE 2.—ANA-ve Lupus

CLINICAL	SEROLOGIC
↓ Nephritis and CNS disease	⅔ Ro ± La
↑ Photosensitive dermatitis	+ve Latex test
Mouth ulcers	
Alopecia	+ve ss DNA
⅓ Systemic features:	↑ Sjogren's syndrome
Arthralgias	↑ Thrombocytopenias
Fevers	± Hemolytic anemia
Malaise, fatigue	
¼ Hematological	↑ Leucopenia
⅕ Pleurisy and pericarditis	

Anti-Ro Antibody and Other Lupus Subsets

The Ro antigen[4] is a predominantly cytoplasmic glycoprotein. It is often accompanied by antibodies to another soluble tissue protein, termed "La."[5]

Anti-Ro antibody has been found in 25% of SLE sera and 75% of sera from patients with primary sicca syndrome.[6] A subset of lupus patients with these antibodies has been identified.[7, 8] These patients characteristically present with a prominent cutaneous component, a severe photosensitive dermatitis. These skin lesions may cover a wide spectrum that may vary from DLE to the butterfly erythema of SLE.[9] However, the most characteristic finding is the rash long recognized by rheumatologists as subacute cutaneous lupus erythematosus (SCLE).[10] Other features are constitutional symptoms, such as arthralgia and fatigue. Patients are usually ANA-negative (although titers may fluctuate in some). They may also have nonscarring alopecia, hypergammaglobulinemia and positive rheumatoid factor.[7] These patients have a more benign course and if renal disease develops, it is seldom severe. Response to antimalarial therapy is usually dramatic and patient's symptoms can often be controlled on this drug alone, without recourse to steroids.

Anti-Ro antibodies may also be found in patients presenting with a primary sicca syndrome, when again they may be accompanied by Anti-La. These patients also have IgG levels above normal in addition to having IgA rheumatoid factor.[11]

A third type of subset found with the anti-Ro antibody is thrombocytopenia. Thrombocytopenia is frequent in both SLE and the primary sicca syndrome, and idiopathic thrombocytopenic purpura may form the prodromal phase of either condition. In SLE, the frequency of anti-Ro antibody is almost doubled in patients with thrombocytopenia. Conversely, 25% of patients with ITP are Ro antibody +ve.[12]

The anti-Ro antibody has been found in about two-thirds of the mothers delivering children with congenital heart block;[13] the babies are positive during the first six months of life, probably because the antibody was passively transferred from the mother to the child. We have recently seen two adults at Hammersmith Hospital with heart block and a maternal history of SLE who had developed anti-Ro positive SLE or sicca syndrome.[14] Most patients with the anti-Ro antibody demonstrate HLA DRw3, which is also seen in other neurological disorders and is often associated with the B8 antigen as well.

Reichlin[15] has also commented on a group of patients with either widespread vasculitis or a vasculitic process that is mainly manifest in the skin in association with anti-Ro antibody. These patients do not satisfy the ARA criteria of SLE, although they share some clinical features with SLE patients. Anti-Ro antibodies were sometimes accompanied by anti-La antibodies, and all had positive tests of rheumatoid factor (with titers above 1/40). None of the sera contained anti-DNA. All patients had a non-thrombocytopenic purpura, and some also had widespread erythematous, scaling, macular lesions or ulcers over the malleoli. In most, evidence of vasculitis was demonstrable.

Reichlin also has postulated a strong link between the production of the anti-Ro antibody and homozygous C2-deficient sera. Twenty sera were studied and 10 of these were found to contain anti-Ro. This association between vasculitis and anti-Ro has also been documented in Sjögren's syndrome.[16] This finding and the DRw3 association previously mentioned implies that strong genetic factors play a role in producing anti-Ro. In a family study (unpublished) of SLE patients, we found a high incidence of null alleles of C4A and C4B.[17] We noted that a number of first degree relatives of these patients also had anti-Ro and other ENA's.

Anti-RNP

These antibodies are found in about one-fourth of all patients with SLE, but less frequently in systemic sclerosis, the sicca syndrome, and dermatomyositis. High titers are found in patients without DNA antibodies and in whom the features of Raynaud's syndrome and swollen fingers, together with varying symptomatology of SLE, scleroderma, myositis, rheumatoid arthritis and the sicca syndrome occur. This syndrome is called mixed connective tissue disease (MCTD), and these patients seem to have a higher incidence of pulmonary hypertension and less renal disease than patients with SLE.[18]

Anti-Sm

This antigen is resistant to RNase and was the first RNP-associated antigen to be described.[19] It has been found to be a component of at least five distinct small nuclear RNP particles, each of which contains a different but specific RNA component.[20] Although found most frequently in SLE, this antibody has also been found in patients with MCTD and is not specific for SLE, as has previously been reported.[19]

Two reports have associated the presence of antibody to Sm with a more benign form of SLE.[21, 22] Winn[22] noted a greater frequency of Raynaud's phenomenon in 135 patients with SLE, but less severe CNS disease. However, Barada[23] could not confirm this finding.

Anti-SL

The incidence of this antibody system has recently been investigated by our department.[24] Apart from a higher incidence of fever and lymphadenopathy/splenomegaly and an increased frequency of anti-Ro, there were no significant differences between SLE patients with or without this antibody. Anti-SL was also found in other diseases, such as rheumatoid arthritis, primary sicca syndrome, idiopathic thrombocytopenia, purpura, and primary biliary cirrhosis. Harmon et al.[25] also identified this antibody in patients with rheumatoid lung disease and autoimmune thyroid disease.

Other Precipitin Systems

Several other precipitin antigen-antibody systems with a frequency of 10% or less occur in SLE,[26] but their numbers are too few to further delineate "subsets" at the present time.

These include PL4, proliferative cell nuclear antigen (PCNA), and the antibodies to RNA antigens—Anti Tm, Anti Mu, and Anti-r-RNP. The antibodies to PM1, M1 and Jo-1, are found predominantly in patients with myositis and Anti-SC1-70 and associated with PSS. "Nuclear Dots" are still undefined clinically. Anti Jo-1 has recently been identified as histidyl-+-RNA transferase,[27] and has been strongly associated with polymyositis accompanied by pulmonary fibrosis.[28]

Compartment Deficient SLE (CD-SLE)

This has been well reviewed recently by Rynes.[29] This type of SLE, often found in the absence of ANA, usually presents after puberty, often during child-bearing years. It has been reported as occurring in a number of patients not yet 15 years of age.

The extensive skin lesions are often discoid in type and photosensitive, and they may be accompanied by alopecia. The lupus band test is often negative (the deposition of immunoglobulins and complement at the dermal-epidermal junction, detectable by immunofluorescent microscopy). Renal disease, where present, has been described as "occult" and only documented on biopsy.

Anti-DNA antibodies are often also present in low titers, like the ANA's, and absent in 75% of these patients. Rheumatoid factor, anti-Sm antibodies, and a false positive test for syphilis have been documented. These patients, like others with complement deficiency may develop severe, recurrent, or unusual infections.

SLE may occur in association with the absence of any of the subsets of C1, C2, C4 or C11NH. But SLE has most often been reported in association with this component deficiency because C2 deficiency is the most prevalent of the homozygous deficiencies. The co-existence of such conditions as angio-edema should lead one to suspect C1 1NH deficiency in particular.

Drug-Induced Lupus

A "lupus-like" syndrome was first associated with drug administration as early as 1945, when sulphadiazine was implicated. Since then hydralazine, procainamide, isoniazid, chlorpromazine, D-penicillamine, and various anti-convulsants have joined the long list of offenders. Despite the length of the list, drug-induced lupus is distinctly, and perhaps surprisingly, rare.[30]

The clinical features of drug LE have been extensively reviewed,[31] and there are important differences between the two forms of SLE. With the exception of anti-convulsant-induced lupus, drug LE occurs in an older age group. There appears to be a low frequency of renal and CNS involvement, with Raynaud's phenomenon being relatively unusual. A higher frequency of pleuro-pulmonary involvement occurs, particularly with procainamide. Skin rashes are distinctly uncommon.

Serological differences also exist between the two groups. The antinuclear antibodies demonstrated are largely directed against nuclear histone. Antibodies to native DNA are usually absent and serum complement values are normal.

Possibly related phenomena reported in patients taking these drugs include a positive Coombs test (occurring in 21% of patients treated with methyldopa).[32] The "lupus anticoagulant" is also a useful marker, occurring particularly in patients on chlorpromazine.[33]

This subject was also recently reviewed by Mueh et al.,[34] who found the "LA" in patients not only on chlorpromazine, but also on hydralazine, procainamide, fluphenazine, and penicillin therapy. Some of these also developed thrombotic complications.

It is apparent that genetic factors seem to be implicated in the development of drug LE. Slow acetylators develop ANA's more rapidly and with a lower drug dosage than fast acetylators. Acetylation is controlled by the hepatic enzyme N-acetyl transferase, and approximately 50% of the non-American and European populations are phenotypically fast acetylators of such drugs as hydralazine, procainamide and isoniazid.[35] In addition, Batchelor et al.[36] recently found an increased frequency of HLA-DR W2 and DR W3 in idiopathic LE. Interestingly, the patients in this series did not have demonstrable ENA's

Subset of Lupus with the Lupus Anticoagulant and Antibodies to Cardiolipin

In the 1950s and 1960s it became obvious that certain patients with SLE possessed anticoagulant activity in serum that was associated with thrombocytopenia, multiple abortions, and the presence of biologically false positive test for syphilis.[37–43] Although many types of anticoagulants were found in SLE patients, it became obvious that the most common was an inhibitor directed against the phospholipid component of the "prothrombin activator complex." A schematic representation of this action is shown in Table 3.

Bowie et al.[44] first drew attention in 1963 to the occurrence of thrombosis in association with this anticoagulant, and this was studied again by Mueh et al. in 1980.[34]

However, the frequency of this association was not fully appreciated until detailed studies from the Hammersmith Hospital recently demonstrated the presence of this anticoagulant activity in such conditions as renal vein thrombosis,[45] pulmonary hypertension,[46] and various other arterial and venous occlusions in SLE that had previously been labelled as "vasculitis." A list of various sites of thrombosis appears in Table 4.

This lupus anticoagulant activity has also been demonstrated in three patients who developed large vessel occlusions resulting in gangrene of the extremities,[47] as well as bowel infarction.[48]

However, the assay for the lupus anticoagulant is a func-

TABLE 3.—Prothrombin Activation Complex

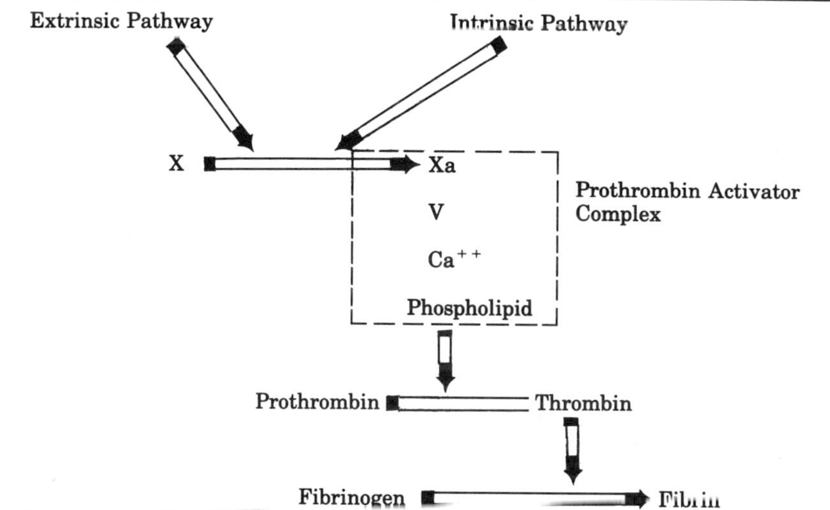

TABLE 4.—LUPUS ANTICOAGULANT
HAMMERSMITH HOSPITAL THROMBOTIC
EVENTS

Deep venous thromboses	11
Pulmonary embolism	3
CVAs	11
Renal vein thromboses	2
Central retinal vein thrombosis	2
Coeliac axis thrombosis	1
Upper/lower limb arterial thrombosis	3
Axillary vein thrombosis	1

tional one and measures other factors besides activity against phospholipid. In addition, observer error is high. Therefore, it was decided to develop another test that might measure the same antibody more precisely.[49]

Carreras and his co-workers[50] suggested that the antibody may cross-react with phospholipids in endothelial cell membranes, thus preventing the release of arachidonic acid. This, in turn, would lower prostacyclin production, causing platelet aggregation.

Alternatively, Angeles-Cano et al.[51] demonstrated a decrease in plasminogen production in SLE patients (Table 5). This results in decreased fibrinolysis, predisposing to thrombus formation. A plasminogen activator is also produced by endothelial cells, and decreased production of this protein could also result in injury by these cross-reacting phospholipid antibodies.

Anticardiolipin Antibodies

Because of the strong association of the anticoagulant activity with a biological false positive serological test for syphilis

TABLE 5.—POSTULATED MECHANISMS FOR THROMBOSIS

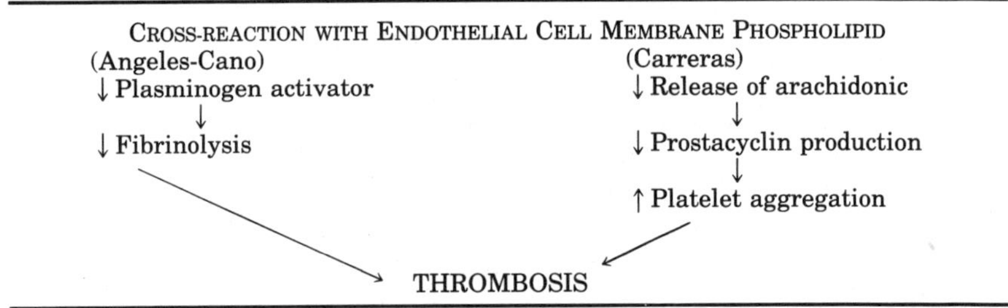

(BFP-STS), it was decided to investigate this phenomenon further. A more sensitive radioimmunoassay than the precipitin assays available was developed for the detection of antibodies against cardiolipin, the antigen used in the standard BFP-STS.[50] This assay was not only strikingly sensitive (1:640), as opposed to the usual very low titers measured in the standard test (1:8), but there was also a strong and significant correlation with the lupus anticoagulant positive sera. It is apparent that there is such a strong association between the two tests, that we are measuring the same antibody systems in both, although the mechanisms for producing thrombosis is unknown.

These antibodies have been demonstrated in all the patients previously reported with "LA" activity. In addition, we have also found a strong correlation in SLE patients presenting with cerebral infarction.[52]

Anticardiolipin antibodies have also been demonstrated in several patients with Behçet's disease[53] and in other autoimmune conditions, such as the Degos' syndrome, where the predominant clinical presenting features (CNS, skin and gastrointestinal) all stem from an underlying small-vessel vasculitis. The titers of antibody levels in the non-SLE group of patients, however, is usually lower than those with SLE. The anticardiolipin antibody assay represents an important addendum to subset of patients summarized in Table 6.

Studies are presently underway to try to detect these antibodies in several patients with so-called "lupoid sclerosis," as well as in patients with "Jamaican neuropathy." In both these conditions the existence of BFP-STS has been remarked on. Antibodies to cardiolipin have in fact been detected in a recent patient with SLE and a Guillain-Barre syndrome.[54]

TABLE 6.—SUBSET OF SLE—
ASSOCIATION WITH LUPUS
ANTICOAGULANT AND
ANTICARDIOLIPIN ANTIBODIES

False positive biological test for syphilis
Thrombosis (arterial venous)
Thrombocytopenia
Multiple abortions
Cerebral disease (stroke, neurological disease)
Pulmonary hypertension
? Others

The cross-reaction between this group of antibodies with complex brain lipids, such as sphingomyelin and cephalin, hint at their possible role in cerebral lupus erythematosus and other demyelinating diseases. Studies of these interactions are also presently being carried out in our department.

This subset of lupus patients has recently been reviewed by Hughes in the *British Medical Journal*.[55]

REFERENCES

1. Holman R., Diecher H.R.: The reaction of the LE cell factor with deoxyribonucleoprotein of the cell nucleus. *J. Clin. Invest.* 38:2059(2), 1959.
2. Lachman P.J., Kunkel H.G.: Correlation of antinuclear antibodies and nuclear staining patterns. *Lancet* 2:436, 1982.
3. Bernstein R.M., Bunn C.C., Hughes G.R.V.: Identification of antibodies to acidic antigens by counterimmunoelectrophoresis. *Ann. Rheum. Dis.* 41:554(1), 1982.
4. Clark G., Reichlin M., Tomasi T.D.: Characterization of a soluble cytoplasmic antigen reactive with sera from patients with systemic lupus erythematosus. *J. Immunol.* 102:117, 1968.
5. Mattioli M., Reichlin H.: Heterogeneity of RNA protein antigens reactive with sera of patients with systemic lupus erythematosus. *Arthritis Rheum.* 17:421, 1974.
6. Bernstein R.M., Bunn C.C., Hughes G.R.V., et al.: A surgery of autoantibodies, recognition of cellular protein and RNA antigens. Submitted for publication.
7. Bell D.A., Maddison P.J.: Serological subsets in systemic lupus erythematosus. *Arthritis Rheum.* 23:1268, 1980.
8. Wechsler H.L., Stavrides A.: Systemic lupus erythematosus with anti-Ro antibodies: Clinical, histological and immunologic findings.
9. Maddison P.J., Provost T.T., Reichlin H.: Serological findings in patients with "ANA-negative" systemic lupus erythematosus. *Medicine (Baltimore)* 60:87, 1981.
10. Sontheimer R.D., Thomas J.R., Gilliam J.N.: Subacute cutaneous lupus erythematosus. A cutaneous marker for a discoid lupus erythematosus subset. *Arch. Dermatol.* 115:1409, 1979.
11. Elkon K.B., Caeiro F., Gharavi A.E., et al.: Radioimmunoassay profile of antiglobulins in connective tissue diseases: Elevated level of 1gA antiglobulin in systemic sicca syndrome. *Clin. Exp. Immunol.* 46:547, 1981.
12. Morley K.D., Bernstein R.M., Bunn C.C., et al.: Thrombocytopenia and anti-Ro. *Lancet* 2:940, 1981.
13. Maddison P.J., Skinner R.P., Esscher E. et al.: Serologic studies in congenital heart block (abstr.) *Ann. Rheum. Dis.* 42:1983 (In press).
14. Lanham J.G., Walport H.J., Hughes G.R.V.: Congenital heart block and familial connective tissue disease. *J. Rheumatol.* 1983. (In press).
15. Reichlin M.: Clinical and immunological significance of antibodies to Ro and La in systemic lupus erythematous. *Arthritis Rheum.* 25:767, 1982.
16. Alexander E.L., Provost T.T., Ainet F.C., et al.: Vasculitis in Sjogren's syndrome: Association with antibodies to Ro (SSA) (abstract). *Arthritis Rheum.* 24:588, 1981.
17. Fiedler A.H.L., Walport M.J., Batchelor J.R., et al.: Family study of the major histocompatibility complex in patients with systemic lupus erythematosus: Importance of null alleles of C4A and C4B in determining disease susceptibility. *Br. Med.* 286:425, 1983.
18. Graziano F.M., Friedman L.C., Grossman J.: Pulmonary hypertension in a patient with mixed connective tissue disease: Clinical and pathological findings, and review of literature. *Clin. Exp. Rheum.* 1:251, 1983.

19. Tan E.H., Kunkel H.G.: Characteristics of a soluble nuclear antigen precipitating with sera of patients with systemic lupus erythematosus. *J. Immunol.* 96:464, 1966.
20. Lerner M., Steitz J.: Antibodies to small nuclear RNA's complexed with proteins are produced by patients with systemic lupus erythematosus. *Proc. Natl. Acad. Sci. USA* 76:5495, 1976.
21. Powers R., Akizuki H., Boehm-Truitt H., et al.: Substantial purification of the SM with a clinical subset of lupus erythematosus. *Arthritis Rheum.* 20:131, 1977.
22. Winn D.H., Wolfe J.F., Lindberg D.A., et al.: Identification of a clinical subset of systemic lupus erythematosus by antibodies to the SM antigen. *Arthritis Rheum.* 22:1334, 1979.
23. Barada F.A., Andrews B.S., Davis J.S.: Antibodies to SM in patients with systemic lupus erythematosus: Correlation with disease activity. *Arthritis Rheum.* 33:652, 1980.
24. Morgan S.H., Bunn C., Bernstein R.H., et al.: Clinical and serological features of patients with precipitating antibodies to the soluble cellular antigen SLC. (In press).
25. Harmon E.C., Portanova J.P.: Drug induced lupus: Clinical and serologic studies. *Clinics in Rheumatic Diseases.* 8:121, 1982.
26. Bernstein R.M., Hughes G.R.V.: Autoantibodies; overlap syndromes in the connective tissue diseases. *Advanced Medicine.* 1983. 184. Ed. Saunders K.B. (Pitman).
27. Mathews H.B., Bernstein R.M.: Myositis autoantibody inhibits histidyl-tRNA synthetase: A model for autoimmunity. *Nature* 304:177, 1983.
28. Bernstein R.M., Morgan S.H., Bunn C.C., et al.: Anti Jo-1 Antibody: A marker for myositic with interstitial lung disease. (In press).
29. Rynes R.I.: Inherited Complement Deficiency States and SLE. *Clinics in Rheumatic Diseases.* (Philadelphia: W.B. Saunders Co., April 1982.)
30. Lee S.L., Ribeiro I., Siegel H.: Activation of systemic lupus by drugs. *Arch. Intern. Med.* 117:620, 1966.
31. Alarcon-Segovia D.: Drug induced lupus and related syndromes. Rothfield N. (ed.): In *Clinics in Rheumatic Diseases.* (Philadelphia: W.B. Saunders Co., p. 573.)
32. Perry H.H., Chaplin H., Carmody S., et al.: Immunologic findings in patients receiving methyldopa: A prospective study. *J. Lab. Clin. Med.* 78:907, 1971.
33. Zarrabi H., Zuckea S., Miller F., et al.: Immunologic and coagulation disorders in chlorpromazine-treated patients. *Ann. Intern. Med.* 91:194, 1979.
34. Mueh J.R., Herbst K.D., Rapaport I.: Thrombosis in patients with the lupus anticoagulant. *Ann. Intern. Med.* 92:156, 1980.
35. Woosley R.L., Drayer D.E., Reidenberg H.H. et al.: Effect of acetylator phenotype on the rate at which procainamide induces antinuclear antibodies and the lupus syndrome. *N. Engl. J. Med.* 298:1157, 1978.
36. Batchelor J.R., Welsh K.I., Tinoco R.H. et al.: Hydralazine-induced systemic lupus erythematosus: Influence of HLA-DR and sex on susceptibility. *Lancet* 1:1107, 1980.
37. Aggeler P.M., Lindsay S., Lucia S.P.: Studies on the coagulation effect in a case of thrombocytopenic purpura complicated by thrombosis. *Am. J. Pathol.* 22:1181, 1946.
38. Conley C.L., Hartmann R.C.: A haemorrhagic disorder caused by circulating anticoagulant in patients with disseminated lupus erythematosus. *J. Clin. Invest.* 31:621, 1952.
39. Hitzig W.H., Labhart A., Uehlinger E.: Transitorische hemmkorperhamophilie bei rheumatismus. *Helvet Med. Acta* 18:410, 1951.
40. Ley A.B., Reader G.G., Sorenson C.W., et al.: Idiopathic hypoprothrombinaemia associated with haemorrhagic diathesis and the effect of Vitamin K. *Blood* 6:740, 1951.

41. Barkhan P.: Observations on a coagulation defect characterized by thrombocytopenia with a circulating anticoagulant. *South Afr. J.M. Sci.* 17:87, 1952.
42. Nilsson I.M., Wenckert A.: Hyperglobulinaemia as the cause of hemophilia-like disease. *Blood* 8:1067, 1953.
43. Frick P.G.: Acquired circulating anticoagulants in systemic "collagen disease." *Blood* 10:691, 1955.
44. Bowie E.J.W., Thompson J.H., Pascuzzi C.A., et al: Thrombosis in systemic lupus erythematosus despite circulating anticoagulants. *J. Lab. Clin. Med.* 62:416, 1963.
45. Asherson R.A., Lanham J.G., Boey H.L., et al.: Renal vein thrombosis in systemic lupus erythematosus: Association with the lupus anticoagulant. *J. Clin. Exp. Rheum.* Jan. 1984 (In press).
46. Asherson R.A., Mackworth Young C.G., Boey M.L., et al.: Pulmonary hypertension in systemic lupus erythematosus. *Br. Med. J.* 287:1024, 1983.
47. Asherson R.A., Mackworth Young C.G., Harris N.: Large vessel occlusion and gangrene in systemic lupus erythematosus: Association with the lupus anticoagulant and antibodies to cardiolipin. (In press).
48. Morgan S.H., Asherson R.A., Hughes G.R.V.: Bowel infarction in systemic lupus erythematosus: Association with the lupus anticoagulant. *Br. J. Rheum.* 1984 (letter) (In press).
49. Harris E.N., Gharavi A.E., Boey M.L., et al.: Anticardiolipin antibodies: Detection by radioimmunoassay and association with thrombosis in systemic lupus erythematosus. *Lancet* 2:1211, 1983.
50. Carreras L.O., De Freyn G., Machin S.J., et al.: Arterial thrombosis, intrauterine death and "lupus anticoagulant": Detection of immunoglobulin interfering with prostacyclin formation. *Lancet* 1:244, 1981.
51. Angeles-Cano E., Sultan Y., Clauvel J.P.: Predisposing factors to thrombosis in systemic lupus erythematosus. *J. Lab. Clin. Med.* 94:213, 1979.
52. Harris E.N., Asherson R.A., Boey M.L., et al.: Cerebral infarction in systemic lupus: Association with anticardiolipin antibodies. (In press).
53. Hull R.G., Harris E.N., Gharavi A.E., et al.: Anticardiolipin antibodies: Occurrence in Behcet's disease. (In press).
54. Harris E.N., Englert H., DeRue G., et al.: Antiphospholipid antibodies in acute Guillain-Barre Syndrome. *Lancet* 2:1361 (letter), 1983.
55. Hughes G.R.V.: Thrombosis, abortion, cerebral disease and the lupus anticoagulant. *Br. Med. J.* 287:1088, 1983.

Membranous Glomerulopathy in Systemic Lupus Erythematosus

HUGO GONZALEZ-DETTONI AND FRANÇOIS TRON

*From Unité de Recherches sur les Maladies Rénales, INSERM U25, Hôpital Necker,
161 rue de Sèvres 75015 Paris - France*

LUPUS GLOMERULONEPHRITIS is among the most severe manifestations of systemic lupus erythematosus (SLE). It occurs in over 50% of patients with clinical evidence of SLE[1-3] and remains the leading cause of death in this disorder.[1, 4-6]

It is generally accepted that lupus glomerulonephritis results from the deposition of immune complexes in the kidney.[7, 8] These deposits may be associated with a spectrum of histologic changes that have been classified by many authors[9-13] and recently by the World Health Organization (WHO)[14] in the hope of finding histologic criteria which may be significant for prognosis.

Membranous lupus glomerulonephritis (MLG), WHO class V, has a frequency ranging from 7% to 26% of all histologic pictures.[15] Its clinical course is generally considered benign,[16, 17] although some authors have stressed the occurrence of renal insufficiency.[11, 18]

A few immunologic studies have suggested that the immunopathology of this histologic group is different from that of others,[19-21] which might explain the stable morphological outcome, since transition to severe histologic forms has only rarely been reported.[2, 13, 22-26]

347

0084-5957/84/0014-0347-0364-$04.00
© 1984, Year Book Medical Publishers, Inc.

Finally, the studies that have concentrated on this population of SLE patients emphasized either morphological[11, 16] or immunologic characteristics.[19, 20] Therefore, we undertook a study of both clinical and immunologic status of the 16 patients with MLG of the 117 patients with SLE referred to Necker Hospital between 1962 and 1982. We compared, in particular, patients with MLG and patients with diffuse proliferative lupus glomerulonephritis (DPLG) referred to us within the same period, and attempted to determine whether MLG constitutes a clinical and immunologic entity among SLE patients.

Patients, Material, and Methods

All the patients included in this study were referred to Necker Hospital as inpatients between 1962 and 1982 and fulfilled the SLE criteria of the American Rheumatism Association (ARA).[27] Sixteen patients with MLG, 33 with DPLG, and 3 patients with systemic lupus vasculitis without renal involvement were studied.

The diagnosis of MLG was established by both light microscopic and immunofluorescent studies of a kidney biopsy specimen. MLG was characterized by diffuse, generalized thickening of the basement membrane and, when deposits were present, by their exclusive intramembranes and/or epimembranous location, with no or only a minimal local increase in the mesangial matrix and no proliferation or mesangial or endothelial cells as determined by light microscopy.

The diagnosis of DPLG was characterized by generalized glomerular hypercellularity due to the proliferation of mesangial, endothelial, and epithelial cells, associated with an exudation of polymorphonuclear cells and areas of glomerular necrosis. Immune deposits were generally intense and present in a subendothelial as well as mesangial location.

The diagnosis of systemic vasculitis was based on histopathologic criteria, including necrosis of vascular walls and surrounding perivascular tissue; the presence of material having the staining qualities of fibrinoid; and a cellular infiltration, composed predominantly of neutrophils in the vessel walls and the perivascular zone.

The following variables were evaluated and defined: (1) sex

and age of the patient and clinical manifestations of SLE (ARA criteria); (2) duration of SLE, from the time of the first symptoms to the time of the first renal biopsy; (3) duration of renal disease, determined as the time between the discovery of proteinuria and/or an abnormal urinary sediment and the time of renal biopsy; and (4) follow-up after the first renal biopsy until renal death or most recent examination.

Renal disease was defined by one of the following: proteinuria higher than 250 mg/24 hours, microscopic hematuria or blood cell casts, serum creatinine above 1.2 mg/dl or BUN above 25 mg/dl, at least, or 20.4 mg/dl rise in serum creatinine above baseline values. Nephrotic syndrome was defined as a 24-hour excretion of urinary protein of 3.5 gm or more; serum albumin, less than 3.0 gm/dl; serum cholesterol, more than 300 mg/dl; and edema. Mild proteinuria was defined as a 24-hour excretion of urinary protein of less than 3.5 gm. Arterial hypertension was included when the diastolic pressure was persistently above 90 mm Hg.

High-dose steroid therapy was arbitrarily defined as the administration of prednisone (or its equivalent) in a daily dose of 40 mg or more for at least 60 days; low-dose steroid therapy, as the administration of prednisone, less than 40 mg/day, for any length of time. Statistical comparisons between the groups were made using the χ^2 test, modified by Yates.

The following immunologic studies were performed:

1. The deoxyribonucleic acid (DNA) binding capacity was assessed by the Farr assay, using [14] C-labeled *E. coli* DNA, as previously described.[28, 29] Normal values were less than 20% binding.

2. Spontaneously precipitating antibodies to DNA were determined according to the method described by Gershwin and Steinberg.[30] Briefly, 0.2 µl of [14] C-labeled *E. coli* DNA was incubated with 10 µl of test serum and borate-buffered saline (BBS), pH 8, in a final volume of 200 µl, for 1 hour at 37° C and 1 week at 4° C. Then, the suspension was centrifuged at 10,000 g for 1 hour. Fifty µl of the supernatant was removed and the radioactivity determined in a β-scintillation counter. One hundred µl of the same supernatant was collected, incubated with 55% ammonium sulfate, and then centrifuged, as in the Farr assay. This procedure allowed a measure of precipitat-

ing and nonprecipitating DNA antibodies. The ratio of precipitating DNA antibodies was calculated according to the formula:

$$\text{Ratio} = \frac{\text{Precipitating DNA antibodies}}{\text{Total DNA binding capacity}}$$

3. Antinuclear antibodies were detected by indirect immunofluorescence using mouse liver sections.

4. *Crithidia luciliae* assay. Anti-double-standard DNA (dsDNA) antibodies were determined by the indirect immunofluorescent technique, as described by Aarden et al.[31] Briefly, *C. luciliae* were dried onto a slide, incubated with 10 µl of undiluted test serum, washed in phosphate-buffered saline (PBS), and then incubated with fluorescein conjugated rabbit antihuman γ-globulin antiserum.

5. Serum complement C3 and C4 levels were evaluated by immunonephelometry. Normal values were C3, 70 mg/dl or above; C4, 15 mg/dl or above.

6. Circulating immune complexes (CIC) were determined by the polyethylene glycol (PEG) assay, described by Digeon et al.[32] Cryoglobulins were evaluated by previously described techniques.[33]

7. Antibodies to saline extractable nuclear antigens (ENA) (lyophilized rabbit thymus extract) were detected by double immunodiffusion in agar.

8. Other autoantibodies were obtained and evaluated by techniques used in our laboratory: antibodies to red blood cells (Coombs), antibodies to phospholipids (VDRL), antibodies to prothrombinase (circulating anticoagulant), and rheumatoid factor (Waaler-Rose, Latex fixation tests).

Results

GENERAL DATA AT THE TIME OF RENAL BIOPSY

Of the 16 patients who fulfilled the diagnosis criteria of MLG, 13 were female. The mean age of the patients was 24.8 years (range, 13–45 years).

Clinical manifestations of SLE were present before renal abnormalities in all patients for a period ranging from 0.1 to 7 years (average, 1.6 years) (Table 1). The duration of renal ab-

TABLE 1.—MEMBRANOUS GLOMERULOPATHY: GENERAL DATA AT THE TIME OF RENAL BIOPSY

PARAMETER	VALUE
Age (yr)	24.8 (13–55)*
Duration of SLE (yr)	1.6 (0.1–7)*
Duration of renal disease (yr)	0.8 (0–3.0)*
No. of patients	16
No. female	13
Renal function	
Normal	13
Mild insufficiency	3
Nephrotic syndrome	10
Mild proteinuria	6
Prior steroid therapy	
High dose	1
Low dose	6
None	9

*Ranges in parentheses; for these parameters, values given represent means.

normalities before renal biopsy ranged from 0 to 3 years (mean, 0.8 years). Only one patient had received high-dose steroid therapy prior to renal biopsy, while 6 patients had received low doses and 9 patients had received no steroid treatment (see Table 1).

RENAL DATA AT THE TIME OF BIOPSY

All patients had proteinuria. Ten (62.5%) had nephrotic syndromes. Microscopic hematuria was present in ten patients (62.5%). Renal function was normal in 13 patients, while the other three subjects had mild renal insufficiencies. The average serum creatinine level was 0.9 mg/dl (range, 0.7 mg–2.0 mg/dl) (see Table 1).

EXTRARENAL CLINICAL MANIFESTATIONS AT THE TIME OF RENAL BIOPSY

Extrarenal clinical manifestations were not different in the MLG group as compared to the DPLG group (Table 2). Both groups had the same frequencies of arterial hypertension and systemic vasculitis.

TABLE 2.—CLINICAL DATA IN 16 PATIENTS
WITH MEMBRANOUS LUPUS
GLOMERULOPATHY (MLG) AND 33 PATIENTS
WITH DIFFUSE PROLIFERATIVE LUPUS
GLOMERULONEPHRITIS (DPLG) AT THE TIME
OF RENAL BIOPSY

FINDING	MLG (%)	DPLG (%)
Facial erythema	47.8	64
Raynaud's phenomenon	12.5	12
Alopecia	18.8	24
Photosensitivity	12.5	6
Oral or nasal ulceration	6.3	6
Arthritis	62.5	73
Lymph nodes	12.5	18
Pleuritis	6.3*	24
Pericarditis	6.3*	24
Myocarditis	6.3*	9
Vasculitis	18.8	18
Arterial hypertension	18.8	15
Nephrotic syndrome	62.5	55

*Not significant.

IMMUNOLOGIC FINDINGS AT THE TIME OF RENAL BIOPSY

DNA BINDING CAPACITY.—The DNA binding capacities were low (mean value, 27.3% ± 19.9%) and ranged from 12% to 83% in the MLG group (Fig 1). Five patients had normal binding capacities. Only two patients had DNA binding capacities over 40%. In contrast, most patients with DPLG had high DNA binding capacities (mean, 77.5% ± 20.2%), ranging from 40% to 99% (see Fig 1).

PRECIPITATING DNA ANTIBODIES.—The precipitating characteristic of anti-DNA antibodies was evaluated in 12 patients with MLG at the time of renal biopsy. An absence or a low ratio ($<$ 0.1) of precipitating DNA antibodies was observed in all patients but two. These two patients with high ratios of precipitating DNA antibodies were the only patients of the MLG group to have systemic vasculitis (Fig 2). Moreover, the anti-DNA antibody profiles of these two patients (low DNA binding capacities and high ratios of precipitating DNA antibody) were identical to those observed in the three lupus patients with systemic vasculitis and no renal involvement. In contrast, in the DPLG group the eight untreated patients tested had high DNA binding capacities and high ratios of precipitating DNA anti-

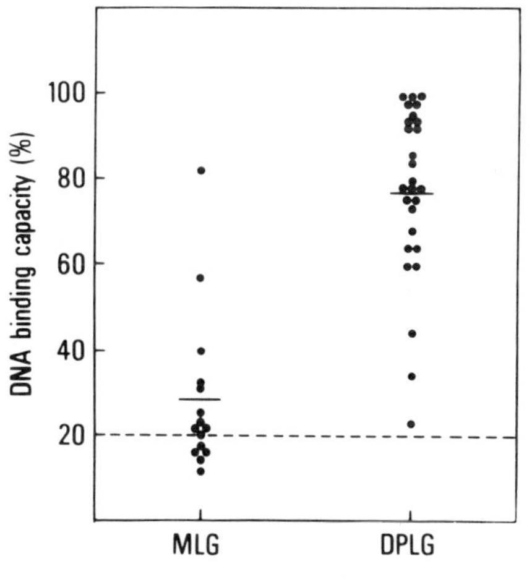

Fig 1.—DNA binding capacity in patients with membranous lupus glomerulonephritis *(MLG)* (27.3% ± 19.9%) and diffuse proliferative lupus glomerulonephritis *(DPLG)* (77.5% ± 20.2%) *(P< .001)*.

bodies. Figure 2 summarizes these data and shows that patients with MLG, DPLG, and systemic vasculitis without renal involvement could be separated into subgroups, according to their anti-DNA antibody properties.

CRITHIDIA LUCILIAE ASSAY.—All sera from patients with MLG

Fig 2.—Relationship between the DNA binding capacity and the ratio of precipitating antibodies in patients with membranous lupus glomerulonephritis *(solid circle)*, and diffuse proliferative lupus glomerulonephritis *(triangle)*. (The serum of the patient with MLG and a high DNA binding capacity was not available for determining the precipitating DNA antibodies.)

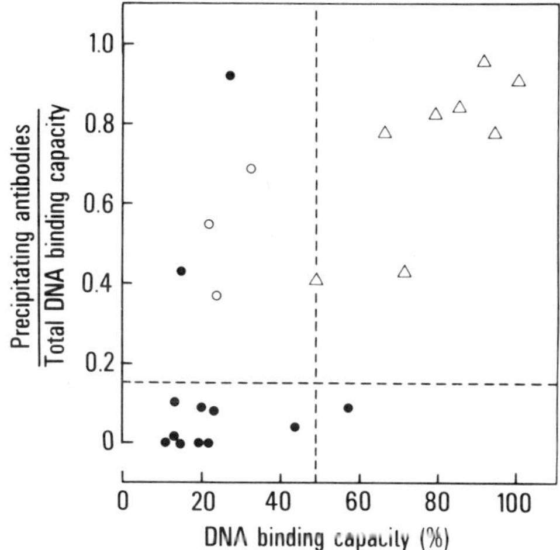

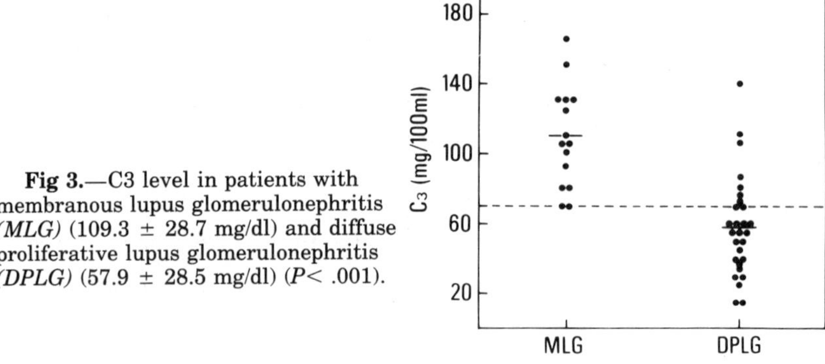

Fig 3.—C3 level in patients with membranous lupus glomerulonephritis *(MLG)* (109.3 ± 28.7 mg/dl) and diffuse proliferative lupus glomerulonephritis *(DPLG)* (57.9 ± 28.5 mg/dl) *(P< .001).*

(12/16) were negative in the *C. luciliae* assay at the time of renal biopsy. In contrast, the 20 sera from patients with DPLG tested in the assay were positive (end point dilution ranged from 1/10 to 1/640).

COMPLEMENT LEVELS.—The C3 and C4 levels were normal in all patients but one from the MLG group (Figs 3 and 4). Conversely, most patients with DPLG had low C3 and C4 levels.

OTHER IMMUNOLOGIC FINDINGS

Table 3 shows the results of the other immunologic tests performed at the time of renal biopsy in patients with MLG and DPLG. No differences were observed between these two groups

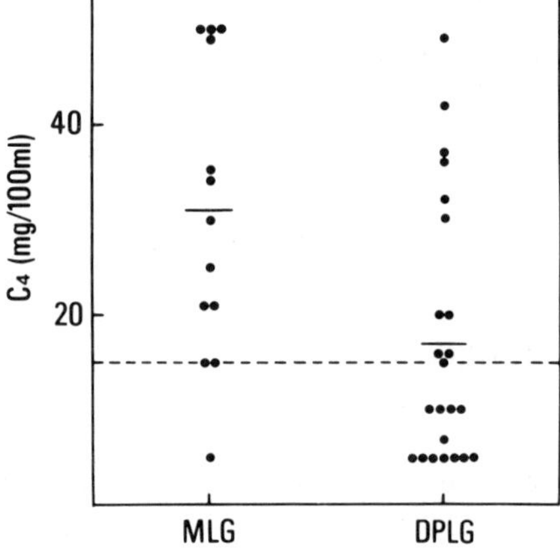

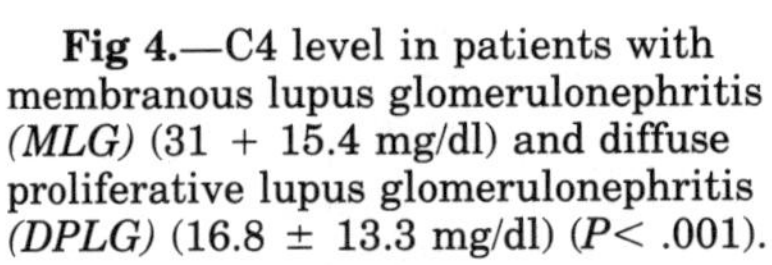

Fig 4.—C4 level in patients with membranous lupus glomerulonephritis *(MLG)* (31 + 15.4 mg/dl) and diffuse proliferative lupus glomerulonephritis *(DPLG)* (16.8 ± 13.3 mg/dl) *(P< .001).*

TABLE 3.—BIOLOGIC AND IMMUNOLOGIC DATA IN 16
PATIENTS WITH MLG AND 33 PATIENTS WITH DPLG AT THE
TIME OF RENAL BIOPSY*

FINDING	MLG	DPLG
Biologic		
Serum creatinine (mg/dl)	0.9 (0.7–2.0)	1.38 (0.7–4.5)
Hematuria (no patients)	10	28
Hemolytic anemia	2	5
Leukopenia	7	12
Thrombocytopenia	2	7
Immunologic		
Antinuclear antibodies	12(12)	33(33)
Anti-extractable nuclear antibodies		
Anti-Sm(+)	5(12)	9(33)
Anti-RNP(+)	6(12)	11(33)
Latex (+)	3(16)	4(22)
Waaler-Rose (+)	1(16)	2(22)
Coombs (+)	2(12)	8(24)
VDRL (+)	3(16)	3(15)
Cryoglobulinemia (+)	0(12)	10(22)
PEG (+)	1(12)	11(22)
Circulating anticoagulant (+)	1(8)	5(29)

*Figures in parentheses represent the number of patients tested.

when antinuclear, anti-ENA antibodies, circulating anticoagulant, Coombs, and false syphilis serology were considered. In
contrast, CIC and cryoglobulinemia were rarely observed in the
MLG group.

RENAL AND MORPHOLOGIC FEATURES DURING THE FOLLOW-UP PERIOD

NEPHROTIC SYNDROME.—Ten patients had nephrotic syndromes. Eight had nephrotic syndrome in remission, with no
persistent proteinuria in six. Of these eight patients, seven received high-dose steroid therapy and in one the disease remit-
ted spontaneously. The nephrotic syndrome persisted in two patients, one of whom received no treatment. The six patients
with mild proteinuria at the time of renal biopsy remained unchanged whether or not they received steroid treatment (Tables
4 and 5).

RENAL FUNCTION.—Four patients developed chronic renal insufficiencies. Of the three patients who had mild renal insufficiency at the time of renal biopsy, one recovered normal renal

TABLE 4.—CLINICAL FEATURES AT THE ONSET AND THE LATEST OBSERVATION IN 16 PATIENTS WITH MEMBRANOUS LUPUS GLOMERULOPATHY

FEATURE	ONSET	LATEST OBSERVATION
Total patients	16	16
No. with:		
Mild proteinuria	6	8
Nephrotic syndrome	10	2
No urinary abnormality	0	6
Hypertension	3	4
Renal insufficiency		
Mild	3	2
End stage	0	2
Years of observation		
<2		5
2–5		4
>5		7
Renal vein thrombosis		1
Transition to DPLG		1
Alive		16
Dead		0

TABLE 5.—STEROID THERAPY AND CLINICAL OUTCOME IN 16 PATIENTS WITH MEMBRANOUS LUPUS GLOMERULOPATHY

FINDING	STEROID THERAPY AFTER KIDNEY BIOPSY	
	High-dose	None
Total No. of patients	12	4
Nephrotic syndrome		
No. of patients	8	2
Persistent	1	1
Mild proteinuria	2	0
Remission	5	1
Mild proteinuria		
No. of patients	4	2
Persistent	4	2
Normal	0	0
Renal insufficiency		
No. of patients	2	2
Mild	1	1
End stage	1	1

function, with remission of the nephrotic syndrome (see Table 4). The two other patients had persistent, moderately impaired renal function. Both patients had arterial hypertension. None of them underwent a second kidney biopsy.

Two patients with normal renal function at the time of renal biopsy showed progressive loss of renal function until end-stage renal failure ensued. These two patients underwent second kidney biopsies. In the first patient, the transition to severe-diffuse proliferative glomerulonephritis was observed on the second kidney specimen obtained 1 year after the initial histologic evaluation. It is of importance that at the time of the first renal biopsy, this patient was the only one in the MLG group to have a very high DNA binding capacity (83%). The second patient had arterial hypertension, and severe tubulointerstitial and vascular lesions were seen in the second biopsy specimen, obtained 2 years after the initial histologic evaluation. Neither of them had received steroid or immunosuppressive therapy at the time of the first biopsy when the diagnosis of MLG was made. The follow-up period for all patients after the renal morphological diagnosis was first established ranged from 0.1 to 11.6 years (mean, 4.5 years). All patients are alive. The patient whose disease underwent morphological change into DPLG on repeated renal biopsy also had extrarenal manifestations (cerebritis). There were recurrent systemic manifestations of SLE in only two of the 16 patients. These two patients, who had systemic lupus vasculitis at the time of renal biopsy, had recurrent episodes of vasculitis (myocarditis, skin necrosis) during the follow-up period. Another patient experienced renal vein thrombosis.

Immunologic Findings During the Follow-up Period

DNA BINDING CAPACITY.—The DNA binding capacities remained low in all patients except the patient who showed histologic transition from MLG to severe DPLG (Fig 5).

PRECIPITATING DNA ANTIBODIES.—The ratios of precipitating DNA antibodies remained low (<0.1) in 11 of 12 patients tested. In one patient, transient increases of the ratio were observed in relation to exacerbations of systemic vasculitis.

CRITHIDIA LUCILIAE.—The *C. luciliae* assay was negative in all patients tested during the period of observation.

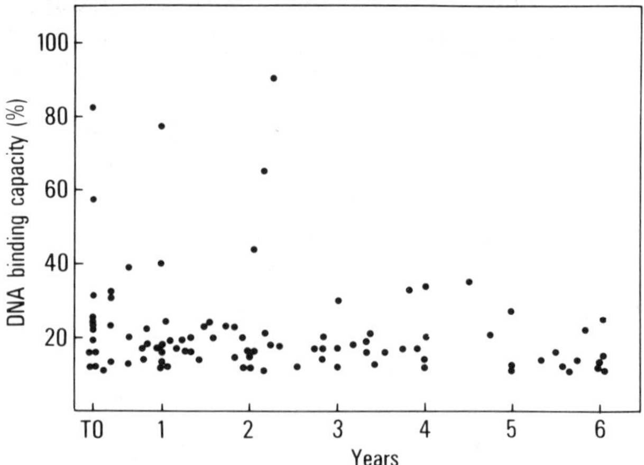

Fig 5.—Evolution of DNA binding capacities during the follow-up study of patients with membranous lupus glomerulonephritis *(MLG)*.

COMPLEMENT LEVELS.—During the course of the study, C3 and C4 levels remained normal in all patients but one; that patient had low complement levels in relation to recurrent episodes of systemic vasculitis.

Comments

Sixteen patients with MLG out of 117 patients with SLE referred to Necker Hospital between 1962 and 1982 were studied. The diagnosis of MLG was made upon the preestablished morphological criteria proposed by Baldwin et al.[11] and incorporated in WHO guidelines, as described by Appel et al.[34] and used by Donadio et al.[16]

All patients but one were untreated or received minimal dose steroid therapy at the time of the first renal biopsy. Despite previous reports[22, 35, 36] showing histologic transitions from focal lupus glomerulonephritis and DPLG to MLG with aggressive steroid therapy, the patient undergoing high-dose therapy was included in the study since therapy was initiated only 2 months before renal biopsy.

We did not insist on the morphological description of MLG since it has been analyzed extensively in previous studies.[11, 16] Our purpose was to investigate the immunologic manifestations that some authors thought to be characteristic[19, 34] and to analyze the clinical aspects and the evolutionary pattern of this histologic SLE group.

In our MLG group, most patients had a similar immunologic status, which included low DNA binding capacities, low or no precipitating DNA antibodies, negative *C. luciliae* assay, normal C3 and C4 levels, and the absence of cryoglobulinemia and CIC, as detected by the PEG assay. The low DNA binding capacity and the absence of precipitating DNA antibodies in patients with MLG have been reported previously.[19, 20] In contrast, and in agreement with the findings of Friend et al.,[19] all untreated patients with DPLG that we tested had high DNA binding capacities and precipitating DNA antibodies. Another striking feature was the negativity of the *C. luciliae* assay, even in untreated patients, at the time of renal biopsy. This is in agreement with a previous study citing either negative or very low titers of anti-dsDNA antibodies detected by this assay in three patients with MLG.[37] These results may be the consequence of either the absence of anti-dsDNA antibodies or the low sensitivity of the method compared to the Farr assay.[38–40] Antinuclear antibodies as detected by indirect immunofluorescence were found in all patients tested. These results, along with the low or normal DNA-binding capacities and the negativity of the *C. luciliae* assay, suggest that the presence of antinuclear antibodies is the best biologic indicator of the disease in patients with MLG. This is of importance, since membranous glomerulonephritis may precede the emergence of SLE by several years, particularly in children.[41]

Most patients had normal C3 and C4 levels. This is in agreement with the results reported by Decker et al.[42] However, other workers have reported low complement levels in most MLG patients tested.[13, 16, 34]

At variance with what is seen in patients with DPLG, CIC and cryoglobulinemia were rarely detected in our patients with MLG. These data may be regarded in a similar light as those obtained for patients with idiopathic membranous glomerulopathy, a disease strongly suspected to be mediated by the glomerular deposition or formation of immune complexes.[43] Thus, the low DNA binding capacities and the absence of CIC suggest that a low formation rate of DNA: anti-DNA complexes involving nonprecipitating DNA antibodies is required for the development of a membranous lesion in lupus patients.

Patients with MLG who had the immunologic profiles described above had almost identical extrarenal manifestations as patients with DPLG, as if the pathogenetic mechanisms reflected in this particular immunologic status modified only the renal histologic pattern. On the other hand, patients with MLG and different serologic features had either particular clinical manifestations or transition to another renal histologic pattern. Precipitating DNA antibodies were observed in two patients. Both had clinical and histologic pictures of systemic lupus vasculitis. This is in agreement with the findings of Edmonds et al.[44] and Cameron et al.,[45] who demonstrated by counterimmunoelectrophoresis the presence of precipitating DNA antibodies in their patients with systemic lupus vasculitis. One of the two patients with systemic lupus vasculitis had low C4 levels. In this regard, it would be of interest to know whether the patients with MLG and low complement levels described in other studies[13, 16, 34] had similar clinical profiles. In addition, a high DNA binding capacity was observed in one patient at the time of renal biopsy. This patient did not receive any treatment and showed histologic progression to severe DPLG within a year and ultimately to end-stage renal failure. Taken together, these results demonstrate that careful follow-up of immunlogic data in patients with MLG may provide adequate information concerning prognosis and therapy.

Of the three other patients with chronic renal insufficiency, one progressed to end-stage renal failure and underwent a second kidney biopsy, which showed tubulointerstitial and vascular lesions quite similar to those seen in idiopathic membranous glomerulopathy.[46] No modification of the patient's immunologic status was observed. Therefore, among the renal lesions that may be responsible for the development of renal insufficiency in MLG patients are the following: vascular lesions,[11] tubulointerstitial damage, renal vein thrombosis,[47] transition to DPLG,[2, 13, 22, 24] and vasculitis.[2, 43] The last two may be anticipated by serial immunologic evaluations.

Most of our patients had stable clinical and immunologic pictures. No deterioration of major crises occurred over several years, except in the two patients with systemic lupus vasculitis. None of them died. In the present study, the favorable renal outcome and good overall survival are similar to results reported by Pollack et al.[17] and Lee et al.[48] but much superior to those reported by others.[13, 16, 46, 48] In most series, in spite of the few deaths occurring as a result of renal insufficiency, MLG has been shown to have a favorable renal outcome and of itself is not an indication for high-dose steroid therapy. However, the differences in the overall prognosis observed between series must be explained. It is probably influenced by patient selection, variations in ethnic group distribution, and especially by the high frequency of complications observed during treatment. For instance, in MLG patients described by Donadio et al.,[16] death occurred in six of 28 patients and recurrent systemic complications manifested in ten of the 22 survivors during the follow-up study. These patients had either myocardial infarctions (3 patients) or sepsis (1 patient) which are suspected to be a consequence of steroid therapy,[50] or else manifestations (cerebrovascular accidents, cerebritis, recurrent pleural effusions) compatible with systemic lupus vasculitis. The frequency of low complement levels observed in Donadio's series might be associated with the frequency of vasculitis. Moreover, one should note the absence, over several years, of recurring major systemic manifestations in our patients, suggesting a lower pathogenic disease level in the MLG group. The relatively benign renal and clinical MLG course in our series demonstrates that an aggressive therapy, including prolonged high-dose steroid and/or cytotoxic agents, may not be clearly indicated in the case of MLG.

Finally, a particular immunologic status and a benign clinical outcome characterize patients with MLG as a distinct group among SLE patients.

Acknowledgments

Work was supported by a grant from the Fondation Day-Solvay.

We thank Mrs. Dominique Droz and Micheline Levy for the selection of patients and Miss Janet Jacobson for reviewing the manuscript.

REFERENCES

1. Pirani C.L., Manaligod J.R.: The kidneys in collagen diseases, in Mostofi F.K., Smith D.E. (eds.): *The Kidney*. Baltimore, Williams & Wilkins Co., 1966, pp. 147–203.

2. Baldwin D.S., Gluck M.C., Lowenstein J., et al.: Lupus nephritis: Clinical course as related to morphologic forms and their tansitions. *Am. J. Med.* 62:12–20, 1977.

3. Wolf L., Sheahan M., McCormick J., et al.: Classification criteria for systemic lupus erythematosus: Frequency in normal patients. JAMA 236:1497–1499, 1976.

4. Estes D., Christian C.L.: The natural history of systemic lupus erythematosus by prospective analysis. *Medicine* 50:85–95, 1971.

5. Dubois E.L., Wierzchowiecki M., Cox M.B., et al.: Duration and death in systemic lupus erythematosus: An analysis of 249 cases. *JAMA* 227:1399–1402, 1974.

6. Karsh J., Klippel J.H., Balow J.E., et al.: Mortality in lupus nephritis. *Arthritis Rheum.* 22:764–769, 1979.

7. Koffler D., Schur P.H., Kunkel H.G.: Immunological studies concerning the nephritis of systemic lupus erythematosus. *J. Exp. Med.* 126:607–623, 1967.

8. Koffler D., Agnello V., Thoburn P., et al.: Systemic lupus erythematosus: Prototype of immune complex nephritis in man. *J. Exp. Med.* 134:1695–1785, 1971.

9. Pollak V.E., Pirani D.L., Schwartz F.C.: The natural history of the renal manifestations of systemic lupus erythematosus. *J. Lab. Clin. Med.* 63:537–550, 1964.

10. Pollack V.E., Pirani C.L.: Renal histologic findings in systemic lupus erythematosus. *Mayo Clin. Proc.* 44:630–644, 1969.

11. Baldwin D.S., Lowenstein J., Rothfield N.F.: The clinical course of the proliferative and membranous forms of lupus nephritis. *Ann. Intern. Med.* 73:929–942, 1970.

12. Spargo B.H., Seymour A.E.: The value of electron microscopy in the study of glomerular disease. Edited by Back D. Oxford, Backwell Scientific Publications, 1973, p. 155.

13. Cameron J.S., Turner D.R., Ogg C.S., et al.: Systemic lupus with nephritis: A long-term study. *Q. J. Med.* 48:1–24, 1979.

14. McCluskey R.T.: Lupus nephritis, in Sommers S.C. (ed.): *Kidney Pathology*. New York, Appleton-Century-Crofts, 1975, pp. 435–460.

15. Morel-Maroger L., Mery J.P., Droz D., et al.: Aspects évolutifs des glomérulonéphrites lupiques: Apport des biopsies rénales itératives, in Hamburger J., Crosnier J., Funck-Brentano J.L. (eds.): *Actualités Néphrologiques, Hôpital Necker*. Paris, Flammarion Médecine-Sciences, 1981, pp. 155–159.

16. Donadio J.B., Burgess J.H., Holley K.E.: Membranous lupus nephropathy: A clinicopathologic study. *Medicine* 56:527–536, 1977.

17. Pollack V.E., Pirani C.L., Dujovne I., et al.: The clinical course of lupus nephritis: Relationship to the renal histologic findings, in Kincaid-Smith P., Mathew T.H., Becker E.L. (eds.): Glomerulonephritis: *Morphology, Natural History, and Treatment*. New York, John Wiley & Sons, 1973, pp. 1167–1181.

18. Decker J.L., Klippel J.H., Plotz P.H., et al.: Cyclophosphamide or azathioprine in lupus glomerulonephritis: A controlled trial. Results at 28 months. *Ann. Intern. Med.* 17:606–615, 1974.

19. Friend P.S., Kim Y., Michael A.F., et al.: Pathogenesis of membranous nephropathy in systemic lupus erythematosus: Possible role of nonprecipitating DNA antibody. *Br. Med. J.* 1:25, 1977.

20. Friend P.S., Michael A.F.: Hypothesis: Immunologic rationale for the therapy of membranous lupus nephropathy. *Clin. Immunol. Immunopathol.* 10:35–40, 1978.

21. Germuth F.G. Jr., Rodriguez E.: Immunopathology of the renal glomerulus: Immune complex disease and antibasement membrane disease. Boston, Little, Brown & Co., 1973, p. 58.

22. Mahajan S.K., Ordonez N.G., Spargo B.H., et al.: Changing histopathology patterns in lupus nephropathy. *Clin. Nephrol.* 10:1–8, 1978.

23. Ginzler E.M., Nicastri A.D., Chen C.K., et al.: Progression of mesangial and focal to diffuse lupus nephritis. *N. Engl. J. Med.* 291:693–696, 1974.

24. Boelaert J., Morel Maroger L., Méry J.P.: L'insuffisance rénale du lupus érythémateux disséminé, in Hamburger J., et al. (eds.): *Actualités Néphrologiques, Hôpital Necker*. Paris, Flammarion Médecine-Sciences, 1981, pp. 155–159.

25. Agnello V.: Immunopathogénie de la néphrite lupique, in Hamburger J., Crosnier J., Funck-Brentano J.L. (eds.): *Actualités Néphrologiques, Hôpital Necker.* Paris, Flammarion Médecine-Sciences, 1976, pp. 117–135.

26. Hill G.S., Hinglais N., Tron F., et al.: Systemic lupus erythematosus: Morphologic correlations with immunologic and clinical data at the time of biopsy. *Am. J. Med.* 64:61–79, 1978.

27. Cohen A.S., Reynolds W.E., Franklin E.C., et al.: Preliminary criteria for the classification of systemic lupus erythematosus. *Bull. Rheum. Dis.* 21:643–648, 1971.

28. Pincus T., Schur P.H., Rose J.A., et al.: Measurement of serum DNA-binding activity in systemic lupus erythematosus. *N. Engl. J. Med.* 281:701–705, 1969.

29. Hughes G.R.V.: Significance of anti-DNA antibodies in systemic lupus erythematosus. *Lancet* 2:861–863, 1971.

30. Gershwin M.E., Steinberg A.D.: Qualitative characteristics of anti-DNA antibodies in lupus nephritis. *Arthritis Rheum.* 17:947–954, 1974.

31. Aarden L.A., DeGroot E.R., Feltkamp T.E.: Immunology of DNA: III. *Crithidia luciliae,* a simple substrate for the determination of anti-dsDNA with the immunofluorescent technique. *Ann. NY Acad. Sci.* 254:505–515, 1975.

32. Digeon M., Laver M., Riza J., et al.: Detection of circulating immune complexes in human sera by simplified assays with polyethylene glycol. *J. Immunol. Methods* 16:165–183, 1977.

33. Brouet J.C., Clauvel J.P., Danon F., et al.: Biologic and clinical significance of cryoglobulins: A report of 86 cases. *Am. J. Med.* 57:775–788, 1974.

34. Appel G.B., Silva F.G., Pirani C.L., et al.: Renal involvement in systemic lupus erythematosus (SLE): A study of 56 patients emphasizing histologic classification; *Medicine* 57:371–410, 1978.

35. Hayslett J.P., Kashgarian L., Cook C.D., et al.: The effect of azathioprine on lupus glomerulonephritis. *Medicine* 51:393–412, 1976.

36. Hecht B., Siegel N., Adler M., et al.: Prognostic indices in lupus nephritis. *Medicine* 55:163–180, 1976.

37. Ballou S.P., Kushner I.: Immunochemical characteristics of antibodies to DNA in patients with active systemic lupus erythematosus. *Clin. Exp. Immunol.* 37:58–67, 1979.

38. Aarden L.A., Lakmaken F., DeGroot E.R., et al.: Detection of antibodies to DNA by radioimmunoassay and immunofluorescence. *Scand. J. Rheumatol. Suppl.* 11:12–19, 1975.

39. Slater N.G., Cameron J.S., Lessof M.H.: The *Crithidia luciliae* kinetoplast immunofluorescence test in systemic lupus erythematosus. *Clin. Exp. Immunol.* 25:480–486, 1976.

40. Crowe W., Kushner I.: An immunofluorescent method using *Crithidia luciliae* to detect antibodies to double stranded DNA. *Arthritis Rheum.* 20:811–814, 1977.

41. Kallen R.S., Lee S.K., Aronsen A.J., et al.: Idiopathic membranous glomerulonephritis preceding the emergence of systemic lupus erythematosus in two children. *J. Pediatr.* 90:72–76, 1977.

42. Decker J.L., Steinberg A.D., Reinertsen J.L., et al.: NIH Conference: Systemic lupus erythematosus. Evolving concepts. *Ann. Intern. Med.* 91:587–604, 1979.

43. Cameron J.S.: Pathogenesis and treatment of membranous nephropathy. *Kidney Int.* 15:88–103, 1979.

44. Edmonds J.P., Johnson G.D., Ansell B.M.: The value of tests for antibodies to DNA in monitoring the clinical course of SLE: A long-term study using the Farr test and the DNA counterimmunoelectrophoretic method. *Clin. Exp. Immunol.* 22:9–15, 1975.

45. Cameron J.S., Lessof M.H., Ogg C.S., et al.: Disease activity in the nephritis of systemic lupus erythematosus in relation to serum complement concentrations: DNA-binding capacity and precipitating anti-DNA antibody. *Clin. Exp. Immunol.* 25:418–424, 1976.

46. Noel L.H., Zanetti M., Droz D., et al.: Long-term prognosis of idiopathic membranous glomerulonephritis. *Am. J. Med.* 66:82–90, 1979.
47. Appel G.B., Williams G.S., Meltzer J.I., et al.: Renal vein thrombosis, nephrotic syndrome and systemic lupus erythematosus. *Ann. Intern. Med.* 85:310–317, 1976.
48. Lee P., Urowitz M.B., Bookman A.A.M., et al.: Systemic lupus erythematosus: A review of 110 cases with reference to nephritis, the nervous system, infections, aseptic necrosis and prognosis. *Q. J. Med.* 181:1–32, 1977.
49. Striker G.E., Kelly M.R., Quadracci L.J., et al.: The course of lupus nephritis: A clinical-pathological correlation of 50 patients. *Perspect. Nephrol. Hypertens.* 1:1141–1144, 1973.
50. Bulkley B.H., Roberts W.C.: The heart in systemic lupus erythematosus and the changes induced in it by corticosteroid therapy. *Am. J. Med.* 58:243–264, 1975.

Immunologic Problems and Perspectives in the Therapeutic Use of Monoclonal Antibodies in Nephrology

JEAN-FRANÇOIS BACH, M.D. AND
LUCIENNE CHATENOUD, M.D.

INSERM U-25, Département de Néphrologie, Hôpital Necker, Paris, France

ANTIBODIES have now been used for therapy in man for more than 60 years. The administration of sera from animals or humans immunized against infectious agents can prevent or even, in some cases, cure the infections caused by these microbes. Polyvalent immunoglobulins (without defined specificity) are used in the same way to restore the anti-infectious defense of some children with humoral immunodeficiency. Antivenom sera effectively prevent severe complications secondary to certain snake bites. Anti-Rhesus antibodies injected into the mother within 48 hours after delivery prevent the maternal immunization which would increase the risk of hemolytic disease of the newborn in subsequent pregnancies. Lastly, antilymphocyte sera are administered to organ graft recipients to prevent or cure rejection.

This long list recalls, if it were necessary, the great interest in and potential of serotherapy in man. It should be recognized, however, that clinical indications for antibody use are limited by difficulties of diverse natures, such as (1) the generally low titer of specific antibodies, requiring the use of large amounts of serum, (2) the practical difficulties of antisera collection or

0084-5457/84/0014-0365-0388-$04.00

production, (3) the cost of immunoglobulin purification, (4) the risk of xenosensitization when xenogeneic serum (originating from a different species) is used, (5) the usual absence of a good definition and standardization of the antibody responsible for the therapeutic effect, and (6) the constant presence of contaminating antibodies prone to generate side effects or sometimes to block the effect of active antibodies.

The problem is to determine whether the use of monoclonal antibodies produced by hybridomas in the place of polyclonal antisera produced by the whole animal would preclude these difficulties and thus leave hope for new clinical uses of antibodies. This is the subject of this review, which will be based both on theoretical data emerging from basic immunologic research and on observations made in the first patients treated by monoclonal antibodies.

Production and Properties of Monoclonal Antibodies

It was in 1975 that Kohler and Milstein described the production of monoclonal antibodies by hybridomas. The immunologic world rapidly realized that this was a major discovery carrying the seeds of a true technological revolution.

DESCRIPTION OF THE TECHNIQUE

The *principle* is simple[43]: the fusion of a plasma cell derived from an animal immunized against a given antigen and of a myelomatous cell gives rise to a hybrid cell, the hybridoma. This cell produces in quasi-unlimited and eternal fashion antibodies that are homogeneous, monoclonal, and strictly specific for the selected antigen. Immunized cells bring the genetic information necessary to the synthesis of the desired antibody; myelomatous plasma cells confer immortality on the fused cells, i.e., their capacity to multiply and survive in culture. After fusing in the presence of polyethylene glycol, myelomatous plasma cells selected as carriers of a metabolic deficiency (HGPRTase deficiency) are eliminated by passage on a selective culture medium, hypoxanthine-aminopterine-thymidine (HAT), in which only hybrids multiply. Myelomatous parental cells die because of their inability to use hypoxanthine. Surviving hybrids synthesize large amounts of monoclonal antibodies.

They can then be selected on the basis of their capacity to synthesize a particular antibody recognized by the systematic study of supernatants by a method using the antigen in question. Selection or cloning is performed by the limiting dilution technique in which relevant hybrids, detected by their supernatants, are cultured at increasingly low cell concentrations (down to one cell per well).

By allowing the unlimited production, so far done only in the mouse and the rat, of monoclonal antibodies with a precise and selected specificity, the hybridoma technique represents one of the most striking successes in immunology in recent years.

Monoclonal antibodies produced by hybridomas are basically identical to antibodies present in polyclonal hyperimmune sera. However, the homogeneity of monoclonal antibodies, which are present as multiple copies of a single and same molecule, give them certain characteristics that distinguish them from a practical standpoint from polyclonal antibodies. First, the monoclonal antibody is derived from a single clone and thus possesses only the properties of this clone. If it is an IgG, the antibody is usually an agglutinator; if it is an IgE or an IgA, it does not fix complement. Additionally, the antibody reacts with a single epitope, i.e., a single antigenic determinant of a single molecule (with the exception of cross reactions). This essential property is often very useful inasmuch as it ensures the strict specificity of the desired effect; but it may in some cases explain a paradoxical inefficacy of the antibody. For example, the molecule recognized by the antibody may be present on the cell surface in amounts too small to allow the close linkage of two antibody molecules that is necessary for complement activation.

The production of monoclonal antibodies for clinical use does not pose problems that differ greatly from those that were met and completely resolved in the production of monoclonals used as in vitro reagents. The main problem is that of quantity. Whereas a limited amount of antibody suffices in in vitro experiments, doses ranging from 1 to 50 mg are administered in man. However, even these much higher doses do not pose a major problem. Practically speaking, the production can remain relatively modest and at moderate cost, fortunately much lower than that estimated from the price of antibodies sold as reagents. Antibodies for use in man must be as pure as possible in order to avoid contamination from oncogenic viruses. The absence of such contaminants is fundamental from the ethical viewpoint. It has been verified for the antibodies already used in man. The choice of the antibody-providing species is so far limited to the mouse and the rat. A striking publication in 1980 raised the hope of producing human monoclonal antibody by fusing immunized human lymphocytes with human myelometous B cells.[34] There is now a consensus that this hope cannot be consistently fulfilled. It is nearly impossible, except in some specific settings such as cancer patients,[55] to obtain stable human-human hybridomas. The alternative solution, which has given interesting results,[23] consists in the production of human-mouse hybrids, more difficult to obtain but more stable when they have been cloned.

The use of such human antibodies would in theory avoid patient sensitization, but perhaps only partially (see below). In addition, it would be much more difficult to obtain the immunized lymphocytes, the antibodies would probably in general have a lower affinity than those produced across the species barrier (essentially being IgM), and the risk of oncogenic virus transmission (often species-specific) would be increased. Finally, all these considerations suggest that it is probably not by modifying the already excellent production methods that progress will be made in the clinical use of monoclonal antibodies.

Therapeutic Trials of Monoclonal Antibodies: Experimental and Clinical Results

We have already mentioned the main circumstances in which polyclonal antibodies are commonly used in the form of traditional serotherapy. Most of these indications have been the subject of experimental and sometimes clinical studies with monoclonal antibodies, particularly antibodies directed against lymphocytes or infectious agents. Other indications, such as autoimmune diseases, tumors, and intoxications, have been studied extensively. It is apparent that numerous other therapeutic applications will rapidly emerge beyond the present indications for serotherapy. We discuss the first results obtained in various laboratories, with particular emphasis on the indications involving renal diseases, and among them those with which we have personal experience.

ANTILYMPHOCYTE ANTIBODIES AND NONSPECIFIC IMMUNOSUPPRESSION

Numerous monoclonal antibodies have been raised in the mouse against human T lymphocytes (Table 1). Some of these antibodies react against all mature T cells (such as OKT3), others against well-defined T cell subsets, notably the inducer subpopulations (such as OKT4), or against the suppressor/cytotoxic subset (such as OKT8). The analysis of the immunologic specificity, serology, and immunochemistry of the antibody and the functional dissection of subpopulations recognized have re-

TABLE 1.—MONOCLONAL ANTIBODIES REACTING WITH CELLULAR DIFFERENTIATION ANTIGENS*

LYMPHOHEMATOPOIETIC CELLS	TYPE	MW (IN KD)
Cortical thymocytes	NA1/34	49
	T6	49
	D47	45–49
All E+ cells	9.6	50
	D66	50
All E+ blood cells	OKT3	19
Inducer	9.3	44
	OKT4	62
	3A1	40
	Leu-3a, 3b	62
Cytotoxic/suppressive	OKT5	30–33
	OKT8	30–33
	Leu-2a, 2b	30–33
B cells	B1	30
	B2	140
T and CLL-B cell	10.2	65–67
	T65	65
	L17	67
	Leu-1	69–71
	A50	65
	OKT1	70
Leukemic non-T, non-B and T cells	D44	. . .
or thymocytes	OKT10	45
	12E7	28
Dividing cells	OKT9	90
	4F2	40–80
Only or mainly on non-T cells	Ia	29–33
	J5	95
	H27	. . .

*After L. Boumsell et al., in Bernard A., Boomsell L., Demeocq F. (eds.): *Biologie des Leucémies et hématosarcomes.* Paris, G. Lachurie, 1983, p. 25.

vealed that most antibodies produced in different laboratories have operationally analogous effects to one of the antibodies OKT3, OKT4, or OKT8, and in fact usually react with the very same molecules on T cells (even if they recognize different sites on the molecule). Conversely, most recent immunologic studies indicate that the subdivision of T cells into two populations with opposed functions probably represents an oversimplification. It has been shown in particular that OKT4+ inducer T cells include T cells that induce suppressor T cell differentiation.[60] Additionally, it does not appear that suppressor and cytotoxic functions, whose inactivation should have opposite effects on immune function, are necessarily carried by distinct cells. No antibody can distinguish them from one another.

The experimental study of the immunosuppressive activity of these antibodies is rendered difficult by the absence of activity of antihuman lymphocyte antibodies in species other than man, with the exception of some antibodies that react with primate lymphocytes. For example, OKT4 binds with good affinity to Macaca Rhesus lymphocytes, at variance with OKT3, which does not recognize them. In addition, no monoclonal antibody has been obtained that reacts with high affinity to mouse lymphocytes. In the absence of hybridomas of species other than mouse and rat, one must use in mice allogeneic monoclonals (mouse antimouse) or xenogeneic (rat antimouse) monoclonals that cross a species barrier insufficient to provide high-affinity antibodies. Interesting data have been reported with anti-Thy-1[50] and anti-Lyt-1[40] antibodies, but one cannot extrapolate directly from these results in those that might be expected in humans receiving high-quality antibodies.

Without going into clinical data, which are the subject of the chapter by H. Kreis in this volume,[38] the immunosuppressive activity of some monoclonals can be firmly accepted, with nevertheless major individual variations.

Two antibodies that react with all T cells have been evaluated in the monkey: OKT11A, which binds to the E rosette receptor, and WT1. OKT11A induces only modest and nonsignificant skin allograft survival and is inactive on renal allografts.[24, 25] T cells are not eliminated because they selectively lose the expression of the antigen recognized by the monoclonal due to the phenomenon of antigenic modulation, which will be discussed below (antigenic modulation represents the active and reversible disappearance of the membrane antigen that is specifically induced by the corresponding antibody). Better immunosuppression is observed with the WT1 antibody, but here again without long-term T cell depletion because of antigenic modulation.[32]

In man, the anti-HuLym-1 antibody directed against the E rosette receptor has been found inactive in allograft recipients having a rejection episode.[61] OKT3 and T12 antibodies react with mature T cells, that is, with the quasi-totality of circulating T cells, but with only a fraction of thymic lymphocytes (those that are the most mature). The immunosuppressive activity of these two antibodies has been evaluated in man. Within minutes following the first injection, both of them induce a nearly complete disappearance of circulating T cells.[8, 10, 12] Nevertheless, T cells reappear after 2–5 days, again because of antigenic modulation. Ultimately, if the treatment is continued long enough, the antibody effect is abrogated by the onset of an antimouse monoclonal immune response. We shall return later to this subject and discuss in more detail the characteristics of their antimonoclonal sensitization. The immunosuppressive effect of OKT3 and T12 is indicated by the rapid cure of rejection episodes induced by each of these two antibodies,[12, 14, 36] as well as by the absence of rejection usually observed with OKT3 when it is used prophylactically in the first weeks after transplantation and before patients are sensitized against the antibody.[38]

Less consistent results have been reported at present (only in monkeys) for antibodies directed against T cell subsets. OKT4 and OKT4A, which are specific for the inducer population, are immunosuppressive, both to skin and to renal allograft rejection,[13, 22] and this relatively independently of their capacity to deplete circulating T cells. One even finds OKT4-coated T cells in the blood of OKT4- or OKT4A-treated monkeys.[32, 33] Modulation occurs with one or the other antibody, particularly when they are used simultaneously.[33] At variance with anti-T cell inducer antibody, antibody directed against cytotoxic/suppressor T cells is little or not immunosuppressive, at least in the monkey. This is true for OKT8, OKT8A,[32] and for a mixture of five antibodies with the same specificity as OKT8.[31] This opposition between immunosuppressive OKT4 and inactive OKT8 antibodies merits confirmation on a large number of antibodies.

If confirmed, it would support the hypothesis that inducer OKT4+ cells, which recognize class II transplantation antigens (Ia in the mouse, DR in man) play the major role in rejection. It should be noted in this respect that an anti-Lyt-1 monoclonal with a specificity analogous to that of OKT4 induces immunosuppression, notably in skin grafts,[40] and that in man rejection episodes are often, although inconsistently, associated with an increase in the number of OKT4+ cells.[9, 12]

Although still preliminary in many respects, these first results already provide important information on the immunosuppressive activity of monoclonal antibodies. The most active antibodies are those reacting with all T cells or their inducer subset. However, the specificity for this subpopulation is not sufficient to render the antibody immunosuppressive since the antibodies OKT11A or anti-HuLym-1, which also recognize OKT4+ T cells (which have an E rosette receptor), are little or not immunosuppressive. In fact, it appears that probably more than the specificity for a functional subset, two other factors control the in vivo immunosuppressive activity of a monoclonal antibody. First, its capacity to give rise to antigenic modulation: an antibody which modulates strongly will not induce the depletion of its target cell. Second, the immunologic function of the antibody-reactive molecule: antibodies specific for molecules essential to lymphocyte function, such as OKT3, which reacts with a membrane structure tightly linked to the T cell antigen recognition receptor, or OKT4, are much better immunosuppressants than are antibodies reacting on the same cells with molecules not having defined functions (such as OKT11A, which recognizes the E rosette receptor). In the former case, even if the antibody induces antigenic modulation, it keeps its immunosuppressive potency, since the disappearance of the target molecule from the cell membrane alters the lymphocyte immunocompetence

In any case, one understands the absence of correlation observed between immunosuppressive activity and lymphocytopenia of individual antibodies. Mechanisms other than lympholysis, such as modulation, may intervene, at least for some antibodies. The lymphocyte depletion at the origin of lymphocytopenia may be due, as was formerly described for conventional antilymphocyte sera, to opsonization, as assessed by the chemiluminescence induced in monocytes in the presence of T cells coated with some anti-T cell monoclonals.[17]

It should also be noted, before closing this section, that OKT3 has been used in the prevention of graft-versus-host reaction by treating the bone marrow cell inoculum with the antibody in vitro at the time of transplantation. First results are discordant: favorable according to Prentice et al.[47] and negative according to Filipovich et al.[22] A lack of effect on the graft-versus-host reaction has also been observed by Thierfelder et al. after monoclonal injection into the graft recipient.[59]

ANTILYMPHOBLAST ANTIBODIES

Takahashi et al. have recently reported the successful use in the treatment of rejection episodes in renal transplantation of a monoclonal antibody directed against human lymphoblasts (and monocytes).[58] Interestingly, this antibody is specific for activated lymphocytes and does not provoke mature cell depletion.

ANTI-IA ANTIBODIES

Major histocompatibility complex genes that code for class II antigens (Ia in the mouse, DR in man) control antigen recognition by T cells and consequently play the central role in the genetic control of antigen-specific immune response. The intimate mechanisms of Ia gene intervention remain uncertain, but probably involve class II antigen recognition on the macrophage surface by the T cell receptor. This basic concept has led to the idea of depressing immune responses by blocking Ia antigen recognition by anti-Ia antibodies. Indeed, anti-Ia antibodies suppress production of antibody directed against synthetic polypeptides under Ia gene control: in the mouse, anti-Ia monoclonals selectively inhibit the production of antibodies against the T, G, A—L polypeptide under control of the corresponding Ia gene.[50] Similarly, anti-Ia antibodies can suppress the development of several autoimmune diseases. Experimental allergic encephalomyelitis induced by the injection of myelin basic protein incorporated in complete Freund's adjuvant may be prevented by monoclonals reacting with disease-associated IA determinants, in both acute and chronic forms.[56, 57] The same result has been obtained for experimental myasthenia gravis induced by the injection of acetylcholine receptor preparations.[67] Of particular interest for the nephrologist, anti-IA antibodies may prevent the onset of the immune complex disease of (NZB × NZW)F$_1$ mice. The mouse survival is statistically increased, even when the treatment is started late, after the clinical onset of the disease.[1] It remains to be determined, however, how survival is prolonged and glomerulonephritis is prevented (without proteinuria), while antinuclear antibody production, including anti-native DNA antibodies, is not depressed. This discrepancy is intriguing since it is generally accepted that the nephritis is due to the deposition of immune complexes formed by these antibodies. Additionally, it is the NZW parent gene products, against which the monoclonal was raised, which control the production of antinuclear antibodies in the (NZB × NZW) hybrids. More generally, the mechanisms of anti-IA monoclonal-mediated immunosuppression remain obscure. Converging experimental arguments indicate, however, that the anti-IA antibodies could induce the production of suppressor factors by macrophages or T cells,[45] but other mechanisms may operate, such as blocking of the recognition of autoantigens presented by macrophages or a direct pharmacologic effect on Ia$^+$ cells (macrophages or B cells). Although it is still preliminary and somewhat confusing, the use of anti-IA monoclonal antibodies seems to represent a promising approach which could easily be applied to human autoimmune diseases.

Monoclonal Autoantibodies: Anti-idiotypic Autoimmunization

The hybridoma technique provides a readily available possibility of obtaining monoclonal autoantibodies by fusing myeloma cells with lymphoid cells from autoimmune animals or patients, without stimulation of the autoreactive lymphocytes. Such autoantibodies have been obtained in several models, particularly DNA in the mouse[3, 62] and in man,[54] RNA in the mouse,[21] acetylcholine receptors in mouse[65] and man,[66] Langerhans islet cells in the mouse by our group (M. Dardenne and M. Sachs), in the rat,[15] and in man,[20] and thyroglobulin in the mouse.[68] The availability of these antibodies has already been at the origin of important basic progress by providing a new approach to the heterogeneity of autoimmune responses. Additionally, it opens a new domain of immunomanipulation based on anti-idiotype autoimmunization.

The study of anti-DNA antibodies in (NZB × NZW)F$_1$ and MRL/1 mice has already provided much information. Monoclonal antibodies strictly selected by their reactivity with native DNA are heterogeneous. In a given anti-DNA specificity, there exist multiple clones producing autoantibodies with different antigenicity (class or subclass) and physicochemical characteristics (pI). Each autoantibody clone also has its own idiotypes (idiotypes are the antigenic determinants present on the variable portion of the immunoglobulin molecule that are characteristic of the antibody specificity). R. Schwartz's group has reported the existence of recurrent idiotypes, that is, idiotypes common to several different monoclonal autoantibodies in the MRL/1 mouse, but these studies were performed on anti-DNA antibodies with wide specificity, reacting with numerous polynucleotides and some phospholipids. Studying strictly DNA-specific monoclonal autoantibodies, we have not found recurrent idiotypes.[4] In spite of this heterogeneity, in both studies the main clones are present in numerous (NZB × NZW)F$_1$ mice, and not only in the mice given the cell used by hybridization.[63]

These data do not allow prediction of the effect of autoimmunization against the idiotypes of a given anti-DNA monoclonal autoantibody. In Schwartz's scheme, one may hope to induce antibody production against the recurrent idiotype and thus decrease the overall leading of anti-DNA antibody, preventing the onset of clinical manifestations, including glomerulonephritis. This is the result obtained by Hahn and Ebling.[26] Conversely, one may fear that the anti-idiotypic autoantibodies will only recognize the antibody identical to the monoclonal used for autoimmunization, which will not decrease the overall production of anti-DNA antibodies, all the more so since according to a well-established mechanism, an idiotypic escape may occur: new clones producing antibody with the same specificity but bearing idiotypes different from those of the suppressed clone substitute for the switched off clone. It is this result that we have personally obtained by autosensitizing 6-week-old (NZB × NZW)F$_1$ mice against the anti-DNA monoclonal autoantibody PM77 (F. Tron et al., unpublished data). One may hope that the numerous studies underway will cast light on this situation and eventually lead to autoimmunization against a mixture of several monoclonal autoantibodies. Other complications could appear. In particular, results obtained by D. Sachs when attempting to suppress the allograft response by autoimmunization against anti-H_2 monoclonal antibody idiotypes indicate that in certain settings, there is paradoxically a stimulation of immune responses under the effect of anti-idiotypes,[4] probably secondary to a direct clonal stimulation by the anti-idiotype, according to a mechanism initially described several years ago by Eichmann for antistreptococcal immune responses. The same difficulty has been met by Zanetti in a model of autoimmune membranous glomerulonephritis induced by sensitizing against renal tubular antigens.

Because of all these uncertainties, it is difficult to predict which autoimmune or immune complex diseases could benefit from such a new approach. As far as renal diseases are concerned, the very interesting studies of Nelson and Phillips[44] may be mentioned. They showed the suppression of an experimental interstitial nephritis by anti-idiotypic autoimmunization, according to the principle described above, although they used a slightly different experimental approach in rats immunized with renal tubular antigens. The onset of the interstitial nephritis was prevented by induction of anti-idiotypic antibodies after immunization with tubular antigen-specific blasts whose receptors bear the same idiotypes as corresponding antibodies.

It is still most difficult to determine when and how this approach could be applied clinically. There should not be, a priori, difficulties in obtaining human monoclonal autoantibodies since it has already been possible to produce human monoclonal anti-DNA[54] and anti-islet cell[20] autoantibodies. Rather, the problem would be to monitor and control the direction of the eventual effect in order to avoid disease exacerbation. Theoretically, the method is also applicable to antigraft immunity. It is in fact in this setting that it was initially described by Binz and Wigzell.[6] It should be recognized, however, that it has proved very difficult to reproduce Binz's and Wigzell's data, and that, as already mentioned, recent results by D. Sachs indicate that in most cases enhancement rather than suppression of alloreactivity is obtained. It would be necessary to find efficient means to immunize patients againt monoclonal antibodies, which has not yet been solved, inasmuch as all anti-idiotypic autoimmunization achieved in the animal has entailed the use of complete Freund's adjuvant, which cannot be injected into man. Perhaps synthetic adjuvants such as the muramyl dipeptide (MDP) would help circumvent this difficulty.

OTHER ANTIBODIES

The therapeutic use of other monoclonals is presently under study in domains more distant to the nephrologist's interest than those just discussed. We shall briefly mention the present status of these studies, which illustrate both the enormous promises of the new "drugs" represented by monoclonal antibodies and the great and sometimes unexpected difficulties that arise in their use.

Antitumoral Antibodies

Considerable effort has been devoted to this field, notably for the treatment of lymphomas and leukemias. Several antibodies have been produced against the common acute lymphoblastic leukemia antigen (CALLA) present in 80% of patients with this type of leukemia and in 40% of those in active phases of chronic myeloid leukemia, as well as in a low percentage of normal bone marrow cells. When the J5 antibody is injected into patients with acute leukemia, there is a very rapid and nearly complete disappearance of circulating leukemic cells.[49] However, the effect is short-lived, since many leukemic cells are not hit. This escape is due to the phenomenon of antigenic modulation. Other trials have been performed, also with transitory success, essentially in animals with antibodies directed against "normal" differentiation antigens, intensely expressed on some leukemic cells such as the TL antigen in the mouse.[5] In man, patients with Sézary's syndrome were treated with the anti-Leu-1 antibody directed, like OKT3, against all mature T cells.[42] Three of the eight patients thus treated had complete remission, terminating when they became immunized against the monoclonal. The same antibody provoked a marked but also transient reduction in the number of leukemic cells in a few cases of acute lymphoblastic leukemia[42] and of chronic lymphoid leukemia.[18] In fact, the only really convincing results are those reported by R.A. Miller and R. Levy in the treatment of a lymphoma where the monoclonal IgM present on the surface of the malignant cell carried idiotypes characteristic of the tumor, thus behaving as a true tumor-associated antigen.[42] Lymphoma cells were fused with a murine myeloma to produce hybrids secreting large amounts of the tumor-derived monoclonals. These immunoglobulins were injected into mice in order to obtain anti-idiotypic hybridomas whose product, shown to be specific for the tumor immunoglobulin idiotypes, was injected into the patient. A complete and long-lasting (18 months) remission was observed in one patient. Only few significant data have been reported in the treatment of solid tumors by monoclonal antibodies, essentially for gastrointestinal tumors.[52]

Multiple difficulties explain the relative failure met in the use of monoclonal antibodies in the treatment of leukemias and cancers: antigenic modulation and xenosensitization, the presence of large amounts of circulating antigen (absorbing the antibody before it reaches its target), and the selection of antibody-resistant variants.

Antibodies Against Infectious and Parasitic Agents

A large number of antibodies have been produced against bacteria, viruses, and parasites, promoting a complete reversal in serodiagnostic methods. Few studies have been published to date on the in vivo use of these antibodies in protection against infection, but positive results have already been obtained in several models. Among results published so far, one may cite the protection obtained against *Hemophilus influenzae* in the mouse using mouse[27] or human[28] antibodies, *Streptococcus pyogenes*,[46] and *Escherichia coli*.[53] An important fact is that not all monoclonal antibodies produced against bacteria are protective. Similar results have been reported for rabies virus,[37] Bluetongue virus,[39] and various parasites, notably *Leishmania mexicana*[2] and *Plasmodium knowlesi*.[11] In all these cases, the production of protective monoclonal antibodies could lead to their clinical use in patients that do not respond or react too late to specific chemotherapy. The could also guide the characterization and the isolation of antigens giving rise to a protective vaccination, as has been done for *Plasmodium* antigens by Cochrane et al.[11]

ANTIDRUG ANTIBODIES

The treatment of some drug-induced intoxications is rendered difficult by the fixation of the drug to certain organs, as in the case of digitalin. The administration of drug-specific monoclonals can stop the effects of the intoxication, first by neutralizing the antibody, and then by accelerating its removal. Promising results have been obtained with an antidigitalin high-affinity monoclonal,[19] which was shown to prevent the lethal effect of digitalin-induced intoxication in the rabbit (own unpublished results).

Two Major Escape Mechanisms: Antigenic Modulation and Antimonoclonal Sensitization

Unlike many drugs, monoclonals may induce host escape reactions that oppose their therapeutic effects. The escape is rapid but inconstant and variable in its effects, depending on the antibody for antigenic modulation, and later but usually complete for sensitization.

ANTIGENIC MODULATION

Antigenic modulation was initially described by Boyse, Old, and Luell in 1963[7]: thymocytes or thymic leukemic cells which normally express the TL differentiation antigen reversibly lose their sensitivity to the cytotoxic action of anti-TL antibodies in the presence of complement when they have previously been exposed, in vivo or in vitro, to anti-TL antibodies. Recently, the concept has been extended to the antibody-induced disappearance of membrane antigens detected by immunofluorescence, a phenomenon closely related to the preceding one and often confused with it, although they are not strictly identical.

Antigenic modulation is linked to the redistribution of membrane antigens after they have bound the monoclonal. At the minimum, there may be a membrane microrearrangement which renders the antigen unable to induce the complement

activation required for cytolysis. At best, the antigen-mono-
clonal antibody complex microprecipitates and, moved by
the cytoskeleton, concentrates at a cell pole before being removed either inside or outside the cell. The phenomenon is reversible since the mere incubation of cells modulated in vitro
for a few hours in the absence of the antibody is sufficient to
let the antigen reappear. In all cases, the membrane alterations involve only the monoclonal-specific antigen, all other
molecules on the membrane (receptors or antigens) keeping a
normal distribution.

Antigenic modulation plays a central role in host susceptibility to monoclonal antibodies. Its effects depend closely on the
target cell, on the functional importance of the molecule recognized by the monoclonal, and on the desired duration of the
therapeutic effect. In the case of tumors or leukomas, in which
one aims at destroying malignant cells, the monoclonal treatment loses all its efficacy as soon as the monoclonal antibody
appears. In the case of anti-T cell monoclonal antibody–induced immunosuppression, the therapeutic effect is lost only
when the target molecule is not necessary to the lymphocyte
function, as discussed above for OKT11A. In the opposite case,
modulation does not abrogate the immunosuppressive effect
and may even contribute to it by rendering the cell immunoin-
competent. We have observed in the case of OKT3 that T cells
from patients showing antigenic modulation (with OKT3 –
OKT4 + or OKT3 – OKT8 + phenotype) simultaneously recovered in vitro in less than 24 hours in the absence of OKT3 the
full expression of the OKT3-defined antigen and their reactivity to phytohemagglutinin. This reversibility is not observed,
however, if the incubation is performed in the presence of
OKT3.

The modulation intensity varies with the antibody, especially in vitro, where it is generally more difficult to induce
than in vivo. We have thus shown for OKT3 that modulation
was only partial in vitro but total in vivo. It is enhanced by the
presence of certain "piggyback" antibodies, notably anti-idiotype class-specific antibodies produced in patients sensitized
against the monoclonal.

Is antigenic modulation an obligatory consequence of the in
vivo use of monoclonal antibodies? Several approaches can be
envisioned to avoid it, independently of the already mentioned

selection of antibodies recognizing functionally important molecules (a solution which is not applicable to tumor therapy). The production of nonmodulating antibodies could obviously represent an ideal solution. It still is difficult to say whether such antibodies really exist. In vitro studies do not suffice to demonstrate the point, for, as just discussed, antibodies modulate much better in vivo than in vitro. It appears, however, that some antibodies induce only a weak or negligible modulation in vivo. This is particularly true of OKT4 and of some antibodies belonging to the already mentioned B9 pool. Monkeys treated by these antibodies keep circulating T cells coated with the injected antibody. Note also that conventional polyclonal antilymphocyte sera do not readily give rise to antigenic modulation, which can be explained, among other hypotheses, by the presence of nonmodulating antibodies. One could also use two or more antibodies in a successive or even alternative fashion, the treatment with the second antibody beginning after some time interval necessary for the target cell to recover from the modulation induced by the first monoclonal. Finally, one may attempt to build univalent antibody by removal of a Fab arm by limited papain proteolytic digestion.[23] Fab/c antibody fragments thus obtained are more able to induce modulation but keep their capacity to activate complement. This approach has been used successfully in the mouse against lymphoid leukemia.[25] A last possibility, which has been widely investigated in antitumor immunotherapy, consists of complexing the antibody to a toxin, most often a chain of ricin, which has lost its cellular binding site but kept its toxicity. These immunotoxins bring the toxin to the target cell of the monoclonal antibody, whose activity is considerably enhanced.[30] This method does not eliminate the modulation problem but in the best cases permits killing of all tumor cells after the first injection(s) before modulation occurs. One may regret that major difficulties still persist in most potential indications for immunotoxins, which have thus not definitively proved their operational efficiency.[30]

Antimonoclonal Sensitization

One of the major drawbacks of traditional serotherapy is linked to the use of xenogeneic (heterologous) proteins. This nearly constant sensitization poses the double problem of the risk of anaphylactic shock and of abrogation of therapeutic activity by neutralization followed by accelerated elimination of the monoclonal antibody. One might have reasonably hoped that the comparatively low doses administered would not involve the risk of this problem. This is not the case. Murine monoclonal antibodies provoke in man an intense and rapid immunization, even after a limited number of intravenous injections containing no more than 50 mg of protein.

The sensitization is not regularly observed but is present in more than 80% of allograft recipients and 5% of leukemic or lymphomatous patients.[18, 42] This difference probably relates to the endogenous immunosuppression present in the latter patients. From the clinical viewpoint, the sensitization, which usually occurs about 10 days after the beginning of treatment in the absence of associated immunosuppressive treatment, is manifested by the brisk cessation of monoclonal therapeutic activity. Inasmuch as the monoclonal antibody–induced immunosuppression is very rapidly reversible because of antigenic modulation, its effects wane as soon as antimonoclonal antibodies become detectable. The antibody-target cells recover full expression of the antibody-reactive antigen. In the case of renal allograft recipients, a rejection occurs. However, no clinical manifestations of serum sickness or anaphylaxis are usually noted. In our own clinical trial, we observed only a mild allergic skin reaction. It would be interesting in this regard to investigate antimonoclonal IgE antibodies, but to our knowledge this has not yet been done on a significant series of patients. The problem is also posed of the predictive value of skin tests performed before the beginning of treatment. Although these tests can be performed effectively, it should be recognized that their interpretation is often difficult.

Antimonoclonal antibodies are heterogeneous, both for their class (initially IgM, then IgG after a few days) and especially for their specificity. We have studied in detail the various categories of antibodies produced against OKT3 in renal allograft recipients treated prophylactically with OKT3 from the day of transplantation. Anti-OKT3 antibodies were studied by four techniques.:

1. An enzyme-linked immunosorbent assay (ELISA) in which OKT3 is fixed on a plastic plate and OKT3 binding is revealed

by the addition of an anti-human Ig serum coupled with peroxidase;

2. An immunofluorescence technique in which the capacity of anti-OKT3 antibody to bind to OKT3-coated cells is evaluated. This fixation is revealed by adding an anti-human Ig fluorescent antibody;

3. and 4. Two techniques, based on the inhibition of the OKT3 fixation on its target, revealed either by immunofluorescence (with an anti-mouse Ig serum) or by the proliferative response to phytohemagglutinin.

The composite use of these four techniques has shown that OKT3-treated patients produce essentially two categories of anti-Ig antibodies. The first is directed against the constant OKT3 region more particularly against Ig2a isotype (class-specific) determinants, best expressed after combination of the monoclonal with its target cell. These antibodies bind to T cells coated with OKT3 or other Ig2a monoclonals but do not react with T cells coated with monoclonals with another isotype. Importantly, these antibodies do not inhibit OKT3 binding to its target and are negative in the ELISA test (probably because the constant part by which the monoclonal is coupled to the plate is no longer accessible). These anti-constant region antibodies have the particularity of intensely augmenting antigen modulation (whereas, paradoxically, goat anti-mouse Ig sera do not). Conversely, these antibodies do not accelerate OKT3 catabolism, as assessed by the presence of high serum OKT3 levels (evaluated by ELISA), as long as the treatment is continued and the total persistence of the therapeutic effect is patients who produce only these antibodies. The second type of anti-OKT3 antibodies is directed against the variable region, and more particularly against the idiotypic determinants that are characteristic of the OKT3 antibody specificity. These antibodies give positive results in the four techniques mentioned above. They may be obtained in purified form by passage of the patient's serum on an immunoadsorbent prepared with an Ig2a monoclonal antibody without the OKT3 antibody specificity and thus without OKT3 idiotypes. Additionally, this immunoadsorption method allows the preparation (by dilution) of the anti-idiotype antibodies.

Similar although less detailed data have been reported for

the anti-OKT3[29] and anti-Leu-1[42] response. Miller and Levy have shown that in patients with Sézary's syndrome treated with the anti-Leu-1 antibody, anti-idiotypic antibodies represented about 5% of the total antimonoclonal antibodies produced.

Efforts have been devoted to slow—or, better to prevent—the antimonoclonal sensitization. Cyclophosphamide administration to anti-Leu-1–treated patients, 12–24 hours before the first injection, was without effect.[42] Conversely, the simultaneous administration of azathioprine (2 mg/kg/day) and low-dose steroids (0.25 mg/kg/day) has been found capable of clearly delaying and diminishing sensitization. Anti-OKT3 antibodies appear only on days 25–30 in patients thus treated, and at clearly lower levels, with a predominance of low-affinity IgM antibodies at titers insufficient to induce accelerated OKT3 clearance or cessation of its therapeutic effect.

Other approaches may be considered. One could use human monoclonal antibodies if they could be produced with good affinity in sufficient quantities, but the risk of anti-idiotypic sensitization (the most harmful) would persist. One may also think of coupling the antibody to a toxin or a radioisotope, with the aim of destroying B and T cell clones that specifically react with the monoclonal. It is in fact possible that OKT3 binding to T cells itself contributes to the patients' hyperreactivity to the monoclonal. One could attempt to induce tolerance to mouse Ig by injecting deaggregated monoclonals since such a technique is capable of inducing tolerance to xenogeneic Ig in the mouse. However, it is difficult to exclude the possibility that some aggregates are not removed or that they reform in vivo after monoclonal binding to their target molecule. The overall result may then be the opposite of the desired effect, that is, enhanced hyperreactivity. A last approach, but probably presently one of the most realistic, consists of using several antibodies consecutively, as is done for conventional antilymphocyte sera (shifting from horse to rabbit sera). One should then take into consideration the possibility of changing species (mouse/rat), as well as isotypes and idiotypes if it is confirmed that anti-constant region antibodies are essentially directed against isotypes, as we have shown to be the case for OKT3.

Conclusions and Perspectives

The production of monoclonal antibodies, now possible on a large scale, has elicited considerable hope for a renewal of indications for serotherapy, particularly in the field of immunosuppression. It is still too early to formulate definitive conclusions as to the interest of these antibodies in the few clinical conditions where they have been used. It appears, however, that these antibodies have a powerful pharmacologic activity, particularly in the immunosuppressive treatment of allograft recipients. The initial enthusiasm has been somewhat tempered by the observation of the major obstacles represented by antigenic modulation and xenosensitization. However, a more detailed analysis has shown that modulation was not necessarily harmful and could intervene fruitfully when one used antibodies directed against molecules essential to cellular function. Additionally, xenosensitization can be delayed for long-term treatment by association with low-dose conventional immunosuppressive agents. There is little doubt that once these problems are definitively solved, monoclonal antibodies should take a growing place in our therapeutic panoply, substituting for and improving antilymphocyte sera (which, after all, are nothing more than a mixture of monoclonal antilymphocyte antibodies). Other indications will appear, particularly in the specific immunomodulation of the autoimmune diseases, in the treatment of infections or intoxications resistant to present specific treatments, and even in the treatment of cancer, where, however, it should be kept in mind that the objective is probably more remote.

REFERENCES

1. Adelman N.E., Watling D.L., McDevitt H.O.: Treatment of (NZB × NZW)F$_1$ disease with anti-I-A monoclonal antibodies. *J. Exp. Med.* 158:1350, 1983.
2. Anderson S., David J.R., McMahon-Pratt D.: In vivo protection against *Leishmania mexicana* mediated by monoclonal antibodies. *J. Immunol.* 131:1616, 1983.
3. Andrzejewski C. Jr., Stollar B.D., Schwartz R.S.: Hybridoma autoantibodies to DNA. *J. Immunol.* 124:1499, 1980.
4. Auchincloss H. Jr., Bluestone J.A., Sachs D.H.: Antiidiotypes against anti-H$_2$ monoclonal antibodies: V. In vivo antiidiotype treatment induces idiotype-specific helper T cells. *J. Exp. Med.* 157:1273, 1983.
5. Bernstein I.D., Tam M.R., Novinski R.C.: Mouse leukemia: Therapy with monoclonal antibodies against a thymus differentiation antigen. *Science* 207:68, 1980.

6. Binz H., Wigzell H.: Antigen-binding idiotypic T cell receptors. *Contemp. Top. Immunobiol.* 2:113, 1977.

7. Boyse E.A., Old L.J., Luell S.: Antigenic properties of experimental leukemias: II. Immunological studies in vivo with C57BL/6 radiation-induced leukemias. *JNCI* 31:987, 1963.

8. Chatenoud L., Baudrihaye M.F., Schindler J., et al.: Human in vivo antigenic modulation induced by the anti-T cell OKT3 monoclonal antibody. *Eur. J. Immunol.* 12:979, 1982.

9. Chatenoud L., Chkoff N., Kreis H., et al.: Interest and limitations of the use of monoclonal anti-T cell antibodies for the follow-up of renal transplant patients. *Transplantation* 36:45, 1983.

10. Chatenoud L., Baudrihaye M.F., Kreis H., et al.: Diversity of the immunization against the monoclonal antibody OKT3 in renal allograft recipients, in Chatterjee S. (ed.): *Proceedings of the International Conference on Monoclonal Antibodies: Diagnostic and Therapeutic Uses in Tumor and Transplantation.* San Francisco, to be published.

11. Cochrane A.H., Santoro F., Nussenzweig V., et al.: Monoclonal antibodies identify the protective antigens of sporozites of *Plasmodium knowlesi. Proc. Natl. Acad. Sci. USA* 79:5651, 1982.

12. Cosimi A.B., Colvin R.B., Burton R.C., et al.: Use of monoclonal antibodies to T cell subsets for immunologic monitoring and treatment in recipients of renal allografts. *N. Engl. J. Med.* 305:308, 1981.

13. Cosimi A.B., Burton R.C., Kung P.C., et al.: Evaluation in primate renal allograft recipients of monoclonal antibody to human T cell subclasses. *Transplant. Proc.* 13:499, 1981.

14. Cosimi A.B.: Anti-T cell monoclonal antibodies in transplantation therapy. *Transplant. Proc.* 15:1889, 1983.

15. Crump M.A., Scearce R., Dobersen M., et al.: Production and characterization of a cytotoxic monoclonal antibody reacting with rat islet cells. *J. Clin. Invest.* 70:659, 1982.

17. Descamps-Latscha B., Golub R.M., Nguyen A.T., et al.: Monoclonal antibodies against T cell differentiation antigens initiate stimulation of monocyte/macrophage oxidative metabolism. *J. Immunol.* 131:2500, 1983.

18. Dillman R.O., Shwaler D.L., Sobol R.E., et al.: Murine monoclonal antibody therapy in two patients with chronic lymphocytic leukemia. *Blood* 59:1036, 1982.

19. Edelman L., Colignon A., Schermann J.M., et al.: Production d'un anticorps monoclonal antidigitaline. *CR Acad. Sci.* 294:421, 1982.

20. Eisenbarth G.S., Linnenbach A., Jackson R., et al.: Human hybridomas secreting anti-islet autoantibodies. *Nature* 300:264, 1982.

21. Eilat D.R., Asofsky, Laskov R.: A hybridoma from an autoimmune NZB/NZW mouse producing a monoclonal antibody to ribosomal RNA. *J. Immunol.* 124:766, 1980.

22. Filipovich A.H., McGlave P.B., Ramsay N.K.C., et al.: Pre-treatment of donor bone marrow with monoclonal antibody OKT3 for prevention of acute graft-versus-host disease in allogeneic histocompatible bone-marrow transplantation. *Lancet* 1:1266, 1982.

23. Garchon H.J., Blancher A., Champonier F., et al.: Production of human monoclonal antibodies against tetanus toxoid. *Rev. Fr. Transfus. Immunohematol.* 26(2):147, 1983.

24. Giorgi J.V., Burton R.C., Barrett L.V., et al.: Immunosuppressive effect and immunogenicity of OKT11A monoclonal antibody in monkey allograft recipients. *Transplant. Proc.* 15:639, 1983.

25. Glennie M.J., Stevenson G.T.: Univalent antibodies kill tumour cells in vitro and in vivo. *Nature* 295:712, 1982.

26. Hahn B.H., Ebling F.: Suppression of NZW/NZW/F$_1$ murine nephritis by adminis-

tration of a syngeneic monoclonal antibody to DNA: Possible role of anti-idiotypic antibodies. *J. Clin. Invest.* 71:1728, 1983.

27. Hansen E.J., Robertson S.M., Gulig P.A., et al.: Immunoprotection of rats against *Haemophilus influenzae* type B disease mediated by monoclonal antibody against a *Haemophilus* outer membrane protein. *Lancet* 1:366, 1982.

28. Hunter K.W., Fischer G.W., Hemming V.G., et al.: Antibacterial activity of a human monoclonal antibody to *Haemophilus influenzae* type B capsular polysaccharide. *Lancet* 2:798, 1982.

29. Jaffers G.J., Colvin R.B., Cosimi A.B., et al.: The human immune responses to murine OKT3 monoclonal antibody. *Transplant. Proc.* 15:646, 1983.

30. Jansen F.K., Blythman H.E., Carriere D., et al.: Immunotoxins: Hybrid molecules combining high specificity and potent cytotoxicity. *Immunol. Rev.* 62:185, 1982.

31. Jonker M., Malissen B., Mawas C.: The effect of in vivo application of monoclonal antibodies specific for human cytotoxic T cells in Rhesus monkeys. *Transplantation* 35:374, 1983.

32. Jonker M., Goldstein G., Balner H.: Effects of in vivo administration of monoclonal antibodies specific for human T cell subpopulations on the immune system in a Rhesus monkey model. *Transplantation* 35:521, 1983.

33. Jonker M., Malissen B., Van Vreeswijk W., et al.: In vivo application of monoclonal antibodies specific for human T cell subsets permits the modification of immune responsiveness in Rhesus monkeys. *Transplant. Proc.* 15:635, 1983.

34. Kaplan H.S., Olsson L., Raubitschek A.: Monoclonal human antibodies: A recent development with wide-ranging clinical potential, in McMichael A.J., Fabre J.W. (eds.): *Monoclonal Antibodies in Clinical Medicine.* New York, Academic Press, 1982, p. 17.

35. Kirch M.E., Hammerling U.: Immunotherapy of murine leukemias by monoclonal antibody: I. Effect of passively administered antibody on growth of transplanted tumor cells. *J. Immunol.* 127:805, 1981.

36. Kirkman R.L., Araujo J.L., Busch G.J., et al.: Treatment of acute renal allograft rejection with monoclonal anti-T12 antibody. *Transplantation,* to be published.

37. Koprowski H., Wiktor T.: Monoclonal antibodies against rabies virus, in Kennett R.H., McKearn T.J., Bechtol K.B. (eds.): *Monoclonal Antibodies Hybridomas: A New Dimension in Biological Analysis.* New York, Plenum Press, 1980, p. 375.

38. Kreis H., Chkoff N., Chatenoud L., et al.: Utilisation des anticorps monoclonaux en transplantation rénale. This volume.

39. Letchworth G.J. III, Appleton J.A.: Passive protection of mice and sheep against Bluetongue virus by a neutralizing monoclonal antibody. *Infect. Immun.* 39:208, 1983.

40. Michaelides M., Hogarth P.M., McKenzie I.F.C.: The immunosuppressive effect of monoclonal anti-Lyt-1.1 antibodies in vivo. *Eur. J. Immunol.* 11:1005, 1981.

41. Miller R.A., Maloney D.G., Warnke R., et al.: Treatment of B-cell lymphoma with monoclonal anti-idiotype antibody. *N. Engl. J. Med.* 306:517, 1982.

42. Miller R.A.: Unpublished findings.

43. Milstein C.: Monoclonal antibodies from hybrid myelomas: Theoretical aspects and some general comments, in McMichael A.J., Fabre J.W. (eds.): *Monoclonal Antibodies in Clinical Medicine.* New York, Academic Press, 1982, p. 5.

44. Nelson E.G., Phillips S.M.: Suppression of interstitial nephritis by auto-anti-idiotypic immunity. *J. Exp. Med.* 155:179, 1982.

45. Perry L.L., Greene M.I.: Conversion of immunity to suppression by in vivo administration of I-A subregion specific antibodies. *J. Exp. Med.* 156:480, 1982.

46. Pinel A.M., Normier G., Dussourd D'Hinterland L., et al.: Hybridoma antibodies against protective and nonprotective antigenic determinants of a *Streptococcus pyogenes* ribosomal vaccine, abstracted, in *5th International Congress of Immunology,* 1983.

47. Prentice H.G., Blacklock H.A., Janossy G., et al.: Use of anti-T cell monoclonal

antibody OKT3 to prevent acute graft-versus-host disease in allogeneic bone marrow transplantation for acute leukaemia. *Lancet* 1:700, 1982.

48. Reinherz E.L., Meuer S., Fitzgerald K.A., et al.: Antigen recognition by human T lymphocytes is linked to surface expression of the T3 molecular complex. *Cell* 30:735, 1982.

49. Ritz J., Pesando J.M., Sallan S.E., et al.: Serotherapy of acute lymphoblastic leukemia with monoclonal antibody. *Blood* 58:141, 1981.

50. Rosenbaum J.T., Adelman N.E., McDevitt H.O.: In vivo effects of antibodies to immune response gene products: I. Haplotype-specific suppression of humoral immune responses with a monoclonal anti-I-A. *J. Exp. Med.* 154:1694, 1981.

51. Seaman W.E., Wofsy D., Greenspan J.S., et al.: Treatment of autoimmune MRL/lpr mice with monoclonal antibody to Thy-1,2: A single injection has sustained effects on lymphoproliferation and renal disease. *J. Immunol.* 130:1713, 1983.

52. Sears H.F., Atkinson B.A., Mattis J., et al.: Phase-I clinical trial of monoclonal antibody in treatment of gastrointestinal tumors. *Lancet* 2:762, 1982.

53. Sherman D.M., Acres S.D., Sadowski P.L., et al.: Protection of calves against fatal enteric colibacillosis by orally administered *Escherichia coli* K99-specific monoclonal antibody. *Infect. Immun.* 42:653, 1983.

54. Shoenfeld Y., Isenberg D.A., Rauch J., et al.: Idiotypic cross-reactions of monoclonal human lupus autoantibodies. *J. Exp. Med.* 158:718, 1983.

55. Sikora K., Alderson T., Phillips J., et al.: Human hybridomas from malignant gliomas. *Lancet* 1:11, 1982.

56. Sriram S., Steinman L.: Anti-I-A antibody suppresses active encephalomyelitis: Treatment model for a disease linked to IR genes. *J. Exp. Med.* 158:1362, 1983.

57. Steinman L., Rosenbaum J.T., Sriram S., et al.: In vivo effects of antibodies to immune response gene products: Prevention of experimental allergic encephalitis. *Proc. Natl. Acad. Sci USA* 78:7111, 1981.

58. Takahashi H., Okazaki H., Terasaki I., et al.: Reversal of transplant rejection by monoclonal antiblast antibody. *Lancet* 2:1155, 1983.

59. Thierfelder S., Hoffmann-Fezer G., Rodt H., et al.: Antilymphocyte antibodies and marrow transplantation: VI. Absence of immunosuppression in vivo after injection of monoclonal antibodies blocking graft-versus-host reactions and humoral antibody formation in vitro. *Transplantation* 35:249, 1983.

60. Thomas Y., Rogozinski L., Irigoyen O.H., et al.: Functional analysis of human T cell subsets defined by monoclonal antibodies: IV. Induction of suppressor cells within the OKT4 population. *J. Exp. Med.* 154:459, 1981.

61. Thurlow P.J., Lovering E., D'Apice A.J.F., et al.: A monoclonal anti-pan-T-cell antibody. *Transplantation* 36:293, 1983.

62. Tron F., Charron D., Bach J.F., et al.: Establishment and characterization of a murine hybridoma secreting monoclonal anti-DNA autoantibody. *J. Immunol.* 125:2805, 1980.

63. Tron F., Leguern C., Cazenave R.A., et al.: Intrastrain recurrent idiotypes among anti-DNA antibodies (NZB × NZW)F$_1$ hybrid mice. *Eur. J. Immunol.* 12:761, 1982.

64. Tron F., Jacob J., Bach J.F.: Murine monoclonal anti-DNA antibodies with an absolute specificity for DNA have a large amount of anti-idiotype antibody. *Proc. Natl. Acad. Sci. USA* 81:1728, 1983.

65. Tzartos S.J., Rand D.E., Einarson B.L., et al.: Mapping of surface structures of electrophorus acetylcholine receptor using monoclonal antibodies. *J. Biol. Chem.* 256:8635, 1981.

66. Vernet der Garabedian B., Morel E.: Monoclonal antibodies against the human acetylcholine receptor. *Biochem. Biophys. Res. Commun.* 113:1, 1983.

67. Waldor M.K., Sriram S., McDevitt H.O., et al.: In vivo therapy with monoclonal anti-I-A antibody suppresses immune responses to acetylcholine receptor. *Proc. Natl. Acad. Sci. USA* 80:2713, 1983.

68. Zanetti M., De Baets M., Rogers J.: High degree of idiotypic cross-reactivity among murine monoclonal antibodies to thyroglobulin. *J. Immunol.* 131:2452, 1983.

Therapeutic Use of Monoclonal Antibodies in Kidney Transplantation

H. KREIS M.D.*, N. CHKOFF M.D.*, PH. VIGERAL
M.D.*, L. CHATENOUD M.D.*, M. LACOMBE M.D.*,
H. CAMPOS M.D.*, A. PRUNA M.D.*,
G. GOLDSTEIN M.D.**, J.F. BACH M.D.*, AND
J. CROSNIER M.D.*

*Département de Néphrologie (Unité de Transplantation Rénale) et INSERM U-25,
Hôpital Necker, Paris, France. **Ortho-Pharmaceutical Corporation,
Raritan, New Jersey

DESPITE recent major advances in various fields of kidney
transplantation, such as tissue typing, organ crossmatching,
and immunosuppression, the success of kidney transplantation
is still hindered by the occurrence of rejection. Leading to graft
destruction, rejection remains an ill-known phenomenon often
resistant to present immunosuppressive agents. Immunologic
rejection of transplanted kidneys is probably triggered by different mechanisms. Circulating antibodies, activated lymphocytes, and release of various mediators, such as lymphokines,
can cooperate to destroy the kidney. Clinical expression of graft
injury is complex and frequently asymptomatic with transient
exacerbation, before progressing to a patent chronic mode. Up
to the present time, an increased serum creatinine level was
the only important criterion for the diagnosis and follow-up of
kidney graft rejection.

However, conventional immunosuppressive agents, azathioprine and especially steroids, used on an empirical basis, have already yielded good results. For many years, efforts have been made to generate antibodies directed against lymphocytes or thymocytes involved in the immune process of rejection and to administer these antibodies either as prophylactic agents to prevent rejection or as therapeutic agents to patients undergoing renal rejection. Unfortunately, no homogeneous results have been reported in the literature, probably because of lot-to-lot variations and reactivity with other blood components, such as human erythrocytes and/or platelets. Even the well-purified fraction of IgG removed from animals immunized with thymocytes can react not only with various T lymphocyte antigens but sometimes also with platelet antigens. Here again clinical results are conflicting.[2, 11, 18, 27, 29] The ideal antibody would possess a unique specificity and be prepared in a high state of purity to avoid lot-to-lot variations so as to guarantee a bare minimum of adverse activity.

It is clear now that the human T cell population contains distinct subsets with perhaps unique functions.[25] During the last stages of their maturation, thymocytes express antigens defined by anti-T4 and anti-T8 antibodies, in addition to the previously expressed T6 antigen. With further maturation, thymocytes lose their T6 antigen and acquire and express the T3 antigen present on all mature T cells. Finally, thymocytes bearing T3, T4, and T8 antigens segregate into distinct T3+,T4+ and T3+,T8+ subsets. T3 antigen is thus present on all peripheral T lymphocytes, whereas the T4 antigen appears as a marker of T lymphocytes having the helper/inducer function and T8 antigen appears as a marker of suppressor but also of cytotoxic T lymphocytes. These antibodies directed against specific subsets of lymphocytes might then be used in vivo as immunosuppressive agents.

Kung and colleagues[20, 21] have produced a panel of monoclonal antibodies specifically reacting with surface antigens of mature T cells. Among them, OKT3 PAN, a murine monoclonal antibody, is secreted by a hybridoma produced by the procedure of Kohler and Milstein.[16] The procedure consists of immunizing a mouse with human peripheral T lymphocytes, fusing the spleen cells of the mouse with myeloma cells, and selecting from the resultant antibody-secreting hybridomas a hybridoma whose product is uniquely reactive with the T cell set of human lymphocytes. This hybridoma is stable and can be grown in vitro or in vivo to produce large amounts of OKT3 PAN. Optimally, it is grown in vivo in mice to produce an ascites from which OKT3 PAN monoclonal antibody is biochemically purified and prepared as a sterile solution suitable for intravenous (IV) administration.

Salient Features of OKT3 PAN Monoclonal Antibody

OKT3 PAN is reactive with over 95% of peripheral T cells, 20% of thymocytes, and 30% of splenocytes. OKT3 PAN is nonreactive with peripheral B cells, monocytes, granulocytes, null cells, and natural killer (NK) cells.[19] Functional studies with an OKT3-depleted cell population did not demonstrate any T cell activity in the following assays: T cell proliferation with mitogen or allogeneic stimulation, T cell–mediated help during pokeweed mitogen–driven antibody responses in vitro, cell-mediated suppression, and the generation of cytotoxic T cells (CTL) in response to allogeneic targets in mixed lymphocyte culture. Therefore, the OKT3 PAN–positive cell population contains all the T cells that are responsible for T cell functions. Since OKT3 PAN is a potent mitogen and blocks T cell cytotoxicity, it appears to recognize an important functional molecule.[4, 23, 28]

OKT3 PAN monoclonal antibody appears to be a unique immunosuppressive agent that can block cytotoxic T cell function. In vitro studies have shown that binding of OKT3 PAN to human T lymphocytes appears to inhibit CTL-mediated cell lysis of alloreactive lymphocytes, B cell lines, and human influenza virus immune cells.[1, 3] This inhibition was found to be as great as 90% of CTL activity when effector cells and target cells were mixed in medium containing 1 μg/ml of OKT3 PAN. The inhibitory effect of OKT3 PAN on CTL is not restricted to the effector phase of cell-mediated lysis (CML), since antibody added 20 hours after the initiation of mixed lymphocyte culture also resulted in a 90% reduction of CTL activity.[3] The ability of OKT3 PAN to functionally inhibit allogeneic CML may be an important factor when OKT3 PAN is used therapeutically as an immunosuppressive agent. Since 1 μg/ml of OKT3 PAN results in maximum inhibition of CTL in vitro, a therapeutic dose of 5 mg/day of OKT3 PAN, which usually results in serum levels of

1.0–2.0 µg/ml, should provide maximum in vivo inhibition of T cell cytotoxic activity.

Monoclonal Antibody for the Treatment of Acute Rejection

In most human studies on monoclonal antibody in renal transplantation, anti-T3 antibody was used. A few groups, however, have used other pan-T monoclonal antibodies: anti-T12 antibody,[15] Leu-1 and Leu-4 antibodies,[13] and CBL-1 antiblast antibody.[26] Antibodies with a specificity restricted to lymphocyte subsets, such as anti-T4 or anti-T8 antibody, have not yet been used in human trials. Following the first reports of Cosimi et al.[9, 10] on the successful use of OKT3 PAN for the treatment of acute allograft rejection, randomized trials were designed to assess the efficacy of pan-T monoclonal antibodies. OKT3 PAN (5 mg IV for 14–21 days) has been used by the majority of groups, either to treat first rejection episodes in comparison with conventional immunosuppressive agents or as rescue treatment for steroids and antithymocyte globulin (ATG)-resistant rejection episodes.[24] Preliminary results do not allow statistically significant conclusions. However, the very first reports mentioned that 93% of OKT3 PAN–treated rejection episodes were totally reversed without any alteration in ongoing doses of steroids. That was also the case for 90% of steroid- and ATG-resistant rejection episodes.[24] A recent attempt to use a monoclonal antibody directed against T12, a determinant present on all postthymic T lymphocytes, for the treatment of established rejection episodes gave less encouraging results (success in 7 of 19 treated patients).[15]

Efficacy of the monoclonal antibody has always been limited by two major factors: (1) Occurrence of re-rejection episodes in about two thirds of cases, necessitating the reintroduction of conventional antirejection treatment. However, the frequency of re-rejection was similar to that seen in patients on high-dose steroids.[24] (2) An antimonoclonal antibody immunization observed in the majority of treated patients. Various classes of antibody were reported[14]: Anti-idiotypic antibody was frequently observed and sometimes as the unique type. However, anti-allotypic, anti-isotypic and anti-light chain antibody were also observed. Although serum sickness has yet never been reported, some of these antibodies were able to block the immunosuppressive effect of OKT3 PAN, thus limiting its usefulness and its subsequent administration.

On the other hand, OKT3 PAN toxicity during the treatment of allograft rejection has always been mild. Severe side effects such as high fever, chills, bronchospasm, and, in rare cases, pulmonary edema were only seen after the first OKT3 PAN injection. Drug-induced toxicity is usually well prevented by antihistaminic agents. It is probably related to a physiologic response to the release of mediators following the abrupt T cell removal and breakdown that occurs after the initial injection. No other such reactions have since been observed.[11]

Finally, OKT3 PAN monoclonal antibody appears to be highly effective in reversing acute cadaver kidney allograft rejection episodes. It also appears to provide a significant benefit in salvaging kidneys that would otherwise be lost in the first rejection. Such an efficacy seems to be confirmed by studies in progress.[11, 22, 24] On the other hand, cyclophosphamide could contribute to a decrease in antimonoclonal antibody immunization.[8]

Prophylactic Use of Monoclonal Antibody in Kidney Recipients

From our present knowledge of the immune phenomenon which leads to allograft rejection, we can hypothesize that it is a permanent phenomenon whose activity reaches a maximum after organ grafting and decreases thereafter. Such a permanent aggression of the graft probably progresses in a wavelike motion, with the waves becoming fewer and farther between and decreasing with time. During each wave of immune response a large amount of antibody, activated cells, and mediators is released, thus increasing graft injury to the clinical aspect usually described as an acute rejection episode. Antirejection treatment initiated at the occurrence of clinical or biologic signs will not be able, in most cases, to prevent or to cure all pathologic lesions of the graft. The later the treatment, the more severe the sequelae. On the other hand, lessening the host immune response as early as possible might decrease both the permanent attack on the target organ and the frequency as well as the severity of the acute waves. It will then be possible to reduce the amount of irreversible graft lesions and thus to postpone the occurrence of chronic graft failure.

It might also happen that after an early but prolonged immunosuppression a state of tolerance easy to control with a low immunosuppressive regimen will be obtained. OKT3 PAN, which is able to clear all T lymphocytes from the blood as long as it is present in the serum, should be a good immunosuppressive agent. We decided, therefore, to use OKT3 PAN for the prophylaxis, and not the treatment, of cadaver kidney rejection.

First Trial (B81-052)

The objective of our first study was to evaluate the ability of OKT3 PAN used as the sole immunosuppressive agent during a period of 2 weeks following surgery to induce a state of tolerance easy to perpetuate with azathioprine alone. Forty patients were to be enrolled in this open, single-center phase II study. Patients who voluntarily signed an informed consent form were divided equally between OKT3 PAN and conventional immunosuppressive treatment according to a randomized schedule (Fig 1). Only first cadaveric grafts were considered. Patients assigned to the control group were given azathioprine, 3 mg/kg-1/day, starting on day -1, and prednisolone, starting with 1 gm IV during surgery, followed by 5 mg/kg-1/day of oral administration for 5 days. Steroids were then tapered to 0.25 mg/kg-1/day. Patients assigned to the OKT3 PAN group were given OKT3, 5 mg/day, by IV push, from day -1 through day 13. No additional immunosuppressive drugs and no steroids were given during this period of time. Azathioprine alone was introduced at day 14 and continued thereafter. In the event of a documented rejection observed during the first 2 weeks, the current treatment was maintained for 5 days before conventional antirejection treatment was introduced and OKT3 was discontinued in the experimental group. From the third week and thereafter, prednisolone was introduced according to the same schedule as in postsurgery period of the control group.

This first study was discontinued before its completion for reasons which will be discussed below. Thirteen patients were enrolled, six in the OKT3 group and seven in the steroid group.

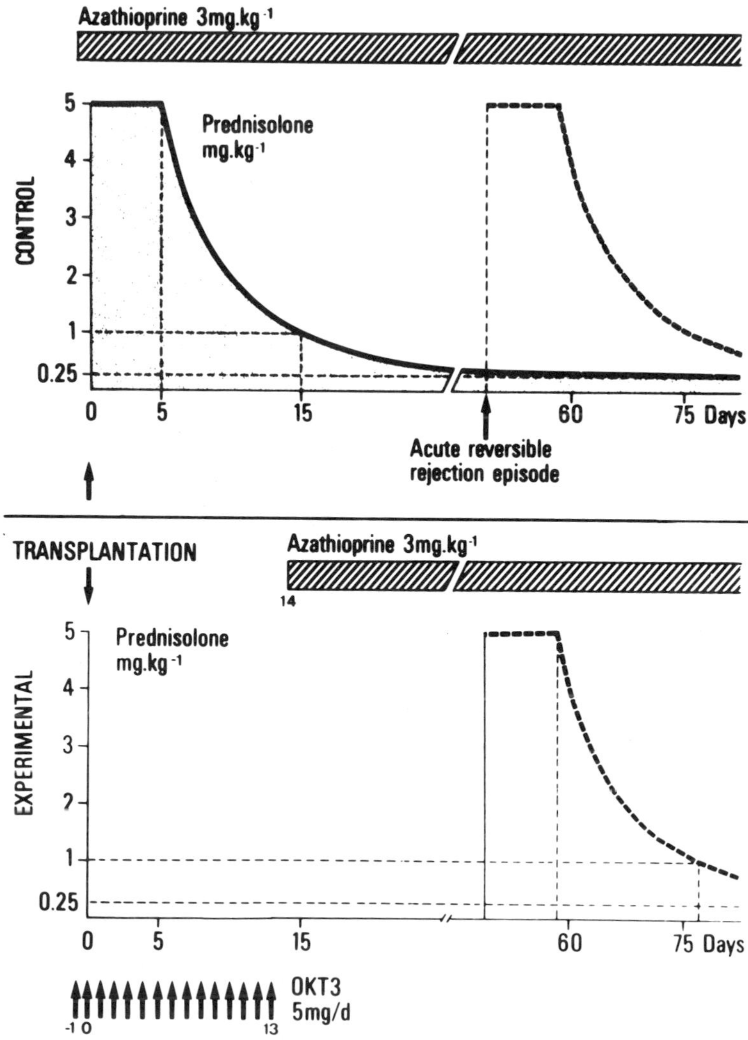

Fig 1.—Treatment protocol in B81-052 experimental and control groups.

There were no differences between the two groups regarding age of patients, sex, duration of hemodialysis, total ischemia of the graft, and HLA compatibility (Table 1).

OKT3 PAN tolerance was excellent despite the lack of steroids. However, as in other studies, all patients had profuse diarrhea, fever, and chills after the first injection.

TABLE 1.—PROTOCOL OKT3 PAN (B81–052): COMPARISON OF GROUPS

GROUP	N	AGE	SEX M/F	TRANSFUSED PATIENTS	HEMODIALYSIS PERIOD (YR)	TOTAL ISCHEMIA (MIN)	HLA-COMPATIBLE RECIPIENTS
OKT3 PAN	6	34.3 ± 9.2	3/3	6	3.9 ± 1.6	$1,444. \pm 346$	3
Steroids + azathioprine	7	35.7 ± 11.2	4/3	7	2.8 ± 0.6	$1,408.3 \pm 299$	2
		NS			NS	NS	NS

Results reported on Table 2 explain why this protocol was discontinued. All six patients in the experimental group developed an acute rejection episode necessitating the introduction of steroids about 12 days after surgery, thus indicating that not only was tolerance not induced by the monoclonal antibody, but also that steroid dosage could not be reduced. Nevertheless, it is noteworthy that no rejection episode occurred before day 13 after transplantation, although no immunosuppressive agent other than OKT3 PAN was used. This proves that OKT3 PAN is certainly a powerful immunosuppressor, otherwise rejection episodes would have developed before day 5.[17] Why then did we observe rejection? At least two explanations can be drawn from studying the first-month posttransplantation course of patients in the experimental group (Fig 2). In fact, as early as 1 hour after the first OKT3 injection, a dramatic and concomitant decrease of T3+, T4+, and T8+ cells was observed. T3+ cell level stayed close to zero up to 10–13 days after transplant and then suddenly rose. Acute rejection was observed immediately thereafter in all cases. There appears to be a very close relationship between blood repopulation by T3+ cells and occurrence of rejection. The reappearance of T3+ cells is explained either by the discontinuation of OKT3 PAN at the end of the treatment period or, when earlier while patients were still on OKT3 PAN, by an immunization against the monoclonal antibody, as observed in five of the six treated recipients. Various types of antibodies, directed either against mouse IgG or against the idiotypic site of the OKT3 PAN molecule, have been isolated.[6] OKT3 PAN level during the therapeutic phase decreases with the appearance of anti-OKT3 immunization (Fig 3). Finally, OKT3 PAN appears to be a good immunosuppressive agent as long as it is present in the blood. Unfortunately, the large majority of patients developed inhibiting an-

TABLE 2.—PROTOCOL B81–052: OKT3 PAN*

| | | | | 1ST REJECTION EPISODE | OUTCOME | | |
| | | | | Time After Transplant | | | |
GROUP	N	ATN	N	(Days)	Good Function	HDC	Died
OKT3	6	5	6	12.8 ± 2.9	5	1	0
Control	8	3	3	33.3 ± 20.5	6	1	1

*Starting January 1982.

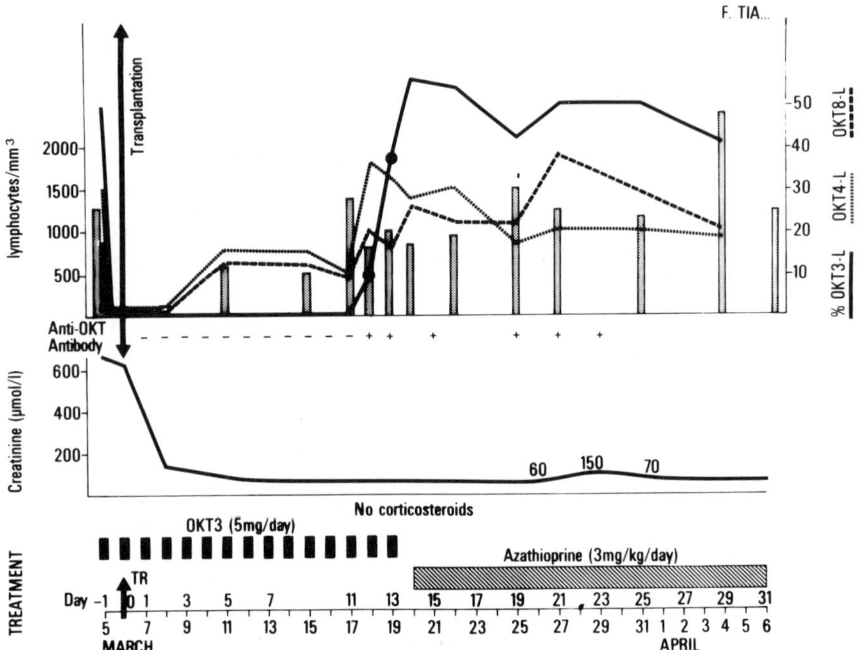

Fig 2.—Typical posttransplantation course after cadaver kidney graft in B81-052 patient receiving OKT3 PAN.

tibodies in the second week following initiation of treatment when OKT3 PAN was given as the sole immunosuppressive agent.

Another explanation[5,7] could be provided by the observation that early in the posttransplant period, a significant proportion of circulating T4+ and T8+ cells was observed while T3+ cells were still not seen (Fig 4), indicating the appearance of OKT3-,4+ and OKT3-,8+ cells. In fact, when these cells were incubated in vitro in the absence of OKT3,[5] they reexpressed the OKT3-defined antigen, which was clearly detected as early as 8 hours of incubation and was at its optimal level after 20 hours.

These data are best explained by the phenomenon of antigenic modulation, according to which the expression of a membrane antigen can be reversibly suppressed by the specific antibody. It must be remembered that even though the absolute number of T cells remains low, it is not known whether modu-

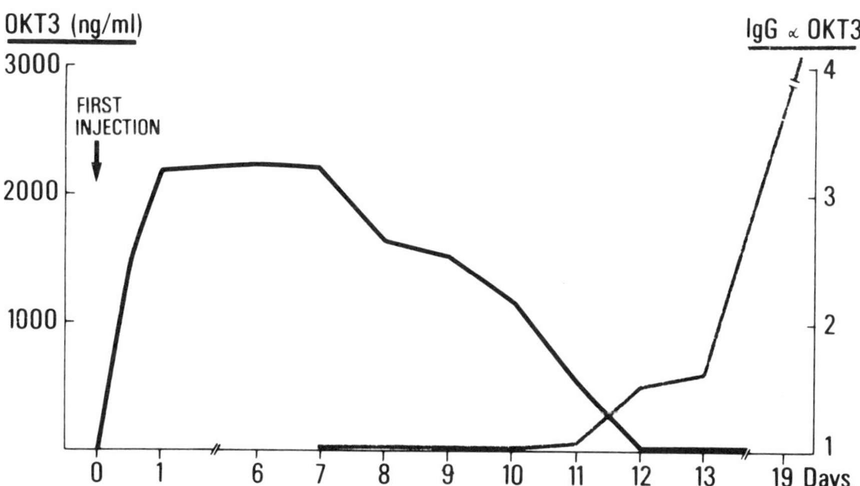

Fig 3.—Circulating OKT3 PAN serum levels before and after immunization against monoclonal antibody during treatment period (B81-052 protocol).

lated cells are immunocompetent. However, it should also be noted that rejection did not occur in the presence of OKT3- T cells. But it was not possible to know whether rejection episodes observed very early after reappearance of T3 + cells were not in fact initiated a few days earlier by modulating cells.

In conclusion, although this first OKT3 PAN trial did not allow graft survival in the absence of steroids for more than 10–15 days, it brought us important knowledge on OKT3 PAN in human transplant recipients. It led us to the conclusion that OKT3 is a powerful and well-tolerated immunosuppressive agent whose major problem is its immunogenicity. A new protocol has therefore been initiated in order to avoid or to decrease anti-OKT3 antibody formation.

Second Trial (C82–054)

This protocol, which was begun on Dec. 19, 1983, and is still in progress, is at present (1/1/84) composed of 30 cadaveric kidney recipients. Results obtained in the first 32 patients having more than 1 month follow-up are reported here. The principal aim of this protocol is to attempt to reduce immunization to OKT3 PAN by associating it with other immunosuppressive

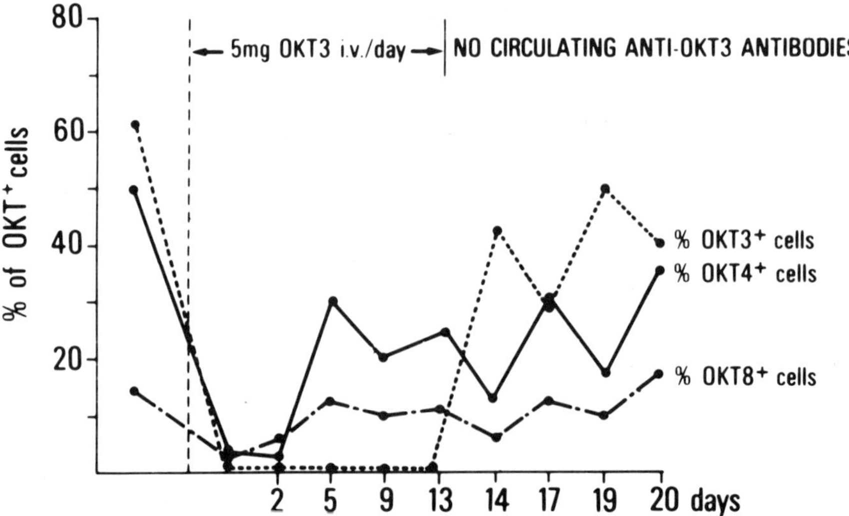

Fig 4.—Percentages of lymphocyte subpopulations during the first posttransplantation month in a patient receiving OKT3 (protocol B81-052).

agents to allow continued administration until the end of the second posttransplantation month. Patients in this group receive the following (see Fig 5): (1) A minimum of 15 IV injections of monoclonal antibody at 5 mg/day. When no immunization is observed after the 15th injection, administration of OKT3 PAN is continued until day 30 following transplantation as long as two consecutive examinations show the T3 marker below or equal to 30%. (2) Azathioprine, continuously, at 3 mg/kg/day. (3) Low-dose steroids at 0.25 mg/kg/day from day 2 to day 9, 1 mg/kg/day from day 10 to day 14, tapering back to 0.25 mg/kg/day at day 30. Between Dec. 19, 1982, and Jan. 1, 1984, 11 patients received this treatment.

Controls were divided into two groups (Fig 5). As of Jan. 1, 1984, 11 patients had been entered into the high-dose control group, receiving the protocol which has been standard in our group since 1973 and which has been described elsewhere.[12] The other 10 patients were placed in the low-dose control group receiving azathioprine and prednisolone in a protocol identical to that of the OKT3 PAN group but without monoclonal antibody.

Patients were randomly assigned to one of the three groups

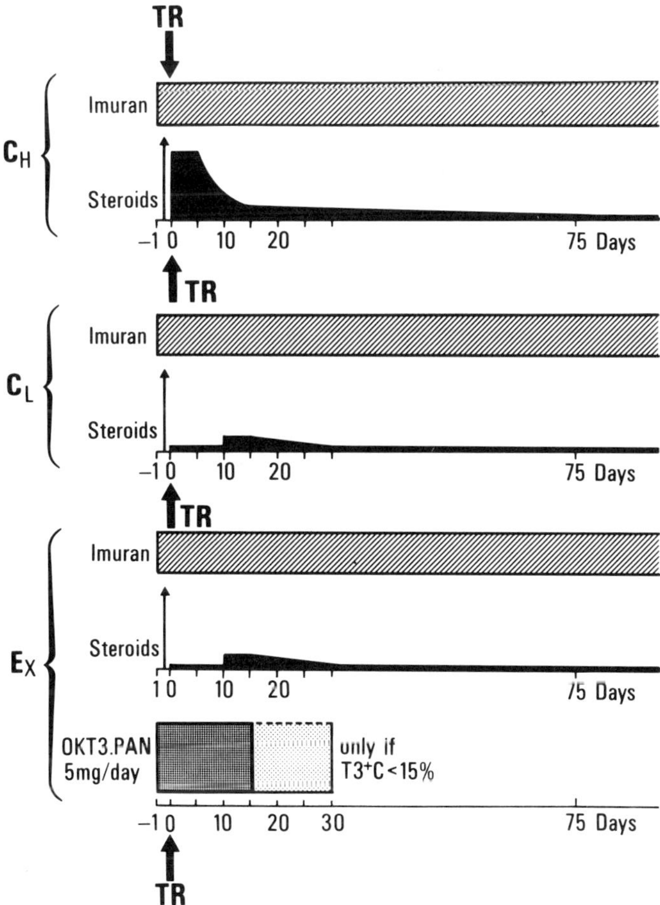

Fig 5.—Treatment protocol in C82-054 experimental and control (high- and low-dose) groups.

after giving written consent. Although only half of the initially scheduled number of patients had received a renal transplant by Jan. 1, 1984, preliminary results are already sufficiently interesting to report.

Anti-OKT3 Immunization

Seven OKT3 PAN patients received monoclonal antibody treatment during the 30-day protocol (Fig 6). Treatment was

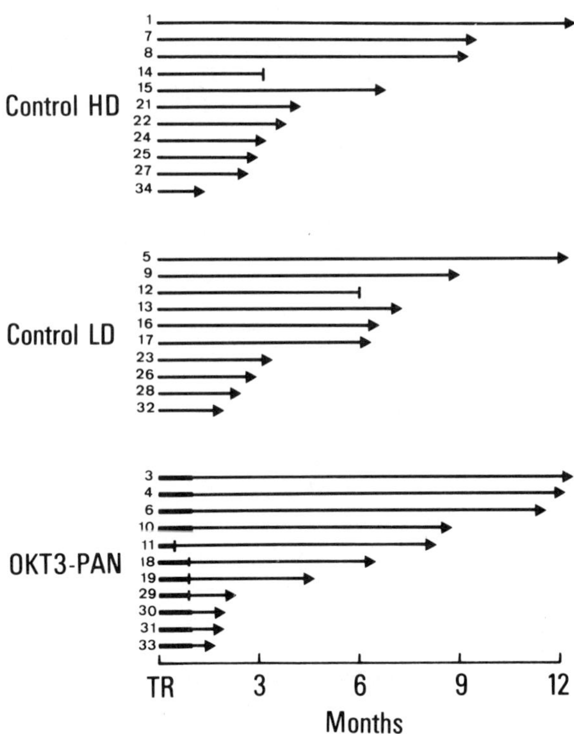

Fig 6.—Status as of 1/1/84 during follow-up period of patients in protocol C82-054. *Arrows* indicate functioning grafts. *Vertical line* indicates return to regular dialysis treatment. In the OKT3 group, *thick lines* indicate period of treatment by OKT3 PAN.

stopped in one (patient 11) at day 14 because of early immunization against OKT3. Pretreatment positive skin test had shown presensitization to mouse immunoglobulin in this patient. In the last three patients, OKT3 PAN had to be stopped at day 28 and 29 because a T3 level above 30% showed immunization against OKT3 PAN. In seven of ten patients no T3+ cells were observed during the treatment protocol; when these cells were observed, it was at the 28th or 29th day, except in the presensitized patient. It would thus appear that the association of azathioprine and low-dose prednisolone with OKT3 PAN considerably modifies, both quantitatively and qualitatively, immune response to monoclonal antibody. IgM response was predominant and early, while IgG response was always late (after day 30) or absent, except in the presensitized patient, in whom anti-OKT3 IgG was observed as early as day 4 at much higher levels than in other patients. IgM-type antibody did not perceptibly affect circulating OKT3 PAN levels.

Rejection Episodes

The number of patients having at least one rejection episode (Table 3) is slightly lower in the OKT3 PAN group; more interestingly, three of the 11 patients in this group had no rejection episode, with a 1-year follow-up in one (patient 6). It is of particular interest that the frequency of rejection episodes per patient (Table 4) is 1.3 in the OKT3 PAN group and 1.5 in the high-dose control group but reaches 1.9 in the low-dose control group. In addition, only two rejection episodes were observed during the first month in the 11 patients in the OKT3 PAN group, whereas all ten of the patients in the low-dose control group ($P<.0002$) and eight of the 11 in the high-dose control

TABLE 3.—PROTOCOL C82–054:
REJECTION EPISODES*

		NO. OF PATIENTS DEMONSTRATING					
GROUP	N	0	1	2	3	>3	Rejection episodes
Control HD	11	1	5	3	2	0	
Control LD	10	0	4	4	1	1	
OKT3 PAN	11	3	4	2	2	0	

*From Dec. 19, 1982, to (as of) Jan. 1, 1984. HD, high dose; LD, low dose.

TABLE 4.—PROTOCOL C82–054: REJECTION
EPISODES*

		NO. OF REJECTION EPISODES		
GROUP	N	Total	1st mo.	Irreversible
Control HD	11	17	8 ($P = .01$)	1
Control LD	10	19	10 ($P < .0002$)	1
OKT3-PAN	11	14	2†	0

*Dec. 19, 1982 to (as of) Jan. 1, 1984. One patient developed anti-OKT3 antibodies on day 28 and rejected the transplant on day 29, HD, high dose; LD, low dose.
†One presensitized patient (positive skin test)

group ($P<.02$) had rejection episodes ($P<.02$). Two of the episodes in the control groups were irreversible, but none in the OKT3 PAN group.

It can thus be stated that OKT3 PAN induced effective immunosuppression precluding the occurrence of rejection episodes while present in patient serum and even after interruption in three patients. In the other cases, the frequency of late rejection (after the first month) is similar in the high-dose control group (0.8), the low-dose control group (0.9), and the experimental group (0.9). There is thus no rebound after stopping monoclonal antibody during repopulation of T3 cells.

Antigen Modulation

Antigen modulation was observed in all group OKT3 PAN patients during days 2–5, as was observed in our first study. It is thus clear that cells whose marker is modulated by monoclonal antibody cannot induce rejection episodes, since they all occurred more than 25 days after appearance of these cells.

Side Effects

Side effects (Table 5) were also mainly observed after the first injection of OKT3 PAN. They were clearly less severe than

TABLE 5.—PROTOCOL C85–054: SIDE EFFECTS OF
TREATMENT*

	CONVENTIONAL TREATMENT		
	High dose (N = 11)	Low dose (N = 10)	OKT3-PAN (N = 11)
SIDE EFFECT	---	---	---
Chills and fever	1	3	9
Skin rash	0	0	3
Arthralgia	0	0	2
Diarrhea	1	1	3
Enlarged lymph nodes	0	0	4
Leukopenia and/or thrombocytopenia	1	0	0
Diabetes	3	0	0
GI pain	2	0	0
↑ Transaminase	3	1	0
Miscellaneous	3	2	2

*From Dec. 19, 1982, to (as of) Jan. 1, 1984.

in our previous protocol. However, two patients had discrete arthralgia associated with transient skin eruption suggesting nonsevere serum sickness. Only three patients had diarrhea, which was also observed in two control group patients. On the other hand, no side effects due to corticosteroids were observed in the low-dose control group or the OKT3 PAN group. A special problem was the appearance of enlarged cervical and axillary lymph nodes in four patients in the experimental group. It persisted for a few days to a few weeks. In all cases, biopsy showed immunoblasts and large multinuclear histiocytes, but lymph node structure remained intact. This complication of adenopathies probably corresponded to viral infections favored by the monoclonal antibody.

Infectious Complications

The overall frequency of infectious complications (Table 6) is similar in the OKT3 PAN and the high-dose control groups. Curiously, this frequency is lower in the low-dose control group, even though these patients received a clearly higher total dose of prednisolone because of their higher rate of rejection episodes. In addition, the type of infectious agent varies greatly according to treatment group. When patients receive monoclonal antibody, viral infections predominate, while in the high-dose control group, bacterial infections predominate. These infections were generally of moderate severity, except for one primary cytomegalovirus infection in a patient in the low-dose control group and one case of Legionnaires' disease in an OKT3 PAN patient. None of these infections was fatal.

In conclusion, it can be stated that OKT3 PAN is a major immunosuppressive agent having low toxicity. However, when

TABLE 6.—PROTOCOL C82–054: INFECTIOUS EPISODES*

		VIRAL			PATIENTS WITHOUT
GROUP	BACTERIAL	CMV	Other	FUNGAL	INFECTIOUS EPISODES
Control HD	6	1	2	0	4/11
Control LD	1	1	3	0	5/10
OKT3 PAN	2†	2	5 + 1‡	1	3/11

*Dec. 19, 1982, to (as of) Jan. 1, 1984.
†Including one case of *Legionella*
‡Herpes simplex virus while on antithymocyte globulin.

given alone for a short time, it does not induce tolerance and its effect is limited by its immunogenicity. It is, however, possible to reduce the antibody response directed against OKT3 by combined treatment with conventional immunosuppressive agents. Treatment can then be continued for at least 30 days to reduce the frequency of rejection episodes and even abolish them in some patients. Clinical use of monoclonal globulins is still experimental, and it is difficult to predict their future role in renal transplantation. Nevertheless, certain improvements ameliorating the conditions of their use may be expected. Among these are further reduction in their immunogenicity, allowing more prolonged administration, and the use of antibodies directed against cell markers, such as T12 markers,[15] lymphoblast markers,[26] or particularly T4 and T8 cytotoxic markers, which may play a more specific role in graft rejection. Such advances would provide a precision in clinical use that is still impossible to attain today with conventional immunosuppressive treatment.

REFERENCES

1. Biddison W.E., Sharrow S.O., Shearer G.M.: T cell subpopulations required for human cytotoxic T lymphocyte response to influenza virus: Evidence of T cell help. *J. Immunol.* 127:487–491, 1981.
2. Butt K.M.H., Zielinski C.M., Parsa I., et al.: Trends in immunosuppression for kidney transplantation. *Kidney Int.* 13(suppl. 8):95–98, 1978.
3. Chang T.W., Gingras S.P.: OKT3 monoclonal antibody inhibits cytotoxic T lymphocyte-mediated cell lysis. *Int. J. Immunopharmacol.* 3:183–186, 1981.
4. Chang T.W., Kung P.C., Gingras S.P., et al.: Does OKT3 monoclonal antibody react with an antigen recognition structure on human T cells? *Proc. Natl. Acad. Sci. USA* 78:1805–1808, 1981.
5. Chatenoud L., Baudrihaye M.F., Chkoff N., et al.: Immunologic follow-up of renal allograft recipients treated prophylactically by OKT3 alone. *Transplant. Proc.* 15:643–645, 1983.
6. Chatenoud L., Baudrihaye M.F., Kreis H., et al.: Diversity of the immunization against the monoclonal antibody OKT3 in renal allograft recipients. *Transplant. Proc.,* to be published.
7. Chatenoud L., Baudrihaye M.F., Kreis H., et al.: Human in vivo antigenic modulation induced by the anti-T cell OKT3 monoclonal antibody. *Eur. J. Immunol.* 12:979–982, 1982.
8. Cosimi A.B.: Personal communication.
9. Cosimi A.B., Burton R.C., Colvin R.B., et al.: Treatment of acute renal allograft rejection with OKT3 monoclonal antibody. *Transplantation* 32:535–539, 1981.
10. Cosimi A.B., Colvin R.B., Burton R.C., et al.: Use of monoclonal antibodies to T-cell subsets for immunologic monitoring and treatment in recipients of renal allograft. *N. Engl. J. Med.* 305:308–314, 1981.
11. Cosimi A.B., Wortis H.H., Delmonico F.L., et al.: Randomized clinical trial of ATG in cadaver renal allograft recipients: Importance of T-cell monitoring. *Surgery* 80:155–163, 1976.

12. Crosnier J.: Indications for kidney transplantation preparation, treatment and supervision of the patients, in Hamburger J., Crosnier J., Bach J.F., et al. (eds.): *Renal transplantation: Theory and practice.* Baltimore, Williams & Wilkins Co., 1981, pp. 146–176.

13. Eastbrook A., Berger C.L., Mittler R., et al.: Antigenic modulation of human T-lymphocytes by monoclonal antibodies. *Transplant. Proc.* 15:651–656, 1983.

14. Jaffers G.F., Colvin R.B., Cosimi A.B., et al.: The human immune response to murine OKT3 monoclonal antibody. *Transplant. Proc.* 15:646–648, 1983.

15. Kirkman R.L., Araujo J.L., Busch G.J., et al.: Treatment of acute renal allograft rejection with monoclonal anti-T12 antibody. *Transplantation,* to be published.

16. Kohler G., Milstein C.: Continuous cultures of fused cells secreting antibody of predefined specificity. *Nature* 256:108, 1975.

17. Kreis H., Lacombe M., Noel L.H., et al.: Kidney graft rejection: Has the need for steroid to be reevaluated? *Lancet* 2:1169–1172, 1978.

18. Kreis H., Mansouri R., Descamps J.M., et al.: Antithymocyte globulin in cadaver kidney transplantation: A randomized trial based on T-cell monitoring. *Kidney Int.* 19:438–444, 1981.

19. Kung P.C., Goldstein G., Reinherz E.L., et al.: Monoclonal antibodies defining distinctive human T-cell surface antigens. *Science* 206–347, 1979.

20. Kung P.C., Talle M.A., Dermaria M.E., et al.: Strategies for generating monoclonal antibodies defining human T lymphocyte differentiation antigens. *Transplant. Proc.* 12(suppl. 1):141–146, 1980.

21. Kung P.C., Talle M.A., Demaria M.E., et al.: Creating a useful panel of anticell monoclonal antibodies. *Int. J. Immunopharmacol.* 3:175–181, 1981.

22. Goldstein G.: Personal communication.

23. Landegren U., Ramstedt U., Axberg I., et al.: Selective inhibition of human T cell cytotoxicity at levels of target recognition or initiation of lysis by monoclonal OKT3 and Leu-2a antibodies. *J. Exp. Med.* 155:1579, 1982.

24. Norman D.J., Bohannon L.L., Barry J.M., et al.: Monoclonal anti-T cell antibody for treatment of acute allograft rejection. *Transplant. Proc.,* to be published.

25. Reinherz E.L., Schlossman S.F.: The differentiation and function of human T lymphocytes. *Cell* 19:821–827, 1980.

26. Takahashi H., Okazaki H., Terasaki P.I., et al.: Reversal of transplant rejection by monoclonal antiblast antibody. *Lancet* 2:1155–1158, 1983.

27. Uittenbogaart C., Robinson B.J., Maleksadch M.H., et al.: Use of antilymphocyte globulin (dose by rosette protocol) in pediatric allograft recipients. *Transplantation* 28:291–293, 1979.

28. Van Wauwe J.P., De Mey J.R., Goosens J.G.: OKT3: A monoclonal anti-human T lymphocyte antibody with potent mitogenic properties. *J. Immunol.* 124:2708–2713, 1980.

29. Wechter W.J. Brodie J.A., Morrel R.M., et al.: Antithymocyte globulin (ATGAM) in renal allograft recipients: Multicenter trials using a 14-dose regimen. *Transplantation* 28:294–381, 1979.

Side Effects Due to Materials Used in Hemodialysis Equipment

JÜRGEN BOMMER, M.D., EBERHARD RITZ, M.D., AND KONRAD ANDRASSY, M.D.

Department Internal Medicine, University of Heidelberg, Heidelberg, West Germany

HEMODIALYSIS is of unquestioned benefit in reversing the uremic syndrome, but concern has been growing about chronic sequelae resulting from this procedure. Only a few complications relating to the material used in hemodialysis equipment have been reported since maintenance hemodialysis was introduced.[1] However, evidence has accumulated recently to suggest that several acute or chronic complications in dialysis patients are related to bioincompatibility problems. Such documented or suggested complications include side effects of ethylenoxide or phthalate, exposure to endotoxin-like material on dialysis membranes, and uptake of spallation products from plastic tubing by macrophages. In addition, such problems in dialysis patients as eosinophilia, hyper-IgE-immunoglobulinemia, pruritus, arthralgia, complement activation and dialysis leucocytopenia, hypoxia, dialysis thrombocytopenia may be related to bioincompatibility. Only some of the many problems of bioincompatibility will be discussed here. They were chosen either because they have not been in the limelight of current interest or because new information has become available recently.

In view of the above appalling list of self-created iatrogenic problems, one is reminded of *Der Zauberlehrling,* the poem of

0084-5957/84/0014-0409-0438-$04.00

Johann Wolfgang von Goethe, in which the sorcerer's apprentice exclaims when the spell has gone out of control: "Herr, die Not ist grob; Die ich rief, die Giester, Werd ich nun nicht los." ("Oh Lord, I cannot rid myself of the spirits whom I called").

However, it is imperative to view the problems in proper perspective. Important though the above complications are, they should not detract from the amazing record of short-term safety of today's hemodialysis procedures; however, the review should illustrate the need to optimize biocompatibility of dialysis procedures to guarantee similar long-term safety.

Ethylene-Oxide (ETO)

In the past, sterilization of dialyzers has been a serious problem. In the "pioneer age" of dialysis, when disposable dialyzers were not available, bacteremia was not uncommon[2, 3] and drastic procedures were adopted to reduce bacteriological hazards. Chemical disinfection with formalin poses toxicological[4] and long-term immunological risks.[5, 6] It was therefore a welcome breakthrough when disposable dialyzers could be sterilized with apparent safety using ETO. However, ETO has recently been suspected of causing both toxic and allergic side reactions in dialyzed patients.

ETO (C_2H_4O) is a volatile liquid (boiling point 10.7°C) that is water-soluble, highly flammable, and explosive in contact with air, so that it must be blunted with inert gases, e.g., freon or CO_2. ETO sterilizes by alkylating protein molecules.[7, 8] However, ETO is avidly taken up by plastic material. Pulmonary venous capillary (PVC) blood lines absorb ETO up to 1.16% of their wet weight.[9] In addition to ETO absorption, ETO-derived reaction products, e.g., 2-chloro-ethanol are generated in PVC, cuprophane, or polyurethane[10, 11] as used in potting and cases of hollow fiber dialysers.

The following clinical observations in dialysis patients point to side reactions secondary to ETO. Nicols et al.[12] reported that 15 dialysis patients who were exposed to various dialyzers experienced sneezing, watering of eyes, urticaria, bronchospasm, hypotension, flushing, headaches, and chest pain at the beginning of hemodialysis. These patients recovered within 30 minutes after dialysis was stopped. One patient who became symptomatic was disconnected from the dialyzer and the symptoms subsided, only to develop again when she was reconnected to the dialyzer. Symptoms recurred immediately when her blood, which had been stored in the dialyzer, was reinfused. Interestingly, such reactions were not observed when the same dialyzer was used again or sterilized with formalin. Such early symptoms could reliably be avoided by intensive rinsing of the dialyzer prior to use.

Another suggestion of ETO-related side effects was the observation of Takajashi et al.,[13] who noted eosinophilia and bronchospasm or various other symptoms when ETO-sterilized dialyzers were used. Eosinophilia and bronchospasm subsided when gamma-X-ray or steam-sterilized dialyzers were used.

Even more tangible proof for the involvement of ETO comes from the study of Poothullil.[14] Some dialysis patients developed breathlessness, generalized itching, a throbbing sensation in the head, tightness of the chest, and hypotension when they were dialyzed using ETO-sterilized devices. The skin prick test for ETO was negative, but was positive for human serum pretreated with ETO. In other dialysis patients or normal subjects, the prick test was negative. The ETO reaction product 2-chloroethanol could be demonstrated in the dialyzer. It was assumed that 2-chlorocthanol formed because of the interaction of ETO with cuprophane, PVC, and polyurethane. The latter are presumably of prime importance, since the highest reported incidence of ETO sensitivity has been noted in repeated plasma donors who are contacted with ETO-sterilized plastics, but not exposed to cellulose et al.[15]

The involvement of histamin in the clinical reaction is suggested by the in vitro observation of Poothullil et al.[14] that ETO-pretreated human serum albumin releases histamin in peripheral leucocytes of dialysis patients, but not of control subjects. This agrees with the observations of Takahashi et al.[13] who noted the release of histamin after contact with ETO gas-sterilized hemodialysis systems in the blood of dialysis patients with eosinophilia and clinical side effects.

The incidence of severe "first use" anaphylactic or pseudoanaphylactic reactions in patients immediately after exposure to a non-reused disposable dialyzer is quite low.[16, 12] The reaction resembles the above described symptoms, but whether all of this is related to ETO has not yet been determined. The low incidence of severe reactions has hampered progress in delineating the causal agent(s) involved.

Concern based on the above side effects in dialysis patients is the more appropriate since both toxic reactions and anaphylactic and delayed type allergic complications have been observed in other medical disciplines. Several children died after open heart surgery from toxic shock unresponsive to volume, vasopressors, or steroids.[9] Similar fatalities were avoided when PVC tubing was used that was sterilized by autoclave instead of gas. The toxic action of ETO was substantiated by experimental studies in which ETO caused irreversible shock in dogs.[9]

Another indication of the toxic effects of ETO is the observation that hemolysis occurred when stored blood was exposed to plastic material containing ETO, so that final ETO blood levels of 5,800 ppm were reached. In addition, subcutaneous implantation of ETO-containing PVC caused concentration-dependent tissue damage in mice.[17] The impurity, 2-(2-hydroxymethylmercapto) benzolthiazole, was found to arise in syringe plungers, when an accelerator compound interacted with ETO.[18] This product has not been shown to cause toxicity in patients, but it is of note that material extracted from rubber syringe tips may be cytotoxic.[19, 20]

Apart from such toxic effects, allergic effects are also well known outside of nephrology. Acute inflammatory dermatitis resulting from ETO-sterilized oxygen mask were reported.[21, 22] Skin tests were positive with ETO-sterilized gauze; positive skin tests were not prevented when gauze was ventilated for up to 72 hours or extensively rinsed with water. In another observation, bullous dermatitis was noted in a patient after contact with a ETO-sterilized reusable canvas and rubber theater lift mat. Patch tests with ETO, ethylenglycol and polyethylenglycol, i.e., polymers of ETO and water, were positive.[22]

The above reports clearly illustrate the need to reduce exposure to ETO. This can be achieved by several simple procedures during the manufacture of dialyzers and during their preparation for clinical use.

After ETO sterilization, ETO is removed by ventilation with freon or CO_2. Although ETO deaerates very quickly, substantial amounts are retained in dialyzers. For instance, when hemofilters were ventilated through bacteria-proved filters for various times, 10 mg ETO was found in the recirculation fluid after ventilation for 10 days and 1 mg after ventilation for 60 days.[11] This example illustrates the need for intensive ventilation and/or packaging of dialysis material in packing material that can be penetrated by gas but is impermeable for bacteria.

The ETO burden can be further reduced by extensive saline rinsing of the dialyzer not only from the blood side, but also from the dialysate side. Although often neglected, the latter is important because polyurethane, which is used for potting of hollow fibers, apparently binds ETO intensely and releases ETO more slowly than PVC.[11]

Those who use ETO should consider the comment of C.V. Bruch: "The gas sterilization process has provided much help and benefit due to decreased incidence of bacterial infections through the availability and the use of sterile disposable supplies . . . . . There is a need for continuing dialogue as to the safe residue limit for all ETO-sterilized supplies."[11]

In the long run, the best sterilization process will be the one that poses no toxicological hazards. Therefore, efforts to use non-chemical methods, particularly steam sterilization, should be pursued and optimized. Currently, there is reluctance to use steam, because filter performance deteriorates due to shrinkage of pore size, because of cost, and because of the necessity to ship dialyzers wet. It is hoped that these impediments can be overcome in the future.

Phthalate

To date, no defined pathology in dialysis patients can unequivocally be attributed to phthalate toxicity. However, given the large body of information on phthalate toxicity, this issue urgently requires clarification. Patients on dialysis are continuously exposed to phthalate because of the high phthalate content of PVC tubing and, to a minor extent, blood bags.

Organic polymers are hard solids due to strong cohesive forces within the crystalline polymer structure. Such hard polymers are transformed into flexible elastomers by the incorporation of polar or polarizable plasticizers that reduce intermolecular forces in the polymerisate by dipol action.[23, 24] The first to propose the diethylester of phthalic acid for use as a plasticizer was Nobel in 1883.[25] In the meantime, diethylhexylphthalate (DEHP) production has continuously increased so that West Germany's annual production reached 300,000 tons in 1977.[26] DEHP dissolves poorly in water, but is readily soluble in organic solvents and lipids. This property is of relevance for the desorption of DEHP from dialysis tubing in aqueous solutions *vs.* blood. Because of its wide ranging use, DEHP can be demonstrated in pbb (part per billion) amounts in soil, river or sea water, and food. Consequently, concern about phthalate toxicity goes far beyond biomedical considerations.

PHARMACOKINETICS AND METABOLISM

There are some species differences in DEHP metabolism; because of this, data in rodents cannot be readily extrapolated to primates. DEHP is hydrolyzed in the liver by a monoesterase to monoethylhexyphthalate (MEHP) and subsequently oxydized in omega and beta position by a microsomal NADP-dependent oxidoreductase,[27,28] although this is not confirmed by all authors.[29] The rate of metabolism of phthalate esters depends on the length of the alkyl-side chain and the water solubility of the compound. In rodents,[30,31] the resulting alcohols—and to a lesser extent sulphate conjugates—are then excreted in urine, whereas DEHP and its metabolites are excreted as glucuronides in primates, including man.[32,33] Apart from MEHP, a large number of other metabolites can be demonstrated in the urine of primates.[32–35] Because of its rapid clearance, the plasma half-life of the parent substance DEHP is extremely short (7–8 minutes). Excretion, primarily in the form of metabolites, occurs preferentially through the kidney, both in animals[32,36–40] and in man.[33,34] In primates, 74% of DEHP can be recovered in urine after eight hours.[34] As a consequence, DEHP levels in the brain, heart, and lung tissues of nephrectomized dogs are higher than those of control dogs, documenting cumulation when renal excretion is compromised.[25] This conclusion is supported by the observation that serum DEHP levels are higher when uremic patients are dialyzed than when non-uremic patients are dialyzed for the treatment of psoriasis.[41] In addition to renal excretion, biliary and intestinal excretion can be demonstrated[28] and some evidence points to the existence of enterohepatic recirculation.[37]

Since DEHP is a highly lipid-soluble substance, it will rapidly partition from plasma into tissues; this has been demonstrated using i.v. injection of ^{14}C-DEHP in the rat.[38] One hour after injection, only 2% of the injected tracer remained in the circulation; 76% was recovered in the liver and the rest in other tissues. In another study, 55% of the dose was recovered after 24 hours in the urine, 25% in feces, and the rest was sequestered in other organs. In organs as well as in the circulation, DEHP will be hydrolyzed to MEHP by tissue lipases or lipoprotein lipase, respectively.

Toxicity

The most important toxic effects of DEHP concern the liver, heart, blood cells and coagulation, macrophages of reticuloendothelial system, the lungs, and testes.

Most disquieting with respect to potential implication for dialysis are the observations of Jacobsen et al.,[42] who transfused monkeys with platelet concentrates or plasma that were stored in DEHP containing PVC bags. During one year, the animals received a cumulative DEHP load of up to 69 mg/kg. Persisting abnormalities of hepatic ^{99}Tc-scan and bromsulfalein excretion were demonstrable in the animals during followup observation that extended over 40 months. Liver biopsies showed disturbances of hepatic architecture and chronic inflammatory cell infiltrates. In addition, foci of parenchymal necrosis and increased Kupffer cells were noted.

Such potential hepatotoxicity in primates is in line with demonstrated changes in liver weight,[31, 43–45] glycogen content,[45] ultrastructure,[46–48] and enzyme activities[47, 48] in rodents acutely or chronically exposed to DEHP. From the large body of literature, several salient features deserve comment. DEHP diminishes cholesterol synthesis[43, 48, 49] and cholesterol content[48] in liver or testis. It also lowers plasma cholesterol concentration.[43, 48] Mitochondrial enzymes such as cytochrome oxidase or succinate dehydrogenase are decreased.[31, 48] Microsomal protein content and microsomal enzymes are apparently first diminished and subsequently increased.[31, 50] The metabolites MEHP or 2-ethylhexanol can also induce stimulation of microsomal enzymes; therefore, the parent substances may not cause at least part of the stimulation.

The clinically important consequences for drug metabolism

are somewhat controversial. In normal rabbits, a dose-dependent diminution of cytochrome P-450, paraxylolhydroxylase and bencphetamin-N-demethylase was found by Patel.[46] The action of DEHP on hepatic drug-metabolizing enzymes in the rat and hexobarbital sleeping time[51–53] are controversial, but there is agreement that DEHP affects these two indices in uremic rats.[54] With respect to hepatotoxicity, the induction of peroxisomes in rat hepatocyte cultures by the DEHP metabolites MEHP and EHA is of note. This observation raises the possibility of hepatic tissue damage by oxygen radicals.[55] This effect is analogous to that of clofibrate and may also be involved in the action described above on sterol synthesis.[43, 48, 49] The effect of DEHP on drug metabolism or lipid metabolism in dialysis patients has not been explored.

Of interest also are reports on cardiotoxicity. Lawrence et al.[56] found a pronounced decrease in inotropy when hearts were exposed to solutions recirculated through dialyzer tubing. In toxicity studies, DEHP was found to reduce palmityl-CoA-oxidation in rat heart mitochondria[57] after feeding as little as 200 mg DEHP/day. In isolated perfused rat hearts, Aronson et al.[58] found that DEHP caused bradycardia, reduction of coronary perfusion, prolongation of PQ and QT-intervals, ectopic beats and delayed conduction, reduction of glycogen content, and concentration of energy-rich nucleotides (ATP, CP). DEHP may also act on peripheral vascular smooth muscles, since several authors commented on hypotension after DEHP.[59]

Furthermore, DEHP causes abnormalities of the hematopoetic and reticuloendothelial systems. Rubin et al.[59] noted significant leucopenia after DEHP. Actions on cell proliferation may be related to the known dose-dependent, DNA-damaging effects on procaryotes,[60] the mutagenic activity,[60, 61, 62] the teratogenic action on mammalian embryos,[60, 63] the inhibitory action on fibroblast and lymphocyte cultures,[42a, 64] and the hypothetical carcinogenic action.[65, 66] Exposure to DEHP also caused changes of macrophage function, e.g., phagocytosis, or the release of lysosomal enzymes.[67] Reticuloendothelial function, as assessed by the clearance of colloidal carbon particles, was either stimulated or depressed, depending on the schedule of administration.[52]

DEHP has also been demonstrated to cause intravascular hemolysis.[57] Furthermore, prolonged exposure of stored blood to plastic bags containing DEHP increased the number of microclots. Apparently platelet clumps resulted from increased platelet adhesiveness.[52, 68] Furthermore, increased fibrin monomers were demonstrated in animals exposed to DEHP.[69] Interactions of DEHP with hemostasis in dialysis patients have not been explored to date.

One component of DEHP toxicity may be related to histamine.[69] DEHP was shown to cause an increase of both histamine and histaminase in serum. When the effect of histaminase was neutralized by administering a histaminase inhibitor, DEHP increased serum histamine concentration. And at the same time, mortality from DEHP increased.

Acute respiratory distress with toxic interstitial pulmonary edema has been found in animal studies after high doses of DEHP were administered.[59, 70, 71] Finally, testicular (but not ovarian) functions are compromised by DEHP—organ weight, testicular zinc content, testicular succinate dehydrogenase, testosterone production, and spermatogenesis.[72–74]

DEHP in Dialysis

Determination of DEHP and its metabolites poses formidable methodological problems. Many data reported in literature must therefore be viewed with the utmost circumspection. In our experience, using gas-chromatography and mass-spectrometry, the detection limit for DEHP is 1 ppm. Reproducibility of measurements below 10 ppm is rather poor. Consequently, some of the following information on blood levels, body burden, and organ levels in dialysis patients may have to be revised later.

Blood Levels in Dialysis Patients

DEHP blood levels in dialysis patients were found to increase to 389 ppb,[75] with a postdialysis fall to low levels. At the end of dialysis, the blood's total phthalic acid content was much higher than the DEHP levels, suggesting rapid metabolism of DEHP. Lewis et al.[76] measured levels of DEHP up to 946 ppb with a rapid postdialysis decrease. Patients on long-term dialysis had higher levels. In our own studies, we found no consistent increase of DEHP blood levels during dialysis. This finding is not surprising, since patients receive a DEHP load of approximately 30 mg DEHP per dialysis (see below). On the other hand, animal studies show that the fraction of DEHP remaining in the circulation after one hour is less than 2%.[38] Consequently, it will be impossible to demonstrate an increase of DEHP, using a method with a detection limit of 1 ppm.

DEHP Body Burden During Dialysis

Estimates of the amount of DEHP transferred into the organism during one dialysis session varied from 0.5 mg[75] to 150 mg.[77] From arteriovenous differences (264–541 ppb.) and blood flow rates, Lewis et al.[76] calculated desorption rates of 3–6.5 mg DEHP per hour. From Ono's data,[75] one can similarly calculate a load of 0.5 mg DEHP per dialysis session. Gibson et al.[77] on the basis of av-differences, calculated a five hour load of 9–150 mg.

Since blood level measurements are delicate, as outlined above, more credence can be given to in vitro measurements using recirculation systems. Fayz et al.[78] found that DEHP was not desorbed from dialysis tubing by aqueous solutions, but by bovine plasma. Gerstrof et al.[79] found a DEHP leakage rate of 3.4 mg/h at 37° C from a dialysis system with a plasma flow rate of 200 ml/min. Using human plasma of 37° C under similar conditions, Easterling found DEHP leakage rates of 10 mg per five hours.[80] In our own studies,[81] we found a linear increase of DEHP release with time, both when PVC and polyurethane-coated PVC tubing was used. Figure 1 shows a typical experiment. We did not observe saturation of DEHP transfer over the observation period. We noted consistent results within individual blood units, but large variations between different blood units. This variability may be related to differences in lipid content, platelet number, rheological factors, etc. When blood was used for recirculation, equal amounts of DEHP were recovered in the plasma and blood cell fractions. However, when cell-free plasma was used for recirculation, considerably less DEHP was released as compared with whole blood.

This might point to an erythrocyte role in promoting DEHP desorption. This may be related to the cholesterol-rich plasma membrane of erythrocytes. However, more detailed kinetic

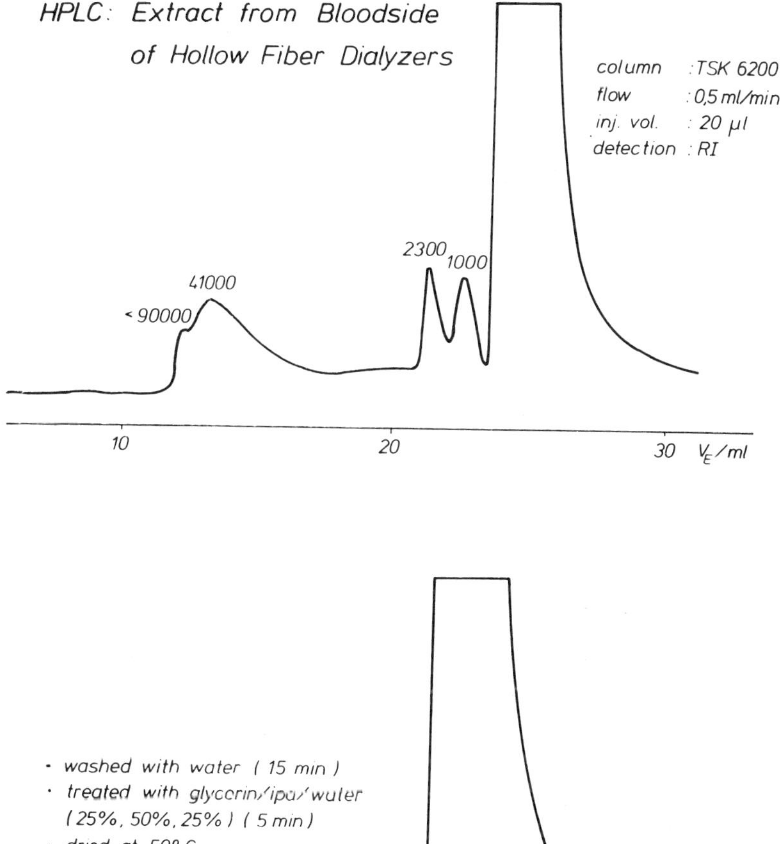

Fig 1.—Demonstration of material in the blood side extract of cuprophane (R) hollow fiber dialyzers. The extract from the blood side of hollow fibers was analyzed with high pressure liquid chromatography (HPLC), using the conditions given in the upper panel. The figure shows some low molecular material 2,3 kDalton and below. In addition, however, material in the molecular weight range 41-90 kDalton tentatively identified as cellulosic fragments is eluated (upper panel). After washing with water for 15 minutes the material is no longer demonstrable in the eluate.

analyses are necessary before this hypothesis can be considered as proved. On the basis of our in vitro studies, approximately 30 mg DEHP are transferred from PVC tubing into the patient's circulation during a five-hour dialysis session using a standard 200 ml/min. blood flow rate.

DEHP Organ Levels in Dialysis Patients

Jaeger et al.[82] examined tissues of patients who had been on cardiopulmonary bypass for several hours. Using gas chromatography with the Gas-chrom-Q, they measured concentrations up to 92 ppm in the lung and 70 ppm in the liver.

Using GC-MS, we found DEHP levels in the liver and spleen of dialysed patients between 5 and 10 ppm; no DEHP was detectable in the liver of non-dialyzed control patients.[83] Our measurements do not exclude substantial amounts of DEHP metabolites. Concomitantly, we found some unidentified sterol material. This observation is of note because dialysis tubing contains filling material other than DEHP.

ENDOTOXIN-LIKE MATERIAL ON CELLULOSIC MEMBRANES

The high prevalence of febrile reactions in the early days of hemodialysis virtually disappeared with the introduction of disposable material and appropriate water purification systems. Indeed, even heavy bacterial colonization of the dialyze compartment has been shown to cause no febrile reaction in hemodialyzed dogs,[84] although species differences in pyrogen reaction must be kept in mind.

When endotoxinemia was demonstrated in febrile patients on hemodialysis, it was thought to result from membrane microleaks.[85] The parent endotoxin molecule with a molecular weight of 10^6 daltons is effectively restricted by the dialysis membranes[84, 86, 87] and ultrafiltration.[88] Degradation products, e.g., lipid A components which may be as small as 2000 daltons are highly water insoluble.[84] Consequently, exogenous infection or endotoxin exposure from the dialysate compartment do not appear to be a hazard of today's hemodialysis procedures. It should be mentioned, however, that some investigators[89] continue to note consistent minor elevations of body temperature in patients on dialysis.

There has been recent concern about the possibility that the cellulosic membrane in itself contains microgram amounts of material that react in the limulus amebocyte lysate test (LAL). This was first noted by Peterson et al.[90] Using static or dynamic leaching, LAL reactive material (LAL-RM) could be eluted from various commercial cellulosic hollow-fiber dialyzers. Such material was LAL-reactive, but did not cause fever in the standard USP rabbit pyrogen test.[90] The doses frequently exceeded 1.0 ng/kg of body weight, i.e., the dose that is considered the threshold pyrogenic dose for human beings when measured with a LAL test standardized against the reference endotoxin lot EC-2. Therefore, it was of note that pyrogenic reactions in patients dialyzed with such dialyzers were only reported when the dialyzers had been reused and apparently contaminated with endotoxin. Although such AL-RM is released rapidly early in the wash-out period,[90] the observation was of great concern because of recent concepts relating various pathological features during hemodialysis to macrophage activation and interleucin I generation during maintenance hemodialysis.[88]

Endotoxin does not cause fever directly; the fever comes via intermediate steps involving genomic depression and de novo production of a family of low molecular-weight polypeptides in macrophages, which then elicit a febrile response through interaction with some nuclei in the anterior hypothalamus.[91-95] These polypeptides are thought to be related to, or identical with, interleucin I. However, various host responses other than fever occur below the febrile threshold. In other words, the febrile reaction is the most noticeable of the host reactions to microbial products, but it is only the tip of the iceberg.[96] At subpyrogenic doses, acute phase reactions—e.g., an increase in circulating neutrophils, decrease in serum zinc and iron concentrations, increasing globulin synthesis, anemia, and synthesis of a series of acute phase hepatic proteins, for example, haptoglobin, fibrinogen, C-reactive protein or serum amyloid A (SAA) protein—are known to occur.[97] Some of these features have also been noted in dialysis patients.

In view of such dire possibilities, it appeared urgent to identify the nature of LAL-RM on cellulosic membranes. Before discussing this problem, some comments on the limulus assay are appropriate. Amebocyte lysate is endowed with a heat labile, pH-sensitive, trypsin-like enzyme that induces LAL gelation as part of a primitive subvertebrate coagulation system. This system can also be activated by thrombin. Although the sensitivity of the LAL test is well established, its specificity is in doubt. Substances other than endotoxin can elicit positive LAL reactions, e.g., thrombin and thromboplastin,[87] polynucleotides (poly-I: poly-D; poly-A: poly-U), although there is some conflict of data in this respect;[70] peptidoglycanes of gram positive bacteria;[98] streptococcal exotoxines;[99] synthetic dextranphosphate and plamitoyl-dextranphosphate; lipoteichoic acids[100] and low molecular weight thiocompounds, e.g., dithiotreiotol and dithioerythritol.[101]

Keeping such non-specificity in mind, it is of note that saline rinses of hemodialyzers, although positive for all LAL systems (with the exception of the commercial LAL system of Malinckrodt Co.)[11] were non-pyrogenic in the USP rabbit pyrogen test at doses up to 2,000 ng/kg. LAL-RM proved also non-toxic in the USP mouse toxicity assay at 5,000 ng/kg and had no influence on hematology, liver function enzymes, coagulation or complement activity at 1,000 ng/kg in rats.[102] One note of caution must be made, however. While lack of pyrogenicity is not typical for endotoxin, so called "environmental pyrogens," in contrast to standard enterobacterial endotoxin preparations, pass the USP pyrogen assay at doses between 2.0 and 100.0 ng when the threshold fever reaction is 1.0 ng/kg with standard endotoxin.[102] This raises the possibility that LAL-RM in capillary flow dialyzers is an extreme case of an "environmental endotoxin." Other possibilities to explain the discrepancy, as suggested in the original Peterson paper,[90] include the presence of environmental endotoxin in raw materials or water used for membrane production, and endotoxin degradation by alkylation during ethylenoxide sterilization.

The production process was carefully examined in extensive studies of the manufacturer, Enka Glanzstoffe Company of Wuppertal, West Germany. It could be excluded with reasonable certainty that endotoxin is present in the water used in the production process and that endotoxin is partially degraded by alkylation during ethylenoxide. The presence of LAL-RM could also be dissociated from dialysis leucocytopenia. LAL-RM appeared when LAL-RM-negative cellulose acetate hollow fibers were saponified with NaOH. This observation also excludes the presence of performed endotoxin on membranes.[11]

Preliminary studies by Watson of the Woods Hole Oceanographic Institution, using gas chromatography and mass spectrometry, indicate that LAL-RM is an endotoxin.[102] However, several other lines of evidence argue against the notion that LAL-RM is an endotoxin. LAL-RM is not inhibited by polymyxin-B when evaluated by LAL, in contrast to endotoxin. LAL-RM does not stimulate the production of endogenous pyrogen at 30 ng/ml, whereas 5 ng/ml of E. coli endotoxin does so in the hands of Dr. Dinarello of Boston.[102] Furthermore, LAL-RM, in contrast to bacterial lipopolysaccharide, does not stimulate the macrophage killing of SV-40-transformed fibroblasts.

Simple polysaccharides are known to cause LAL gelation, as shown by Mikami et al.[103] Morita et al.[104] demonstrated the presence of a (1→3-B-D-glykan)-mediated coagulation pathway in LAL that is not activated by endotoxin. This raises the possibility of carbohydrate induction of lysate gelation by non-endotoxin products of the cellulosic membranes. This speculation is also of interest because cellulose-derived membranes could possibly activate the alternative complement pathway by a similar glycan.[102, 105–107] Indeed, the HPLC chromatogram in Figure 1, kindly provided by Dr. Henne of Enka Glanzstoffe demonstrates that the bloodside extract of Cuprophane (R) hollow-fiber dialyzers contains material in the 40 90 kD range (upper panel). Such material can be readily removed by a brief rinsing of a dialyzer (lower panel). The concentration of this 40–90 kD cellulosic material was in the ppm range.

On balance, the weight of the evidence argues against the notion that LAL-RM is an endotoxin. The biologic consequences of exposure to presumably non-endotoxic LAL-RM have not yet been defined. Consequently, whether or not the presence of LAL-RM in cellulosic membranes necessitates the introduction of fully synthetic membranes cannot be decided from the data currently available.

Silicone Particle Thesaurismosis

General Particle-Related Problems in Medicine

Introducing particles into the circulation is a recognized hazard in procedures involving access to the vascular system. In the past, a great number of particles was detected in infusion fluids, e.g., rubber particles, bast, cellulose fibers, etc. Injection of such particles, especially of cellulose fibers, into experimental animals caused pulmonary granuloma.[108] This observation led to the introduction of rigorous standards for particle content in intravenous fluids.[108] Dialyzers are not free of debris and cellulosic extrables in the 40–90 kD range. Although cellulosic material can be recovered from the rinsing fluid of dialyzers, no related pathology has been recognized in humans.

Particulate material in the dialysate used for peritoneal dialysis was shown to cause peritoneal reactions.[109] Winchester et al.[109] demonstrated particulate material ($\sim$ 200 particles > 5 μm in 2 1 dialysate) that could be removed effectively by filtration through the 0.2 μm filter. The relation of such particulate material, if any, to sclerosing peritonitis on CAPD remains to be established.

It has been reported that particles are generated from wearable insulin pumps as a result of fatigue from unfinished surfaces of plastic tubing, but this led to no severe consequences.[91, 110, 111] In artificially perfused cultures of liver cells maintained within capillary systems and perfused via silicone tubing, Wolf et al.[112, 113] noted clogging of the capillaries by silicone debris generated by the roller pump. During bypass surgery, emboli may enter the brain from various sources—debris from the circuit and the prime, flakes coming off plastic from the pump, silicone antifoam and precipitates from added drugs, as discussed by Wildevuur.[114] Particle-related brain dysfunction after open heart surgery is also suggested by the observation of Arberg et al.[111] Taylor[115] noted an increase of cerebrospinal fluid (CSF) and creatine kinase (CK) after open heart surgery; such an increase was prevented when a micropore filter was added to the extracorporeal circuit to prevent microembolism.

Other authors[116] noted that the difficulty to resuscitate hearts after cardiac standstill was related to particle content in the perfusion fluid; micropore filtration eliminated this problem.

Silicone Particle Related Pathology

Systemic dispersion of silicone particles is a known hazard of aortic ball valves. As described by Fiegenberg et al.[117] and Ridolfi et al.,[118] silicone debris may come off defective aortic ball valves when their surface is roughened by fatigue and fissures. Associated pathology included hepatomegaly with granuloma formation. This was accompanied by elevation of serum transaminases.

In dialysis patients, both we[83] and other investigators[118–121] noted deposition of refractile material in macrophages or giant foreign-body cells within various organs, e.g., lung, liver, spleen, bone marrow, skin, and lymph nodes. By energy dispersive X-ray fluorescence microanalysis, it could be established that the material contained the element silicone (Si), which is virtually absent in biological tissue. It was concluded that the particles represented silicone, i.e., the inorganic polymer polydimethylsiloxane. We recently substantiated this finding by our studies, using laser-activated micromass analysis (LAMMA), which unequivocally gave fragment masses indicative of polymethylsiloxane. There is now consensus that the refractile particles illustrated in Figure 2 result from spallation of silicone tubing in the pump segment of dialysis tubing when such tubing is mechanically damaged by the roller pump.

Although Mikuz et al.[122] concluded that silicone is degraded within phagocytes by hydrolytic attack on the Si-O-Si-bonds, most authors agree that the material is not biodegradable. This holds at least for eucaryotic cells, although some exceptional procaryotes degrade silicone.[123] In archaeological and environmental research, the presence in sediments of silicone, because of its virtual non-destructibility, is used as an index of contemporaneous civilization.[124]

It is known from experimental studies that any inert non-biodegradable material may activate macrophages and cause granulomatous inflammation.[108] The clinical consequences of silicone-related pathology depend largely on the physical nature of the polymer. The consistency of the silicone technically available varies from oil to hard rubber. The former is paramedically used for cosmetic purposes,[125–127] the latter is used medically for dialysis tubing,[83, 119] ball valve prostheses,[117, 129, 130] or joint prostheses.[127, 131–134] Silicone oil has been used for augmentation mammoplasty in women and by homosexuals to acquire feminine hip contours. After subcutaneous injection of silicone oil, Ellenbogen et al.[126] noted a chronic syndrome characterized by granulomatous hepatitis with elevated transaminases. Several

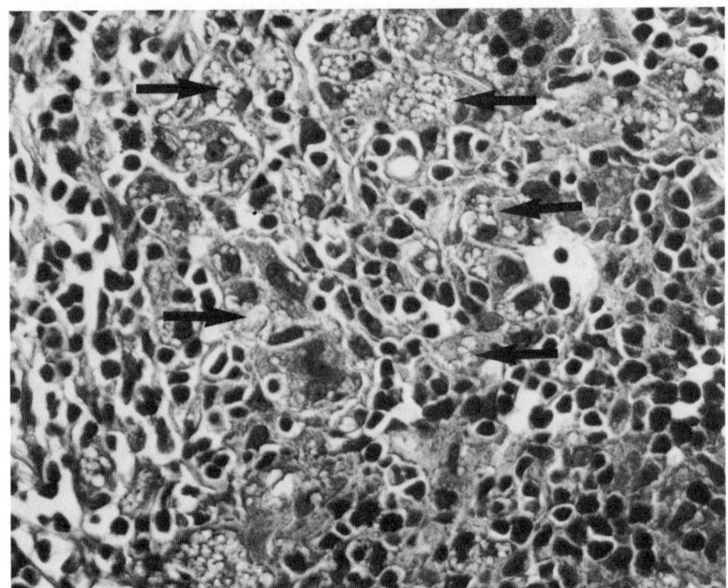

Fig 2.—Demonstration of refractile silicone particles in macrophages from the splenic tissue of a dialysis patient. (Paraffin section, Masson-Trichrome stain, magnification x 500.) As indicated by the arrow, the cytoplasm of the macrophages contains numerous translucent, non-crystalline, refractile particles.

authors observed an acute fatal syndrome of fever, respiratory distress, and acute renal failure after accidental intravenous injection.[125] Furthermore, acute respiratory distress resulting from alveolitis was noted in homosexuals who had injected huge amounts of silicone oil into the subcutaneous fat of the pelvic region. Their alveolar lavage fluid revealed numerous macrophages studded with silicone oil granules.

TABLE 1—CLINICAL CONSEQUENCES OF SILICONE
PARTICLE DEPOSITION IN DIALYSIS PATIENTS

Hepatomegaly[83, 118, 119]
Granulomatous hepatitis[83, 119, 121]
Elevated transaminases (non A-non B-hepatitis)?[83, 119, 121]
Splenomegaly[136]
Splenogenic pancytopenia[135]
Impaired microbial resistance?[138]
Carcinogenesis?, i.e., lymphoma formation as in non-dialyzed
  patients[127, 131, 136, 140]

In contrast to the syndromes resulting from silicone oil, the clinical consequences, if any, resulting from silicone particles are less obtrusive. Similar to what has been noted in patients with aortic ball valves,[128] the main clinical features in dialysis patients relate to hepatosplenomegaly. Table 1 lists the major clinical consequences discussed in literature. For details, the reader is referred to numerous original articles[118, 119, 131, 135] and reviews.[136, 137]

Mechanism of Silicone-Induced Damage

The mere presence of silicone material in organs does not necessarily imply abnormal organ function. In order to clarify the function of macrophages with silicone particle ingestion, we recently administered silicone particles to Wistar rats by either intravenous or intraperitoneal injection. To elucidate whether other polymers shared the properties of silicone, parallel studies with polyvinylchloride (PVC) and polyurethane (PU) were also carried out. As shown in Figure 2, intraperitoneal injection of silicone, PVC, or PU particles increased PGE_2 release from peritoneal macrophages, both under basal conditions and after stimulation with bacterial lipopolysaccharide (LPS) and zymosan. Similar results were obtained with peritoneal macrophages of animals with chronic intravenous injection of particles. Increased PGE_2 release was paralleled by similarly increased thromboxane (TXB_2) release.

For obvious reasons, human material is not readily available. However, we have limited observations on two dialysis patients who had been splenectomized for pancytopenia.[138] Large amounts of silicone particles could be shown in their spleens. As demonstrated in Table 2, the patients' splenic cells released more PGE_2, TXB_2 and 6-keto-PGF-1-alpha than those obtained from a cadaver kidney donor used as control. These studies document that cellular storage of plastic particles is not inert with respect to macrophage function, and demonstrate increased prostanoid release as an index of macrophage activation. Although the mechanism by which activated macrophages may induce organ damage is still unknown, several possibilities exist—e.g., enzyme release and oxygen radical generation, which must be tested in further studies. The observation of high fever in patients exposed to great amounts of silicone

TABLE 2—Prostanoid Release from Spleen Cells
of Dialysis Patients

	PGE$_2$ (ng/ml)	TXB$_2$ (ng/ml)	6-keto-PGF$_{1\alpha}$ (ng/ml)
Control patient			
spontaneous release	0.05 ± 0.01	2.54 ± 0.30	0.34 ± 0.04
+ Zymosan	0.05 ± 0.02	3.26 ± 0.40	0.49 ± 0.08
+ Con A	0.13 ± 0.02	3.73 ± 0.16	0.62 ± 0.08
Patient 1			
spontaneous release	0.54 ± 0.08	2.50 ± 0.28	1.12 ± 0.13
+ Zymosan	0.59 ± 0.05	4.81 ± 0.56	1.21 ± 0.12
+ Con A	0.93 ± 0.04	6.18 ± 0.53	1.52 ± 0.03
Patient 2			
spontaneous release	0.08 ± 0.02	3.82 ± 0.51	1.39 ± 0.05
+ Zymosan	0.55 ± 0.08	15.20 ± 2.23	3.56 ± 0.52
+ Con A	0.21 ± 0.03	8.53 ± 1.22	1.67 ± 0.11

Spleen cells were incubated at a concentration of 3×10^6/ml for 24 h, with or without Zymosan particles or Con A.

Values represent the mean ± SD of 4 identical and simultaneous incubations.

nil[125, 139] would be compatible with the notion that macrophages activated by silicone produce interleucin I. Long-term consequences of such interleucin I production would be of some concern, particularly given some recent suggestions of interleucin I production in dialysis patients as a result of contact with dialysis membranes. Further concerns relate to disturbance of immune function[83] and even possible carcinogenicity.[83, 127, 131, 140]

Mechanism of Spallation and Possibilities of Its Prevention

Figure 3 shows the luminal surface of dialysis tubing that had been exposed to a roller pump for five hours. The surface, no longer smooth, is fractured by numerous fault lines. In addition, many meandering protuberances are visible that were evidently cast up by tangential shearing forces. The surface is covered by debris consisting of large particles, i.e., elongated 100-μm-long flakes resembling rollers, and of small nondescript particles presumably derived from ground-up large particles. Similar fissuring and fracturing of the luminal surface, with generation of debris, has also been demonstrated for the tubing used in cardiopulmonary bypass surgery.[37] Luminal damage is the combined result of shearing and compression

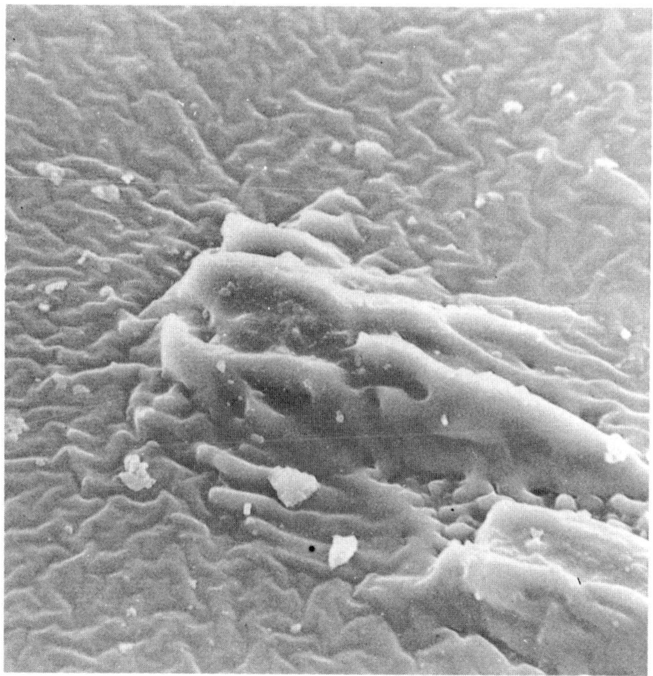

Fig 3.—Scanning electron micrograph of luminal surface of dialysis PVC tubing. Commercial silicone dialysis tubing was exposed to a roller pump in an in vitro system for five hours. The luminal surface was examined with SEM, using a jeol-1 apparatus. The surface is fractured and fissured. Numerous protuberances are visible in the middle of the electron micrograph.

forces exerted by the pump, which acts on the tubing wall like a fulling mill.

To further elucidate the amount of material released and the factors determining such release, in vitro fragmentation of silicone tubing was evaluated in a recirculation system (300 ml saline) using a commercial hemodialysis roller pump (Fresenius Co.) and silicone tubing (internal diameter 8 mm; wall thickness 1.8 mm). At 25 rpm = 280 ml/min, silicone particle release, as determined by microscopically counting particles in aliquots subjected to quick filtration on millipore filter (Fig 4), was a function of the occlusion force in the range of 5–22 kp (kilopond). Silicone release into the recirculation fluid was also quantitated using flameless atomic absorption spectrophotometry.[141] Previous estimates, using chloroform extraction, as-

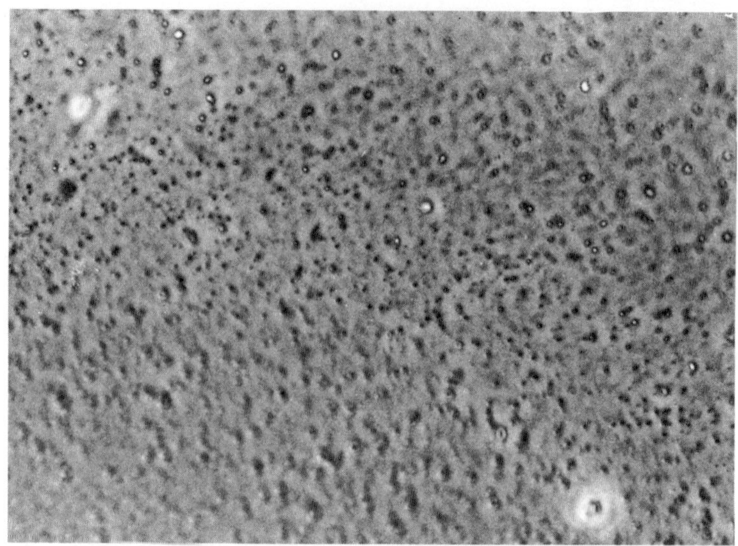

Fig 4.—Microscopic demonstration of silicone particles on a Millipore filter. Commercial dialysis tubing was exposed to a roller pump as described for Figure 3 in a recirculation system. The recirculation fluid was quick-filtered, using a Millipore filter membrane. Microscopic examination of the filter membrane shows numerous refractile particles of several μ diameter (⊢——⊣ corresponds to 0.04 mm).

sessed only soluble silicone oligomers and yielded unrealistically low figures (50 μg/5 h of dialysis).[119] When occlusion forces are reduced from 22 to 5 kp by using different spring coils, silicone release decreases to one fourth of the original value. With low occlusion pressures, our figures yield a silicone load of 0.24 mg silicone per session, equivalent to 36 mg silicone per year.

How can we avoid exposing patients to silicone filings? The above studies show that careful adjustment of the occlusion pressure by controlling the distance between roles and abutment are effective in reducing silicone load. Excessive occlusion in the pump segment is the major factor in generating silicone debris.

Since macrophage function was equally altered in experimental studies by silicone, PVC and polyurethane particles,[138, 142] substituting alternate plastic material for silicone does not appear to be a promising approach. Only the future can tell whether better handling of existing technology is sufficient to avoid clinical problems, or whether more radical changes of the pump system will be required to control spallation.

Conclusions

Side effects caused by some of the material used in hemodialysis equipment have recently generated much concern. Some selected topics were discussed in this review.

ETHYLENOXIDE (ETO).—Halogenated reaction products are generated from ETO when this alkylating sterilizing agent is exposed to polyurethane and PVC. Experimental and clinical studies demonstrate that both allergic and toxic reactions occur to such products. Allergic side effects are either of the anaphylactic or delayed type. In particular, controlled studies suggest that bronchospasm, eosinophilia, hyper-IgE-immunoglobulinemia, and other acute problems in dialysis patients are related, at least in part, to ETO sterilization.

PHTHALATE.—This plasticizer in PVC tubing and its metabolites are excreted via the kidneys so that it accumulates in anephric patients. Recent methodologic improvements gave realistic estimates of the phthalate load during one dialysis session (approximately 30 mg) and allow the demonstration of phthalate in the organs of dialysis patients. Although no pathology in dialysis patients can unequivocally be ascribed to phthalate, a considerable body of evidence in animals, including primates, points to substantial toxicity of phthalate—e.g., hepatotoxicity, cardiotoxicity, effects on the hematopoietic and macrophage/reticuloendothelial system, and testicular function.

LAL-RM.—Limulus assay lysate reactive material has recently been demonstrated on cellulosic dialysis membranes. Paradoxically, the material was devoid of pyrogenicity in the USP rabbit test. Although an unusual endotoxin is not finally excluded, the weight of evidence favors direct interaction of membrane (carbohydrate) components with the intrinsic coagulation system of limulus hemolymph. The biological consequences, if any, of exposure to such material are uknown.

SILICONE THESAURISMOSIS.—The uptake of silicone filings by macrophages throughout the body is a well-recognized and characterized complication in dialysis patients. Recently physical studies unequivocally show that the refractile particles consist of polymethylsiloxane. In the past, it was controversial whether this storage of particles was bland or caused organ dysfunction. Our recent experimental studies demonstrate that plastic particle uptake by macrophages in vivo activates prostanoid metabolism as one indicator of macrophage activation. Preliminary evidence also shows activation of the spleen cells of dialysis patients and provides a rationale for the genesis of organ dysfunction. Furthermore, recent quantitative studies illustrate the overriding importance of occlusion pressure in the generation of debris in the roller pump segment, and suggest ways of avoiding filing by reducing occlusion pressure.

REFERENCES

1. Bommer J., Ritz E., Andrassy K.: Necrotizing dermatitis resulting from hemodialysis with polyvinylchloride tubing. *Ann. Intern. Med.* 91:869, 1979.
2. Robinson P.J.A., Rosen S.M.: Pyrexial reactions during hemodialysis. *Brit. Med. J.* 1:528, 1971.
3. Jones D.M., Tobin B.M., Harlow G.R., et al.: Bacteriological studies of the modified Kiil dialyser. *Br. Med. J.* 3:135, 1970.
4. Ogden D.A., Myers L.E., Eskelson C.D., et al.: Iatrogenic administration of formaldehyde to hemodialysis patients. *Proc. Clin. Dial. Transplant Forum* 5:141, 1973.
5. Belzer F.O., Kountz S.L., Perkins H.A.: Red cell cold autoagglutinins as a cause of failure of renal allotransplantation. *Transplantation* 11:422, 1971.
6. Fassbinder W., Koch K.: A specific immunohemolytic anemia induces by formaldehyde sterilisation of dialysers. *Contrib. Nephrol.* 36:51, 1983.
7. Fisher A.A.: Postoperative ethylene oxide dermatitis. *Cutis.* 12:177, 1973.
8. Glaser Z.R.: Ethylene oxide: Toxicology review and field study results of hospital use. *J. Environ. Pathol. Toxicol.* 2:173, 1979.
9. Stanley P., Bertranou E., Forest F., et al.: Toxicity of ethylene oxide sterilization of polyvinyl chloride in open heart surgery. *J. Thorac. Cardiovasc. Surg.* 61:309, 1971.
10. Gutch C.F., Eskelson C.D., Ziegler Z., et al.: 2-Chloroethanol as a toxic residue in dialysis supplies sterilized with ethylene oxide. *Dial. & Transpl.* 1976, 5, 21–25.
11. Henne W., Dietrich W., Pelger M., et al.: Biocompatibility of cuprophane. II. Residual ethylene oxide in hollow fiber dialysers. *Artif. Organs* (in press) 1983a.
12. Nicholls A.J., Platts M.M: Anaphylactoid reactions due to haemodialysis, haemofiltration, or membrane plasma separation. *Br. Med. J.* 285:1607, 1982.
13. Takahashi S., Ohsima H., Watanabe H., et al.: Eosinophilia observed in regular hemodialysis patients. *Jap. J. Nephrol.* 9, 1979.
14. Poothullil J., Shimizu A., Day R.P., et al.: Anaphylaxis from the product(s) of ethylene oxide gas. *Ann. Intern. Med.* 82:58, 1975.
15. Hiner E.E.: Report on plasmapheresis donor reactions. FDA-Office of Biologics. *Plasma Quarterly.* 1983.
16. Ing T.S., Daugirdas I.T., Ivanovich P.T., et al.: Severe reactions to cuprammonium cellulose dialyzers. *Am. Soc. Nephrol.* 1983 (Abstr.)
17. Shupack J.L., Andersen S.R., Romano S.J.: Human skin reactions to ethylene oxide. *J. Lab. Clin. Med.* 98:723, 1981.
18. Peterson M.C., Vine J., Ashley J.J., et al.: Leaching of 2-(2-hydroxyethylmer-

capto) benzothiazole into contents of disposable syringes. *J. Pharm. Sci.* 70:139, 1981.

19. Howell R.T., McDermott A., Gregson N.M.: Syringe toxicity in amniotic fluid cultures. *Lancet* 1:1099, 1983.
20. Burles J.V., Huxley M.P., Kennedy T.S.: Syringe toxicity in amniotic fluid cultures. *Lancet* 1:1336, 1983.
21. Alomar A., Camarasa J.M.G., Noguera J., et al.: Ethylene oxide dermatitis. *Contact Dermatitis* 7:205, 1981.
22. Romaguera C., Grimalt F.: Irritant dermatitis from ethyle oxide. *Contact Dermatitis.* 7:205, 1981.
23. Buttrey D.N.: *Plasticizers.* London 1950, Cleaver-Hume Press Ltd.
24. Gnamm H.: Die Lösungsmittel und Weichmachungsmittel, 1950. Wiss. Verlagsges. GmbH, Stuttgart
25. Kerkay J., Nakamoto S.: Plasticizers and the uremic patients. *Int. J. Artif. Organs.* 2:107, 1979.
26. Batelle-Institut: Bewertung von organisch-chemischen Stoffen. Di-2-äthylhexylphthalat, 1978.
27. Rowland I.R.: Metabolism of di-)2-ethylhexyl) phthalate by the contents of the alimentary tract of the rat. *Food Cosmet. Toxicol.* 12:293, 1974.
28. Rubin R.J., Miller J.: Metabolism of a plasticizer, di(2-ethyl-hexyl) phthalate (DEHP) in the rat. *Fed. Proc.* 33:499, 1974.
29. Travenol Laboratory: Toxicity of components of plastic having contact with blood. Final technical progress report, September 1975.
30. Lake B.G., Philips J.C., Linnell J.G., et al.: The in vitro hydrolysis of some phthalate diesters by hepatic and intestinal preparations from various species. *Toxicol. Appl. Pharmacol.* 39:239, 1977.
31. Lake B.G., Gangolli S.D., Grasso P., et al.: Studies on the hepatic effects of orally administered di-(2-ethylhexyl) phthalate in the rat. *Toxicol. Appl. Pharmacol.* 32:355, 1975.
32. Albro P.W., Hass J.R., Peck C.C., et al.: Identification of the metabolites of di (2-ethylhexyl) phthalate in urine from the African green monkey. *Drug. Metab. Dispos.* 9:223, 1981.
33. Albro P.W., Corbett J.T.: Distribution of di-(3-ethylhexyl) phthalate and mono-(2-ethylhexyl) phthalate in human plasma. *Transfusion* 18:750, 1978.
34. Peck C.C., Albro P.W., Hass J.R., et al.: Metabolism and excretion of the plasticizer di-2-ethylhexyl phthalate in man. *Clin. Res.* 26:101, 1978.
35. Peck C.C., Bailey F.J., Odom D.G., et al.: Plasticizer disposition in a (conscious) primate. *Pharmacologist* 18:195, 1976.
36. Booth G.M., Rhees R.W., Petersen R.V., et al.: Metabolism and autoradiographic localization of di-2-ethylhexyl phthalate (DEHP) in mice and a model ecosystem. *Proc. Int. Congr. Pharmacol.*, Oxford. 6:225, 1976.
37. Chu I., Villeneuve D.C., Secours V., et al.: Metabolism and tissue distribution of mono-2-ethylhexylphthalate in the rat. *Drug Metab. Dispos.* 6:146, 1978.
38. Tanaka A., Adachi T., Takahashi T., et al.: Biochemical studies on phthalic esters; elimination, distribution and metabolism of di(2-ethylhexyl) phthalate in rats. *Toxicology* 4:253, 1975.
39. Williams D.T., Blanchfield B.J.: Retention, excretion and metabolism of di-(2-ethylhexyl) phthalate administered orally to the rat. *Bull. Environ. Contam. Toxicol.* 11:371, 1974.
40. Williams D.T., Blanchfield B.J.: Retention, excretion, and metabolism of phthalic acid administered orally to the rat. *Bull. Environ. Contam. Toxicol.* 12:109, 1974.
41. Chen W.S., Kerkay J., Pearson K.H., et al.: Bis(2-ethylhexyl) phthalate levels in nonuremic patients treated with extracorporeal devices. *Proc. Clin. Dial. Transplant Forum.* 9:189, 1981.
42. Jacobsen M.S., Parkman R., Dutton L.N., et al.: The toxicity of human serum

stored in flexible polyvinyl chloride containers on human fibroblast cell cultures: An effect of di-2-ethylhexyl-phthalate. *Res. Commun. Chem.: Pathol. Pharmacol.* 9:315, 1974.

42a. Jones A.E., Kahn R.H., Groves J.T., et al.: Phthalate ester toxicity in human cell cultures. *Toxicol. Appl. Pharmacol.* 31:283, 1975.

43. Bell F.P., Patt C.S., Brundage B., et al.: Studies on lipid biosynthesis and cholesterol content of liver and serum lipoproteins in rats fed various phthalate esters. *Lipids* 13:666, 1978.

44. Nikonorow M., Mazur H., Piekacz H.: Effect of orally adminstered polyvinylchloride stabilizers in the rat. *Toxicol. Appl. Pharmacol.* 26:253, 1973.

45. Sakurai T., Miyazawa S., Hashimoto T.: Effects of di-(2-ethylhexyl) phthalate administration on carboanhydrate and fatty acid metabolism in rat liver. *J. Biochem. (Tokyo)* 83(1):313, 1978.

46. Patel J.M.: The destruction of pulmonary and hepatic cytochrome p-450 by phthalaldehyde. *Toxicol. Appl. Pharmac.* 48:337, 1979.

47. Srivastava S.P., Seth P.K., Agarwal D.K.: Biochemical effects of di-2-ethylhexyl phthalate. *Environ. Physiol. Biochem.* 5:178, 1975.

48. Srivastava S.P., Agarwal D.K., Mushtaq M., et al.: Effects of di-(2-ethylhexyl) phthalate (DEHP) on chemical constituents and enzymatic activity of rat liver. *Toxicology* 11:271, 1978.

49. Moody D.E., Reddy J.K.: Hepatic peroxisome (microbody) proliferation in rats fed plasticizers and related compounds. *Toxicol. Appl. Pharmacol.* 45:497, 1978.

50. Carter D.E., Feldman B., Sipes I.G.: Liver and lung toxicity of diallylphthalate. *Toxicol. Appl. Pharmacol.* 45:219, 1978.

51. Calley D., Autian J., Guess W.L.: Toxicology of a series of phthalate esters. *J. Pharm. Sci.* 55:158, 1975.

52. Rubin R.J., Jaeger R.J.: Some pharmacological and toxicologic effects of di-2-ethylhexyl phthalate (DEHP) and of plasticizers. *Environm. Health Perspect.* 3:53, 1973.

53. Swinyard E.A., Woodhead J.H., Petersen R.V.: Nonspecific effect of bis-(2-ethylhexyl) phthalate on hexobarbital sleep time. *J. Pharm. Sci.* 65:733, 1976.

54. Leber H.W., Uviss T., Prenter A.: Influence of the plasticizer di-2-ethylhexyl-phthalate on drug metabolising enzymes in the liver of uraemic rats. *Proc. Eur. Dial. Transplant. Assoc.* 16:232, 1979.

55. Gray T.J., Beamand J.A., Lake B.G., et al.: Peroxisome proliferation in cultured rat hepatocytes produced by clofibrate and phthalate ester metabolites. *Toxicol. Lett.* 10:273, 1982.

56. Lawrence W.H., Autian J.: Cardioactive substances leached from a commercial hemodialysis set. *N. Engl. J. Med.* 292:1356, 1975.

57. Bell F.P., Gillies P.J.: Effect of dietary di-2-ethylhexylphthalate on oxidation of 14 C-palmitoyl CoAmitochardia from mammalian heart and liver. *Lipids* 12:581, 1977.

58. Aronson C.E., Serlick E.R., Preti G.: Effects of di-2-ethylhexylphthalate on the isolated perfused rat heart. *Toxicol. Appl. Pharmacol.* 44:155, 1978.

59. Rubin R.J., Chang J.C.F.: The phthalate plasticizer, di-(2-ethylhexyl) phthalate (DEHP) and shock lung in rats. *Tox. Appl. Pharmacol.* 37:154, 1976.

60. Tomita I., Nakamura Y., Aoki N., et al.: Mutagenic/carcinogenic potential of DEHP and MEHP. *Environ. Health Perspect.* 45:119, 1983.

61. Singh A.R., Lawrence W.H., Autian J.: Mutagenic and antifertility sensitivity of mice to DEHP and DMEP. *Tox. Appl. Pharmacol.* 29:35, 1974.

62. Yagi Y.K., Shimoi N.: Tetratogenicity and mutagenicity of phthalate esters. *Teratology* 14:259, 1976.

63. Yagi Y., Nakamura Y., Tomita I., et al.: Tetratogenic potential of di- and mono-(2-ethylhexyl) phthalate in mice. *J. Environ. Pathol. Toxicol.* 4:533, 1980.

64. Turner J.H., Petricciani J.C., Crouch M.L., et al.: An evaluation of the effects of di-ethylhexyl-phthalate (DEHP) on mitotically capable cells in blood packs. *Transfusion* 14:560, 1974.
65. Grasso P.: DEHP and other phthalate esters: An appraisal of toxicological data and recent studies on carcinogenicity, mutagenicity and teratogenicity. Occup. and Health Memorandum 25–70–0037. *BP Res.*
66. NTP Technical Report Series 212: Carcinogenesis bioassay of di(2-ethylhexyl) adipate (CAS no. 103–23–1) F344 rats and B6C 3F1 mice (feed study). NIH publication No. 81–1768.
67. Bally M.B., Opheim D.J., Shertzer H.G.: Di-(2-ethylhexyl) phthalate enhances the release of lysosomal enzymes from alveolar macrophages during phagocytosis. *Toxicology* 18:49, 1981.
67a. Hirose T., Goldstein R., Bailey C.P.: Hemolysis of blood due to exposure to different types of plastic tubing and the influence of ethylene-oxide sterilization. *J. Thorac. Cardiovasc. Surg.* 45:245, 1963.
68. Swank R.L.: Screen filtration pressure method and adhesiveness and aggregation of blood cells. *J. Appl. Physiol.* 19:340, 1964.
69. Chang J.C.F., Rubin R.J.: Studies on the mechanism of the pulmonary and lethal effects of intravenous di-(2-thylhexyl)phthalate (DEHP). *Toxicol. Appl. Pharm.* 48:46, 1976.
70. Rubin R.J., Chang J.C.F.: Effect of the intravenous administration of the solubilized plasticizer di-(2-ethylhexyl) phthalate on the lung and on survival of transfused rats. *Tox. Appl. Pharmacol.* 45:230, 1978.
70a. Siegel S.E., Nachum R.: Use of the limulus lysate assay (LAL) for the detection and quantitation of endotoxin, in: *Perspectives in Toxicology,* Bernheimer A.W. (ed.): John Wiley & Sons, (New York, pp. 61–86, 1977).
71. Schulz C.O.: Acute lung injury from the interaction of a plasticizer di-(2-ethylhexyl) phthalate (DEHP) and a polysorbate surfactant, Tween-80. *Fed. Proc.* 33:234, 1974.
72. Cater B.R., Cook M.W., Gangolli S.D.: Zinc metabolism and dibutyl phthalate-induced testicular atrophy in the rat. *Biochem. Soc. Trans.* 4:652, 1976.
73. Cater B.R., Cook M.W., Gangolli S.D., et al.: Studies on dibutyl phthalate-induced testicular atrophy in the rat: Effect on zinc metabolism/toxicol. appl. *Pharmacology* 41:609, 1977.
74. Seth P.K., Srivastava S.P., Agarwal D.K., et al.: Effect of di-2-ethylhexyl phthalate (DEHP) on rat gonads. *Environ. Res.* 12:131, 1976.
75. Ono K., Tatsukawa R., Wakimoto T.: Migration of plasticizer from hemodialysis blood tubing. *J.A.M.A.* 234:948, 1975.
76. Lewis L.M., Flechtner Th.W., Kerkay J., et al.: Bis(2-thylhexyl) phthalate concentrations in the serum of hemodialysis patients. *Clin. Chem.* 24:741, 1978.
77. Gibson Th.P., Briggs W.A., Boone B.J.: Delivery of di-2-ethylhexyl phthalate to patient during hemodialysis. *J. Lab. Clin. Med.* 87:519, 1976.
78. Fayz S., Herbert R., Martin A.M.: The release of plasticizer from polyvinyl chloride haemodialysis tubing. *J. Pharm. Pharmacol.* 29:407, 1977.
79. Gerstof J., Christiansen E., Nielsen I.L., et al.: The migration of plasticizers from PVC haemodialysis tubes. *Proc. Eur. Dial. Transplant. Assoc.* 16:739, 1980.
80. Easterling R.E., Johnson E., Napier E.A., Jr.: Plasma extraction of plasticizers from "medical grade" polyvinylchloride tubing (38389). *Proc. Soc. Exp. Biol. Med.* 147:572, 1974.
81. Bommer J., v.Sonntag C., Büchler N., et al.: DEHP leakage from dialysis tubing. 4th Congress of the Internat. Soc. Artif. Organs 1983
82. Jaeger R.J., Rubin R.J.: Migration of a phthalate ester plasticizer from polyvinyl chloride blood bags into stored human blood and its localization in human tissues. *N. Engl. J. Med.* 287:1114, 1972.

83. Bommer J., Waldherr R., Gastner M., et al.: Iatrogenic multiorgan silicone inclusions in dialysis patients. *Klin. Wochenschr.* 59:1149, 1981.

84. Port F.K., Bernick J.J.: Pyrogen and endotoxin reactions during hemodialysis. *Contrib. Nephrol.* 36:100, 1983.

85. Dinarello C.A.: Pathogenesis of fever during hemodialysis. *Contrib. Nephrol.* 36:90, 1983.

86. Bernick J.J., Port F.K.: Absence of bacteremia and endotoxemia despite contaminated dialyzate. *Clin. Nephrol.* 14:13, 1980.

87. Elin R.J., Wolff S.M.: Nonspecificity of the limulus amebocyte lysate test: Positive reactions with polynucleotides and proteins. *J. Infect. Dis.* 128:349, 1973.

88. Henderson L.W., Beans E.: Successful production of sterile pyrogen-free electrolyte solution by ultrafiltration. *Kidney Int.* 14:522, 1978.

89. Maggiore Q., Pizzarelli F., Sisca S.: Blood temperature and vascular stability during hemodialysis and hemofiltration. *Trans. Am. Soc. Artif. Intern. Organs.* 28:523, 1982.

90. Petersen N.J., Carson L.A., Favero M.S.: Bacterial endotoxin in new and reused hemodialyzers: A potential cause of endotoxemia. *Trans. Am. Soc. Artif. Intern. Organs* 27:155, 1981.

91. Atkins E., Bodel P., Francis L.: Release of an endogenous pyrogen in vitro from rabbit mononuclear cells. *J. Exp. Med.* 126:357, 1967.

92. Atkins E., Francis L., Bernheim H.A.: Pathogenesis of fever in delayed hypersensitivity: role of monocytes. *Infect. Immun.* 21:813, 1978.

93. Jackson D.L.: A hypothalamic region responsive to localized injection of pyrogens. *J. Neurophysiol.* 30:586, 1967.

94. Jackman W.S., Lougheed W., Marliss B., et al.: For insulin infusion: A miniature precision peristaltic pump and silicine rubber reservoir. *Diabetes Care.* vol. 3, pp. 322–331, 1980.

95. Rosendorff C., Money J.J.: Central nervous system sites of action of a purified leukocyte pyrogen. *Am. J. Physiol.* 220:597, 1971.

96. Henderson L.W., Koch K.M., Dinarello C.A., et al.: Hemodialysis hypotension: The interleukin hypothesis. *Blood Purification.* 1:3, 1983.

97. Dinarello C.A., Wolff S.M.: In *Handbook of Experimental Pharmacology*. Milton A.S. (ed.): Exogenous pyrogens, chap. 4, vol. 60 (Berlin-Heidelberg: Springer Verlag, pp. 73–112, 1982).

98. Wildefeuer A., Heymer B., Schleifer K.H., et al.: Investigations on the specificity of the limulus test for the detection of endotoxin. *Appl. Microbiol.* 28:867, 1974.

99. Brunson K., Watson D.W.: Limulus amebocyte lysate reaction with streptococcal pyrogenic exotoxin. *Infect. Immun.* 14:1256, 1970.

100. Fine D.H., Kessler R.E., Tabak L.A., et al.: Limulus lysate activity of lipoteichoic acids. *J. Dent. Res.* 56:1500, 1977.

101. Platica M., Harding W., Hollander V.P.: Dithiols stimulate endotoxin in the limulus reaction. *Experientia.* 34:1154, 1978.

102. Pearson F.C., Weary M., Bohon J.: Detection of limulus amebocyte lysate reactive material in capillary flow hemodialyzers, in *Endotoxins and Their Detection with the Limulus Amebocyte Lysate Test.* (New York: Riss A.R., pp. 247–260, 1982.)

103. Mikami T., Nagase T., Matsumoto T., et al.: Gelation of limulus amoebocyte lysare by simple polysaccharides. *Microbiol. Immunol.* 26(5):403, 1982.

104. Morita T., Tanaka S., Nakamura T., et al.: A new (1 3)-β-D-glucan-mediated coagulation pathway found in limulus amoebocytes. Elsevier/North Holland Biomedical Press. *FEBS Lett.* 129(2)318, 1981.

105. Chaddock P.R., Rehr J., Dalmasso A.P., et al.: Hemodialysis leukopenia. Pulmonary vascular leukostasis resulting from complement activation by dialyzer cellophane membranes. *J. Clin. Invest.* 59:879, 1977a.

106. Craddock P.R., Fehr J., Brigham K.L., et al.: Complement and leukocyte-mediated pulmonary dysfunction in hemodialysis. *N. Engl. J. Med.* 296:769, 1977b.

107. Jacob A.I., Gavellas G., Zarco R., et al.: Leukopenia, hypoxia, and complement function with different hemodialysis membranes. *Kidney Int.* 18:505, 1980.
108. Garvan J.M., Gunner B.W.: The harmful effects of particles in intravenous fluids. *Med. J. Aust.* 2:1, 1964.
109. Winchester J.F., Ash S.R., Bousquet G., et al.: Successful peritonitis reduction with a unidirectional bacteriologic CAPD filter. *Trans. Am. Soc. Artif. Intern. Organs.* 24:611, 1983.
110. Albisser A.M.: Minimizing silicone cell inclusions from peristaltic pumps. *Lancet* Letter, 563, 1981.
111. Arberg T., Ronquist G., Tyden H., et al.: Release of adenylate kinase during open-heart surgery and its relation to postoperative intellectual function. *Lancet* 1139–1142, 1982.
112. Wolf C.F.W., Minick C.R., McCoy C.H.: Morphologic examination of a prototype liver assist device composed of cultured cells and artificial capillaries. *Int. J. Artif. Organs* 1:45, 1978.
113. Wolf C.F.W.: Cells cultured on artificial capillaries and their use as a liver assist device. *Int. J. Artif. Organs* 4:279, 1980.
114. Wildevuur R.H.: Towards safer cardiopulmonary bypass. In: *Towards Safer Cardiac Surgery.* Longmore D.B., (ed.): (Lancaster: MTP, pp. 287–293, 1981.)
115. Taylor K.M., Devlin B.J., Mittra S.M., Assessment of cerebral damage during open heart surgery—a new experimental model. *Scand. J. Thorac. Cardiovasc. Surg.* (in press)
116. Robinson L.A., Braimbridge M.V., Hearse D.J.: Particulate contamination: A potential hazard of cardioplegia. *Lancet* 1:995, 1983.
117. Fiegenberg D.S., DeColli J.A., Lisan P.R.: Fracture of a Starr-Edwards aortic ball valve with systemic embolism of ball fragments. *Am. J. Cardiol.* 23:458, 1969.
118. Laohapand T., Morley A.R., Ward M.K., et al.: Accumulation of silicone elastomer in patients on regular hemodialysis. *Proc. Eur. Dial. Transplant. Assoc.* 19:143, 1982.
118a. Ridolfi R.L., Hutchins G.M.: Detection of ball variance in prosthetic heart valves by liver biopsy. *Johns Hopkins Med. J.* 134:131, 1974.
119. Leong A.S.Y., Disney A.P.S., Grove D.W.: Spallation and migration of silicone elastomer in patients on regular hemodialysis. *N. Engl. J. Med.* 306:135, 1982.
120. Morales J.M., Colina F., Artega J., et al.: Clinical implications of the presence of refractile particles in liver of hemodialysis patients. *Proc. Eur. Dial. Transplant. Assoc.* 14:265, 1982.
121. Parfrey P.S., Paradinas F.J., O'Driscoll J.B., et al.: Chronic liver disease in hemodialysis patients. *Proc. Eur. Dial. Transplant. Assoc.* 14:265, 1982.
122. Mikuz G., Probst A., Hoinkes G., et al.: Granulomatöse Gewebsreaktion bei intrazellulärem Kunststoff-(Silikongummi-) Abbau. *Verh. Dtsch. Ges. Pathol.* 64:279, 1980.
123. Bayer Co.: Leverkusen, personal communication
124. Pellenberg R.: Silicones as tracers for anthropogenic additions to sediments. *Marine Poll. Bulletin* 10:267, 1979.
125. Chastre J., Basset F., Viau F., et al.: Acute pneumonitis after subcutaneous injections of silicone in transsexual men. *N. Engl. J. Med.* 308:764, 1983.
126. Ellenbogen R., Ellenbogen R., Rubin L.: Injectable fluid silicone therapy. Human morbidity and mortality. *J.A.M.A.* 234:308, 1975.
127. Digby J.M., Wells A.L.: Malignant lymphoma with intranodal refractile particles after insertion of silicone prostheses. *Lancet* 2:580, 1981.
128. Symmers W.S.C.: Silicone mastitis in "topless" waitresses and some other varieties of foreign-body mastitis. *Br. Med. J.* 3:19, 1968.
129. Roberts W.C., Morrow A.G.: Fatal degeneration of the silicone rubber ball of the Starr-Edwards prosthetic aortic valve. *Am. J. Cardiol.* 22:614, 1968.

130. Starr A., Pierie W.R., Raible D.A.: Cardiac valve replacement: Experience with the durability of silicone rubber. *Circulation* 33:1, 34:1–123, 1966.
131. Benjamin E., Ahmed A.: Silicone lymphadenopathy: A report of two cases, one with concomitant malignant lymphoma. *Diagn. Histopathol.* 5:133, 1982.
132. Swanson A.B.: Finger joint replacement by silicone rubber implants, and the concept of implant fixation by encapsulation. *Ann. Rheum. Dis.* (suppl.) 28:47, 1969.
133. Swanson A.B.: Flexible implant arthroplasty for arthritic finger joints. *J. Bone Joint Surg.* [*Am.*] 54A:435, 1972.
134. Swanson A.B., Meester W.D., Swanson GDeG, et al.: Durability of silicone implants: An in vivo study. *Orthop. Clin. North. Am.* 4:1097, 1973.
135. Bommer J., Ritz E., Waldherr R.: Silicone-induced splenomegaly. Treatment of pancytopenia by splenectomy in a patient of hemodialysis. *N. Engl. J. Med.* 305:1077, 1981.
136. Bommer J., Waldherr R., Ritz E.: Silicone storage in long-term hemodialysis patients. *Contrib. Nephrol.* 36:115, 1983.
137. Bommer J.: Silikonablagerungen in den Organen von Dialysepatienten-derzeitiger Stand der Untersuchungen. *Nieren- und Hochdruckkrankheiten.* 12:250, 1983.
138. Bommer J., Gemsa D., Waldherr R., et al.: Plastic filing from dialysis tubing induces prostanoid release from macrophages. (Submitted for publication)
139. Uretsky B.F., O'Brien J.J., Courtiss E.H., et al.: Augmentation mammaplasty associated with a severe systemic illness. *Ann. Plast. Surg.* 3:445, 1979.
140. Bommer J., Digby J.M., Wells A.L., et al.: Immunoblastoma formation—a late consequence of filing from silicone articular prosthesis? *Z. Rheumatol.* 41:130, 1982.
141. Bommer J., Ritz E., Waldherr R., et al.: Fremdmaterial-ablagerungen im RES bei Dauerdialysepatienten. *Verh. Dtsch. Ges. Inn. Med.* 1235, 1983.
142. Bommer J., Gemsa D., Waldherr R., et al.: Macrophage activation by particles released from dialysis tubing. *Kidney Int.* 23:143, 1983.

Prevention and Treatment of Aluminum Intoxication in Chronic Renal Failure

P. SIMON*, P. ALLAIN**, K.S. ANG*, G. CAM*, AND
Y. MAURAS**

*Service of Medicine E - Nephrology, La Beauchée Hospital, Saint-Brieuc, France.
**Laboratory of Pharmacology, C.H.U. Angers, France.

AS EARLY as 1970, Berlyne et al.[15] drew the attention of nephrologists to the potential hazards of aluminum toxicity in uremic patients who were taking aluminum compounds for hyperphosphatemia. Ever since then, a great number of articles in the literature have presented evidence that the warning was well-founded. Clinical manifestations of aluminum intoxication have been described in recent reports in which the role of aluminum-contaminated dialysate and orally administered aluminum-containing phosphate binders was demonstrated.[47, 121, 150, 172] At present, prevention of serious complications of aluminum toxicity should be possible by rigorous removal of aluminum from the dialysis fluid. Henceforth, every dialysis patient should benefit from dialysis fluid containing water that has been deionized or treated by reverse osmosis. Besides prophylactic treatment, aluminum tissue depletion by a chelating agent might be an interesting treatment for tissue aluminum overload. In 1980, Ackrill et al.[1] reported that deferoxamine (DFO), a chelating agent for iron, has a high affinity for aluminum and that its timely administration causes the

439

complete disappearance of neurologic disorders in a patient with dialysis encephalopathy. Thus, a new therapeutic era of aluminum intoxication started.

This chapter discusses the value of serum aluminum monitoring in evaluating aluminum intoxication and the status of current knowledge on the prevention and treatment of aluminum intoxication.

Significance of Hyperaluminemia in Evaluating Aluminum Intoxication

Aluminum is widely found in the environment. It may be absorbed through the respiratory and gastrointestinal tracts. Aluminum is excreted in the urine, and its clearance is about half that of creatinine.[5] In normal healthy subjects, mean serum aluminum levels have been found to be less than 10 μg/ L in England[123] and the United States[79] and between 15 and 30 μg/L in France,[8, 68, 140] Germany,[179] and Japan.[165] Aluminum is measured in biologic fluids by flameless atomic absorption spectrophotometry. Blood must be handled carefully with special tubes to avoid contamination by aluminum that could result in erroneous results.[68]

In patients with chronic renal failure, loss of renal function results in a positive aluminum balance.[33] Tissue aluminum levels are consistently increased, especially in bone, liver, spleen, and brain.[6] Aluminum tissue overload progresses during chronic renal failure and dialysis treatment; the greatest overload is found in patients with dialysis encephalopathy.[6] The mechanism of aluminum transfer from plasma to tissues is not known.

HYPERALUMINEMIA AS A REFLECTION OF ALUMINUM LOADING

In a study using various oral aluminum gels, Kaehny et al.[80] reported increased plasma and urine aluminum values in normal subjects. During 2.2 gm ingestion of aluminum in the form of aluminum hydroxyde, aluminum carbonate, and dihydroxy-aluminum aminoacetate, plasma aluminum concentration was found to be elevated to 2.5 times control values. Urinary excretion of aluminum also increased 20- to 40-fold (200–500 μg/24 hours) following the ingestion of these three gels, compared to normal excretion.[80, 136] Thus, gastrointestinal absorption of aluminum exists in normal man during ingestion of several aluminum compounds, but high individual variations can be seen.[98] In contrast, plasma aluminum levels did not increase significantly in subjects taking aluminum phosphate.[80, 163] At acid pH, aluminum phosphate gel was virtually insoluble. This evidence indicates that aluminum may be mainly absorbed in the stomach and proximal duodenum.[80]

Serum aluminum levels in nondialyzed uremic patients not taking aluminum compounds were found to be similar to those in normal subjects.[17, 179] We have confirmed this finding in six patients with end-stage renal failure who had never taken aluminum compounds. In these patients, serum aluminum levels were lower than 10 µg/L. In contrast, in nondialyzed uremic patients taking aluminum-containing phosphate binders, serum aluminum concentrations were higher.[15, 122] Interestingly, average serum aluminum values below 100 µg/L were observed in most patients: 84 µg/L in four patients described by Boukari et al.,[17] 77 µg/L in 11 patients described by Zumkley et al.,[179] 62 µg/L in six patients described by Tsukamoto et al.[165]

In dialyzed uremic patients, predialytic aluminemia was higher (300–400 µg/L) in patients treated in centers using dialysis fluid with a high concentration of aluminum than in patients treated in centers where city tap water was purified by reverse osmosis (90 µg/L).[8] Cartier et al.[29] showed that changes in intradialysis plasma aluminum correlate with dialysate aluminum concentrations ($P = .74; P < .001$). In centers where reverse osmosis water treatment was installed after a period of dialysis with contaminated water, hyperaluminemia in dialyzed patients slowly dropped to below 100 µg/L within a few months.[118, 165] In our unit, a similar assessment was made after installation of reverse osmosis in July 1978. Thirteen patients who had been dialyzed against high concentrations of aluminum and who had serum aluminum levels above 200 µg/L were checked during 5 years of reverse osmosis water treatment (Fig 1). Each patient was taking 2–6 gm of aluminum gels every day. After 30 months, aluminemia had stabilized at an average value of 60 µg/L. In patients who had always been dialyzed against very low concentrations of aluminum, the role of orally administered aluminum-based phosphate binders in maintain-

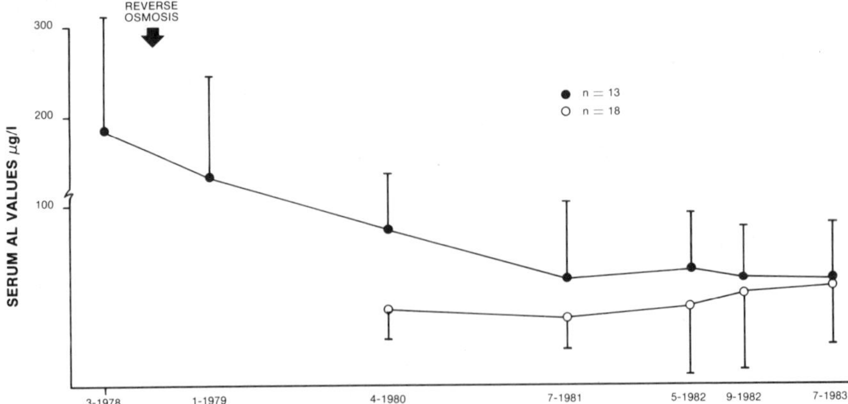

Fig 1.—Evolution of serum aluminum levels in 13 patients who were dialyzed against high concentrations of aluminum (> 100 µg/L) and who had serum aluminum levels above 200 µg/L, who were then checked during 5 years when reverse osmosis water treatment was available. They were compared with another 18 patients in whom hemodialysis had always been performed with reverse osmosis (Al < 10 µg/L). All the patients took aluminum gels (2–6 gm/L) for this period.

ing serum aluminum levels between 50 and 60 µg/L was demonstrated by a rapid drop of aluminum levels to near-normal values when aluminum gels were stopped.[18, 54, 179] In contrast, in 18 dialyzed patients in our unit who were taking aluminum gels and who started hemodialysis treatment after July 1978, aluminemia slowly rose and stabilized after some months at average values of 60 µg/L (see Fig 1). In 16 patients who were dialyzed against purified water, Kaehny et al.[79] reported average serum aluminum levels of 58 µg/L. In a multicenter study, Debroe et al.[41] demonstrated that most chronic hemodialysis patients (70%–80%) had plasma aluminum levels below 100 µg/L. Centers where dialysis therapy was started only recently and where reverse osmosis water treatment was available had the highest proportions of patients with plasma aluminum levels below 100 µg/L.[41] Gilli et al.[61] selected 38 hemodialysis patients chosen for their good compliance in taking aluminum hydroxide and measured serum aluminum levels twice, at 30- to 36-month intervals. The posttreatment mean (38.2 µg/L) was higher than the baseline mean (32.8 µg/L) but there was no consistent pattern. The conclusion of these authors was that serum aluminum monitoring was not useful in evaluating aluminum intoxication.

Thus, it appears from many works and from our experience that most chronic hemodialysis patients who were dialyzed against a dialysate containing water purified by reverse osmosis or by deionization had aluminemia below 100 µg/L, in spite of the regular ingestion of aluminum-containing phosphate binders. Similar data were reported in patients on continuous ambulatory peritoneal dialysis (CAPD).[36, 141, 176] Stability of serum aluminum levels in these conditions may be attributable to these features: the component of the plasma protein that binds aluminum appears to be saturable,[79] and the aluminum load from gastrointestinal absorption increases less the amount of ultrafiltrable aluminum[64] than does the acute aluminum load received during hemodialysis with contaminated dialysate.[88] Elliot et al.[50] reported that 60%–70% of aluminum was bound to a high molecular weight protein, 10%–20% was bound to albumin, and 10%–30% was ultrafiltrable.[50] The amount of ultrafiltrable aluminum would be lower when the plasma aluminum level falls below 200 µg/L. In hemodialysis patients whose serum aluminum levels before dialysis were below 100 µg/L, ultrafiltrable aluminum has been evaluated to be between 5% and 9%.[75, 144] This fraction was not demonstrated in normal subjects. Five major aluminum peaks were observed in chromatographic separation of serum in hemodialysis patients: four were associated with high molecular weight protiens and albumin and one was associated with non-identified molecules, probably inorganic anions.[85] Aluminum could be bound to transferrin and thus be in competition with iron.[164]

In patients with dialysis dementia, such binding with transferrin was not found by Raghavan et al.[134] In contrast, they showed that aluminum had a specific liaison with a low molecular weight protein (10,000 daltons) and increased after administration of DFO.[134] Thus, ultrafiltrable aluminum would not be "free"[66] but complexed with low molecular weight species which might cross the blood-brain barrier.[84] In rats, aluminum increases the permeability of the blood-brain barrier and could contribute to passage of small active peptides or other substances.[13] Acute and brief hyperaluminemia following accidental contamination of dialysate[26] is compatible with this aspect of aluminum metabolism.

The demonstration of a correlation between serum aluminum

levels and the duration of hemodialysis therapy or the total dose of aluminum ingested[17, 25, 65] in patients who were always dialyzed against low concentrations of aluminum was considered proof that only ingested aluminum gels could cause a graduated and constant rise in aluminemia.[17, 140] That opinion was at variance with the data reported by Gilli et al.,[63] Debroe et al.,[41] and us. These conflicting results might be explained by two reports: one of Cannata et al.,[25] in which not all patients were dialyzed against purified water, and one of Boukari et al.[17] in which dialyzed patients were exposed to aluminum dialysate concentrations on the order of 20–60 µg/L, which cannot be considered negligible since they can produce effective intradialysis aluminum uptake,[88] which would explain the rise of aluminemia above 100 µg/L after 3 years of hemodialysis therapy. pH values in the dialysate were not specified in these reports, and a small change in dialysate or tap water pH can make a large difference in the amount of aluminum in dialyzable form, explaining hyperaluminemia in some patients.[57] In a recent paper, Shimada et al.[147] showed that a significant relationship between serum aluminum levels and the time of hemodialysis therapy existed only in patients who were dialyzed against low concentrations of aluminum (23 ± 9 µg/L), not in those who were dialyzed in the same unit against water purified by reverse osmosis. Similar data were reported in a recent paper by Tahiri et al.[161] In a multicenter study, Debroe et al.[41] showed that 20%–25% of patients who were dialyzed against purified water by reverse osmosis of deionization had hyperaluminemia above 100 µg/L. Hyperaluminemia was observed in centers where patients had been dialyzed against high concentrations of aluminum before reverse osmosis.[41] In that report, the duration of hemodialysis treatment with reverse osmosis or with deionization before the determination of aluminemia was not noted. Accidental contamination of dialysate can sometimes occur, by various means: aluminum anodes, which were part of a cathodic protection system against corrosion in the boilers,[53] the Redy cartridge dialysis system,[20, 126] contaminated dialysate on CAPD,[26, 36] or insufficient purification by a deionizer or reverse osmosis.[122]

However, higher gastrointestinal absorption of aluminum could exist in some uremic patients. This is probably exemplified in children who develop "dialysis encephalopathy" without ever being dialyzed.[60, 104, 115, 135] Gastrointestinal hyperabsorption of aluminum could be due to self-medication,[91] hypophosphatemia,[82] hyperparathyroidism,[100] B or non-A, non-B (NANB) hepatitis,[152] or diabetes.[147] We have demonstrated that at equivalent total doses of aluminum hydroxide gels, patients with viral hepatitis have higher baseline aluminemia than other patients without hepatitis (Table 1). Risk factors involved in digestive hyperabsorption of aluminum in uremic patients taking aluminum hydroxide gels must be better understood.

In summary, one practical notion for the physician can be drawn from these data. Most uremic patients receiving aluminum gels over long periods and being dialyzed against water purified by reverse osmosis or a deionizer have serum aluminum levels below 100 μg/L. If hyperaluminemia above 100 μg/L occurs, accidental contamination of the dialysate must first be suspected, then in some patients digestive hyperabsorption must be considered.

HYPERALUMINEMIA AS A REFLECTION OF TISSUE OVERLOAD

In 1978, McDermott et al.[103] showed in three patients who had received functional kidney transplants an overload of aluminum in the brain 4 years after transplantation. Hourmant et al.[76] showed serum aluminum levels near normal values some weeks after successful kidney transplantation. Recently, attention was drawn to the existence of dialysis osteomalacia due to aluminum intoxication in uremic patients whose baseline aluminemia was below 100 μg/L.[37, 41] Boyce et al.,[19] study-

TABLE 1.—HYPERALUMINEMIA TEST IN 20 CHRONIC DIALYSIS PATIENTS WITH OR WITHOUT B OR NANB HEPATITIS*

PATIENTS	DURATION OF HEMODIALYSIS (months)	TOTAL DOSE (Al gels; gm)	T_1 (μg/L)	T_3 (μg/L)	$\Delta T_3 - T_1$ (μg/L)
B- and NANB-negative Ag	57.50	6505.00	31.40	82.30	50.90
(N = 10)	±27.58	±3774.91	±5.95	±30.19	±13.99
B- and NANB-positive Ag	53.68	7088.00	65.80	185.20	119.30
(N = 10)	±23.34	±4050.10	±9.29	±33.88	±26.91
	NS	NS	$P < .01$	$P < .05$	$P < .01$

*The duration of treatment by hemodialysis and the total dose of aluminum hydroxide gels were not different in the two groups. Predialysis aluminemia value (T_1) is significantly higher ($P < .01$) in the hepatitis group. Aluminum overload ($\Delta T_3 - T_1$) is higher in patients with hepatitis.

ing osteomalacia in dialyzed patients with aluminum intoxication, reported high aluminum bone accumulation in patients whose aluminemia values ranged from 62 to 700 µg/L. Since it has been demonstrated that DFO is efficient in chelating aluminum,[1] we studied the value of the DFO mobilization test for evaluating tissue aluminum stores in chronic hemodialysis patients.[151]

The test was performed by infusion of DFO in doses of 2 gm during a 4-hour hemodialysis session. Serum aluminum levels were measured before (T_1) and after (T_2) dialysis, then before (T_3) and after (T_4) the next session (without DFO infusion), 2 days later. A peak of hyperaluminemia at T_3 varied among patients, and no correlation existed with baseline aluminemia (at T_1).[151] The difference between T_3 and T_1 (Δ) reflects the degree of tissue aluminum accumulation.

Fig 2.—Hyperaluminemia test by deferoxamine (DFO) in 25 patients who were dialyzed with tap water purified by reverse osmosis. All were taking 2–6 gm/day of aluminum hydroxide gel. This test was made at two periods, A and B, at an interval of 14 months. DFO (2 gm) was injected during a dialysis session (T_1–T_2) and the peak of hyperaluminemia appeared at the next one (T_3).

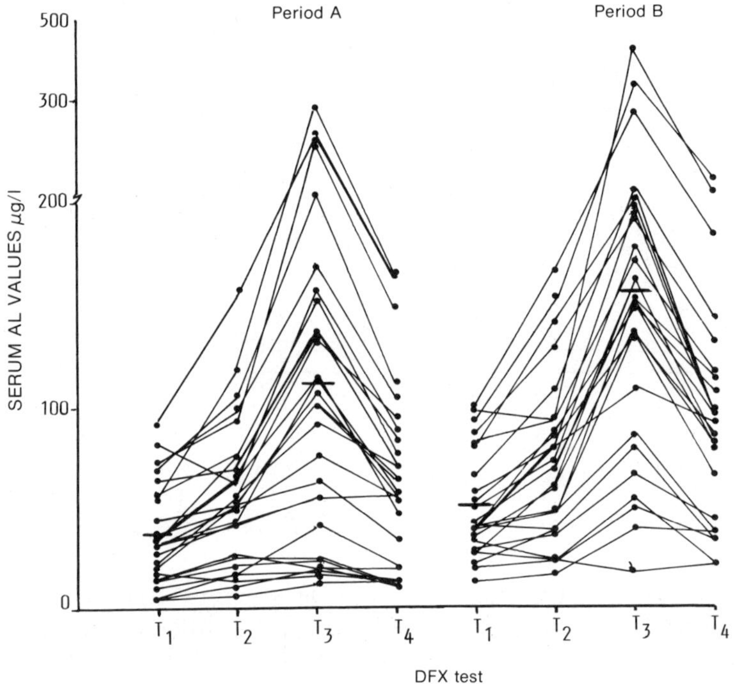

TABLE 2.—CHANGE IN SERUM ALUMINUM LEVELS FOLLOWING HYPERALUMINEMIA TEST AT 14 MONTHS*

DFO TEST (Al, µg/L)	PERIOD	GROUP I (N = 13)	GROUP II (N = 12)	P
T_1	A	60	22	NS
		41	21	
	B	64	40	NS
		27	25	
$\Delta(T_3 - T_1)$	A	117	32	<.05
		15	21	
	B	137	50	<.05
		14	22	

*DFO, 2 gm, was given at an interval of 14 months (period A: July 1981; period B: September 1982). Patients in group I had been dialyzed with tap water with high aluminum concentration for 6–42 months, then by reverse osmosis. Patients in group II had been treated by reverse osmosis in the preceding 12–36 months. All patients were taking aluminum gels (2–6 gm/day).

VALUE OF Δ AND TISSUE OVERLOAD.—We performed this DFO test twice at a 14-month interval in 25 patients taking aluminum hydroxide gels (2–6 gm/day) and dialyzed against dialysate purified by reverse osmosis (Fig 2). Thirteen patients (group I) had been dialyzed prior to July 1978 against dialysate aluminum concentrations (> 100 µg/L) for 6–42 months. Other patients (group II) had started hemodialysis treatment after the installation of reverse osmosis and had been treated for 12–36 months. As detailed in Table 2, Δ value was significantly higher in group I than in group II, both in period A (July 1981) and in period B (September 1982), whereas baseline aluminum (T_1) did not differ between two groups and the two periods. Thus, aluminum tissue stores were higher in group I than in group II. Fourteen months after the first test, a second test showed that tissue stores tended to increase (Fig 3), whereas in all patients aluminum hydroxide gels represented the only source of intoxication.

VALUE OF Δ AND BONE ACCUMULATION.—In six patients, two of whom had clinical and biologic signs of osteomalacia, we demonstrated that the Δ value correlated with the amount of aluminum in trabecular bone (Fig 4). Aluminum present at the junction of mineralized and osteoid bone was measured by trac-

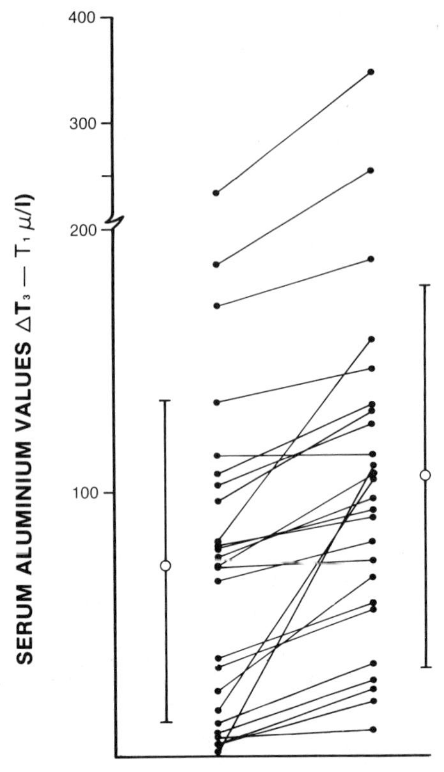

Fig 3.—Values of $\Delta\ T_3 - T_1$ during hyperaluminemia test with 2 gm of DFO. This test was made in 25 patients at an interval of 14 months (periods A and B).

ing the stained area and was expressed as a percentage of total bone surface.[44] The value of Δ was above 150 µg/L in two patients with osteomalacia. The significance of the test for the diagnosis of aluminum osteomalacia or bone accumulation has been confirmed.[55, 107] Milliner et al.[107] demonstrated in 28 hemodialyzed patients with osteomalacia a significative correlation between Δ value (> 180 µg/L) and aluminum bone content. Fohrer et al. obtained the same results in 24 patients with aluminum bone accumulation due solely to the intake of aluminum gels.

VALUE OF Δ AND TOTAL DOSE OF ALUMINUM GELS.—Δ value also correlated with total dose of aluminum gels.[152] In 25 patients that we studied at an interval of 14 months, we demonstrated a positive correlation between $\Delta(B - A)$ and the amount

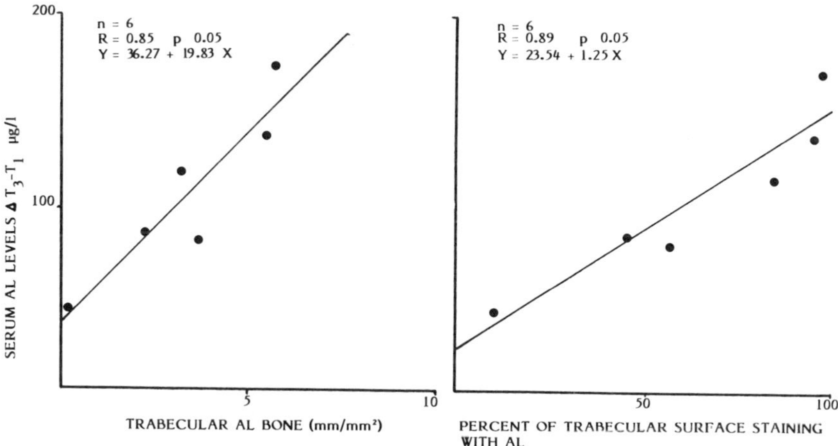

Fig 4.—Relationship between $\triangle$ value and bone aluminum according to aluminum procedure in six patients.

of aluminum hydroxide gels ingested between period A and period B (Fig 5).

CRITICAL DISCUSSION OF DFO TEST.—This noninvasive method could provide a means of determining cumulative aluminum, of following its progression solely due to the intake of phosphate binders, and of confirming the diagnosis of aluminum osteomalacia if clinical and biologic signs are suggestive. To improve the significance of this test, we propose standardizing the dose of DFO at 40 mg/kg, making the IV injection at the end of the hemodialysis session, and measuring the T_3 value 40–48 hours after injection, at a time when the hyperaluminemia peak is the highest. Under these conditions, a $\triangle$ value above 180 µg/L is strongly suggestive of aluminum osteomalacia.[107]

Thus, aluminum bone overload and mineralization disorders[38] may be caused solely by orally administered aluminum hydroxide gels.[2, 9] Recently Prichard et al.[133] showed a significant correlation between the total ingested dose of aluminum and aluminum bone accumulation. Patients who are "good compliers" could be more exposed to risk.[54, 114] The toxic effects of aluminum overload on organs other than bone and brain are still unknown. Liver overload could be particularly important in patients who received high dialysate concentrations of aluminum.[6] Aluminum liver accumulation could be closely corre-

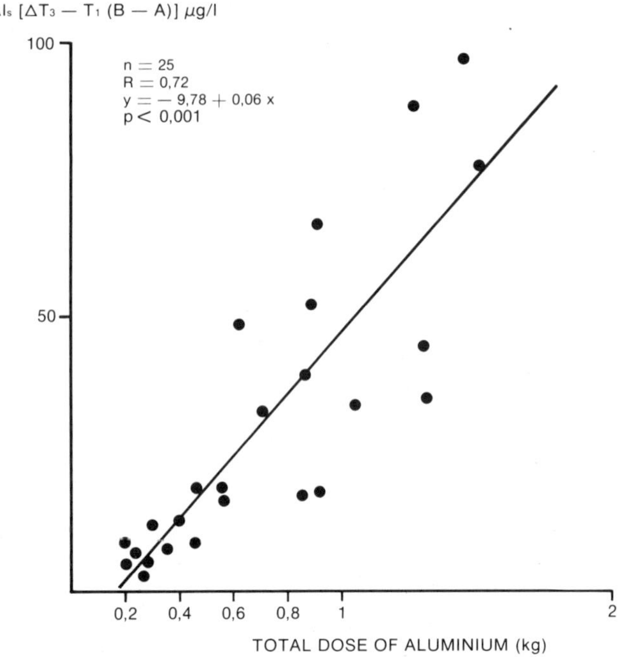

Fig 5.—Relationship between total dose of aluminum gel ingested during 14 months and the increase in aluminum tissue overload [Δ T$_3$ − T$_1$(B − A)].

lated with brain aluminum accumulation.[6] However, contrary to experimental data, aluminum hepatotoxicity remains hypothetical in man.[89, 146] The role of aluminum liver overload in porphyria cutanea tarda–like syndrome in hemodialyzed patients remains to be demonstrated.[21, 124] Preferential stocking of aluminum in the liver lysosomes was considered by Debroe et al.[41, 168] to be the most appropriate way to protect the cell from toxicity. Aluminum overload of parathyroid glands could lead to a secondary decrease in parathyroid gland mass.[105] In their study, Mendes et al.[105] found a positive correlation between parathyroid aluminum concentration and that in bone.

In summary, predialytic baseline aluminemia does not reflect aluminum tissue overload, and only measurements in bone[44, 93] or liver[6] could be indicative. Less invasive and easy to practice regularly, the DFO test would permit following the progressive overload, but its specificity for the degree of osteomalacia remains to be demonstrated.

Hyperaluminemia as a Reflection of Risks for Complications of Aluminum Intoxication

Although osteomalacia can exist when aluminemia is below 100 µg/L, it appears that the risk of dialysis encephalopathy and microcytic anemia exists only if aluminemia is above 100 µg/L. All cases of dialysis encephalopathy which have been reported in the literature had higher serum aluminum values, often above 300 µg/L.[138, 150] Also, when microcytic anemia occurred, aluminemia values were above 200 µg/L.[162] The decrease in serum aluminum levels when tap water was purified by reverse osmosis was followed by correction of anemia after a few weeks.[49, 119, 149] In centers where epidemics of dialysis encephalopathy and osteomalacia existed, most patients had microcytic anemia.[49, 122] Rapid correction of anemia when aluminemia was decreasing was suggestive of direct and rapidly reversible aluminum toxicity. Aluminum has been shown to interfere with an enzyme of the heme biosynthetic pathway[106] and also with an intermediary enzyme in iron metabolism.[77] Trapp[164] suggests that aluminum may cause anemia by entering pathways of iron distribution and metabolism. Also, acute dialysis encephalopathy which shows continuing regression when aluminemia values decrease, should be differentiated from chronic dialysis encephalopathy[29] and could be due to direct and reversible interference of aluminum with enzymes implicated in the production of neuromediators[90] or other enzymatic systems.[171, 177] Absence of a massive brain overload during the course of slow intoxication by aluminum gels[6] could be an explanation of the lack of correlation between the intake of aluminum gels and the observation of chronic dialysis encephalopathy[138] as well as the rapid reversibility of acute dialysis encephalopathy after stopping intake of aluminum.[24] The ultrafiltrable fraction of plasma aluminum, binding probably to inorganic anions, probably increases tremendously in the presence of a large dialysate supply of aluminum, since the fraction binding to plasma proteins is quickly saturable. This ultrafiltrable fraction might increase the permeability of the blood-brain barrier[117] and allow fixation of aluminum in the brain.[84]

In summary, even if aluminemia does not reflect aluminum overload, high aluminum serum levels are strongly correlated with dialysis encephalopathy or microcytic anemia. Rapid increase of aluminemia when accidental contamination occurs[26] justifies regular checking of serum levels in hemodialyzed patients and those on CAPD. The critical value of 3.7 μmol/L (100 mg/L) beyond which exists a risk of neurologic and hematologic complications of aluminum intoxication, a value that was suggested in an international workshop held in Luxembourg in July 1982, appears to us fully justified.[144] However, it is likely that bone aluminum overload and the risk of osteomalacia exist in most patients taking aluminum gels regularly by reverse osmosis or deionization and who are dialyzed against decontaminated dialysate.

Prevention of Aluminum Intoxication

The prevention of aluminum intoxication in chronic renal failure patients would consist of removing each important aluminum source in these patients, not only the aluminum that contaminates the dialysate, but also the aluminum-containing phosphate binders taken to control hyperphosphatemia. Although spectacular results have already been obtained by purification of water in centers where dialysis encephalopathy previously occurred,[30, 39, 122] there exists today a real risk of aluminum accumulation, particularly in bone, due solely to orally administered aluminum-containing phosphate binders. The suppression of aluminum hydroxide gels without replacement by drugs efficient for hyperphosphatemia would be disastrous in the population of dialyzed patients because severe hyperparathyroidism could occur.[82] Also, it is dangerous to suggest stopping orally administered aluminum gels[18] before the research for a new phosphate binder[129, 143, 145] is successful. Thus, total prevention of aluminum intoxication is a further hope, but it is already possible to prevent its complications, or to delay their occurrence.

The Control of Aluminum-Containing Food Intake

The amount of aluminum intake through food has been estimated as 20 mg/day.[91] However, variations in the choice of food, method of food preparation, the use of aluminum cookware, intake of beverages sold in aluminum-lined cans, and the degree of contamination of city tap water explain the variations that have been observed.[91]

We suggest careful evaluation of the intake of aluminum-containing foods in dialyzed patients. Prophylactic reduction of aluminum intake may be particularly advisable for geriatric patients. People of this age group may inadvertently be exposed to high aluminum intake from several sources, especially from nonprescription drugs containing aluminum.[91] This can readily increase the intake of aluminum to several thousand milligrams per day,[91] and existing reports demonstrate that geriatric patients experience a high incidence of metabolic bone disease[43] and Alzheimer-type dementia.[81] The pathogenesis of Alzheimer dementia is controversial, but high aluminum brain accumulation has been shown.[35]

The Control of Hyperphosphatemia

The dose of aluminum gels required to decrease hyperphosphatemia varies among patients. Some patients spontaneously have phosphatemia at near-normal values or just above and so can avoid taking aluminum gels. Recognition of these patients is important because hypophosphatemia due to inappropriate treatment could increase gastrointestinal absorption of aluminum.[82] Aluminum gel intake outside of meals must be avoided.[82] Cannata et al.[27] showed that the suppression of morning intake did not modify the phosphatemia level but, in contrast, significantly improved anemia, indicating that low doses of aluminum could be toxic to red cells. Moriniere et al.[112] showed that high doses of orally administered calcium carbonate could control hyperphosphatemia and allow stopping of aluminum gel intake, consequently normalizing aluminemia. However, the use of this treatment is limited because it could cause hypercalcemia and metastatic calcifications.[112] The use of magnesium-containing phosphate binders in association with a dialysate without this cation has been recommended.[69] In fact, their use should be limited because of the risk of bone disease with prolonged use.[23] Severe secondary hyperparathyroidism still occurs in 5%–10% of hemodialyzed patients and requires surgical correction. A spectacular drop in hyperaluminemia occurs,[47, 140] allowing stopping or decreasing aluminum gel intake. Surgical correction of secondary hyperparathyroidism should be performed early in these patients since parathormone could increase digestive absorption of aluminum[100] and its tissue accumulation,[102] particularly in brain.[101]

The prevention of aluminum intoxication also includes the use of dialyzers with high phosphate clearance.[130, 148] An in vivo study of 14 hollow fiber dialyzers shows that phosphate clearance can range from 90 to 160 ml/minute, according to dialyzer.[70] Thus, in patients taking high doses of aluminum gels to control hyperphosphatemia, doses can be reduced when a dialyzer with high phosphate clearance is used. However, such a concept may be questioned. In fact, it has been demonstrated that after 3 hours of hemodialysis or hemofiltration, a balance exists between the amount of cellular phosphorus transferred into the blood compartment and the amount of phosphate eliminated by epuration.[94] Thus, the use of dialyzers with high phosphate clearance might cause postdialytic hypophosphatemia. It is important in clinical practice today to revise routine habits[140] and adjust the doses of aluminum gels according to other possible treatments for hyperphosphatemia such as increased dialysis time or early surgical correction of secondary hyperparathyroidism, so as to obtain a predialytic phosphoremia between 50 and 58 mg/L.[148] The daily dose of aluminum gels in uremic children should not be above 100 mg/kg.[148]

The Control of Hyperaluminemia by Dialysis

Aluminum may be transferred during hemodialysis or CAPD. The transfer depends on three main factors: dialysate aluminum concentration, dialysate pH, and plasma aluminum levels. It was demonstrated that 70%–95% of aluminum is bound to a high molecular weight protein and to albumin, and 5%–30% is ultrafiltrable.[50, 51, 75, 85, 148] Berlyne et al.[15] first demonstrated a transfer of aluminum from dialysate to blood during dialysis. Dialysate at that time contained high levels of aluminum. In patients with dialysis encephalopathy, Alfrey et al.[6] found no evidence of net aluminum transfer across the dialyzer membrane during dialysis. However, in an experiment conducted in vitro using a hollow fiber dialyzer with tap water as dialysate and deionized water on the blood side, these authors obtained an aluminum clearance of approximately 45 ml/minute.[7]

The study of aluminum kinetics during hemodialysis has given conflicting results. Kaehny et al.[79] reported that aluminum is not removed from plasma by dialysis because serum aluminum is not free but is combined with protein so that aluminum is diffused into the blood from even low aluminum dialysates. In their patients, they reported an increase in serum aluminum from 58 to 63 μg/L during one hemodialysis session with a low aluminum dialysate. Graf et al.[65] found opposite results. They studied aluminum transfer during dialysis with low aluminum dialysates in 24 patients whose predialytic aluminemia averaged 86 μg/L and showed that aluminum could readily cross the dialyzer. At the end of the dialysis session mean serum aluminum level dropped to 72 μg/L, confirming the results reported by Allain et al.[8] Recently, Hosakawa et al.[75] reported identical results. In 55 patients who were hemodialyzed against dialysate containing less than 5 μg/L of aluminum, aluminemia decreased from 55.0 ± 27.6 μg/L before to 46.5 ± 20.1 μg/L after a 5-hour dialysis. They also demonstrated that the ultrafiltrable fraction, averaging 9%, was inversely related to the serum aluminum concentration. Thus, the dialyzance of aluminum should be dependent on the concentration gradient across the membrane between the ultrafiltrable plasma aluminum and the dialysate aluminum concentration.[66] When dialysate aluminum concentration was below the plasma ultrafiltrable aluminum concentration, a negative balance was obtained during hemodialysis.[65, 75] Dialysate aluminum concentration should not be above 5 μg/L.[46, 66] However, a concentration between 10 and 15 μg/L has sometimes been recommended.[73, 148] In France, in 1980 the Health Ministry fixed the limit of 30 μg/L.[36] Since most chronic hemodialysis patients treated by reverse osmosis had serum aluminum levels below 100 μg/L[41] and thus an ultrafiltrable fraction below 10%,[75, 148] dialysate aluminum concentration should be below 10 μg/L. It is likely, but again not demonstrated, that for the first months of treatment by hemodialysis, a period when most patients have near normal levels of aluminemia (10–20 μg/L), a transfer of aluminum from the dialysate to the blood may exist during the dialysis session until the gradient is reversed.

Gacek et al.[57] have shown that variation in dialysate pH contributes to dialyzance of aluminum. In an in vitro experiment, they showed that over the pH range of 6.5 to 7.6, average aluminum clearance is 2.1 ml/minute, and outside this range, aluminum clearance increases dramatically, ranging from 73.6 to 44.3 ml/minute at low and high pH, respectively. These data could explain why patients dialyzed at high pH (bicarbonate dialysate) have significantly higher predialysis serum aluminum levels than those dialyzed at neutral pH (acetate dialysate). In a multicenter study in the United States, aluminum exposure was greater and dialysis encephalopathy occurred more frequently among patients dialyzed against dialysate prepared with tap water having high alkalinity and extreme pH.[57] Van Waeleghen et al.[166] showed the role of blood pH in aluminum clearance in hemodialysis patients. When patients were dialyzed against bicarbonate dialysate, blood pH was 7.35 and the highest aluminum clearances were observed.[166] However, such variation of clearance according to blood pH was not demonstrated in another study.[108]

Since most dialysis centers treat water by reverse osmosis or deionizer, the risk of aluminum intoxication with contaminated dialysate should be virtually nonexistent. However, in home hemodialysis patients whose water is treated by deionizers, the risk of aluminum intoxication can exist, as the following observation proves. A 50-year-old woman whose initial disease was analgesic nephropathy had been hemodialyzed at home for 4 years when microcytic anemia and hypercalcemia suddenly developed. The patient had taken aluminum hydroxide gels (2 gm/day) for even longer and did not take vitamin D derivatives. Her serum aluminum level had recently increased to 192 μg/L, compared to 87 μg/L six months earlier, which had been an average stable value for 2 years. We learned that the deionizer resins had not been changed for 4 months, while they should have been changed every 3 months. Her tap water constantly had an aluminum concentration of 80–100 μg/L. Two months after the resins were changed, anemia improved and hypercalcemia disappeared. Our local tap water may be strongly contaminated, and we have observed that the time limit of deionizer efficacy can vary among areas. Charton et al.[32] showed that high amounts of aluminum could be released from deionizer resins when resins are saturated. To avoid such accidents the alarm system should be set at 1 megaohm.[33] Parkinson et al.[122] demonstrated that the proportion of tap water aluminum in colloidal form varies with pH, being maximum at about pH 6. Colloidal aluminum passes through mixed bed deionizers but redissolves in the dialysis fluid. Individual water supplies may vary in their response to treatment and twin bed deionizers probably behave differently from mixed bed deionizers.[122]

Patients receiving peritoneal dialysis can also present with acute aluminum intoxication.[26, 36] These intoxications are due to the use of dialysate bags with high concentrations of aluminum (620–1,460 μg/L). In these patients, there is a rapid decrease of hyperaluminemia when uncontaminated dialysate bags are used. An aluminum concentration below 27 μg/L in CAPD dialysate bags was recommended in England. Set limits of 27 μg/L are again too high.[95] In France, aluminum concentration in CAPD dialysate bags varies from 4.2 to 20.4 μg/L.[110] Gilli et al.[61, 62] demonstrated a transfer of aluminum from dialysate to blood in patients who were treated on intermittent peritoneal dialysis against dialysate with aluminum concentrations of 19 ± 6.3 μg/L. Dialysate aluminum levels were significantly lower in outlet than in inlet dialysate. Patients on peritoneal dialysis had higher serum aluminum levels than those on hemodialysis.[62] The reason for this positive balance during peritoneal dialysis would be the acid pH of the dialysate (< 5.5), confirming the results of Gacek et al.[57] However, Rottembourg et al.[141] showed an aluminum extraction of 2–5 μmol (54–135 μg/L) each day in patients on CAPD (aluminum concentration in dialysate bags was below 10 μg/L) who were taking aluminum hydroxide gels and whose average aluminemia values were 2–2.4 μmol/L (54–65 μg/L). Hercz et al.[72] showed in 18 patients on CAPD using dialysate bags whose aluminum concentration was below 6 μg/L that daily extraction of aluminum averaged 206 ± 23 μg, with a mean level of serum aluminum of 103 ± 15 μg/L. Weekly CAPD removed 4–5 times more aluminum than did three hemodialysis sessions of 4 hours each.[72] The amount of aluminum removed on CAPD was proportional to the levels of serum aluminum.[110] In patients treated by hemofiltration, a negative balance was obtained when aluminum concentration in the replacement fluid was below 15 μg/L. In contrast, the aluminum balance was always positive when the replacement fluid contained more than 20 μg/L of aluminum.[110]

Some practical advice for avoiding aluminum intoxication

from dialysate emerges from these data. (1) Today, each uremic patient hemodialyzed in a center or at home should be dialyzed against city tap water which is purified by reverse osmosis or deionizer, which is the only way to obtain a dialysate aluminum concentration below 10 μg/L. The lack of such systems for the purification of tap water in countries where tap water is considered to have low aluminum concentration could lead to accidental contamination. In countries where tap water is particularly contaminated, treatment of water by deionizer or by reverse osmosis can be ineffective if the frequency of replacement of resins is insufficient and the alarm system levels are too low. (2) It is necessary to pay close attention to the pH in dialysate and blood, particularly if bicarbonate dialysate is used. A system for evaluating dialysate pH might be incorporated into future dialysis machines. (3) For patients treated by CAPD, manufacturers must furnish dialysate bags of less acid pH and aluminum concentrations below 10 μg/L. (4) Serum aluminum levels must be measured every month in all dialysis patients, whether treated in a center or at home.[175] If a rapid increase in aluminemia above 100 μg/L occurs, accidental contamination of dialysate due to breakdown or failure of the water purification system or contamination of CAPD bags or hemofiltration solution[95] should be sought. De Wolff[46] recommends verification of dialysate aluminum each week, whatever the system of tap water verification.

Treatment of Aluminum Intoxication

The accumulation of aluminum in the body, when it is high and of long duration, may cause organic complications which sometimes are responsible for death. Acute or chronic dialysis encephalopathy, osteomalacia, and microcytic anemia are better known than are other causes of morbidity and mortality in dialysis patients which might be due to aluminum toxicity, such as porphyria cutanea tarda–like syndrome,[21, 124] some types of arthritis,[117] arterial and visceral calcifications,[172] and sudden cardiac arrest.[48] Aluminum tissue overload can persist for several months or years after the end of intoxication or after successful transplantation.[103, 120] While Ihle et al.[78] reported a 50% decrease in bone aluminum accumulation 6 months after successful transplantation, spontaneous mobilization of aluminum from tissue to plasma was not proved and remains to be demonstrated. Therefore, when aluminum intoxication occurs, it seems logical to use tissue chelating agents to deplete the aluminum tissue fixed in the body.

When the brain toxicity of aluminum was recognized, numerous trials of conservative therapy were attempted to achieve improvement of encephalopathy by depletion: increased dialysis time with purified water,[14, 45] hemofiltration,[4] plasmapheresis,[50, 51] and short-term charcoal hemoperfusion.[174] None of these methods resulted in sustained clinical improvement. Renal transplantation was another potential treatment. Serum aluminum levels normalized during the first weeks following successful renal transplantation and greater amounts of aluminum were excreted in the urine.[76] However, clinical results did not prove effective. While complete recovery from dialysis encephalopathy occurred following cadaver kidney transplantation in some cases,[111] others died several months after transplantation,[97] and some developed irreversible dialysis encephalopathy after successful transplantation.[128] The results are too conflicting to indicate rapid renal transplantation in dialysis patients with encephalopathy.[150] In a few patients who had acute dialysis encephalopathy attributed to the intake of aluminum hydroxide gels, stopping intake was sufficient to obtain remission.[24, 96, 132]

Ackrill et al.[1] reported success with the use of the chelating agent DFO in the treatment of a patient with advanced dialysis encephalopathy. The patient was on dialysis for some 8 years preceding the encephalopathy symptoms, with a water supply containing 100–500 µg of aluminum per liter. Treatment was begun several months after the appearance of first symptoms. Once a week, 6 gm of DFO was injected into the arterial line. The dialysate contained less than 20 µg of aluminum per liter, and dialysis was performed for 4 hours thrice weekly for some 250 days, until the neurologic symptoms gradually resolved. Increased amounts of aluminum were removed (6–7 µg at each session) as the serum aluminum level rose between 500 and 1,000 µg/L. Total amounts of aluminum removed during 10 months of treatment were estimated at 500–600 mg. Other cases of encephalopathy treated by DFO were later reported.[11, 109, 131, 153] Dramatic effects of this treatment were confirmed in all but two patients, who died in spite of utilization of water purified by reverse osmosis and treatment by DFO.[109] In our patient, before trying DFO we used another chelating agent, EDTA, at a dose of 1 gm each session. Serum aluminum level increased after injection but the attempt was unsuccessful after 6 weeks of treatment.[153] Delavelle et al.[42] reported similar results in one patient. In 1982, Brown et al.[22] reported results of treatment by DFO in two patients on dialysis who had had severe osteomalacia for 3 years, associated with multiple fractures and progressive deformities of the chest and spine. Bone disease was resistant to vitamin D derivatives, which produced only greater hypercalcemia. The DFO treatment protocol was the same as that used in dialysis encephalopathy.[1] These patients improved rapidly and reported a decrease in bone pain within 2 weeks. After 6 months, they were able to stop taking analgesics and to return to normal activities. The changes in trace metals after DFO treatment were not consistent, and atomic absorption analysis showed no significant change in the aluminum content of bone with treatment. Ihle et al.[78] treated four patients with a different protocol (1 gm of DFO after each dialysis session). The effect of DFO was compared with that in four other patients who received a successful renal transplant. All patients showed dramatic subjective improvement in bone pain and fractures and all histologic parameters studied improved, with bone closer to normal in the patients who had received a transplant. In the two populations, bone aluminum fell by at least 50%. The three cases reported by Ackrill et al.[3] had dialysis osteomalacia and encephalopathy. They also demonstrated the possibility of bone aluminum removal by DFO che-

TABLE 3.—RESULTS OF PROLONGED TREATMENT BY DFO ON REMOVAL OF BONE ALUMINUM

| STUDY | N | BONE ALUMINUM (μg/gm) | | | DOSE OF DFO (gm/week) | DURATION OF TREATMENT (Months) |
		Before DFO	After DFO	Difference		
Ackrill et al.[3]	3	372	116	(−68%)	4–6	10
		360	210	(−42%)	. . .	14
		163	51	(−68%)	. . .	5
Brown et al.[22]	2	156	153	(−2%)	6	4,5
		112	101	(−10%)	. . .	6
Ihle et al.[78]	4	340 ± 88	125 ± 68	(−63%)	3	6
Malluche et al.[92]	3	107 ± 14	53 ± 13	(−50%)	6	8
Pierides et al.[127]	2	415	159	(−62%)	4	12
		162	72	(−55%)	. . .	12
Van De Vyver	1	44,9	32,9	(−26%)	2	9

lation. In one patient who developed severe osteomalacia on CAPD, fractures consolidated only after administration of DFO.[86] In Table 3 we have listed some results of prolonged treatment by DFO in 15 patients with aluminum osteomalacia, where these observations are particularly clear. It thus seems proved that DFO chelation can be an efficient therapy for encephalopathy and bone disease in aluminum intoxication.

CHARACTERISTICS OF DESFERRIOXAMINE

May and Williams[99] defined six major requirements which a chelating agent must ideally satisfy. It must (1) bind the metal strongly enough to compete with biologic ligands, especially proteins; (2) discriminate against the relatively abundant calcium and zinc cations in vivo; (3) be sufficiently lipophilic to penetrate membranes and reach the site of heavy metal deposition; (4) form a lipophilic complex in the body compartment where the metal has accumulated; (5) change to a hydrophilic complex in plasma so that the metal is eliminated in urine and not redistributed into other tissues; and (6) have a low renin toxicity. Although the characteristics of DFO for iron are known, they remain to be demonstrated for aluminum.

The methane sulfonate of DFO B (Desferal) is a hydroxamic acid produced by *Streptomyces pilosis*. In a recent review, Hoffbrand[74] recalls the principal characteristics of DFO in the treatment of iron overload. Its molecular weight is 613. It has three functional hydroxamic acid groups forming a multidentate ligand which binds iron in a 1:1 complex. The binding affinity of DFO for iron is stable. While DFO is lipophilic, feroxamine B becomes hydrophilic due to a salified amine acid. Therefore feroxamine B can be filtered by the glomeruli and excreted in the urine. The half-life of DFO after a single intravenous injection is 5–10 mn, clearance being due to renal excretion, to penetration into extracellular and possibly intracellular spaces, especially in the pancreas, liver, and brain, and to destruction by a plasma enzyme. The distribution volume in the body is greater than the extracellular fluid volume and approaches total body water. In chronic hemodialysis patients with transfusional iron overload, the half-life of ^{14}C DFO was 38.4 ± 3.8 hours in the interhemodialysis period and 4.9 ± 0.6 in the intrahemodialysis period.[56] These results suggest that extradialytic excretion through the stool may be an important excretion route. In the dialyzed patient without iron or aluminum tissue overload, the half-life of ^{59}Fe DFO could be similar to that in normal subjects.[142] DFO chelates iron from three metal-binding proteins, transferrin, ferritin, and hemosiderin. Feroxamine B is little or not excreted in bile. The distribution of feroxamine B volume in the body is smaller than DFO, which approaches the distribution volume of inulin. Therefore, its distribution volume is extracellular. Plasma concentrations of feroxamine B are stable and it does not seem that the hydrophilic molecule is rapidly metabolized. In animals, acute and chronic toxicity tests showed no effects. In contrast, in man some adverse effects were reported, such as digestive disorders, visual acuity disorders, cataract, skin rash, neutropenia, and hypotension. In normal subjects, DFO did not modify the elimination of metals such as Al, Zn, Co, Ni, Mn, Sn, Pb, and Hg. In contrast, in patients with iron overload, the urinary excretion of Cu and Zn would be increased following administration of DFO.[178] In uremic patients on hemodialysis with aluminum overload, blood levels of Ca, Mg, Zn, Cu, Mn, Si, Pb and Ba were not modified by the injection of 2 gm of DFO.[10, 156]

Although the clinical results in patients with aluminum intoxication strongly suggest tissue aluminum chelation by DFO, no experimental study has yet provided answers to the following questions: (1) What are the target organs of DFO activity in aluminum intoxication? (2) What is the site of chelation within organs? The deposition of aluminum in brain[58] and liver lysosomes[59, 168] has been demonstrated. (3) What is the biochemistry of chelation? (4) Is aluminum mobilized only as feroxamine B–aluminum complex? Does DFO also provoke mobilization of free aluminum, as suggested by some authors[67] and by the occurrence of neurologic signs in one patient following administration of DFO[169]? The answer to this question is particularly decisive because if nonchelated aluminum is mobilized by DFO, this drug might cause a new distribution of aluminum in other tissues and a risk of toxicity. (5) Does chelation affect only tissues with aluminum overload or does it also affect plasma protein binding? The lack of answers to these questions at the present time calls for caution in utilizing DFO. The need for such caution is reinforced by the lack of an easy assay for DFO and feroxamine B–aluminum complex in the serum.

Methods of Dialysis and Clearance of Chelated Aluminum

The dialysance of the feroxamine B–iron complex has been measured in vitro through four membranes: regenerated cellulose, cellulose acetate, cuprophane, and acrylonitrile N–methallylsulfonate copolymer (RP610).[137] There was no appreciable difference between dialysance with cellulose acetate and cuprophane membranes (18.6 ± 5.9 and 16.8 ± 1.8 ml/min/m^2, respectively). Dialysance with regenerated cellulose was lowest (14.7 ± 3.1 ml/min/m^2). In contrast, dialysance with RP610 membrane was highest, averaging 50 ml/min/m^2, approximately three times higher than with cuprophane. Wide variance in dialysance among several dialyzers of any one type was found. There was no measurable dialysance of iron when DFO was not present. Therefore, the dialysance which was measured represented the real dialysance of the feroxamine B–iron complex.

We measured in vivo the clearance of aluminum following the injection of 2 gm of DFO during the last hour of dialysis. Several types of dialyzers were studied: cuprophane hollow fibers (Discap), acrylonitrile copolymer (Biospal), and the association of cuprophane hollow fibers and a cartridge of encapsulated charcoal (Dialaid) were utilized with an open circuit system and ultrafiltration control. Sequential measurements of clearance were made at the next dialysis session after the session with DFO injections. Clearance was calculated by Cl =

$$\frac{\text{CBi QB - CBe (QB - Quf)}}{\text{CBi}}$$ where QB is blood flow rate (ml/min),

CB is aluminum concentration in blood influx (CBi) or efflux (CBe), and Quf is ultrafiltration flow rate (ml/min).

The results shown in Fig 6 evoke the following comments. (1) the clearance of aluminum by the three types of dialyzers was significantly higher after DFO than without DFO. The ultrafiltrable fraction after administration of the chelating agent was above 50%.[153] (2) After DFO, the high permeability membrane (Biospal) and Dialaid with coated activated charcoal had clearances higher than that with cuprophane membrane. (3) The clearance curve with Dialaid was suggestive of rapid saturation of charcoal with chelated aluminum early during the hemodialysis session. (4) Without DFO, the clearance of alumi-

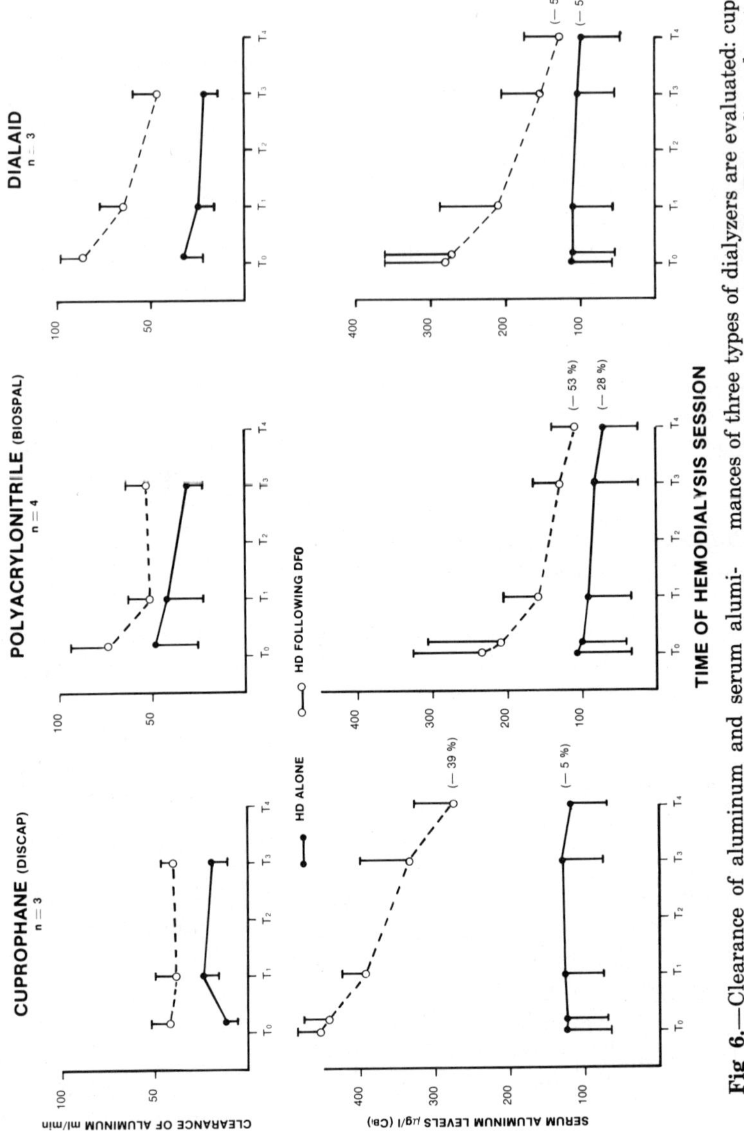

Fig 6.—Clearance of aluminum and serum aluminum levels during a hemodialysis session without DFO (*black circles*), then in the next 48 hours following the IV injection of 2 gm of DFO (*white circles*). Performances of three types of dialyzers are evaluated: cuprophane (Discap), polyacrylonitrile (Biospal), and coat-activated charcoal (Dialaid).

num was not zero, contrary to other studies,[31] but was higher with Biospal than with other dialyzers. A hypothesis to explain such a variation could be that a large fraction of ultrafiltrable aluminum had been fixed on the polyacrylonitrile membrane, as has been demonstrated with the cuprophane membrane.[71] (5) The value of chelated aluminum clearance was higher than that of chelated iron reported by Rembold et al.,[137] suggesting that chelated and nonchelated aluminum were eliminated. Several studies on aluminum clearance have been published (Table 4) and confirm our results. However, some appreciable variations in clearance during dialysis were observed. The dose of DFO[158] and the alteration of blood pH according to dialysate pH (acetate or bicarbonate)[166] could explain some differences in the results reported in the literature. The interpretation of aluminum clearance after DFO remains difficult as long as an easy method of assessing DFO and feroxamine B is not available.

We evaluated the amounts of aluminum removed at each dialysis session according to dialysis method (Table 5). The highest clearances were obtained with open circuit dialysis systems

TABLE 4.—ALUMINUM CLEARANCE WITH THREE
TYPES OF DIALYZERS BEFORE AND AFTER DFO

DIALYZER	IN VIVO CLEARANCE OF ALUMINUM (ML/MIN)	
	Without DFO	After DFO
Cuprophane		
Baldamus et al.[27]	—	85
Chang and Barre[31]	zero	40 ± 178
Milliner et al.[108]	56 ± 08	314 ± 21
Pierides et al.[127]	—	375
Simon et al.[154, 157]	84 ± 21	405 ± 97
Van Waeleghen et al.[166]	165	405
Polyacrylonitrile		
Chang and Barre[31]		
Rhodial	zero	446 ± 137
Monitral	zero	358 ± 110
Simon et al.[154, 157]		
Rhodial	95 ± 23	348 ± 42
Monitral	427 ± 199	584 ± 199
Van Waeleghen et al.[166]	—	309
Dialaid		
Chang and Barre[31]	zero	653 ± 110
Simon et al.[154]	260 ± 80	663 ± 120

TABLE 5.—AMOUNT OF ALUMINUM EXTRACTED
IN EACH DIALYSIS SESSION ACCORDING TO
DIALYSIS METHOD

METHOD	ALUMINUM (mg)
Closed circuit ANH_{12-10}	0.150
Closed circuit cuprophane + DFO, 2 gm	0.525
Closed circuit ANH_{12-10} + DFO, 2 gm	0.675
Open circuit ANH_{12-10}	0.240
Open circuit cuprophane + DFO, 2 gm	1.320
Open circuit ANH_{12-10} + DFO, 2 gm	8.200
Hemofiltration—filtral	0.690
Hemofiltration—filtral + DFO, 2 gm	6.210

utilizing high permeability membrane and with hemofiltration. The high amounts of aluminum removed during hemofiltration alone probably were due to low molecular weight protein aluminum binding which was extracted with the ultrafiltrable fraction by hemofiltration.[139] DFO has also been used in patients on peritoneal dialysis.[78, 141] Removal of not insignificant amounts of feroxamine B–aluminum have been reported, but dialysance values were not given. The recent demonstration of the higher effectiveness of CAPD than of hemodialysis in the treatment of hemosiderosis by DFO[52] should stimulate future work in patients with aluminum intoxication. CAPD could prove to be the more efficient method for removal of aluminum chelated by DFO.[72]

INDICATIONS FOR AND METHODS OF CHELATING TREATMENT IN ALUMINUM INTOXICATION

The indications for DFO treatment when the complications of aluminum intoxication occur cannot be debated since DFO is currently the only depletive therapy that may be depended on to give reliable results. Although neurologic complications may no longer be seen in the future, thanks to prophylactic methods, osteomalacia risks becoming a common complication in dialyzed patients until new phosphate binders without aluminum can be used. Other disorders, whose origin is still unknown, may be shown to be due to aluminum intoxication within the next few years[172] and can be treated by DFO. Pogglitsch et al.[130] suggest beginning chelating treatment when aluminemia is above 200 μg/L. Such a decision seems consistent since there is a risk of neurologic and hematologic disorders when aluminemia increases to such levels. However, before chelating treatment is begun, it must be ascertained whether the increase in serum aluminum levels was due to accidental contamination of the dialysate, in which case this correction alone could decrease aluminemia below 100 μg/L. In the absence of clinical signs of intoxication, chelating treatment could be justified to prevent bone disease due to aluminum since it has been demonstrated that patients with proved aluminum osteomalacia have serum aluminum values below 100 μg/L.[19, 37, 41] It is still unclear whether all patients taking aluminum gels or only those who are considered at risk of overload should receive prophylactic treatment, for two reasons. The first is that diagnosis of aluminum overload before clinical disorders occur requires invasive investigations such as bone or liver biopsy, and tissue aluminum determination must be performed by a specialized laboratory. The second is that in daily clinical practice only a few dialyzed patients regularly taking aluminum gels for several years develop signs of toxicity. Therefore, risk factors which are perhaps of genetic origin and HLA linked, as has been well documented for iron,[41] are strongly suspected but not yet defined. Our approach is based on regular assessment of tissue overload by a DFO mobilization test, as described above. When the amount of aluminum mobilized attains a peak such as Δ (T_3-T_1) above 150 μg/L, we begin the chelating treatment. That such a practice is well founded is illustrated by the case illustrated in Figure 7. In September 1982 chelating treatment was indicated for this patient. Bone biopsy showed severe aluminum osteomalacia. Two gm of DFO at the rate of two injections each month was administered for 8 months. One month after interruption, a new test showed greater mobilization, which led to resumption of treatment. This patient, who had been on dialysis for 9 years, of which 4 were with purified water, took aluminum hydroxide gels (4 gm/day) and probably had a high tissue overload, justifying the maintenance of treatment during several months. This case also illustrates the limited value of plasma aluminum concentration for determination of tissue aluminum overload.

The procedures of chelating treatment in aluminum intoxication are not yet well defined. Considering the amount of

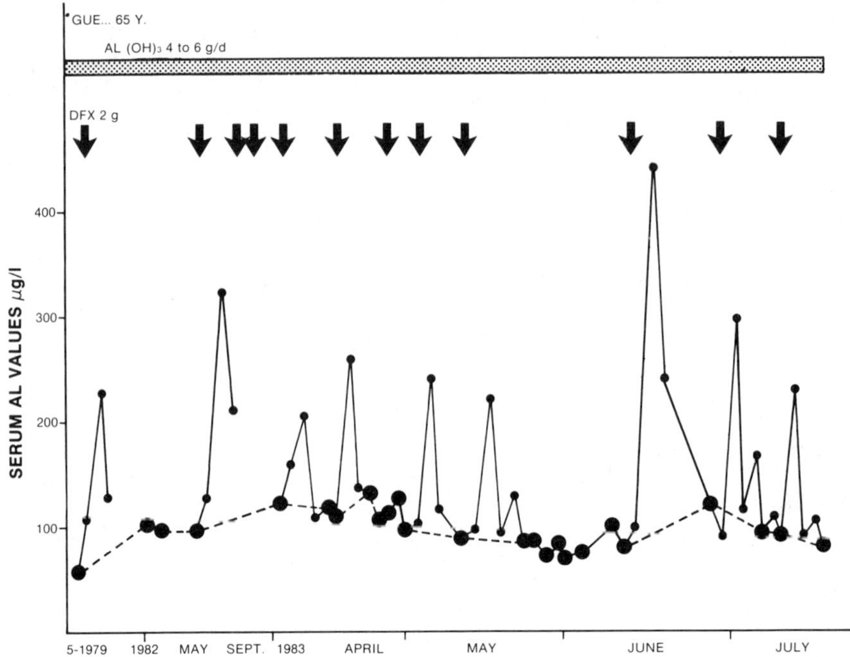

Fig 7.—Evolution of baseline aluminum levels *(black circles)* and the peak of hyperaluminemia (T₃) after injection of 2 gm of DFO *(white circles)* in a chronic hemodialysis patient.

aluminum which might be accumulated in the body of a patient with encephalopathy (3.3 gm)[173] and the amount removed in each dialysis session following 2 gm of DFO (6–8 mg), it would be necessary to treat for 2–3 years. However, clinical improvement in patients with osteomalacia can be obtained after a shorter treatment time. Results in the literature show that 6–10 months of treatment might be sufficient to obtain over 50% decrease in bone aluminum (see Table 3). This length of treatment is close to that which has been reported in the treatment of hemosiderosis in dialyzed patients.[159] In our experience, uremic patients with iron overload showed no signs of intolerance to the prolonged administration of DFO. To our knowledge, no severe complication due to chronic chelating treatment in dialyzed patients has so far been reported. The injection of 2–6 gm of DFO each week seems an adequate and efficient dose to avoid adverse effects of the drug, particularly visual acuity disorders.[40] The amount of aluminum removed after chelation by DFO is dependent on the dose.[158] A single administration each week seems justified until the effect and the kinetics of DFO in uremic patients with aluminum intoxication are known. Dialyzers with high permeability membranes or with charcoal should be preferred to cuprophane, which is less efficient.

The possible simultaneous presence in a dialyzed patient of both iron and aluminum overload[125] suggests the following comments. It is held that binding feroxamine B–iron is stronger (Kd 31) than binding feroxamine B–aluminum (Kd 24). There may be competition between chelation of iron and of aluminum, with iron chelation theoretically stronger. In fact, the first clinical studies showed that both iron and aluminum could be removed by administration of DFO.[12, 16] The administration per os of iron therapy for treatment of aluminum intoxication by DFO should be recommended when plasma ferritin is below 80 ng/L.

Conclusions

The treatment of aluminum intoxication in patients with chronic renal failure must be primarily prophylactic. The effectiveness of the treatment of dialysis water in the prevention of dialysis encephalopathy is now proved and indicates that each dialysis center and each patient on dialysis at home should have a system of water treatment by reverse osmosis or deionizer. Very low concentrations of aluminum in dialysate commercially furnished for CAPD or hemofiltration must henceforth be required. Use of dialyzers with high phosphorus clearance and precise dosage of aluminum hydroxide gels in cases of hyperphosphoremia might lead to maintenance of aluminemia below 100 μg/L. However, potential risks of aluminum osteomalacia will persist as long as aluminum gels are not replaced by new phosphate binders. The tissue depletion of aluminum by DFO is now an alternative therapy which can prevent or cure bone disease due to this metal. Considering the wide indication for this chelating agent, it is urgent to know its mode of action and its kinetics so that it can be put into clinical use, particularly in dialyzed patients who cannot receive a kidney transplant.

Acknowledgments

The authors thank professors F. Cartier, M.E. Debroe, T. Drueke, N.K. Man, A. Meyrier, and Dr. Rottembourg for reviewing the manuscript and providing constructive criticism, Dr. M.C. Devernejoul for assaying aluminum in bone, all persons working in the hemodialysis unit of Saint-Brieuc Hospital, and R. Lemesle for secretarial help.

REFERENCES

1. Ackrill P., Ralston A.J., Day J.P., et al.: Successful removal of aluminum from patient with dialysis encephalopathy. *Lancet* 2:692, 1980.
2. Abreo D., Faugere M.C., Smith A., et al.: Prevalence and etiology of aluminum intoxication in non-dialysed (D−) and dialysed (D+) patients with renal failure. *Kidney Int.* 23:141, 1983.
3. Ackrill P., Day J.P., Garstang F.M., et al.: Treatment of fracturing renal osteodystrophy by desferrioxamine. *Proc. Eur. Dial. Transplant Assoc.* 19:203, 1982.
4. Adhemar J.P., Laederich J., Jaudon M.C., et al.: Removal of aluminum from patients with dialysis encephalopathy. *Lancet* 2:1311, 1980.
5. Alfrey A.C.: Aluminum and tin, in Bronner F., Cobern J.W. (eds.): *Disorders of Mineral Metabolism.* New York, Academic Press, 1981, vol. 1, pp. 353–369.
6. Alfrey A.C., Hegg A., Craswell P.: Metabolism and toxicity of aluminum in renal failure. *Am. J. Clin. Nutr.* 33:1509, 1980.
7. Alfrey A.C., Kaehny W.D.: Letter to the editor. *N. Engl. J. Med.* 294:1131, 1976.
8. Allain P., Thebaud H.E., Dupouet L., et al.: Etude des taux sanguins de quelques métaux (Al, Mn, Cd, Pb, Cu, Zn) chez les hémodialysés chroniques avant et après dialyse. *Nouv. Presse Med.* 7:92, 1978.
9. Andress D.L., Ott S.M., Milliner D., et al.: Diagnosis of aluminum bone disease in long-term dialysis patients using desferioxamine and zero-calcium dialysis. *Kidney Int.,* to be published.
10. Ang K.S., Allain P., Mauras Y., et al.: Etude des taux sanguins du calcium, du magnésium et de quelques métaux (Mn, Pb, Cu, Zn, Si, Ba) au cours du test d'hyperaluminémie provoquée par la desferrioxamine chez les hémodialysés chroniques. *Nephrologie* 4:143, 1983.
11. Arze R.S., Parkinson I.S., Cartlidge N.E.F., et al.: Reversal of aluminum dialysis encephalopathy after desferrioxamine treatment. *Lancet* 2:1116, 1981.
12. Baldamus C.A., Schmidt H., Schevrmann E.H., et al.: Iron and aluminum removal in ESRD patients treated with desferrioxamine, abstracted. *Am. J. Kidney Dis.,* 1984.
13. Banks W.A., Kastin A.J.: Aluminum increases permeability of the blood-brain barrier to labelled DSIP and β-endorphin: Possible implications for senile and dialysis dementia. *Lancet* 2:1227, 1983.
14. Baratt L.J., Lawrence J.R.: Dialysis associated dementia. *Aust. NZ J. Med.* 5:62, 1975.
15. Berlyne G.M., Pest D., Ben Ari J., et al.: Hyperaluminaemia from aluminum resins in renal failure. *Lancet* 2:494, 1970.
16. Bonsdorff M.V., Sipila R.: Iron and aluminum removal during hoemodialysis using desferrioxamine. *Clin. Nephrol.,* to be published.
17. Boukari M., Rottembourg J., Jaudon M.C., et al.: Influence de la prise prolongée de gels d'alumine sur les taux sériques d'aluminium chez les patients atteints d'insuffisance rénale chronique. *Nouv. Presse Med.* 7:85, 1978.

18. Bournerias F., Monnier N., Reveillaud R.J.: Risks of orally administered AlOH$_3$ in hemodialysed patients and results of withdrawal. *Proc. Eur. Dial. Transplant Assoc.* 20:207, 1983.

19. Boyle B.F., Elder A.Y., Elliot H.L., et al.: Hypercalcaemic osteomalacia due to aluminum toxicity. *Lancet* 2:1009, 1982.

20. Branger B., Ramperez P., Marigliano N., et al.: Aluminum transfer in bicarbonate dialysis using a sorbent regenerative system: An in vitro study. *Proc. Eur. Dial. Transplant Assoc.* 17:213, 1980.

21. Brivet F., Drueke T., Guillemette J., et al.: Porphyria cutanea tarda–like syndrome in hemodialysed patients. *Nephron* 20:258, 1978.

22. Brown D.J., Dawborn J.K., Ham K.N., et al.: Treatment of dialysis osteomalacia with desferrioxamine. *Lancet* 2:343, 1982.

23. Brunner F.P., Thiel G.: The use of magnesium-containing phosphate binders in patients with end stage renal disease on maintenance hemodialysis. *Nephron* 32:266, 1982.

24. Buge A., Poisson M., Masson S., et al.: Encéphalopathie réversible des dialysés après arrêt de l'apport d'aluminum. *Nouv. Presse Med.* 34:2729, 1979.

25. Cannata J.B., Briggs J.D., Junor B.J.R., et al.: Aluminium hydroxide intake: Real risk of aluminum toxicity. *Br. Med. J.* 286:1937, 1983.

26. Cannata J.B. Briggs J.D. Junor B.J.R., et al.: Effect of acute aluminum overload on calcium and parathyroid-hormone metabolism. *Lancet* 1:501, 1983.

27. Cannata J., Ruitzalegria P., Cuesta V., et al.: Influence of aluminum hydroxide intake of haemoglobin levels and blood transfusion requirements in hemodialysis patients. *Proc. Eur. Dial. Transplant Assoc.* 20:719, 1983.

28. Cartier F., Allain P., Gary J., et al.: Encéphalopathie progressive des dialysés: Rôle de l'eau utilisée pour l'hémodialyse. *Nouv. Presse Med.* 7:97, 1978.

29. Cartier F., Chatel M., Allain P.: Aluminum toxicity in renal failure, in Zunukzoglu W., Papadimitriou M., Pyrpasopoulos M., et al. (eds.): *Proceedings of the Eighth International Congress of Nephrology.* Basel, Karger, 1981, pp. 1022–1028.

30. Cartier F., Guenel J., Chatel M.: Aluminum et encéphalopathie des dialysés. *Nephrologie* 2:89, 1981.

31. Chang T.M.S., Barre P.: Effect of desferrioxamine on removal of aluminum and iron by coated charcoal hoemoperfusion and haemodialysis. *Lancet* 2:1051, 1983.

32. Charton B., Jehenne G., Man N.K.: Conception et réalisation d'une chaîne de traitement d'eau pour centre d'hémodialyse. *Journées Eau-Insuffisance Rénale,* Toulouse, 17–18 Sept. 1982, p. 5.1.

33. Clarkson E.M., Luck V.A., Hynson W.V., et al.: The effect of aluminum hydroxide on calcium, phosphorus, and aluminum balance: The serum parathyroid hormone concentration and the aluminum content of bone in patients with chronic renal failure. *Clin. Sci.* 43:519, 1972.

34. Crapper D.R., Krishman S.S., Dalton A.J.: Brain aluminum distribution in Alzheimer's disease and experimental neurofibrillary degeneration. *Science* 180:511, 1973.

35. Crapper-McLachlan D.R., Deboni V.: Etiologic factors in senile dementia of the Alzheimer type, in Amaducci A., Davison A.N., Antuono P. (eds.): *Aging of the Brain and Dementia.* New York, Raven Press, 1980, vol. 13, pp. 173–181.

36. Cumming A.D., Simpson G., Bell D., et al.: Acute aluminum intoxication in patients on continuous ambulatory peritoneal dialysis. *Lancet* 1:103, 1982.

37. Cundy T., Kanis J.A.: Serum aluminum measurements in renal bone disease. *Lancet* 1:1168, 1983.

38. Courmot-Witmer G., Zingraff J., Plachot J.J., et al.: Aluminum localisation in bone from hemodialyzed patients: Relationship to matrix mineralisation. *Kidney Int.* 20:375, 1981.

39. Davidson A.M., Walker G.S., Oli H., et al.: Water supply aluminum concentra-

tion, dialysis dementia and effect of reverse-osmosis water treatment. *Lancet* 2:785, 1982.

40. Davies S.C., Marcus R.E., Hungerford J.L., et al.: Ocular toxicity of high-dose intravenous desferrioxamine. *Lancet* 2:181, 1983.

41. Debroe M.E., Van de Vyver F.L., Bekaert A.B., et al.: The correlation of serum aluminum values with tissue aluminum concentration, to be published.

42. Delavelle F., Richalet B., Malvy F., et al.: Le traitement par l'EDTA des encéphalopathies "pseudo-démentielles" chez les hémodialysés. *Nouv. Presse Med.* 6:941, 1977.

43. Dequeker J.: *Bone Loss in Normal and Pathological Conditions.* Lenven, Lenven University Press, 1972, p. 6.

44. De Vernejoul M.C., Belenguer R., Halkidou H., et al.: Histomorphometric evidence of deleterious effect of aluminum on osteoblasts. Unpublished manuscript.

45. Dewberry F.L., McKinney T.D., Stone W.J.: The dialysis dementia syndrome: Report of fourteen cases and review of the literature. ASAIO J. 3:102, 1980.

46. De Wolff F.A.: A toxicologist's new on aluminum poisoning in clinical nephrology. *Clin. Nephrol.,* to be published.

47. Drueke T.: Dialysis osteomalacia and aluminum intoxication. *Nephron* 26:207, 1980.

48. Elliot H.L., MacDougall A.L., Fell G.S.: Aluminum toxicity syndrome. *Lancet* 1:1203, 1978.

49. Elliot H.L., MacDougall A.L.: Aluminum studies in dialysis encephalopathy. *Proc. Eur. Dia. Transplant Assoc.* 15:157, 1978.

50. Elliot H.L., MacDougall A.L., Fell G.S., et al.: Plasmapheresis, aluminum and dialysis dementia. *Lancet* 2:1255, 1978.

51. Elliot H.L., MacDougall A.L., Haase G., et al.: Plasmapheresis in the treatment of dialysis encephalopathy. *Lancet* 2:940, 1978.

52. Falk R.J., Mattern W.D., Lamanna R.W., et al.: Iron removal during continuous ambulatory peritoneal dialysis using defroxamine. *Kidney Int.* 24:110, 1983.

53. Flendrig J.A., Kruis H., Das H.A.: Aluminum intoxication: The cause of dialysis dementia? *Proc. Eur. Dial. Transplant Assoc.* 13:355, 1976.

54. Fleming L.W., Stewart W.K., Fell G.S., et al.: The effect of oral aluminum levels in patients with chronic renal failure in an area with low water aluminum. *Clin. Nephrol.* 17:222, 1982.

55. Fohrer P., Leflon A., Moriniere P., et al.: Assessment of the value of plasma concentrations of aluminum before and after desferrioxamine in the prediction of bone aluminum load induced by phosphate binders in uremic patients. *Clin. Nephrol.,* to be published.

56. Fosburg M., Hakim R.M., Schulman G., et al.: Pharmacokinetics of desferrioxamine during treatment of transfusional iron overload in chronic hemodialysis patients. *Kidney Int.,* to be published.

57. Gacek E.M., Babb A.L., Fry D.L., et al.: Dialysis dementia: The role of dialyzate pH in altering the chalizability of aluminum. *Trans. Am. Soc. Artif. Intern. Organs* 25:409, 1979.

58. Galle P., Chatel M., Berry J.P., et al.: Encéphalopathie myoclonique progressive des dialysés: Présence d'aluminum en forte concentration dansles lysosomes des cellules cérébrales. *Nouv. Presse Med.* 8:4091, 1979.

59. Galle P., Giudicelli C.P.: Toxicité de l'aluminum pour l'hépatocyte: Localisation ultrastructurale et microanalyse des dépots. *Nouv. Presse Med.* 11:1123, 1982.

60. Geary D.F., Feunell R.S., Andriola M., et al.: Encephalopathy in children with chronic renal failure. *J. Pediatr.* 97:41, 1980.

61. Gilli P., Debastiani P., Fagioli F., et al.: Positive aluminum balance in patients on regular peritoneal treatment: An effect of low dialysate pH? *Proc. Eur. Dial. Transplant Assoc.* 17:219, 1980.

62. Gilli P., Farinelli A., Fagioli F., et al.: Serum aluminum levels in patients on peritoneal dialysis. *Lancet* 2:742, 1980.
63. Gilli P., Malacarne F., Fagioli F.: Is serum aluminum monitoring useful in evaluating aluminum intoxication? *Lancet* 1:956, 1983.
64. Gorsky J.E., Dietz A.A., Spencer H., et al.: Metabolic balance of aluminum. *Clin. Chem.* 25:1739, 1979.
65. Graf H., Stummvoll H.K., Meisinger V., et al.: Aluminum removal by hemodialysis. *Kidney Int.* 19:587, 1981.
66. Graf H., Stummvoll H.K., Meisinger V.: Dialysate aluminum concentration and aluminum transfer during haemodialysis. *Lancet* 1:46, 1982.
67. Graf H., Stummvoll H.K., Meisinger V.: Desferrioxamine induced changes of aluminum kinetics during haemodialysis. *Proc. Eur. Dial. Transplant Assoc.* 18:674, 1981.
68. Guillard O., Piriou A., Mura P., Precautions necessary when assaying aluminum in serum of chronic hemodialysed patients. *Clin. Chem.* 28:1714, 1982.
69. Guillot A.P., Hood V.L., Rungis C.F., et al.: The use of magnesium-containing phosphate binders in patients with end stage renal disease on maintenance hemodialysis. *Nephron* 30:114, 1982.
70. Haas T., Meyrand B., Dongradi G.: Etude comparative des performances in vivo de 15 dialyseurs à fibres creuses. *RBM* 3:39, 1981.
71. Henriquez M., Burnatowska-Hledin M.A., Clark M.J., et al.: Evaluation of aluminum binding to hollow fiber dialyzers. *Kidney Int.*, to be published.
72. Hercz G., Milliner D.S., Shimaberger J.H., et al.: Aluminum metabolism and removal during CAPD. *Kidney Int.* to be published.
73. Hodge K.C., Day J.P., O'Hara M., et al.: Critical concentration of aluminum in water used for dialysis. *Lancet* 2:802, 1981.
74. Hoffbrand A.V.: Transfusion siderosis and chelation therapy, in Jacobs A., Worwood M. (eds.): *Iron in Biochemistry and Medicine.* New York, Academic Press, 1980, vol. 2, pp. 499–527.
75. Hosakawa S., Konira S., Tomoyoshi T · Aluminum transfer in chronic renal failure patients during hemodialysis. *Blood Purification* 1:62, 1983.
76. Hourmant M., Soulillou J.P., Boiteau H.L., et al.: Cinétiques des taux sanguins ot urinaires de l'aluminum après transplantation rénale. *Nephrologie* 2:125, 1981.
77. Huber C.T., Frieden E.: The inhibition of ferroxidase by trivalent and other metal ions. *J. Biol. Chem.* 245:3979, 1970.
78. Ihle B.U., Buchanan M.R.C., Stevens B., et al.: The efficacy of various treatment modalities on aluminum associated bone disease. *Proc. Eur. Dial. Transplant Assoc.* 19:195, 1982.
79. Kaenhy W.D., Alfrey A.C., Holman R.E., et al.: Aluminum transfer during hemodialysis. *Kidney Int.* 12:361, 1977.
80. Kaehny W.D., Arlene P., Hegg B.S., et al.: Gastro-intestinal absorption of aluminum from aluminum-containing antacids. *N. Engl. J. Med.* 296:1389, 1977.
81. Katzman R.: The prevalence and malignancy of Alzheimer disease. *Arch. Neurol.* 33:217, 1976.
82. Kerr D.M.S.: Le système nerveux central: Anomalies cliniques et physiopathologiques observées chez les malades en dialyse chronique, in Hamburger J., Crosnier J., Funck-Brentano J.L. (eds.): *Actualités Néphrologiques de l'Hôpital Necker.* Paris, Flammarion Medecine-Sciences, 1979, pp. 133–155.
83. King S.W., Savory J., Wills M.R.: The clinical biochemistry of aluminum. *Crit. Rev. Clin. Lab. Sci.* 14:1, 1981.
84. King S.W., Savory J., Wills M.R.: Aluminum distribution in serum following hemodialysis. *Ann. Clin. Lab. Sci.* 12:143, 1982.
85. King S.W., Wills M.R., Savory J.: Serum binding of aluminum. *Res. Commun. Chem. Pathol. Pharmacol.* 26:161, 1979.

86. Kingswood C., Banks R.A., Bunker T., et al.: Fracture osteomalacia, CAPD, and aluminum. *Lancet* 1:70, 1983.
87. Klein G.L., Alfrey A.C., Miller N.L., et al.: Aluminum loading during total parenteral nutrition. *Am. J. Clin. Nutr.* 35:1425, 1982.
88. Kovalchik M.T., Kaehny W.D., Hegg A.P., et al.: Aluminum kinetics during hemodialysis. *J. Lab. Clin. Med.* 92:712, 1978.
89. Kushelevsky A.L., Yagil R., Alfazi Z., et al.: Uptake of aluminum ion by the liver. *Biomedicine* 25:59, 1976.
90. Leeming R.J., Blair J.A.: Dialysis dementia, aluminum, and tetrahydrobioptern metabolism. *Lancet* 1:556, 1979.
91. Lione A.: The prophylactic reduction of aluminum intake. *Food Chem. Toxicol.* 21:103, 1983.
92. Malluche H.H., Smith A.J., Abreo K., et al.: Successful removal of aluminum from bone of dialyzed patients treated with desferrioxamine. *Kidney Int.*, to be published.
93. Maloney N.A., Ott S.M., Alfrey A.C., et al.: Histological quantification of aluminum in iliac bone from patients with renal failure. *J. Lab. Clin. Med.* 99:206, 1982.
94. Man N.K., Funck-Frentano J.L.: L'hémofiltration, nouvelle méthode d'épuration extra-rénale, in Hamburger J., Crosnier J., Funck-Brentano J.L. (eds.): *Actualités Néphrologiques de l'Hôpital Necker*. Paris, Flammarion Médecine-Sciences, 1977, pp. 387–404.
95. Mason J.C., Jones N.F., Hilton P.J.: Aluminum in haemofiltration solutions. *Lancet* 1:762, 1983.
96. Masselot J.P., Adhemar J.P., Jaudon M.C., et al.: Reversible dialysis encephalopathy: Role for aluminum containing gels. *Lancet* 2:1386, 1978.
97. Mattern W.D., Krigman M.R., Blythe W.B.: Failure of successful renal transplantation to reverse the dialysis-associated encephalopathy syndrome. *Clin. Nephrol.* 7:725, 1977.
98. Mauras Y., Allain P., Riberi P.: Etude de l'absorption digestive de l'hydrocarbonate d'aluminum chez l'individu sain. *Therapie* 37:593, 1982.
99. May P.M., Williams D.R.: The inorganic chemistry of iron metabolism, in Jacobs A., Worwood M. (eds.): *Iron in Biochemistry and Medicine*. New York, Academic Press, 1980, vol. 2, pp. 1–28.
100. Mayor G.H., Keiser J.A., Makdani D., et al.: Aluminum absorption and distribution: Effect of parathyroid hormone. *Science* 197:1187, 1977.
101. Mayor G.H., Remedi R.E., Sprague S.M., et al.: Central nervous system manifestations of oral aluminum: Effect of parathyroid hormone, in Liss L. (ed.): *Aluminum Neurotoxicity*. Park Forest South, Ill., Pathotox Publishers, 1980, pp. 33–39.
102. Mayor G.H., Sprague S.M., Sanchez T.V.: Determinants of tissue aluminum concentration. *Am. J. Kidney Dis.* 1:141, 1;981.
103. McDermott J.R., Smith A.J., Ward M.K., et al.: Brain-aluminum concentration in dialysis encephalopathy. *Lancet* 1:901, 1978.
104. Metha R.P.: Encephalopathy in chronic renal failure appearing before the start of dialysis. *CMA J.* 120:1112, 1979.
105. Mendes V., Jorgetti V., Nemeth J., et al.: Secondary hyperparathyroidism in chronic haemodialysis patients: A chronic pathologic study. *Proc. Eur. Dial. Transplant Assoc.* 20:731, 1983.
106. Meredith P.A., Elliot H.L., Campbell B.C., et al.: Changes in serum aluminum, blood zinc, blood lead and erythrocyte delta-aminoloevulinic acid dehydratase activity during haemodialysis. *Toxicol. Lett.* 4:419, 1979.
107. Milliner D.S. Nebeker H.G., Ott S.A., et al.: Desferrioxamine infusion test for diagnosis of aluminum osteomalacia. *Kidney Int.*, to be published.
108. Milliner D.S., Shinaberger J.H., Miller J.H., et al.: Removal of aluminum during hemodialysis: Effect of desferrioxamine, abstracted. *Am. J. Kidney Dis.*, 1984.

109. Milne F.J., Sharf B., Bell P.D., et al.: Low aluminum water, desferrioxamine, and dialysis encephalopathy. *Lancet* 2:502, 1982.
110. Mion C.: Aluminum in continuous ambulatory peritoneal dialysis and post-dilutional hemofiltration: A review of the literature. *Clin. Nephrol.*, to be published.
111. Mittal V.K., Sharma M.J., Toledo-Pereyra L.H., et al.: Complete recovery from dialysis dementia following kidney transplantation. *Dial. Transplant.* 10:41, 1981.
112. Moriniere P.H., Roussel A., Tahiri Y., et al.: Substitution of aluminum hydroxide by high doses of calcium carbonate in patients on chronic haemodialysis: Disappearance of hyperaluminaemia and equal control of hyperparathyroidism. *Proc. Eur. Dial. Transplant Assoc.* 19:784, 1982.
113. Mudde A.H., Roodvoets A.P.: Desferrioxamine and osteomalacia. *Lancet* 2:608, 1982.
114. Mudde A.H., Roodvoets A.P., Gasthuis E., et al.: Aluminum intoxication in haemodialysis patients: Which patients are at risk? *Eur. Dial. Transplant Assoc.*, vol. 93, 1983.
115. Nathan E., Pedersen S.E.: Dialysis encephalopathy in a non-dialysed uroemic boy treated with aluminum hydroxide orally. *Acta Paediatr. Scand.* 69:793, 1980.
116. Nebeker A.G., Milliner D.S., Ott S.A., et al.: Aluminum-related osteomalacia: Clinical response to desferrioxamine. *Kidney Int.*, to be published.
117. Netter P., Burnel D., Hutin M.F., et al.: Aluminum in joint tissue of patients taking aluminum hydroxyde. *Lancet* 1:1056, 1981.
118. O'Hare J.A., Callaghan N.M., Murnaghan D.J.: Dialysis encephalopathy. *Medicine* 62:129, 1983.
119. O'Hare J.A., Murnaghan D.J.: Reversal of aluminum induced hemodialysis anemia by a low-aluminum dialysate. *N. Engl. J. Med.* 306:654, 1982.
120. Ott S.M., Maloney N.A., Klein G.L., et al.: Aluminum is associated with low bone formation in patients receiving chronic parenteral nutrition. *Ann. Intern. Med.* 98:910, 1983.
121. Parkinson I.S., Ward M.K., Feest T.G., et al.: Fracturing dialysis osteodystrophy and dialysis encephalopathy: An epidemiological survey. *Lancet* 1:406, 1979.
122. Parkinson I.S., Ward M.K., Kerrd, N.S.: Dialysis encephalopathy, bone disease and anoemia: The aluminum intoxication syndrome during regular haemodialysis. *J. Clin. Pathol.* 34:1285, 1981.
123. Parkinson I.S., Ward M.K., Kerr D.N.S.: A method for the routine determination of aluminum in serum and water by flameless atomic absorption spectrometry. *Clin. Chim. Acta* 125:125, 1982.
124. Peserico A., Antonello A., Baggio B., et al.: Pseudoporfiria cutanea tarda in pazienti con insufficienza renal cronica e in pazienti con trapianto di rene. *Minerva Nefrol.* 27:495, 1980.
125. Pierce-Myli M., Pierides A.: Iron and aluminum osteomalacia during hemodialysis: A new syndrome. *Kidney Int.*, to be published.
126. Pierides A.M., Frohnert P.P.: Aluminum related dialysis osteomalacia and dementia after prolonged use of the redy cartridge. *Trans. Am. Soc. Artif. Intern. Organs* 27:629, 1981.
127. Pierides A., Van Den Berg C., Pierce-Myli M., et al.: Resolution of aluminum osteomalacia with IV desferioxamine followed by vitamin-D. *Kidney Int.*, to be published.
128. Platts M.M.: Dialysis encephalopathy. *Lancet* 2:1035, 1980.
129. Pogglitsch H., Knopp C.H., Petek W., et al.: Prevention of aluminum intoxication by administration of acid-resistant aluminum hydroxide. *Eur. Dial. Transplant Assoc.*, 1983, p. 103.
130. Pogglitsch H., Knopp C.II., Wawschlnek O., et al.: Aluminum intoxication in dialysis patients. *Int. J. Artif. Organs* 5:293, 1982.

131. Pogglitsch H., Petek W., Wawchinek O., et al.: Treatment of early stages of dialysis encephalopathy by aluminum depletion. *Lancet* 2:1344, 1981.
132. Poisson M., Maşhaly R., Lebkiri B.: Dialysis encephalopathy: Recovery after interruption of aluminum intake. *Br. Med. J.* 2:1610, 1978.
133. Prichard S., Barre P., Hodsman A., et al.: Bone aluminum content related to Al ingestion. *Eur. Dial. Transplant Assoc.* 1983, p. 104.
134. Raghavan S.R.V., Khalil-Manesch F., Gonick H.C.: Aluminum-binding proteins in dialysis dementia. *Kidney Int.*, to be published.
135. Randall M.E.: Aluminum toxicity in an infant not on dialysis. *Lancet* 1:1327, 1983.
136. Reckerr R.R., Blotcky A.J., Leffler J.A., et al.: Evidence for aluminum absorption from the gastro-intestinal tract and bone deposition by aluminum carbonate ingestion with normal renal function. *J. Lab. Clin. Med.* 90:810, 1977.
137. Rembold C.M., Krumlovsky F.A., Roxe D.M., et al.: Treatment of hemodialysis hemosiderosis with desferrioxamine. *Trans. Am. Soc. Artif. Intern. Organs* 28:621, 1982.
138. Report from the Registration Committee of the European Dialysis and Transplant Association (1980): Dialysis dementia in Europe. *Lancet* 2:190, 1980.
139. Rockel A., Gilge V., Ohl B., et al.: Elimination of low molecular weight proteins during hemofiltration. *Contrib. Nephrol.* 32:40, 1982.
140. Rottembourg J., Jaudon M.C., Legrain M., et al.: Les gels d'alumine chez les insuffisants rénaux chroniques: Un risque potentiel d'encéphalopathie et d'ostéopathie. *Ann. Med. Intern.* 131:71, 1980.
141. Rottembourg J., Gallego J.L., Jaudon M.C., et al.: Evolution des taux d'aluminum sérique et étude des transferts péritonéaux d'aluminum au cours de la DPCA. *Neprhologie,* to be published.
142. Ruiz J.C., Picart X.P., Levy C.L.: Desferrioxamine pharmacokinetics in hemodialysed patients. *Clin. Nephrol.,* to be published.
143. Rutherford E., King S., Perry B., et al.: Use of a new phosphate binder in chronic renal insufficiency. *Kidney Int.* 17:528, 1980.
144. Savory J., Berlin A., Courtoux C., et al.: Summary report of an international workshop on the role of biological monitoring in the prevention of aluminum toxicity in man: Aluminum analysis in biological fluids. *Ann. Clin. Lab. Sci.* 13:444, 1983.
145. Schneider H., Kulbe K.D., Weber H., et al.: High effective aluminum free intestinal phosphate binder: In vitro and in vivo studies. *Proc. Eur. Dial. Transplant Assoc.,* to be published.
146. Sears W.G., Eales L.: Aluminum induced porphyria in rats. *IRCS* 30:35, 1973.
147. Shimada H., Nakamura M., Marumo F.: Influence of aluminium on the effect of 1 (OH)D$_3$ on renal osteodystrophy. *Nephron* 35:163, 1983.
148. Sherrard D.J.: Role of aluminum in bone disease. Introductory lecture, the American Society of Nephrology 16th Annual Meeting, Washington, D.C., Dec. 4–7, 1983.
149. Short A.J.K., Winney R.J., Robson J.S.: Reversible microcytic hypochronic anaemia in dialysis patients due to aluminum intoxication. *Proc. Eur. Dial. Transplant Assoc.* 17:226, 1980.
150. Sideman S., Manor D.: The dialysis dementia syndrome and aluminum intoxication. *Nephron* 31:1, 1982.
151. Simon P., Ang K.S., Tanquerel T., et al.: Surcharge tissulaire en aluminum chez les hémodialysés: Test à la desferrioxamine. *Nouv. Presse Med.* 11:209, 1982.
152. Simon P., Allain P., Mauras Y., et al.: Hyperaluminemia test by desferrioxamine for the determination of tissue aluminum overload in hemodialysis patients. *Kidney Int.* 21:900, 1982.

153. Simon P., Allain P., Mauras Y., et al.: Chélation de l'aluminum tissulaire au cours de l'encéphalopathie du dialysé: Supériorité de la desferrioxamine sur l'éthylène-diamine tetra acétique (EDTA) et de l'hémodialyse sur l'hémofiltraiton. *Nephrologie* 3:145, 1982.

154. Simon P., Allain P., Ang K.S., et al.: Higher performance of polyacrylonitrile dialyser than cuprophane hollow fiber dialyser to remove aluminum by hemodialysis alone and following chelation with desferrioxamine. *Clin. Nephrol.*, to be published.

156. Simon P., Ang K.S., Meyrier A., et al.: Desferrioxamine ocular toxicity and trace metals. *Lancet* 2:547, 1983.

157. Simon P., Ang K.S. Cam G., et al.: Etude comparative de la clairance de l'aluminum sérique en fonction de la méthode d'épuration et de la membrane utilisées au cours du test d'hyperaluminémie provoquée par la desferrioxamine chez les hémodialysés chroniques. *Nephrologie*, to be published.

158. Simon P., Ang K.S., Cam G., et al.: Desferrioxamine, aluminum and dialysis. *Lancet* 2:1489, 1983.

159. Simon P., Bonn F., Guezennec M., et al.: La surcharge en fer chez les patients hémodialysés: Critères diagnostiques, indications et résultats du traitement par desferrioxamine. *Nephrologie* 2:165, 1981.

160. Simon P., Meyrier A., Allain P., et al.: Evaluation of Al tissue stores by a desferrioxamine test in chronic hemodialysis patients. *Kidney Int.*, to be published.

161. Tahiri J., Moriniere P., Jaudon M.C., et al.: Hyperaluminémie des hémodialysés chroniques: Evaluation du rôle respectif de l'aluminum du dialysat et de celui de la prise orale d'hydroxyde d'alumine. *Nephrologie* 4:129, 1983.

162. Touam M., Martinez F., Lacour B., et al.: Aluminum-induced reversible microcytic anemia in chronic renal failure: Clinical and experimental studies. *Clin. Nephrol.* 19:295, 1983.

163. Toulemonde F., Vilotte J., Etienne J., et al.: Etude de la résorption digestive de l'aluminum à partir d'un pansement gastro-intestinal. *Therapie* 34:649, 1979.

164. Trapp G.A.: Plasma aluminum is bound to transferrin. *Life Sci.* 33:311, 1983.

165. Tsukamoto Y., Iwanami S., Marumo F.: Disturbances of trace element concentrations in plasma of patients with chronic renal failure. *Nephron* 26:174, 1980.

166. Van Waeleghen, D'Haese P., Verpooten G.A., et al.: The effect of pH on aluminum clearance in hemodialysis before and after desferrioxamine administration. *Clin. Nephrol.*, to be published.

167. Verbeelen A.H., Smeyers-Verbeke J., Sennesael J., et al.: Serum aluminum measurements in renal bone disease. *Lancet* 1:1168, 1983.

168. Verbueken A.H., Vandevyver F.L., Vangrieken R.E., et al.: Ultrastructural localisation of aluminum and iron in the liver and the bone of patients with haemodialysis osteomalacia. Unpublished manuscript.

169. Viron B., Mignon F.: Personal communication.

170. Ward M.K., Feest T.G., Ellis H.A., et al.: Osteomalacia dialysis osteodystrophy: Evidence for a water-borne oetiological agent probably aluminum. *Lancet* 1:841, 1978.

171. Wardle E.M.: Aluminum intoxication. *Nephron* 33:67, 1983.

172. Wills M.R., Savory J.: Aluminum poisoning: Dialysis encephalopathy, osteomalacia and anaemia. *Lancet* 2:29, 1983.

173. Williams E.D., Elliott H.L., Boddy K., et al.: Whole body aluminum in chronic renal failure and dialysis encephalopathy. *Clin. Nephrol.* 14:198, 1980.

174. Winchester J.F., Ratcliffe J.G., Carlyle E., et al.: Solute aminoacid and hormone changes with coated charcoal hemoperfusions in uremia. *Kidney Int.* 14:74, 1978.

175. Winney R.J., Cowie J.F., Smith G.D., et al.: What is the value of plasma/serum aluminum in patients with chronic renal failure? *Clin. Nephrol.*, to be published

176. Wolf A., Graf H., Pinggera W.F., et al.: Serum aluminum and continuous ambulatory peritoneal dialysis. *Ann. Intern. Med.* 92:130, 1980.
177. Womack F.C., Colowick S.P.: Proton-dependent inhibition of yeast and brain hexokinases by aluminum in ATP preparation. *Proc. Natl. Acad. Sci. USA* 76:5080, 1979.
178. Zaino E.C.: Desferrioxamine and trace metal excretion in chelation therapy in chronic iron overload, in Zaino E.C., Roberts R.H. (eds.): *Chelation and Chronic Iron Overload*. New York, CIBA Medical Horizons Symposia, 1977, pp. 95–107.
179. Zumkley H., Bertram H.P., Lison A., et al.: Aluminum zinc and copper concentrations in plasma in chronic renal insufficiency. *Clin. Nephrol.* 12:18, 1979.

Calcium, Parathyroid Hormone, and Hypertension

DAVID A. McCARRON, M.D. AND CYNTHIA D. MORRIS, PH.D.

Division of Nephrology and Hypertension, Oregon Health Sciences University, Portland, Oregon

DIVALENT CATIONS and related hormonal systems are emerging as critical factors in the regulation of arterial pressure in animals and human beings. This review will assess the current data that associates calcium and its regulatory hormone, parathyroid hormone, to normal and abnormal states of blood pressure control. For several reasons, primarily related to clinical observations from the past, the current interpretation of calcium's and PTH's net effects on cardiovascular physiology is essentially opposite to what they were once thought to be.

For both calcium and PTH, data from physiologic, pharmacologic, animal intervention, and clinical research studies indicate that both the cation, calcium, and the hormone, PTH, exert protective actions on cardiovascular tissue. Their influence appears to be related in both cases to direct effects on vascular smooth muscle cells. The evidence suggests that for both of these physiologic factors, their primary effect is to promote smooth muscle cell relaxation and thereby a reduction in peripheral resistance. In this article, the recent evidence supporting that interpretation of calcium's PTH's effects on blood pressure is presented. In addition, the earlier data, derived principally from clinical observations, is reassessed in light of

479

the newer findings. In this manner, the previous association between acute and chronic hypercalcemia and an elevation in mean arterial pressure can be reconciled with the mounting evidence that, under physiologic conditions, calcium administration is associated with the reduction in mean arterial pressure. Likewise, the long-standing clinical observation that hyperparathyroidism is associated with mild elevations of blood pressure in human beings may not be inconsistent with parathyroid hormone's apparent vasodilating actions in human beings and animals.

In summarizing the accumulated data, a theoretical integration of the past and present information surrounding calcium's and parathyroid hormone's vascular effects is provided. As our understanding of these two factors' cellular actions are expanded in the future, a consistent and logical relationship among calcium, PTH, and normal blood pressure regulation should emerge.

Calcium—A Vasodilator

PHYSIOLOGIC BASIS

Calcium is critical to the normal function of vascular smooth muscle.[1] While the cation is essential for contractility,[1] a membrane stabilizing vasorelaxing action of Ca^{2+} has also been well established.[1-3] The ion in its free state and through its binding to calmodulin,[1,4] therefore, contributes to the regulation of both vascular smooth muscle contraction and relaxation.[1] In vitro, maximal vasoconstrictor response has been demonstrated under conditions of modest reductions in the exposure of Ca^{2+} to the vascular tissue,[3,5] while maximal relaxing responses occur at higher levels of tissue exposure to calcium.[2,3,5,6] This dual effect of Ca^{2+}, while well established in the physiology literature, has been overlooked in terms of clinical application, in part, because of the narrow focus on the cation's role in initiating contraction. This simplistic assessment has been fostered by hypotheses that have equated all increases in intracellular Ca^{2+} with vasoconstriction and a rise in blood pressure.[7] These theoretical postulates have ignored not only this "dual" effect of Ca^{2+} and the observations that span 25 years that Ca^{2+} administration is associated with vascular relaxation[2,3,5,6] and vasodilation,[8,9] but also the more recent observations that have delineated the regulation of intracellular calcium. The consideration of calcium's role in vascular smooth muscle (VSM) function and its impact on blood pressure control is, however, appropriate regardless of one's perception of the ion's "net" effect on vascular tone. Hypertension is principally a disorder of peripheral vascular resistance whether primary in origin or secondary to a regulatory dysfunction such as altered CNS control, or peripheral sympathetic dysfunction. To the extent peripheral vascular tone can be reduced, blood pressure control should be improved. Ca^{2+} and Na^+, as well as K^+ and Mg^{2+}, clearly all modify VSM function in a highly integrated fashion. The influence of one of these cations on VSM tone cannot be separated from the others. This cation interaction has been demonstrated for Ca^{2+}, as its vasorelaxant effects have been shown to be Na^+-,[3, 10, 11] K^+-,[3] and Mg^{2+}-dependent.[12] The lack of further consideration of these other cations is not intended to imply that they are not, in their own right, important.

Pharmacologic Basis

Two prototypical antihypertensive agents exert distinctive and differential effects on Ca^{2+} metabolism. Thiazide diuretics lower blood pressure in 30%–60% of patients and are associated with the induction of positive Ca^{2+} balance in many subjects.[13, 14] There are no substantive data, however, that the antihypertensive action of thiazides is dependent on the compound's systemic effects on calcium balance. It is noteworthy that thiazides do behave as mild vasodilators, consistent with their influence on calcium metabolism.

At the other end of the spectrum of pharmacologic agents, the calcium channel blockers are emerging as potent antihypertensives that lower blood pressure in most subjects via systemic arterial vasodilation and a reduction in both systolic and, to a lesser extent, diastolic pressure.[15] The cellular basis for their induction of vasorelaxation is believed to be secondary to the inhibition of "slow" Ca^{2+} fluxes, and, thereby, calcium activation of smooth muscle contraction.[15] With the current, rapid expansion of interest in the calcium antagonists, there has not been sufficient emphasis placed on the parallel work that has characterized calcium channel inhibition by calcium itself.[16–18] The cation regulates its own fluxes as well as its membrane and intracellular compartmentalization.[19] Functionally, Ca^{2+} acts as a calcium channel blocker, such that, under conditions of adequate cellular exposure, vascular tissue fluxes are reduced and smooth muscle relaxation prevails.

Ca^{2+} METABOLISM ABNORMALITIES IN HUMAN AND EXPERIMENTAL HYPERTENSION

In both human and experimental hypertension disordered Ca^{2+} metabolism has been noted in a variety of organ functions, biochemical parameters, and cellular fractions. Organ involvement in experimental models has included the peripheral vasculature, kidney, intestines, adipose tissue, red blood cells, and bone. In the laboratory, animal vascular tissue has been reported to exhibit increased membrane permeability to calcium, altered binding kinetics of the cation in the cell membranes, and accumulation of calcium in subcellular fractions.[20, 21] Both Na^+-dependent and genetic models of hypertension have been reported to possess one or all of these abnormalities.[21] The renal defects include enhanced urinary calcium excretion in the adult spontaneously hypertensive rat (SHR), a failure of the young animal to diminish appropriately his urinary calcium excretion when placed on a Ca^{2+} deficient intake and a blunted stimulation of urinary cAMP generation under conditions of metabolic stress.[20, 22] Table 1 demonstrates the SHR's inability to respond to the need to maintain calcium status. After two weeks on a low Ca^{2+} diet, cAMP failed to rise appropriately compared to the WKY. Intestinal handling of calcium and vitamin D metabolism have also been noted to be abnormal in the SHR.[23, 24]

Disturbances of calcium metabolism linked to human hypertension include altered renal and bone metabolism.[25–27] The latter encompasses increased urinary calcium excretion, enhanced excretion of an acutely administered calcium load, increased urinary cAMP excretion and an elevated phosphate clearance.[25, 26] Bone disturbances have been implied by the increased prevalence of hypertension reported in osteoporotic women.[27] Serum total calcium is normal, but free or ionized calcium is decreased.[28] Parathyroid hormone values are elevated and serum phosphorus concentrations are low.[25]

TABLE 1.—URINARY cAMP AND CALCIUM EXCRETION

Diet Ca^{2+}	SHR		WKY	
(gm/kg)*	4%	0.02%	4%	0.02%
UcAMP, pmole/24°	$4.8 \pm 0.4 \times 10^4$	$8.4 \pm 1.0 \times 10^4$	$16.7 \pm 4.8 \times 10^4$	$19.4 \pm 3.3 \times 10^4$
U$_{Ca}$V, mEq/24°	0.8 ± 0.2	0.2 ± 0.04	0.56 ± 0.1	0.04 ± 0.01
N =	8	8	8	8

*16- to 18-week-old animals raised on a 1.0% Ca^{2+} diet, then switched to either a Ca^{2+}-supplemented (4%) or Ca^{2+}-restricted (0.02%) diet.

RELATIONSHIP OF DIETARY Ca^{2+} TO BLOOD
PRESSURE IN HUMANS

The functional importance of disordered calcium homeostasis
in the pathogenesis of high blood pressure was originally suggested by the epidemiologic observations in the human beings
that decreased dietary[29, 30] and environmental exposure[31, 32] to
calcium is associated with an increased risk of developing hypertension and hypertensive cardiovascular disease. In the two
prospective studies reported to date, dairy product consumption
was the identified source of reduced calcium intake.[29, 30] Both
fluid milk and nonfluid milk dairy products have been shown
to be consumed less in subjects with either borderline or fixed
hypertension.[29, 30] Based on the National Center for Health Statistics data, reduced dietary calcium consumption is the nutritional pattern that most closely follows the demographics of hypertension in the United States.[33] Published data have
indicated that age, race, sex, weight, and alcohol consumption

Fig 1.—Prevalence of hypertension as defined as a systolic blood pressure >160
mmHg adjusted for age, race and sex based upon daily dietary Ca^{2+} intake. Data derived from the HANES Survey I—National Center for Health Statistics.[34]

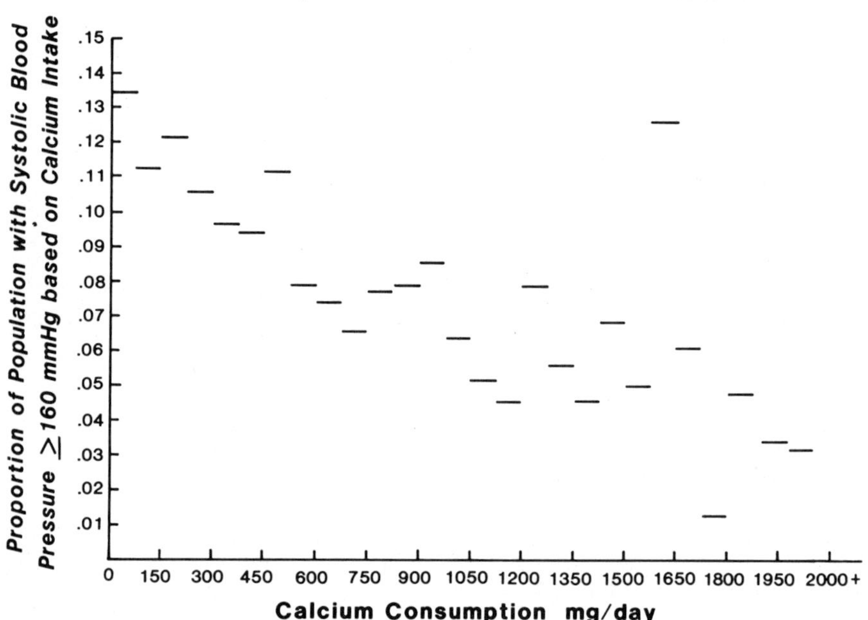

do not account for these differences[29, 30, 34] in calcium consumption between normal and hypertensive subjects. Figure 1 portrays the relative risk of an individual being hypertensive in the United States, based on dietary calcium intake. This analysis is adjusted for age, race, and sex. Similar relationships exist regardless of the level of blood pressure used to define hypertension or the use of diastolic, systolic, or mean arterial pressures.

RESPONSES OF HUMAN AND EXPERIMENTAL ANIMALS TO MODIFICATION OF Ca^{2+} INTAKE

Acute and chronic studies in the SHR and its genetic,[36] normotensive control, the Wistar-Kyoto rat (WKY),[37] have provided additional evidence that calcium homeostasis and its maintenance is a factor in blood pressure control. Supplementing the diet of the SHR with calcium results in marked attenuation of what had been previously called "fixed" hypertension in this laboratory model (Fig 2).[20] In contrast, removal or re-

Fig 2.—Tail-cuff, systolic blood pressure (mmHg) in the SHR-fed normal (0.25% or 0.5%) Ca^{2+} diets versus high (4%) Ca^{2+} diets. Diets introduced at 10 weeks of age after hypertension.

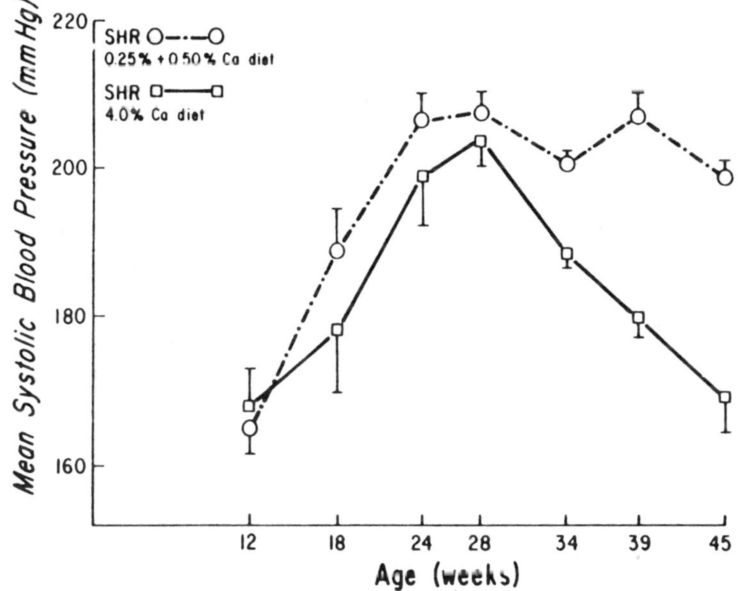

duction of dietary calcium in the SHR results in an acceleration of the animal's hypertension. In the adult SHR, modifying dietary exposure can change blood pressure within two weeks. Reducing calcium in the diet will result in a further rise in the animal's blood pressure while supplementation with calcium will lower the animal's pressure significantly within two weeks.[38] Observations in the WKY are consistent with those in the SHR. The normotensive rat's blood pressure will track inversely depending on the calcium content of the diet. Increased diet exposure results in a lower pressure in the adult animal, while calcium restriction produces borderline hypertension in this putative normotensive animal.[37] Again, dietary calcium manipulations of as short a duration as two weeks will modify the adult WKY's arterial pressure. For the SHR, the reversal of fixed hypertension simply by the supplementation of its diet by Ca^{2+} represents the only reported nonpharmacologic, physiologically relevant maneuver that lowers its blood pressure.[20]

Two reports suggest that comparable effects of Ca^{2+} supplementation on blood pressure are achievable in both normotensive and hypertensive humans.[39, 40] Belizan et al. demonstrated a 6%–10% reduction in the blood pressure of normotensive males and females given 1,000 mg of Ca^{2+} as the carbonate salt for 6 to 20 weeks. A more recent, preliminary report involving 100 subjects indicates that approximately 44% of hypertensive subjects will achieve an excellent therapeutic response with calcium repletion. In this double-blind, placebo-controlled study, 1,000 mg Ca^{2+} for 8 weeks produced an average 21 mm Hg reduction in systolic blood pressure. A more modest reduction (7 mm Hg) in diastolic blood pressure was achieved.

In summary, calcium exerts a dual effect on cardiovascular physiology with the potential to mediate both smooth muscle contraction and relaxation and thereby modify peripheral vascular resistance and blood pressure. In vitro, animal and human investigations indicate that the availability or provision of adequate calcium is associated with a membrane stabilizing action on the VSM and a consequent relaxation of that cell, reduction in vascular resistance in animals, and a lowering of blood pressure in experimental animals and in humans.

Parathyroid Hormone—A Vasodilator

PHYSIOLOGIC BASIS

With Collip's initial report of the isolation of parathyroid hormone in 1925, one of the principal physiologic effects he ascribed to the hormone was a reduction in arterial pressure when the purified extract was administered to laboratory animals.[42] However, this cardiovascular action of the peptide was largely ignored or attributed by other investigators to impurities resulting from the extraction of the hormone.[42] Parathyroid hormone's vasodilating actions reemerged in 1968 with the report of Charbon that characterized both a hypotensive and diuretic effect of the hormone extract.[43] In a series of papers that followed, Charbon and co-workers extensively described the vasodilating, hypotensive action of the peptide in a variety of animal species when the intact, highly purified hormone was infused either systemically or regionally into both renal and hepatic arteries.[44-46] These investigators proposed that the vasodilating action of the hormone could be used as a bioassay.[47]

Pang and associates have since extended these earlier observations concerning PTH's direct vasodilating actions to demonstrate that the hormone lowered blood pressure in a number of both vertebrate and nonvertebrate species.[48, 49] Their most recent reports have demonstrated that PTH's vasodilating effects in the coronary arteries is a specific property of the peptide that is not modified by adrenergic, cholinergic, or histaminergic agonists or antagonists.[50] Additional studies by these researchers have documented that the hypotensive response is principally the result of arterial vasodilation with little or no impact on cardiac output.[51]

Experiments from our laboratory have recently characterized the log-dose dependence of PTH's vasodilating action in the SHR and WKY.[52] In addition, we have characterized the timecourse of the hypotensive response in the animals (Fig 3). The maximal reduction in mean arterial blood pressure occurs between 30 and 60 seconds post injection with a duration of action of 9 to 15 minutes.[52] The duration of the vasodilation is consistent with the half-life of the peptide in the circulation.

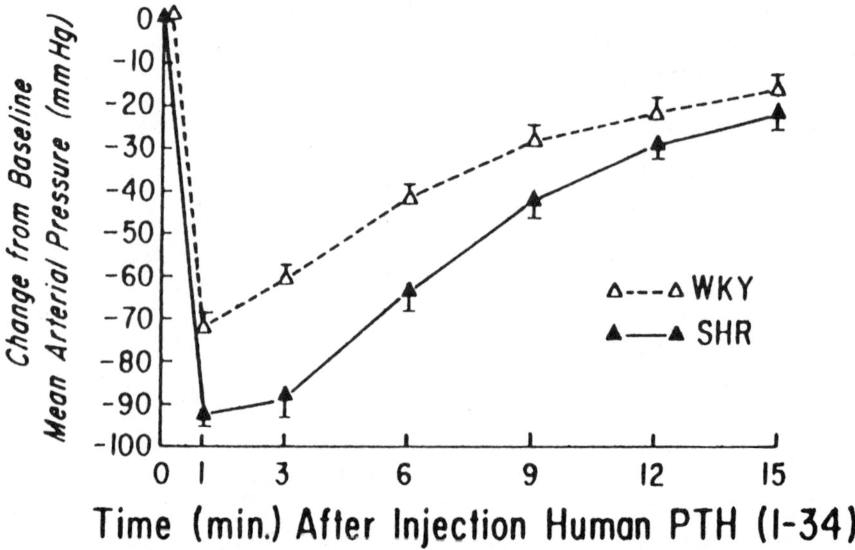

Fig 3.—Time-course and magnitude of the vasodepressive response of the SHR and WKY to hPTH (1–34) administered IV at 18 to 20 weeks of age on a 1% (by weight) Ca^{2+} diet.[52]

Pharmacologic Basis

Utilizing available analogs of PTH, we have defined the structural prerequisites for the peptide's hypotensive action. Both bovine and human PTH (1–34) exhibit virtually identical log-dose curves.[53] Substituting in the 8th and 18th positions of these synthetic analogs does not modify the hormone's vascular potency (Fig 4); although, removal of the first two amino acid residues produces an analog that is devoid of any vasodepressive action.[53] Prior administration of an inactive analog fails to alter the subsequent response to the intact, active analog. The C-terminal portion of the peptide is also inactive.

Parathyroid hormone's vasodepressive effects are critically dependent on the animal's calcium status. Short-term dietary depletion blunts the hypotensive response, whereas calcium supplementation enhances the peptide's vascular actions (Fig 5).[54] This dependence on calcium suggests that PTH's mode of action requires the mobilization of the cation to affect the vasodilating response. An ionophoric mechanism has been postulated in the mediation of other end-organ responses to the pep-

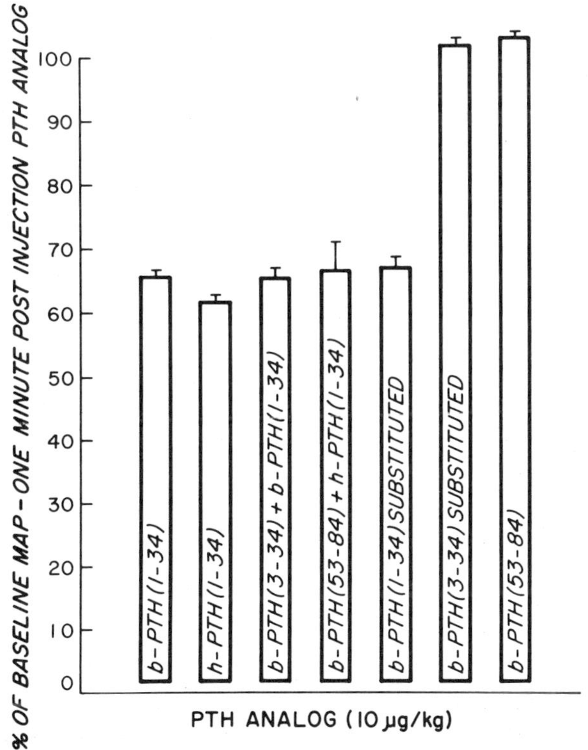

Fig 4.—Maximal blood pressure response of the Wistar–Kyoto rat to IV human and bovine PTH (1–34) and related analogs. Active analogs administered alone and following pretreatment with inactive analogs.[53]

tide.[55] Other calcium inophores have recently been described as systemic vasodilators.[56]

If PTH exerts its hypotensive actions via an ionophoric effect on the vascular smooth muscle membrane, then the peptide's vasodilation is in contradistinction to that of the widely studied calcium channel blockers. From recent work in our laboratory, that indeed appears to be the case.[57] Calcium supplementation in the SHR produces the previously noted enhancement of PTH's vasodilation, but results in blunting of the vasodilation induced by the calcium channel blocker, nifedipine. Precisely the reverse occurs when the animal is provided a calcium-deficient diet for two weeks. Nifedipine's vascular action is increased while PTH's action decreases. Importantly, the optimal

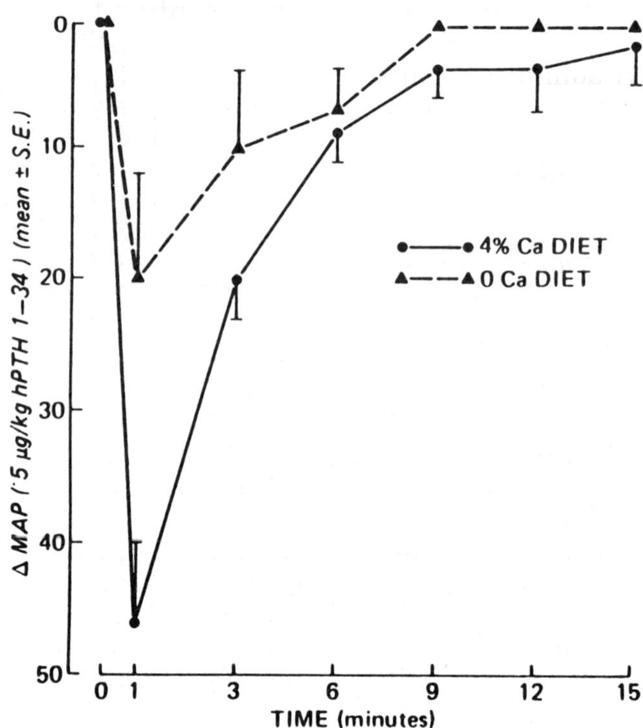

Fig 5.—Time-course of supplemented (4% dietary Ca^{2+}) SHRs' and restricted (0.02% dietary Ca^{2+}) SHRs' blood pressure response (W MAP) to IV hPTH (1–34) −5 μg/kg dose.[54]

blood pressure response is observed in the calcium-supplemented SHR ingesting the higher calcium diet.

Besides an apparent dependence on available calcium, the cellular mechanisms that PTH modifies in its induction of smooth muscle relaxation include two other primary intracellular regulation factors, cyclic AMP and calcium-binding protein, calmodulin. Incubation of isolated, cultured vascular smooth muscle cells with PTH produces an immediate reduction (<30 seconds) in the tissue cAMP content. This inhibition parallels in magnitude and time-course the peptide's systemic vasodilating effects.[58] Both in vitro and in vivo PTH effects on cAMP and mean arterial pressure are inhibited by the concurrent administration of trifluoperazine.[59] This compound represents a relatively specific inhibitor of intracellular calcium-binding protein. These observations regarding the role of calcium, the effect on cAMP and the interaction with calmodulin with PTH administration suggest a theoretical cascade of cellular events. Following PTH's binding to its putative membrane receptor, membrane calcium is mobilized, which, in turn, binds to calmodulin and then modifies cAMP turnover with a resultant decrease in the concentration of the cyclic nucleotide. Presumably the latter event then initiates intracellular pathways that favor smooth muscle relaxation.[1]

BLOOD PRESSURE AND MODIFICATION OF PTH STATUS IN ANIMALS

The data summarizing PTH's acute vasodilating actions do not provide direct evidence that, at physiologic concentrations and under chronic conditions, the hormone directly contributes to blood pressure regulation. Two reports, however, are consistent with a sustained influence on arterial pressure of the peptide at physiologic concentrations. The first study (Fig 6) assessed the response of the SHR and the WKY to the acute administration of angiotensin in the presence and absence of a continuous infusion of PTH at a dose that did not in itself mod-

Fig 6.—Dose-dependent pressor response to IV angiotensin II in the SHR and WKY without sustaining PTH infusion and with pretreatment with bovine PTH (1–34) −15 units/hr.[66]

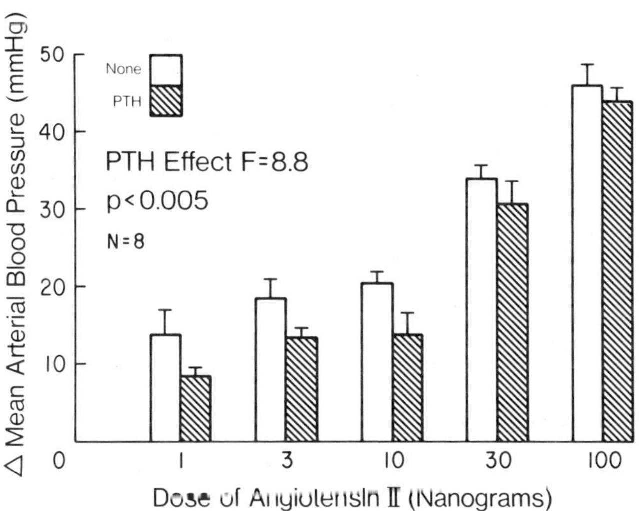

492   D. A. MCCARRON AND C. D. MORRIS

ify blood pressure.[60] Under these conditions the addition of a background infusion of PTH significantly attenuated the animal's vasoconstrictor response to the angiotensin II.

In the second experiment, SHRs were subjected to a total parathyroidectomy after having been raised on either a low/normal calcium-containing diet (0.25% by weight) or a supplemented calcium diet (4%) from 10 weeks of age until 22 to 24 weeks of age.[61] The diets were selected to stimulate endogenous parathyroid function in the case of the 0.25% diet or to suppress the parathyroid axis with the 4% diet. By the seventh day after the surgical ablation of parathyroid function, both diet groups had achieved a significant reduction in their serum ionized calcium concentrations; however, only the SHRs chronically maintained on the low intakes of calcium experienced a significant change in their systolic blood pressures (Fig 7). The animals in whom the high-calcium diet had functionally suppressed PTH activity experienced no effect on their blood pressures after the parathyroidectomy. When the diet was supplemented for both groups between days 7 and 21, postsurgery blood pressure returned toward baseline values but still remained elevated. The pressor effect seen in the presumed hyperparathyroid low-calcium animals may have reflected the removal of the protective action of the circulating endogenous vasodilator, PTH. In the 4% SHR, no such response would have

Fig 7.—Mean tail-cuff systolic blood pressure in dietary Ca^{2+} supplemented (4%) and low/normal (0.25%) SHRs before PTX, 7 days post-PTX and 14–21 days post-PTX.[61]

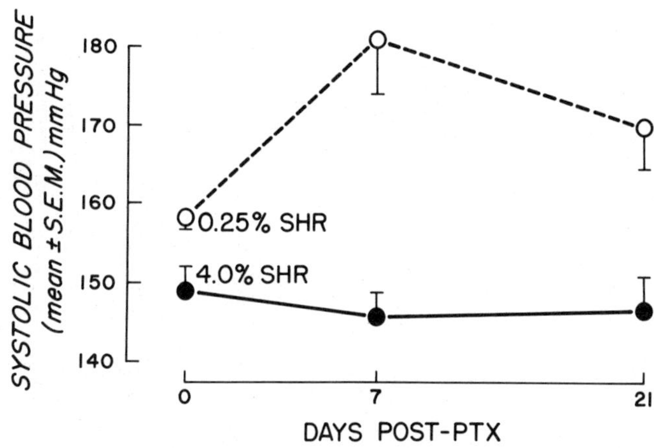

been anticipated, nor was seen, as the animals were presumably already maximally protected by the chronic vasodilating action of dietary calcium supplementation.

BLOOD PRESSURE AND MODIFICATION OF PTH STATUS IN HUMANS

From the limited reports of parathyroid hormone infusions in human beings, there is essentially no data regarding cardiovascular responses. This limitation principally reflects the previous lack of appreciation that vascular smooth muscle cells and resistance arterioles may represent another target organ for the hormone. Acute suppression of endogenous PTH secretion and its relationship to blood pressure control has been assessed by us in an earlier study.[62] Successful long-term survivors of renal transplantation with persistent hyperparathyroidism were examined. All the patients had good to excel-

Fig 8.—Correlation of change in systolic blood pressure with change in serum PTH levels in hyperparathyroid transplant recipients given IV calcium, 15 mg/kg, over four hours.

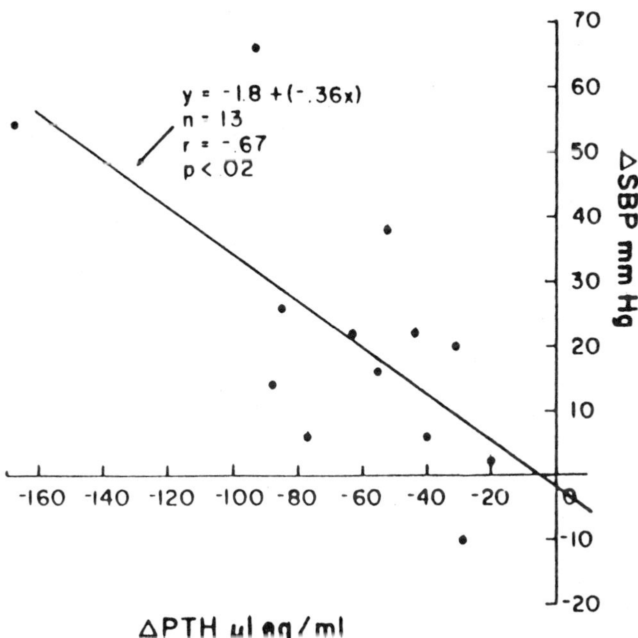

lent graft function and remarkably normal blood pressures for such a population. All the subjects had surgically documented diffuse enlargement of the parathyroid glands.[63] When the subject received a four-hour calcium infusion (15 mg/kg), arterial pressure, principally the systolic component, increased immediately. The pressor response in these patients was not related to degree of hypercalcemia induced, nor to other standard parameters such as changes in volume status. The hyperparathyroid patients increased their blood pressure in proportion to the degree of parathyroid hormone suppression that was induced (Fig 8).[61]

These observations combined with the fact that blood pressure did not change in a normotensive control group who received calcium in the same protocol suggest that the pressor response to hypercalcemia is related to the removal of an endogenous vasodilator, PTH, and not a direct vasoconstrictor effect of the calcium. Consistent with that interpretation were these same transplant recipients' vascular response to another intervention that was also intended to inhibit the release of PTH.[62] When administered isoproterenol, a vasoactive compound itself, the observed increase in arterial pressure again correlated with the measured reduction in circulating PTH. Furthermore, the slope of the "change in blood pressure" and "change in PTH level" relationship was essentially identical to that observed during the calcium infusions.

Hypercalcemia and Hypertension

Increased arterial pressure has been associated in several studies with the induction of acute hypercalcemia.[64, 65] Those human studies involved subjects with mild to moderate renal insufficiency. As with our experience noted above, the blood pressure response was not directly related to the degree of hypercalcemia or to observed variations in catecholamine production, aldosterone excretion, changes in renin concentrations, or hemodynamics. Importantly, PTH levels were not measured in these experiments, but the blood pressure response was correlated in one of the reports with the degree of renal failure (serum creatinine), suggesting once again the possibility that suppression of the parathyroid axis may have accounted for the pressor response seen in the individual patients.[64, 65]

We have recently provided a preliminary report of the blood pressure changes seen in the course of acute calcium administration to normotensive and hypertensive subjects.[66] In spite of comparable and marked degrees of hypercalcemia, no change in the normals' arterial pressure was observed. In contrast, the hypertensive patients transiently, but significantly, increased their blood pressure. Again, the blood pressure increase was dissociated from the induced changes in serum total and ionized calcium concentrations. Since a number of reports have now characterized increased parathyroid gland function in subjects with essential hypertension, the likely possibility exists that the hypertensives' pressor response we observed in this study may also have been related to the suppression of PTH release. This would, in part, account for the transient nature of the blood pressure increase and the return to baseline blood pressures in the face of progressive hypercalcemia.

Hypertension has been encountered in other clinical settings related to hypercalcemia. Tumor-associated hypercalcemia is probably the most common situation, where new onset of hypertension is seen in conjunction with acute and chronic elevations of blood pressure. However, no reports have ever carefully documented what the role is of the concurrent additional hormonal, hemodynamic, and electrolyte disturbances in these subjects. Before a direct pressor action can be ascribed to calcium in these clinical states, data supporting that interpretation must be provided and the other obvious metabolic perturbations excluded as the pressor factors.

HYPERPARATHYROIDISM AND HYPERTENSION

High blood pressure has been associated with hyperparathyroidism. This association has been based on the observation from several reports that the incidence of hypertension is increased in subjects with surgically proved hyperparathyroidism.[67, 68] In addition, several studies have suggested that blood pressure control improves after correction of the hyperparathyroidism.[67–69] A variety of more recent observations suggest that, rather than the functional state of hyperparathyroidism inducing hypertension, factors that predispose an individual to the development of hypertension also predispose selected patients to the later emergence of parathyroid dysfunction.[25]

In a prospective assessment of newly diagnosed hyperparathyroid patients with asymptomatic disease, the principal reason for their identification was a referral for evaluation of high blood pressure.[70] Furthermore, early evidence of parathyroid overactivity has now been characterized in patients with mild essential hypertension.[25, 26] These subjects do not necessarily have hyperparathyroidism, but do have evidence of stimulation of parathyroid gland function in the setting of established elevations in their blood pressure. These data are consistent with the hypothesis that hypertension precedes the onset of hyperparathyroidism in many of the patients with both disorders. In that context, and consistent with the vasodepressive actions of parathyroid hormone, the emergence of hyperparathyroidism may represent a homeostatic response intended to protect calcium balance of individuals with essential hypertension and to attenuate the rise in blood pressure that might otherwise occur.

Consistent with that interpretation of the available data is a prospective study by Lafferty.[71] In an evaluation of 100 consecutive patients with surgically documented parathyroid hypertrophy, this investigator demonstrated that the demographic pattern of the disorder followed that of hypertension in the United States, i.e., more prevalent in older subjects, black individuals, and those with associated cardiovascular risk factors. Most importantly, these patients received follow-up over a two-year period after their surgery, and no improvement in blood pressure control could be documented. In fact, the trend was just the reverse. The likely explanation for the disparity between this report and earlier ones that suggested an improvement in arterial pressure may reflect the fact that all previous studies had reported blood pressure values in only the immediate postoperative period. The patients had not been adequately followed after discharge allowing for a return to their normal lifestyles.

There is not necessarily any inconsistencies between the earlier interpretations of the relationship between these two clinical disorders and this reassessment based on the expanded data base now available. Simply put, other possibilities existed and they have now emerged. The development of additional data that will clarify whether or not hypertension is related to hyperparathyroidism and which clinical entity represents the primary condition must be pursued further.

Theoretical Relationship of Altered Ca^{2+} and Parathyroid Hormone Metabolism to the Pathogenesis of High Blood Pressure

The metabolic pathways by which disturbed calcium homeostasis produces a rise in arterial pressure remain conjectural. The simplest interpretation of the available data suggest that factors that reduce vascular smooth muscle cells' exposure to calcium or impair the cell's storage and mobilization of calcium result in increased peripheral resistance and vascular reactivity. These perturbations of cellular Ca^{2+} make the vascular membrane less stable, calcium permeability is increased ("slow channels" are open), and there is an increase in transmembrane fluxes of calcium. As a consequence, smooth muscle tone, reactivity, and contractility are all enhanced.

An alteration in the membrane binding of calcium might be one such mechanism contributing to vascular smooth muscle dysfunction. The observation that as serum total calcium levels are normal in hypertensives, but ionized values are decreased in a subset of hypertensives is consistent with such a defect.[28, 72] Thus, increased binding of calcium does exist in the extracellular space of some hypertensive humans and animals. A defect in the transport of calcium across cell membranes is a second pathogenetic mechanism that might serve to alter the kinetics of calcium compartmentalization and, thereby, smooth muscle function.[3, 73–75] Reduced dietary exposure to calcium by depleting calcium from its membrane storage sites may effectively produce similar metabolic consequences in the smooth muscle cell, i.e., enhanced calcium fluxes and an increase in vascular tone and reactivity.[1, 3]

Parathyroid hormone's role in this theoretical construct may be to facilitate the mobilization of membrane calcium or to increase the calcium availability to the vascular smooth muscle cells from nonintracellular sources. The data summarized in this article provide substantive evidence that parathyroid hormone is a direct vasodilator working through mechanisms involving cellular calcium with the peptide exerting an ionophoric action. By providing more calcium to the VSM, under conditions where inadequate quantities of the cation would otherwise exist, calcium may then exert its membrane-stabilizing effects and induce the resultant smooth muscle cell relaxation.

Summary

Both calcium and parathyroid hormone appear to be involved in the acute and chronic regulation of arterial pressure in experimental animals and humans. While the direct evidence is still preliminary, the net effect of calcium and parathyroid hormone under normal physiologic conditions is to favor a reduction in blood pressure. The implications of this assessment for common medical disorders, such as essential hypertension, and less common but oftentimes more challenging clinical conditions, such as end-stage renal disease, are potentially substantial.

Acknowledgments

The authors' original research cited in this manuscript was supported in part by grants-in-aid from the American Heart Association, the National Dairy Council, R. Blaine Bramble Trust, and the M.J. Murdock Charitable Trust, as well as Fellowship Training Grants from the National Kidney Foundation and the Oregon Affiliate of the American Heart Association. We would like to express our appreciation to Sharon Anderson, David Ellison, James Grady, and Cindy Wegener who collaborated with us in many of the studies cited. We are also indebted to Joni Utterback for the preparation of the manuscript.

REFERENCES

1. Kuriyama H., Yushi I., Suzuki H., et al.: Factors modifying contraction-relaxation cycle in vascular smooth muscles. *Ann. J. Physiol.* 243:H641, 1982.
2. Bohr D.F.: Vascular smooth muscle: dual effect of calcium. *Science* 139:597, 1963.
3. Webb R.C., Bohr D.F.: Mechanism of membrane stabilization by calcium in vascular smooth muscle. *Am. J. Physiol.* 235:C227, 1978.
4. Cheung W.Y.: Calmodulin plays a pivotal role in cellular regulation. *Science* 207:19, 1980.
5. Lee C.O., Vassalle M.: Modulation of intracellular Na^+ activity and cardiac force by norepinephrine and Ca^{2+}. *Am. J. Physiol.* 244:C110, 1983.
6. Breeman C.V., Aaronson P., Loutzenhiser R.: Sodium-calcium interactions in mammalian smooth muscle. *Pharmacol. Rev.* 30:167, 1979.
7. Blaustein M.P.: Sodium ions, calcium ions, blood pressure regulation and hypertension: a reassessment and a hypothesis. *Am. J. Physiol.* 232:C165, 1977.
8. Scott J.B., Frohlich E.D., Hardin R.A., et al.: Na^+, K^+, Ca^{2+} and Mg^{2+} action on coronary vascular resistance in the dog heart. *Am. J. Physiol.* 201:1095, 1961.
9. Feinberg H., Boyd E., Katz L.N.: Calcium effect on performance of the heart. *Am. J. Physiol.* 202:643, 1962.
10. Lee C.O., Uhm D.Y., Dresdner K.: Sodium-calcium exchange in rabbit heart muscle cells: direct measurement of sarcoplasmic Ca^{2+} activity. *Science* 209:699, 1980.

11. Sitrin M.D., Bohr D.F.: Ca^{2+} and Na^+ interactions in vascular smooth muscle contraction. *Am. J. Physiol.* 220:1124, 1971.

12. Altura B.M., Altura B.T., Carella A., et al.: Ca^{2+} coupling in vascualr smooth muscle: Mg^{2+} and buffer effects on contractility and membrane Ca^{2+} movements. *Can. J. Physiol. Pharmacol.* 60:459, 1982.

13. Brickman A.S., Massry S.G., Coburn J.W.: Changes in serum and urinary calcium during treatment of hydrochlorothiazide: studies on mechanisms. *J. Clin. Invest.* 51:945, 1972.

14. Popovtzer M.M., Subryan V.L., Alfrey A.C., et al.: The acute effect of chlorothiazide on serum-ionized calcium: evidence for a parathyroid hormone-dependent mechanism. *J. Clin. Invest.* 55:1295, 1975.

15. Pedersen O.L.: Calcium blockade in arterial hypertension. (Review). *Hypertension* 5:I174, 1983.

16. Eckert R., Ewald D.: Residual calcium ions depress activation of calcium-dependent current. *Science* 216:730, 1982.

17. Hurwitz L., McGuffee L.J., Smith P.M., et al.: Specific inhibition of calcium channels by calcium ions in smooth muscle. *J. Pharmacol. Exp. Ther.* 220:382, 1982.

18. Larsen F.L., Vincenzi F.F.: Calcium transport across the plasma membrane: stimulation by calmodulin. *Science* 204:306, 1979.

19. Belizan J.M., Villar J.: The relationship between calcium intake and edema-, proteinuria and hypertension-gestosis: an hypothesis. *Am. J. Clin. Nutr.* 33:2202, 1980.

20. McCarron D.A., Yung N.N., Ugoretz B.A., et al.: Disturbances of calcium metabolism in the spontaneously hypertensive rat. *Hypertension* 3:I162, 1981.

21. Webb R.C., Bohr D.F.: Recent advances in the pathogenesis of hypertension: consideration of structural, functional, and metabolic vascular abnormalities resulting in elevated vascular resistance. *Am. Heart J.* 102:251, 1981.

22. Grady J.R., Dorow J., McCarron D.A.: Urinary calcium excretion and cAMP response of the spontaneously hypertensive rat of Ca^{2+} deprivation. *Clin. Res.* 31:330A, 1983.

23. Toraason M.A., Wright G.L.: Transport of calcium by duodenum of spontaneously hypertensive rat. *Am. J. Physiol.* 241:G344, 1981

24. Scheld H., Miller D., Pape J., et al.: Vitamin D metabolism and intestinal calcium transport are abnormal in the spontaneously hypertensive rat. *Clin. Res.* 31:488A, 1983.

25. McCarron D.A., Pingree P., Rubin R.J., et al.: Enhanced parathyroid function in essential hypertension: A homeostatic response to a urinary calcium leak. *Hypertension* 2:162, 1980.

26. Strazzullo P., Nunziata V., Cirillo M., et al.: Abnormalities of calcium metabolism in essential hypertension. *Clin. Sci.* 65:137, 1983.

27. McCarron D.A., Chestnut C.H. III, Cole C., et al.: Blood pressure response to the pharmacologic management of osteoporosis (Abstract). *Clin. Res.* 29:274A, 1981.

28. McCarron D.A.: Low serum concentrations of ionized calcium in patients with hypertension. *N. Engl. J. Med.* 307:226, 1982.

29. McCarron D.A., Morris C.D., Cole C.: Dietary calcium in human hypertension. *Science* 217:267, 1982.

30. Ackley S., Barrett-Connor E., Suarez L.: Dairy products, calcium and blood pressure. *Am. J. Clin. Nutr.* 38:457, 1983.

31. Stitt F.W., Crawford M.D., Clayton D.G., et al.: Clinical and biochemical indicators of cardiovascular disease among men living in hard and soft water areas. *Lancet* 1:122, 1973.

32. Neri L.C., Johansen H.L.: Water hardness and cardiovascular mortality. *Ann. N.Y. Acad. Sci.* 304:203, 1978.

33. McCarron D.A., Stanton R.J., Henry H.J., et al.. Assessment of nutritional correlates of blood pressure. *Ann. Intern. Med.* 98:715, 1983.

34. McCarron D.A., Morris C.D., Henry H.J., et al.: Blood pressure and nutrient intake in the United States. *Science* (in press).

35. Lau K., Chen S., Eby B.: Evidence for the role of PO_4 deficiency in antihypertensive actions of a high-Ca diet. *Am. J. Physiol.* 246:H324, 1984.

36. McCarron D.A.: Calcium, magnesium, and phosphorus balance in human and experimental hypertension. *Hypertension* 4:III27, 1982.

37. McCarron D.A.: Blood pressure and calcium balance in the Wistar-Kyoto rat. *Life Sci.* 30:683, 1982.

38. Anderson S., Grady J.R., Ellison D.H., et al.: Calcium balance and parathyroid hormone-mediated vasodilation in the spontaneously hypertensive rat. *Hypertension* 5:I59, 1983.

39. Belizan J.M., Villar J., Pineda O., et al.: Reduction of blood pressure with calcium supplementation in young adults. *JAMA* 249:1161, 1983.

40. Morris C.D., Henry H.J., McCarron D.A.: Randomized, placebo-controlled trial of oral Ca^{2+} in human hypertension. Abstract presented at 16th Annual Meeting of the American Society of Nephrology, December 1983.

41. Collip J.B.: The extraction of a parathyroid hormone which will prevent or control parathyroid tetany and which regulates the level of blood calcium. *J. Biol. Chem.* 63:395, 1925.

42. Handler P., Cohn D.V.: Effect of parathyroid extract on renal function. *Am. J. Physiol.* 169:188, 1952.

43. Charbon G.A., Brummer F., Reneman A.: Diuretic and vascular action of parathyroid extracts in animals and man. *Arch. Int. Pharmacol.* 171:1, 1968.

44. Charbon G.A.: A rapid and selective vasodilator effect of parathyroid hormone. *Eur. J. Pharmacol.* 3:275, 1968.

45. Charbon G.A., Pieper E.E.M.: Effect of calcitonin on parathyroid hormone-induced vasodilation. *Endocrinol.* 91:828, 1968.

46. Charbon G.A., Hulstaert P.F.: Augmentation of arterial hepatic and renal flow by extracted and synthetic parathyroid hormone. *Endocrinol.* 95:621, 1974.

47. Charbon G.A.: Vasodilator action of parathyroid hormone used as a bioassay. *Arch. Int. Pharmacodyn.* 178:296, 1969.

48. Pang P.K.T., Sawyer W.H.: Parathyroid hormone preparations, salmon calcitonin, and urine flow in the South American lungfish. *Lepidociren. Paradoxa. J. Exp.* 193:407, 1975.

49. Pang P.K.T., Tenner T.E., Yee J.A., et al.: Hypotensive action of parathyroid hormone preparations on rats and dogs. *Proc. Natl. Head. Sci. (USA)* 77:675, 1980.

50. Cross M.F., Pang P.K.T.: Parathyroid hormone: a coronary artery vasodilator. *Science* 217:1087, 1980.

51. Pang P.K.T., Janssen H.F., Yee J.A.: Effects of synthetic parathyroid hormone on vascular beds of dogs. *Pharmacol.* 21:213, 1980.

52. McCarron D.A., Ellison D.H., Anderson S.: Increased sensitivity of the SHR to human PTH (1–34)-mediated vasodilation. *Am. J. Physiol.* 246:F96, 1984.

53. Ellison D.H., McCarron D.A.: Structural prerequisites of parathyroid hormone's hypotensive action. *Am. J. Physiol.* (in press).

54. Anderson S., Grady J.R., Ellison D.H., et al.: Ca^{2+} balance and parathyroid hormone-mediated vasodilation in the SHR. *Hypertension* 5:I59, 1983.

55. Marcus R., Orner F.B.: Parathyroid hormone as a calcium ionophore in bone cells: tests of specificity. *Calcif. Tissue Int.* 32:207, 1980.

56. Osborne M.W., Kovzelove F., Cohen M.R., et al.: Bromol asalacid (Ro 20–0006) antihypertensive ionophore. *Fed. Proc.* 42:191, 1983.

57. Grady J.R., McCarron D.A.: Divergent effects of Ca^{2+} balance on the vasodilating response to PTH and nifedipine in the SHR. *Clin. Res.* 32:36, 1984.

58. McCarron D.A., Plant S.B., Stanton R., et al.: Vascular smooth muscle cell cAMP response to bPTH (1–34) incubation: Correlation with hypotensive action. *Endocrin. Soc.* June 1982.

59. Stanton R., Plant S.B., McCarron D.A.: PTH-induced suppression of vascular smooth muscle cell cAMP content: The influence of trifluoperazine pretreatment. *Endocrin. Soc.* 1983.

60. Ellison D.H., McCarron D.A.: Infusion of bovine parathyroid hormone 1–34 attenuates the pressor response to angiotensin II in spontaneously hypertensive rats. *Clin. Exp. Hyperten.* A4:1637, 1982.

61. Ellison D.H., Dorow J., McCarron D.A.: Cardiovascular response to parathyroidectomy (PTX) in the spontaneously hypertensive rat (SHR): The effect of calcium (Ca) balance. *Kidney Int.* 21:167, 1982.

62. McCarron D.A., Muther R.S., Plant S.B., et al.: Parathyroid hormone: A determinant of post-transplant blood pressure regulation. *Am. J. Kid. Dis.* 1:38, 1981.

63. McCarron D.A., Muther R.S., Krutzik S., et al.: Dynamics of parathyroid function in persistent hyperparathyroidism: Relationship to gland size. *Kidney Int.* 22:662, 1982.

64. Weidman P., Massry S.G., Coburn J.W., et al.: Blood pressure effect of acute hypercalcemia. *Ann. Intern. Med.* 76:741, 1972.

65. Maroni C., Berctta-Picolli C., Weidmann P.: Acute hypercalcemia hypertension in man: Role of hemodynamics, catecholamines, and renin. *Kidney Int.* 22:662, 1982.

66. Ellison D.H., McCarron D.A.: Renal and cardiovascular response to Ca^{2+} infusion at varying Na^+ intakes in hypertensive humans. *Kidney Int.* 23:169, 1983.

67. Hellstrom J., Birke G., and Edvall C.A.: Hypertension in hyperparathyroidism. *Br. J. Urol.* 30:13, 1958.

68. Rosenthol F.D., Roy S.: Hypertension and hyperparathyroidism. *Br. Med. J.* 42:396, 1972.

69. Scholtz D.A.: Hypertension and hyperparathyroidism. *Arch. Int. Med.* 137:1123, 1977.

70. Heath H., III, Hodgson, S.F., Kennedy M.A.: Primary hyperparathyroidism - Incidence, morbidity and potential economic impact in a community.

71. Lafferty F.W.: Primary hyperparathyroidism: Changing clinical spectrum, prevalence of hypertension, and discriminant analysis of laboratory test. *Arch. Intern. Med.* 141:1761, 1981.

72. Resnick L.M., Laragh J.H., Sealey J.E., et al.: Divalent cations in essential hypertension: Relations between serum ionized calcium, magnesium, and plasma renin activity. *N. Engl. J. Med.* 309:888, 1983.

73. Noon J.P., Rice P.J., Baldessarini R.J.: Calcium leakage as a cause of the high resting tension in vascular smooth muscle from the spontaneously hypertensive rat. *Proc. Natl. Acad. Sci.* 75:1605, 1978.

74. Webb R.C., Bhalla R.C.: Altered calcium sequestration by subcellular fractions of vascular smooth muscle from spontaneously hypertensive rats. *J. Mol. Cell. Cardiol.* 8:651, 1976.

75. Bhalla R.C., Webb R.C., Singh D., et al.: Calcium fluxes, calcium binding and adenosine cyclic 3; 5-monophosphate-dependent protein kinase activity in the aorta of spontaneously hypertensive and Kyoto Wistar normotensive rats. *Mol. Pharmacol.* 14:468, 1978.

Subject Index

A

Abdominal bruit: in renovascular hypertension, 290–291

Acetazolamide: and prostaglandins, 281

Acid-base disorders, 67–85
  adaptive responses
    extent of, 70–79
    three observations about, 69–70
  life-threatening, 67–85
  simple, 68
    combinations of, 79–82
  whole body titration curve, 69, 70

Acidosis
  metabolic, 71–72
    alkali therapy in, 82–83
    respiratory acidosis and, 80
    respiratory alkalosis and, 81
  respiratory, 74–77
    acute, 75
    chronic, 75–77
    metabolic acidosis and, 80
    metabolic alkalosis and, 81–82
    treatment of, 84–85

Acylamino penicillins: in prostatic infections, 58

Adenosine
  triphosphatase (see Na-K-ATPase)
  triphosphate synthesis, and Na-K-ATPase activity, 107–108

ADH: and Na-K-ATPase, 135

Adrenergic receptors, activation by catecholamines
  alpha, 182–183
  beta, 183

Adrenocorticosteroids: and regulation of Na-K-ATPase, 128–133

Age: and liver cysts, 4, 5

Agenesis: bilateral renal, prenatal diagnosis, 29

Aldosterone
  indomethacin and, 270

Na-K-ATPase development and, 142

plasma, and calcium antagonists, 206–207

Alkali therapy: in metabolic acidosis, 82–83

Alkalosis
  metabolic, 72–74
    respiratory acidosis and, 81–82
    respiratory alkalosis and, 80–81
    treatment of, 83–84
  respiratory, 77–79
    acute, 77–78
    chronic, 78–79
    metabolic acidosis and, 81
    metabolic alkalosis and, 80–81

Aluminum
  chelated, clearance, and dialysis methods, 463–466
  -containing food intake, control of, 452–453
  gels, 448–449, 450
  intoxication, 439–478
    (See also Hyperaluminemia)
    chelating agent in (see Desferrioxamine, in aluminum intoxication)
    desferrioxamine in (see Desferrioxamine, in aluminum intoxication)
    from dialysis, control of, 454–458
    dietary intake control and, 452–453
    hyperphosphatemia control and, 453–454
    prevention of, 452–458
    treatment of, 458–469
  loading, hyperaluminemia as reflection of, 440–445

Amino acid transport: and Na-K-ATPase, 115–116

Aminoglycosides: in pyelonephritis, 59

Ammonium chloride: in metabolic alkalosis, 83